CANCER SOURCEBOOK

CANCER SOURCEBOOK

Basic Information on Cancer Types, Symptoms,
Diagnostic Methods, and Treatments, Including
Statistics on Cancer Occurrences Worldwide
and the Risks Associated With Known
Carcinogens and Activities

Volume One

Edited by
Frank E. Bair

Omnigraphics, Inc. • Penobscot Building • Detroit, MI 48226

BIBLIOGRAPHIC NOTE:

This volume compiles 37 individual booklets, papers, and bulletins issued by the National Institutes of Health and its subagency, the National Cancer Institute, between January 1986 and July 1989. These documents are identifiable as NIH publications: 86-1136; 86-2227; 86-2685; 86-2706; 87-171; 87-526; 87-528; 87-657; 87-658; 87-659; 87-621; 87-722; 87-1178; 87-1847; 87-2059; 87-2342; 87-2400; 87-2675; 87-2706; 87-2709; 87-2877; 88-95; 88-172; 88-329; 88-2038; 88-2151; 88-2378; 88-2685; 88-2941; 88-2977; 88-2978; and 88-3020. The compilation includes one publication issued by the National Institute of Neurological and Communicative Disorders and Strokes bearing the number 82-504. Other documents in the compilation are unnumbered fact sheets and bulletins, also issued by the National Cancer Institute.

Frank E. Bair
Editor

This book is printed on acid-free paper meeting the ANSI Z39.48 Standard. The infinity symbol that appears above indicates that the paper in this book meets that standard.

ISBN 1-55888-888-8

Printed in the United States of America

CONTENTS

INTRODUCTION

The public information documents assembled in this *Cancer Sourcebook* have been created specifically for the understanding of the lay public. Offered as separate reports and bulletins by the National Cancer Institute, the agency which carries responsibility within the federal government for the development and support of cancer research, the advisories are unified here into a single reference tool encompassing data on most major categories of the illness. The information is direct and precise, although nontechnical, and covers facts about symptoms, diagnostic procedures, treatments, and known risks.

The wide range of this body of knowledge has suggested arrangement of *Cancer Sourcebook* into five major divisions:

Section One comprises a core of reports that closely examine, from diagnosis to prognosis, 20 of the most common forms of cancer. Seven chapters are devoted to the numerous investigative methods and treatments for breast cancer, among these self-examination, radiation, surgical alternatives, reconstruction, and follow-up care.

Section Two defines treatment techniques. Radiation therapy is described in detail, the science of chemotherapy is clarified, and bone-marrow transplantation is explored in lay terms. Cancer recurrence and pain control also are topics addressed here.

Section Three deals with the problems and difficulties that beset both patient and caregiver. Six chapters identify and interpret the anxieties that arise during diagnosis and treatment, and other chapters discuss emotional support, cancer in the young person, and dietary concerns for children in various stages of medical treatment.

Cancer Rates and Risks, the content of Section Four, is a broad overview of what is known about cancer today. It includes a summary of significant statistics and a study of situations that identify the risks of both hereditary and environmental factors.

The final section is a comprehensive index of all key elements treated in the volume. Glossaries are featured throughout, and most of the chapters provide references and bibliographies.

Because research and medical application continue to advance in the fight against cancer, an annual update is planned for *Cancer Sourcebook*. Comments are invited on improvement in style or scope that would make subsequent editions more useful.

PART I—

CANCER INFORMATION FOR THE PATIENT

Research Reports and
Special Texts Developed
by the
National Cancer Institute

Chapter 1

Cancer Types

Differentiating Between Them

Types of Cancer

Generally, cancers can be described by the part of the body in which they originate (for example, breast cancer) or by the way cancer cells look under a microscope (for example, histiocytic lymphoma). The number of types depends on the system of classification used. *The International Classification of Diseases for Oncology*, a World Health Organization publication, identifies 46 body sites that can be affected by cancer. Each site can develop several types of cancers in two broad categories, carcinoma and sarcoma. From this point of view, there are at least 112 types of cancer. But within each subtype there are further histologic subdivisions that behave differently clinically. Cancer of the lung, for example, has four major types, oat cell, epidermoid, large cell and adenocarcinoma.

Following is a list of the major histologic types within 46 anatomic sites. In reviewing the list, the following points should be considered:

■ These cancers were selected on the basis of histological differentiation and not patterns of growth. Many cancers are further classified by growth patterns, such as papillary, solid or cribiform. To include growth patterns in addition to the histological types would greatly extend the list.

■ Some of the childhood cancers are included, such as Wilms' tumor and Letterer-Siwe's disease. Although these cancers are not common compared to cancers in adults, they form an important segment of the practice of pediatric oncology.

■ Cancers of the tooth structures also are included. Listed under bones, these cancers are not common, but they are an essential part of oral medicine.

■ As apparent from the list, some cancers, such as sarcomas, can arise almost anywhere in the body. To conserve space, the various types of sarcomas are listed under "Connective Tissue" and the term "sarcomas" is added to sites where they commonly occur. Often, mixed or combined types of sarcomas are found, such as osteochondro-sarcoma or myxofibrosarcoma. It would be impractical to list all of the combinations that have been reported.

■ Classification schemes and terminology are constantly changing in light of new knowledge. The lymphomas, for example, have been classified several different ways in the past few years. Because of constant changes, the different classification schemes have not been included.

- Many cancers are further divided into "acute" and "chronic" based on clinical considerations. For example, the various types of leukemias are often classified as acute, subacute, or chronic, depending on laboratory and clinical observation.

- Many tumors, particularly those growing in closed spaces, are potentially fatal not in their behavior, but by their location. This is especially true of many brain and spinal cord tumors. Rhabdoinyoma in the heart, for example, can kill by interfering with heart function and the circulatory system.

- Benign tumors have not been included.

- There are many common synonyms used for these terms that may be more popular elsewhere in the country and in other countries. Therefore, the preferred terms will vary considerably in different institutions. As much as possible, the attached list includes those most commonly used in the United States.

Histologic Types Within 46 Anatomic Sites

Lip
adenocarcinoma
mucoepidermoid carcinoma
squamous cell carcinoma

Tongue
adenocarcinoma
adenoidsquamous carcinoma
squamous cell carcinoma

Salivary Glands
acinar cell carcinoma
adenocarcinoma
malignant mixed tumor
mucoepidermoid carcinoma
oncocytic carcinoma
squamous cell carcinoma
adenocystic carcinoma

Floor of Mouth
adenocarcinoma
squamous cell carcinoma

Oropharynx
adenocarcinoma
adenoid cystic carcinoma
squamous cell carcinoma

Nasopharynx
adenocarcinoma
squamous cell carcinoma
transitional cell carcinoma
undifferentiated cell carcinoma

Hypopharynx
adenocarcinoma
squamous cell carcinoma
transitional cell carcinoma

Esophagus
adenocarcinoma
sarcoma
squamous cell carcinoma

Stomach
adenocarcinoma
adenosquamous carcinoma

intestinal type adenocarcinoma
leiomyosarcoma
mucin-producing adenocarcinoma
signet ring cell carcinoma

Small Intestine
adenocarcinoma
leiomyosarcoma
malignant carcinoid tumor

Large Intestine
adenocarcinoma
malignant carcinoid tumor
mucin-producing adenocarcinoma
sarcomas

Rectum and Anus
adenocarcinoma
cloacogenic carcinoma
malignant carcinoid tumor
mucin-producing adenocarcinoma
squamous cell carcinoma
transitional cell carcinoma

Liver and Intrahepatic Bile Ducts
angiosarcoma
cholangiocarcinoma
hepatoblastoma
hepatocellular carcinoma
Kupffer cell sarcoma

Gallbladder and Extrahepatic Bile Ducts
adenocarcinoma
adenosquamous carcinoma
cystadenocarcinoma
mucinous adenocarcinoma

Pancreas
acinar cell carcinoma
cystadenocarcinoma
duct adenocarcinoma
islet cell carcinoma
mucin-producing adenocarcinoma
pleomorphic carcinoma

Retroperitoneum and Peritoneum
malignant mesenchymoma
malignant mesothelioma
malignant papaganglioma
neuroblastoma
sarcomas

Nasal Cavities, Accessory Sinuses, Middle Ear and Inner Ear
adenocarcinoma
adenoid cystic carcinoma
esthesioneurocytoma
malignant mixed tumor
sarcoma
squamous cell carcinoma
transitional cell carcinoma

Larynx
adenocarcinoma
squamous cell carcinoma

Trachea, Bronchus and Lung
acinar cell carcinoma
adenocarcinoma
adenoid cystic carcinoma
adenosquamous carcinoma
bronchiolar carcinoma
giant cell carcinoma
malignant carcinoid tumor
mucin-producing adenocarcinoma
oat cell carcinoma
papillary carcinoma
sarcoma
undifferentiated cell carcinoma

Pleura
malignant mesothelioma
sarcomas

Heart
rhabdomyoma
sarcoma

Mediastinum
gaglioneuroblastoma
Hodgkin's disease
malignant teratoma
sarcoma

Hematopoietic System
basophilic leukemia
eosinophilic leukemia
erythroleukemia
hairy cell leukemia
lymphocytic leukemia
mast cell leukemia
megakaryocytic leukemia
monocytic leukemia
myeloid leukemia
myelosclerosis with myeloid
 metaplasia
plasma cell leukemia
polycythemia vera

Lymph Nodes and
Reticuloendothelial System
Hodgkin's disease
Burkitt's tumor
immunoblastic sarcoma
malignant lymphoma, diffuse
malignant lymphoma, nodular
malignant histiocytosis
histiocytic medullary reticulosis
Letterer-Siwe's disease

Thymes
carcinoma
malignant thymoma
malignant lymphoma

Spleen
angiosarcoma

Bones, Joints and Articular
Cartilage
adamantinoma
ameloblastic odontosarcoma
chondrosarcoma

chordoma
Ewing's sarcoma
malignant ameloblastoma
malignant chondroblastoma
malignant giant cell tumor
malignant odontogenic tumor
osteogenic sarcoma
other sarcomas
parosteal osteogenic sarcoma
synovial sarcoma

Connective, Subcutaneous and
Other Soft Tissues
alveolar soft part sarcoma
angiosarcoma
fibro-sarcoma
Kaposi's sarcoma
leiomyosarcoma
liposarcoma
lymphangiosarcoma
malignant fibrous histiocytoma
malignant hemangioendothelioma
malignant hemangiopericytoma
myxosarcoma
neurofibrosarcoma
rhabdomyosarcoma

Skin
basal cell carcinoma
carcinoma-ln-situ
ceruminous carcinoma
extramammary Paget's disease
malignant melanoma
sarcoma
sebaceous gland carcinoma
squamous cell carcinoma
sweat gland carcinoma

Breast
carcinosarcoma
duct adenocarcinoma
inflammatory carcinoma
lobular carcinoma
malignant cystosarcoma phyllodes
medullary carcinoma

mucinous carcinoma
Paget's disease of the breast
secretory carcinoma
signet rign cell carcinoma
stromal sarcoma
tubular carcinoma

Uterus
adenocarcinoma
adenoacanthoma
endometrial stromal sarcoma
leiomyosarcoma
malignant mixed Mullerian tumor

Cervix Uteri
adenocarcinoma
adenosquamous carcinoma
carcinoma-in-situ
sarcoma
squamous cell carcinoma

Vagina
adenocarcinoma
squamous cell carcinoma
sarcoma

Ovary, Fallopian Tube and Broad Ligament
arrhenoblastoma
choriocarcinoma
dysgerminoma
embryonal carcinoma
endodermal sinus tumor
endometroid carcinoma
granulosa cell carcinoma
malignant Brenner tumor
malignant mesonephroma
malignant mixed Mullerian tumor
malignant struma ovarii
malignant teratoma
mucinous cystadenocarcinoma
sarcoma
serouscystadenocarcinoma
Sertoli cell carcinoma
theca cell carcinoma

Vulva
basal cell carcinoma
squamous cell carcinoma

Placenta
choriocarcinoma

Prostate Gland
adenocarcinoma
sarcoma

Testis
choriocarcinoma
embryonal carcinoma
malignant androblastoma
malignant Leydig cell tumor
malignant teratoma
sarcoma
semonoma
Sertoli cell carcinoma

Penis and Other Male Genital Organs
adenocarcinoma
squamous cell carcinoma

Kidney and Other Urinary Organs
adenocarcinoma (renal cell carcinoma)
angiomyoliposarcoma
sarcoma
squamous cell carcinoma
transitional cell carcinoma
Wilms' tumor

Urinary Bladder
adenocarcinoma
squamous cell carcinoma
transitional cell carcinoma

Eye and Lacrimal Gland
adenocarcinoma
malignant melanoma
retinoblastoma

Brain, Meninges and Spinal Cord
astrocytoma
ependymoma
ganglioglioma
glioblastoma multlforma
glioma
malignant menigioma
malignant neurilemmoma
medulloblastoma
microglioma
neuroblastoma
oligodendroglioma
sarcoma

Thyroid Gland
follicular carcinoma
giant cell carcinoma
medullary carcinoma
papillary carcinoma

Adrenal Gland
adrenal cortical carcinoma
malignant pheochromocytoma

Other Endocrine Glands
adenocarcinoma
craniophryngioma
parathyroid gland carcinoma
pinealoblastoma
pituitary Gland carcinoma

For additional information on this subject, write to the Office of Cancer Communications, National Cancer Institute, Bethesda, MD 20205, or call the toll-free telephone number of the Cancer Information Service at 1-800-4-CANCER *

* In Alaska, call 1-800-638-6070; in Washington, D.C. (and suburbs in Maryland and Virginia), call 636-5700; in Hawaii, on Oahu call 524-1234 (neighbor islands call collect).

Spanish-speaking staff members are available to callers from the following areas (daytime hours only): California (area codes 213, 619, 714, 805 and 818), Florida, Georgia, Illinois, Northern New Jersey, New York City, and Texas.

Chapter 2

Cancer of the Bladder

Introduction

This report describes current research on the causes, prevention, symptoms, diagnosis, and treatment of bladder cancer. The Information presented here was obtained from medical textbooks and recent articles in the medical literature, discussions with National Cancer Institute (NCI) scientists and other researchers, and various scientific meetings.

Description and Function of the Urinary Bladder

The urinary system, which includes the bladder, urethra, ureters, and kidneys, eliminates liquid waste products and helps maintain stable chemical conditions in the body. The bladder, a muscular chamber located in the lower abdomen, is the body's reservoir for urine. Two narrow tubes called ureters carry urine from the kidneys to the bladder. From the bladder, urine is emptied through another tube, the urethra. In females, the urethra is approximately 3 inches long and exits the body in front of the vagina. The male urethra is approximately 8 inches long; it passes through the prostate gland to an opening at the end of the penis.

The wall of the bladder is composed of several layers of tissues. The first layer on the inside of the bladder is made of transitional epithelial cells. (Epithelial cells line many parts of the body, including the digestive tract, the lungs, and the urinary tract. The epithelium is also referred to as the mucosa.) The next layer of tissue, called the lamina propria or submucosa, is made of connective tissue—collagen fibers mixed with a few elastic fibers. A deeper layer of the bladder is made of smooth muscle. The bladder also contains nerves and lymph and blood vessels.

Types of Bladder Cancer

Like all other tissues and organs, the bladder is composed of individual cells. Normally, cells divide and reproduce in an orderly, controlled way as they carry out their proper functions. Cancers of the bladder, as in other organs, result from the abnormal, uncontrolled growth of defective cells. The growing mass of abnormal tissue eventually crowds out and destroys nearby healthy tissue.

Not all growths in the bladder are cancerous (malignant). Benign tumors tend to remain localized and usually do not spread or become life threatening. Once removed by surgery, they seldom recur.

Cancerous tumors invade and destroy neighboring tissue and can spread, or metastasize, to other parts of the body. If cancer cells from the bladder spread through the blood or lymphatic systems, they can form secondary tumors. Even though these new tumors may grow in different organs, the disease is still called bladder cancer.

Nearly 90 percent of bladder cancers arise from transitional epithelial cells, the cells that line the inside of the bladder wall. Called transitional cell carcinomas, these tumors are typically papillary, or nipple-shaped. Often, more than one tumor is present.

About 6 to 8 percent of bladder cancers are squamous cell cancers. Even less common are adenocarcinomas, accounting for 1 to 2 percent of all cases. Bladder sarcomas, arising from connective tissue, make up less than 1 percent of all cases.

Incidence

Cancer of the bladder accounts for 6 percent of all cancers in men and 2 percent of all cancers in women. In 1986 approximately 40,500 cases of bladder cancer were diagnosed in the United States (29,000 cases in men and 11,500 in women).

Cancer of the bladder affects whites twice as often as blacks. Data collected and analyzed by the National Cancer Institute's Surveillance, Epidemiology, and End Results (SEER) Program show that the annual, age-adjusted incidence rates per 100,000 people in the United States for bladder cancer in 1984 (the most recent data available) are 31 for white men, 15 for black men, 7 for white women, and 4.5 for black women.

In general, the risk of bladder cancer increases with age. In the United States, incidence peaks after age 50 and begins to decline after age 80. Based on the SEER data, about 10,600 Americans will die from bladder cancer in 1986, making it the eighth leading cause of cancer deaths in men and the fourteenth in women.

Scientists have also found geographic differences in bladder cancer incidence. Incidence rates in northern sections of the U.S. were approximately 40 percent higher than those in the south.

In addition, the bladder cancer geographic pattern for whites does not parallel the pattern for blacks. Black mortality rates are not as elevated in the north, and the heavy male predominance observed for bladder cancer in whites is less evident in blacks. Scientists have postulated that industrial exposure may account for these differences.

Causes and Prevention

The most important known risk factor for bladder cancer is cigarette smoking. Cigarette smokers develop bladder cancer two to three times more often than nonsmokers; areas in the United States where cigarette sales are high also have high death rates from bladder cancer. Smoking is estimated to be responsible for about 40 percent of bladder cancers among men and 29 percent among women.

As early as 1895, workers in the dyestuffs industry showed a high risk of bladder cancer that was later associated with exposure to aromatic amines, a class of chemical compounds used to make dyes. Two of these compounds, benzidine and 2-naphthylamine, are now known to be potent bladder carcinogens.

Workers in the rubber and leather industries also have an increased risk of developing bladder cancer. Other occupations considered to be at elevated risk for bladder cancer include printers, painters, chemical workers, metal workers, hairdressers, textile workers, machinists, and truck drivers. Occupational exposures in these high-risk industries contribute between 18 and 40 percent of bladder cancer in males and about 20 percent of bladder cancer in females. Among the carcinogens known to cause human bladder cancer are:

3,3 '-dichlorobenzidine
4-aminodiphenyl
2-acetylaminofluorene
soots
magenta
tars and oils.

Heavy use of the pain killer phenacetin is also believed to raise the risk of bladder cancer. Moreover, phenacetin use and smoking appear to act synergistically; that is, the combination increases bladder cancer risk more than either would do alone. In 1983, the Food and Drug Administration banned phenacetin as an over-the-counter drug.

For many years scientists have suspected that infection of the bladder by the parasitic flatworm

Schistosomiasis haematobium leads to increased bladder cancer risk. A thorough study of this association has not been carried out, but the medical literature generally confirms the increased risk in areas of Africa where schistosomiasis infections are common.

The metabolism of tryptophan has also been studied in relation to bladder cancer risk. This amino acid is freed in the process of digestion and transformed into energy by a series of chemical reactions. Tryptophan metabolites, the chemical products of digestion, have been implicated as bladder carcinogens in animals, although dietary tryptophan alone has not been implicated. While the scientific literature contains reports of bladder cancer patients with abnormalities of tryptophan metabolism, this connection is not well understood.

Reports in the literature have linked pelvic irradiation for the treatment of gynecologic cancers with the later development of bladder cancer. The length of time between exposure to the radiation and the development of cancer appears to be greater than 15 years. Overall, the contribution of pelvic irradiation to the total number of cases of bladder cancer in women is very small.

The possible risk of bladder cancer associated with widely used artificial sweeteners received much attention when the Food and Drug Administration removed cyclamates from the market in 1969. It was later reported that the sweetener saccharin caused bladder cancer in male laboratory rats when the animals were exposed to the chemical before birth. Recent epidemiological studies show that, overall, people who use artificial sweeteners do not appear to have a higher incidence of bladder cancer than nonusers.

Although early studies showed a possible link between bladder cancer and coffee drinking, recent studies based on large numbers of individuals found little or no increase in bladder cancer among coffee drinkers compared with those who do not drink coffee.

Detection and Diagnosis

Symptoms

Hematuria, or blood in the urine, is the most common symptom of bladder cancer. The amount of blood does not reflect the stage of the disease (how far cancer cells have spread).

Bladder cancer may cause pain during urination, a feeling of urgency, or need to urinate frequently, but all of these symptoms also signal noncancerous conditions like infection, benign tumors, or bladder stones.

Diagnosis

Before diagnosing bladder cancer, a physician takes the patient's medical history and performs a complete physical examination. A bladder tumor can sometimes be felt during a rectal or vaginal exam performed under local anesthesia. This manual exam may be helpful in determining if the bladder mass is fixed to the pelvic wall. Various x-ray and laboratory tests are also used to help diagnose bladder cancer:

Urinary cytology is the examination of urine samples under a microscope to determine if cancerous or precancerous cells are present. This test is usually more accurate when done with bladder washing using a saline solution that is inserted and collected through a catheter.

The *cystoscope* is an instrument made of a hollow tube with several lenses and a light source allowing visual examination of the bladder's inside surface. While the patient is anesthetized, a physician inserts the cystoscope through the urethra into the bladder, taking a small sample of suspicious tissue (a biopsy) for microscopic study by a pathologist. Sometimes the physician takes several small tissue samples for analysis.

An *intravenous pyelogram* (IVP) or excretory urogram gives x-ray images of the bladder, kidneys, and ureters. An opaque dye visible on x-ray film is injected into a vein, and a series of x-rays are taken. The film shows an outline of the urinary tract, and tumors larger than 1 centimeter can sometimes be seen.

Computed tomographic (CT) *scans* give cross-sectional x-ray images of the body's organs along with information about the size, location, density, and extent of tumors. CT scans can show tumors that have spread beyond the bladder into the pelvic lymph nodes and help define the extent of tumor spread. The CT scan is limited, however, in its ability to identify superficial thickenings in the bladder wall.

A new diagnostic tool called *magnetic resonance imaging* (MRI) has potential for improving the diagnosis and staging of bladder tumors. MRI produces cross-sectional images similar to CT scans but does not expose the patient to x-rays or to contrast agents.

Physicians may also use *ultrasonography* to help diagnose bladder cancer. Ultrasound waves (waves at a higher frequency than sound waves) are emitted by a crystal placed on the skin's surface. The waves, reflecting off internal structures, are reproduced as an image.

Scientists are studying immunological techniques such as monoclonal antibodies to aid in the diagnosis and potential therapy of bladder cancer. Monoclonal antibodies are tailor-made proteins that can selectively attach themselves to specific cells. Scientists are now studying ways of tagging monoclonal antibodies with radioactive materials to identify small secondary tumors. In the future, these antibodies may be used to track the progress of patients after surgery for bladder cancer.

A diagnosis of bladder cancer is confirmed by a pathologist after examining a sample of suspicious tissue under a microscope. The pathologist determines how deeply the cancer cells have penetrated the bladder wall and grades the cancer cells according to their cellular features. Both factors play a major role in selecting treatment and gauging prognosis.

Once bladder cancer is diagnosed, other tests may be performed to help determine the stage or extent of disease. These include chest x-rays, liver function tests, and radioactive liver and bone scans. Newer imaging tools like CT scans, MRI, and ultrasonography are improving the accuracy of staging.

Stages of Bladder Cancer

Different staging systems are used for bladder cancer. Recently, the American Joint Committee on Cancer proposed a staging system that takes into account the major factors influencing prognosis. This system is based on coded descriptions of tumor size (T), lymph node involvement (N), and degree of metastasis (M).

Primary Tumor (T). In the TNM system, the extent of tumor is designated TX (if it cannot be assessed), T*is* (carcinoma *in situ*), Ta (papillary noninvasive carcinoma), or T with a number from 0 to 4 to describe the extent of the tumor's growth through the layers of the bladder wall. If there are multiple cancerous growths, the suffix "m" is added in this category.

Nodal Involvement (N). The site and degree of spread to lymph nodes is indicated by NX or N with a number from 0 to 3.

18

Distant Metastases (M). Finally, M with X, 0, or 1 indicates whether or not the cancer has spread to different parts of the body.

Another staging system, which does not describe nodal involvement as precisely as TNM, is also widely used:

Stage 0:   Cancer cells are found in the epithelium (the most superficial layer of tissue) but have not invaded the bladder wall itself. This includes carcinoma *in situ* and noninvasive papillary carcinomas. (T*is* and Ta)

Stage A: Cancer cells have microscopically spread to the lamina propria (beyond the surface of the bladder wall). (T1)

Stage B1:   The tumor has microscopically invaded the muscle of the bladder wall. (T2)

Stage B2:   The tumor has deeply invaded segments of the muscle of the bladder wall. (T3a)

Stage C: Cancer has invaded the bladder wall and extends into the fat surrounding the bladder. (T3b)

Stage D1:   Cancer has spread through the bladder wall to nearby organs (e.g., the rectum), or has entered the pelvic lymph nodes. (T4, N1-3)

Stage D2:   Cancer has spread through the bladder wall into the tissues beyond the pelvic area to the upper abdomen or more distant sites. (T4, N1-3, M1)

Treatment

In the past 20 years, survival rates for cancer of the bladder have improved steadily. White patients diagnosed between 1960 and 1963 had a 53 percent chance of 5-year survival compared to 75.6 percent for those diagnosed between 1977 and 1983, according to the most recent data available. For blacks, 5-year survival rose from 24 percent in patients diagnosed from

1960 to 1963 to 53.2 percent for those diagnosed in the years 1977-1983.

Treatment for bladder cancer may involve surgery, chemotherapy, immunotherapy, radiation therapy, or a combination of these, depending on the stage of disease, the pathologic grade of the tumor, and the age and health of the patient.

Stages 0 and A bladder cancer may be treated by various methods, although tumors often recur. Patients with recurrent tumors often have various growths at diagnosis, carcinoma *in situ,* or high-grade tumors.

First, doctors use the cystoscope to remove superficial bladder tumors (transurethral resection) or destroy them with electrical current (fulguration). Patients with extensive recurrent disease may also be treated with intravesical chemotherapy (bladder washings with anticancer drugs) or intravesical immunotherapy (bladder washings with an immune stimulant called BCG). The goal of these treatments, usually given as a followup to transurethral resection and fulguration, is to kill any cancer cells remaining in the bladder after surgery. The most common anticancer drugs are thiotepa (TESPA or TSPA) and mitomycin (Mitomycin C). Bleomycin (Blenoxane) and doxorubicin (Adriamycin) have also been used.

BCG *(bacillus Calmette-Guérin),* like chemotherapy, is applied directly to the bladder through the urethra. Originally used to immunize against tuberculosis, BCG stimulates the body's immune system, although its precise mechanism of action against cancer cells is not well understood. Cancer researchers have found that BCG treatment for superficial bladder cancer effectively prevents or delays cancer growth and the need for surgical removal of the bladder.

Patients with stage A bladder cancer who have widespread involvement of the bladder lining may be treated with radiotherapy in the form of external beam irradiation or radiation implants (or both). In some patients with extensive superficial disease, it may be necessary to remove the bladder entirely in an operation called radical cystectomy. (Only select patients benefit from parital cystectomy, since bladder cancer tends to arise on various parts of the bladder at once.) Patients who have received treatment for superficial bladder cancer should be followed up closely with regular cystoscopy.

Stage B1 treatment generally involves radical cystectomy, often with preoperative radiation. External beam irradiation or partial removal of the bladder may be used in selected circumstances.

Patients with *stages B2 and C* are teated with (1) radical cystectomy, often with preoperative radiotherapy; or (2) radiotherapy with external beam radiation. Clinical trials now under way in various cancer centers will help determine whether adjuvant chemotherapy—anticancer drugs given after primary treatment—prevents cancer recurrence in this group of patients.

In stages D1 and D2, secondary tumors are often found in the lungs or bones. Systemic chemotherapy is under investigation using agents like doxorubicin (Adriamycin), cisplatin (Platinol), methotrexate, and vinblastine (Velban). Combination chemotherapy with cisplatin, methotrexate, and vinblastine was recently reported to be among the most effective chemotherapies for advanced transitional cell cancer of the bladder. Studies suggest that this regimen may be useful as a followup to radiation therapy if the latter treatment is not effective.

Advances in Bladder Surgery

In women a radical cystectomy involves removal of the bladder, uterus, fallopian tubes, ovaries, and part of the vaginal wall. In men the bladder, prostate gland, and seminal vesicles are removed during surgery.

In the past, nearly all men undergoing a radical cystectomy were rendered impotent by the surgery. Recent refinements in surgical techniques can often spare the nerves responsible for erection; with this procedure, more than 80 percent of male patients retain sexual function. A study of female sexual function found that counseling helps alleviate many sexual problems following radical cystectomy.

After cystectomy, patients require urinary diversion or a substitute for the bladder. In one of the most common methods, an ileal conduit is fashioned from a piece of the small intestine (the ileum) to make a passageway for urine. The ureters are connected to one end of the conduit, while the other end is brought out through the wall of the abdomen near the navel. A small bag (referred to as an appliance) is the placed over the stoma, or opening, in the abdomen to collect the urine. Most patients adjust well to this technique because it is easy to maintain and preserves kidney function with few complications. Trained health professionals, usually enterostomal therapists or nurse specialists, teach patients how to manage their appliances.

New techniques have been developed to bypass the need for external appliances. One is an artificial urine reservoir formed from a piece of the ileum. The ureters are attached to one end, and the opposite end is connected to a lower abdominal stoma. Since an actual internal reservoir is formed instead of a canal, the patient may drain the pouch with a catheter as needed without having to rely on an external appliance.

The Camey procedure is another method of urinary diversion. A section of the ileum is removed during surgery; one end is attached to the ureters, while the other is connected to the remainder of the urethra, forming a type of canal for urine. The patient must urinate frequently to avoid leakage, but an appliance is not necessary. Reports of combining these two procedures to form an artificial internal urine reservoir have also been described in the medical literature.

Lasers are under investigation as a possible tool for treating urologic cancers. A laser is an instrument that transmits light at a particular energy and wavelength. In one type of laser, the light can be directed through a fiberoptic tube, and when the beam strikes tissue, enough heat is absorbed to destroy the tumor. Since the light energy may be sharply focused, little damage occurs to surrounding normal tissue and blood vessels. The preliminary results of several recent scientific studies found that the neodymium-yttrium-aluminum-garnet (nd:YAG) laser was effective in treating superficial bladder cancer. The laser may help treat invasive cancer as well, but more work needs to be done to assess its potential.

Photodynamic therapy is an experimental form of cancer treatment combining a photosensitizing drug with light of a specific wavelength, which destroys localized tumors while leaving the surrounding tissue unharmed. The drug (either hematoporphyrin derivative or dihematoporphyrin ether) is injected into a vein and selectively absorbed by cancerous or precancerous tissues. When tumors are exposed to the proper wavelength of light (usually in the form of a laser), a chemical reaction occurs, killing the cancer cells. Thus far, this treatment appears to be most effective in eradicating diffuse, resistant carcinoma *in situ.*

Suggestions for Additional Reading

Except as noted, the following materials are not available from the National Cancer Institute. They can be found in medical libraries, and some public libraries.

Benson, R.C. "Treatment of Diffuse Transitional Cell Carcinoma In Situ by Whole Bladder Hematoporphyrin Derivative Photodynamic Therapy," *The Journal of Urology,* 134 (4), 1985, pp. 675-678.

Cancer Rates and Risks. 3rd edition, prepared by the Office of Cancer Communications, National Cancer Institute, NIH Publication No. 85-691.

Chemotherapy and You: A Guide to Self-Help During Treatment, prepared by the Office of Cancer Communications, National Cancer Institute. NIH Publication No. 85-1136.

Connolly, J.G., ed. *Progress in Cancer Research and Therapy Vol 18: Carcinoma of the Bladder.* New York: Raven Press, 1983.

DeVita, V.T., Jr. et al., eds. *Cancer: Principles and Practice of Oncology.* Second edition. Philadelphia: Lippincott, 1985.

Javadpour, N., ed. *Principles and Management of Urologic Cancer,* Second edition. Baltimore: Williams and Wilkins, 1983.

Johnson, D.E. "Bladder Cancer: When to suspect it, how to confirm it, what treatments to recommend." *Your Patient and Cancer,* August, 1982, pp. 62-68.

Kakizoe, T. et al. "Significance of Carcinoma In Situ and Dysplasia in Association with Bladder Cancer," *The Journal of Urology,* 133 (3), 1985, pp. 395-398.

Lilien, O. and Camey, M. "25-Year Experience with Replacement of the Human Bladder (Camey Procedure)," *The Journal of Urology,* 132 (5), 1984, pp. 886-891.

Morales, A. "Long-Term Results and Complications of Intracavitary Bacillus Calmette-Guerin Therapy for Bladder Cancer," *The Journal of Urology,* 132 (2), 1984, pp. 457-460.

Morrison, A. et al. "An International Study of Smoking and Bladder Cancer," *The Journal of Urology,* 131 (2), 1984, pp. 650-654.

Pinsky, C.M. et al. "Intravesicular Administration of Bacillus Calmette-Guerin in Patients with Recurrent Superficial Carcinoma of the Urinary Bladder: Report of a Prospective Randomized Trial," *Cancer Treatment Reports,* vol. 69, No. 1, Jan. 1985, pp. 47-53.

Radiotherapy and You: A Guide to Self-Help During Treatment, prepared by the Office of Cancer Communications, National Cancer Institute. NIH Publication No. 85-2227.

Schottenfeld, D. and Fraumeni, J., eds. *Cancer Epidemiology and Prevention.* Philadelphia: W.B. Saunders Company, 1982.

Schover, L. and von Eschenback, A. "Sexual Function and Female Radical Cystectomy: A Case Series," *The Journal of Urology,* 134 (3), pp. 465-68, 1985.

Walsh, P.C. et al., eds. *Campbell's Urology.* 5th edition, vol 2. Philadelphia: W.B. Saunders Company, 1986.

Walsh, P. and Mostwin, J. "Radical Prostatectomy and Cystoprostatectomy with Preservation of Potency. Results Using a New Nerve-Sparing Technique," *British Journal of Urology,* 56, pp. 694-97, 1984.

* *What Are Clinical Trials All About?,* prepared by the Office of Cancer Communications, National Cancer Institute. NIH Publication No. 86-2706.

---

* *The mentioned text is reprinted within this book. See CONTENTS for location.*

Chapter 3

Bone Cancer
and Other Sarcomas

Introduction

This *Research Report* describes current research on the causes, incidence, symptoms, diagnosis, and treatment of bone cancer and soft tissue sarcomas. The information presented here came from medical textbooks, recent articles in the scientific literature, discussions with National Cancer Institute (NCI) scientists and other researchers, and various scientific meetings.

Types of Sarcomas

Sarcomas are cancers that begin in the body's connective tissues. Scientists writing about sarcomas often divide them into two groups: "bone cancers," which begin in the hard substance of bones and "soft tissue sarcomas," which start in muscle, fat, fibrous tissue, blood vessels, nerves, or other supporting tissue of the body.

Bone marrow, blood, and lymph are also forms of connective tissue, but the cancers that arise in them—multiple myeloma, leukemias, and lymphomas—are classed separately from sarcomas and treated differently.

Like other tissues of the body, bones and soft tissues are made up of individual cells. Laboratory studies have shown that a cancerous tumor of bone or soft tissue—a sarcoma—can result from the transformation of a single cell into a cancer cell.

The process of cell transformation has not been clearly defined. Research suggests that it occurs in a series of steps and stages. Scientists hope to learn what triggers the changes and find ways of preventing or interrupting the process.

A cancer cell has an unexplained defect that makes it divide excessively and persistently. The defect is passed on to the newly formed cells resulting from its division. The first cancer cell becomes two cancer cells, the two become four, four become eight, and so on—the mass repeatedly doubling as the cancer cells divide. This growing mass, a cancerous tumor, eventually crowds out and destroys neighboring healthy tissue. Cancer cells may break off and spread (metastasize) to other parts of the body, forming new tumors. Sarcomas tend to metastasize to the lungs.

Not all tumors of bone and soft tissue are cancerous. In fact, benign tumors are far more common. Benign tumors do not invade surrounding tissue or spread to other parts of the body. Once removed by surgery, they seldom recur. In contrast, sarcomas can recur after they have been treated and apparently eradicated.

Incidence

Sarcomas are relatively rare. About 2,000 new cases of bone cancer and 5,000 new cases of soft tissue sarcoma are diagnosed each year in the United States. Together they account for less than 2 percent of all new cancer cases per year.

By comparison, carcinomas—cancers that begin in the skin and the linings of inner organs—account for about 85 percent of all cancers. Carcinomas originate in organs like the lung or colon and often spread to form secondary tumors (metastases) in

Major Types of Soft Tissue Sarcoma

Type	Usual Age Range	Ages of Peak Occurrence	Major Locations in the Body	Average Number of New Cases Per Year
Liposarcoma	25-79	60-74	Fat in extremities* or trunk*	906
Fibrosarcoma of soft tissue	25-79	55-69	Fibrous tissue of extremities or trunk	508
Leiomyosarcoma	40-79	45-54	Smooth muscle of uterus or digestive tract	298
Rhabdomyosarcoma	30-84	55-69	Muscle of extremities	256
Embryonal rhabdomyosarcoma	0-19	0-4	Muscle of head and neck or genitourinary tract	66
Blood vessel sarcoma	20-84	70-74	Blood vessels of extremities or trunk	276
Synovial sarcoma	15-69	15-24	Tissue near joints of extremities	150
Mesenchymoma	10-74	60-69	Mixed tissue of extremities	72

*The word "extremities" refers to legs, feet, arms, and hands. The word "trunk" refers to the body apart from the head and extremities.

bones. These secondary or metastatic bone tumors are treated with methods used to treat the original cancer—they should not be confused with cancers that originate in the bone.

The accompanying tables list the major types of bone cancer and soft tissue sarcoma, the ages at which they are most likely to occur, their most common locations in the body, and the average number of new cases per year.

Cause and Prevention

Scientists do not fully understand why some people develop sarcomas while others do not. But by identifying common characteristics in groups having unusually high occurrence rates, they have been able to single out some factors that play a part in causing these diseases.

Years ago, for example, radium workers were found to have a high rate of bone cancer. Scientists suspected that the radiation given off by radium caused the disease. Later, scientists found that heavy doses of radiation given as treatment caused some cases of bone cancer and soft tissue sarcoma.

It is important to note that radiation has accounted for only a small fraction of sarcoma cases. In the future, the number is expected to be even smaller due to the growing use of megavoltage radiotherapy, which increases penetration of radiation to diseased tissue but spares surrounding bone and soft tissue from high doses.

Paget's disease, a noncancerous disorder resulting in bone deformity, leads to bone cancer in some cases. Researchers have found 13 times the average rate of bone cancer among patients with Paget's disease.

The peak occurrence of osteogenic sarcoma among teenagers appears related in some way to the growth spurt at the time of puberty. Osteogenic sarcoma tends to arise in bones that grow very rapidly.

A link between soft tissue sarcoma and occupational exposure to herbicides was suggested in a recent Swedish study. In this country, a link has been found between angiosarcoma of the liver (a rare blood vessel sarcoma) and occupational exposure to vinyl chloride, a substance used in the manufacture of certain plastics. The plastics themselves are not a cancer hazard.

Scientists have found several families that are prone to sarcomas of bone and soft tissue. However, family clusters of sarcomas represent only a small proportion of all cases.

Injuries are often suggested as causes of bone and soft tissue sarcomas. But available evidence suggests that injuries only call attention to preexisting tumors.

Certain viruses can cause sarcomas in laboratory animals, but there is no evidence that viruses are a direct cause of human sarcomas. Researchers believe, however, that a retrovirus plays an indirect role in the development of Kaposi's sarcoma when it is associated with AIDS, the acquired immune deficiency syndrome. (Kaposi's sarcoma is a rare cancer of the endothelial cells, the cells that line blood vessels.) The symptoms and treatment of this disease are not discussed here, but that information is available from sources listed at the end of this report.

Detection and Diagnosis

The symptoms of sarcomas vary depending upon the type and location of the tumor. In general, however, the symptoms develop very gradually. Pain, awareness of a mass, inability to move a part of the body nor-mally, or an unexpected fracture are the complaints that usually bring the patient to the doctor.

The doctor begins by asking questions about symptoms and past health problems, and by examining the affected site. The doctor also arranges for x-rays of that area of the body. If these suggest the presence of bone or soft tissue sarcoma, further diagnostic studies are indicated. These include chest x-rays to check for lung metastases and laboratory tests of urine and blood. Elevation of alkaline phosphatase in the blood can be a sign of osteogenic sarcoma, but that enzyme can also be elevated in various noncancerous conditions.

An x-ray technique called tomography may be used to obtain clearer pictures of the suspect area and the lungs. With tomography, shadows of structures in front of and behind the section under scrutiny do not show.

A CT scan (computed tomography scan), a highly sophisticated x-ray technique introduced in the 1970's, can show a tumor in even finer detail and detect lung metastases much earlier than conventional chest x-rays.

A conclusive diagnosis of sarcoma is made by means of a biopsy—the removal and microscopic examination of a sample of the suspect tissue. The tissue sample may be obtained through a needle or by a surgical incision. Sometimes a needle biopsy does not withdraw enough tissue for a definite diagnosis. Incisional biopsy is usually best.

The pathologist who examines the tissue actually makes the diagnosis, and not only determines the type of sarcoma present but also determines its grade, or degree of malignancy.

X-ray pictures of the entire skeleton may be made to determine whether any other areas of bone appear abnormal. Cancers that spread to the bones from other parts of the body often appear in more than one area, but bone sarcoma usually appears in only one site.

A bone scan is another method of finding abnormalities in any part of the skeleton. In this procedure a harmless amount of the radioactive isotope technetium-99 is injected into a vein and then tracked by a special camera. The isotope will collect in any area of bone where there is increased cellular activity.

An arteriogram, a special x-ray examination of blood vessels in and near the tumor, may be helpful in planning the best surgical approach to treatment.

Treatment

It is best for a sarcoma patient to begin treatment in a hospital that has an expert staff and resources to apply all forms of effective therapy. Surgery, chemotherapy (treatment with anticancer drugs), and radiation are often used in the initial treatment of sarcoma. It is important for specialists in these fields to decide jointly upon the treatment plan.

A doctor may refer a patient to a hospital that has a research program on sarcomas. In such programs, cancer specialists are trying new combinations, sequences, and amounts of treatment in an effort to improve the outcome for patients.

Treatment of Bone Cancer

Osteogenic sarcoma or *osteosarcoma,* the most common form of bone cancer, occurs mainly in teenagers. The tumor usually develops in a leg or arm bone, and cells from the tumor tend to spread to the lungs. Osteogenic sarcoma used to be rapidly fatal in most cases because of lung metastasis. Now, with better ways of killing cancer cells before they can form secondary tumors, as well as better methods of detecting early metastasis, patients are living longer and many are cured.

After diagnosis, a surgeon removes the primary tumor. Besides surgery, chemotherapy is now recommended to destroy any cancer cells that may have strayed beyond the tumor. Results of clinical trials have shown that patients with high-grade, localized osteosarcoma who are given anticancer drugs in addition to surgery have a significantly higher rate of disease-free survival than those who have not received chemotherapy.

Several drugs are known to kill osteosarcoma cells. These drugs, used in various combinations, include doxorubicin (Adriamycin), high-dose methotrexate, cisplatin (Platinol), cyclophosphamide (Cytoxan), bleomycin, vincristine, and dactinomycin. Clinical studies are attempting to determine the best timing of chemotherapy—whether before or after surgery or both.

Frequent tomographic examinations of the lungs are important to detect any metastasis in an early, operable stage. Surgeons have found that by removing lung metastases as they develop, they can prolong survival of their patients. Chemotherapy is continued or increased after this surgery. When lung metastases cannot be surgically removed, radiation therapy is sometimes helpful if chemotherapy alone is not successful.

Before the advent of chemotherapy, amputation of the affected limb was considered necessary because lesser surgery usually resulted in return of the cancer at its original site. Now clinical investigators are finding that when anticancer drugs are given before and/or immediately after the operation, limb-sparing surgery can be performed without increasing the risk of local recurrence in about 50 percent of cases. In the other 50 percent, amputation remains necessary because of the size or location of the tumor, its involvement with major blood vessels or nerves, the presence of infection, or other factors.

In clinical research programs where limb-sparing surgery is being tried, surgeons often replace diseased bone with a prosthesis made of the metal vitallium. In some cases, bone from another part of the patient's body is used. When only small segments of nonweight-bearing bones are removed, replacement is often unnecessary.

Parosteal osteosarcoma, a rare type of osteosarcoma, involves both the outer part of a limb bone and the membrane called the periosteum that covers the bone. Patients are usually cured by surgery that removes the tumor and a margin of healthy tissue. Amputation is seldom required.

Chondrosarcoma occurs mainly in persons of middle age and usually begins in cartilage of a leg, hip, or rib. Generally, it grows slowly and does not spread to other parts of the body for many years, if at all. Lung metastases are uncommon.

Chondrosarcoma is treated surgically. Depending on the tumor's size and location, either part of the bone or the entire

bone is removed. In many cases, adequate surgery requires amputation. Following appropriate surgery, long-term survival can be expected in at least 60 percent of all patients.

Ewing's sarcoma, a cancer of young people, usually begins in bone of the leg, hip, rib, or arm. It is a fast-growing cancer that quickly spreads to the lungs. It may also spread to other bones.

Until recently, 20 to 40 percent of patients with Ewing's sarcoma were free of disease 5 to 10 years after treatment. Now studies show that more than 50 percent of patients without

Major Types of Bone Cancer

Type	Usual Age Range	Ages of Peak Occurrence	Major Locations in the Body	Average Number of New Cases Per Year
Osteogenic sarcoma (also called osteosarcoma)	10-55	10-20	Bone of leg, arm, or hip	520
Chondrosarcoma	25-65	50-60	Cartilage of leg, hip, or rib	428
Ewing's sarcoma	10-30	10-20	Bone of leg, hip, or arm	234
Fibrosarcoma of bone	25-60	30-40	Bone of leg, arm, or hip	66
Malignant giant cell tumor	40-60	40-55	Bone of leg or arm	58
Chordoma	40-70	55-65	Spinal column or skull	56
Parosteal osteosarcoma	20-45	30-40	Bone of leg or arm	26

widespread disease at diagnosis have long-term, disease-free survival.

Ewing's sarcoma is very sensitive to radiation. Therefore, patients are usually treated with radiation beamed at the affected bone, plus chemotherapy to kill cancer cells that may have spread to the lungs. The combination of anticancer drugs most commonly used consists of vincristine, dactinomycin, cyclophosphamide, and doxorubicin.

Before chemotherapy began to be used in the initial treatment of Ewing's sarcoma, lung metastasis killed most patients within 2 years. Now 70 percent of patients are alive 2 years after diagnosis and treatment.

If metastases do develop in the lung, chemotherapy is continued or resumed with the original drugs or different drugs. This treatment often results in regression or disappearance of the lung metastases. When there is a single persistent metastatic growth in the lung, surgery may be performed to remove it.

In some cases, surgery is performed following initial radiotherapy and chemotherapy to remove the affected part of a bone or an entire limb.

Fibrosarcoma of bone is a very rare cancer that arises in the ends of major limb bones and spreads into soft tissues. Amputation is the standard method of treatment. Although this sarcoma is not as responsive as others to radiation and chemotherapy, these methods may be of help if the tumor cannot be removed surgically or if metastases develop in the lungs.

Giant cell tumor is a benign tumor that sometimes becomes cancerous. Its most common location is in the thigh bone near the knee. If benign, the tumor and a margin of normal tissue should be removed surgically. If cancerous, the tumor and a wider margin of normal tissue may be removed, but in some cases amputation is necessary.

Chordoma, a very rare cancer, occurs in the spinal column or skull and is usually treated with radiation.

Treatment of Soft Tissue Sarcomas

There are many different types of soft tissue sarcoma (cancers that arise in muscle, fat, fibrous tissue, blood vessels, nerves, and other supporting tissues of the body). But to physicians planning a patient's treatment, the type is not as important as the cancer's size, its location and extent of spread, and whether the patient is an adult or a child. Another factor playing an important role in the choice of treatment is the grade of the cancer cells, which is determined by the pathologist in analyzing the structure of the cancer cells. High-grade tumors have a greater potential for spread than low-grade tumors.

Soft tissue sarcomas of the extremities occur mainly in adults. According to a consensus development conference sponsored by the National Institutes of Health, limb-sparing surgery for patients with high-grade soft tissue sarcomas of the extremities is often possible. Frequently, radiation, chemotherapy, or both are also given in an effort to kill any stray cancer cells. Clinical trials now under way are attempting to determine how each of these therapies can best enhance disease-free survival. Some of the investigational approaches being used to treat soft tissue sarcomas involve preoperative infusion of chemotherapy to the affected limb,

followed by limb-sparing surgery; postoperative chemotherapy with various regimens; and trials investigating the role of radiation therapy delivered in different ways.

One NCI trial, conducted between 1975 and 1981, suggested that the use of chemotherapy immediately after surgery may lead to improvement in freedom from disease recurrence, but further study is needed to define the role of chemotherapy as a backup to surgery in treating soft tissue sarcomas of the extremities.

Soft tissue sarcomas in the trunk of adults are usually treated with surgery and postoperative radiation therapy. In some research centers, radiation is being used before surgery to reduce the size of the tumor.

So far, chemotherapy seems less effective against these sarcomas than against those of the extremities. But in clinical research programs, new drugs and combinations are being tried that may prove more promising.

Children with soft tissue sarcoma are usually treated with a combination of surgery, radiation therapy, and chemotherapy. The drugs most often used are vincristine, actinomycin D, cyclophosphamide, and doxorubicin. The surgery performed on children is more conservative than that employed for adults. If surgery is not advisable because of a tumor's location, radiation and chemotherapy are often effective.

Embryonal rhabdomyosarcoma is the most common soft tissue sarcoma in children. With a combination of surgery, radiation therapy, and multidrug chemotherapy, more than 60 percent of all patients are cured. Embryonal rhabdomyosarcoma occurs mainly in the head and neck area or in the genitourinary tract. The surgery for these cancers is limited in order to preserve the normal appearance of the head and neck and the normal function of genital and urinary organs.

The next most common site of embryonal rhabdomyosarcoma is the eye socket. If the cancer has not spread beyond the eye socket, radiation therapy alone can control the disease in 90 percent of cases while preserving good-quality vision. In some cases, however, surgery is performed to remove the tumor and the eye. If the cancer has spread, multidrug chemotherapy is recommended.

PDQ

The National Cancer Institute has developed PDQ (Physician Data Query), a computerized database designed to give doctors quick and easy access to:

- the latest treatment information for most types of cancer;
- descriptions of clinical trials that are open for patient entry; and
- names of organizations and physicians involved in cancer care.

To get access to PDQ, a doctor may use an office computer with a telephone hookup and a PDQ access code, or the services of a medical library with online searching capability. Most Cancer Information Service offices (1-800-4-CANCER) provide a physician with one free PDQ search, and can tell doctors how to get regular access to the database. Patients may ask their doctor to use PDQ or may call 1-800-4-CANCER themselves. Information specialists at this toll-free number use a variety of sources, including PDQ, to answer questions about cancer prevention, diagnosis, and treatment.

Suggestions for Additional Reading

Except as noted, the following materials are not available from the National Cancer Institute. They can be found in medical libraries, many college and university libraries, and some public libraries.

Chemotherapy and You: A Guide to Self-Help During Treatment, prepared by the Office of Cancer Communications, National Cancer Institute. NIH Publication No. 85-1136.

DeVita, V.T., Jr., Hellman, S., and Rosenberg, S.A., eds. *Cancer: Principles and Practice of Oncology,* second edition, Philadelphia: Lippincott, 1985.

Eilber, F.R. et al. "Advances in the Treatment of Sarcomas of the Extremity: Current Status of Limb Salvage," Supplement to *Cancer,* Dec. 1, 1984, pp. 2695-2701.

Holland, J. and Frei, E., III, eds. *Cancer Medicine,* Philadelphia: Lea and Febiger, 1982.

Link, M.P., Goorin, A.M. et al., "The Effect of Adjuvant Chemotherapy on Relapse-Free Survival in Patients with Osteosarcoma of the Extremity," *The New England Journal of Medicine,* June 19, 1986, pp. 1600-1605.

Mitsuyasu, R.T. and Groopman, J.E. "Biology and Therapy of Kaposi's Sarcoma," *Seminars in Oncology,* March 1984, pp. 53-59.

NIH Consensus Development Conference Statement on Limb-Sparing Treatment of Adult Soft-Tissue and Osteosarcomas, Dec. 3-5, 1984.

Radiation Therapy and You: A Guide to Self-Help During Treatment, prepared by the Office of Cancer Communications, National Cancer Institute. NIH Publication No. 85-2227.

Rosenberg, S.A. et al. "The Treatment of Soft-Tissue Sarcomas of the Extremities," *Annals of Surgery,* vol. 196, no. 3, Sept. 1982, pp. 305-15.

Schottenfeld, D. and Fraumeni, J., *Cancer Epidemiology and Prevention,* Philadelphia: W.B. Saunders Co., 1982.

Volberding, P. "Therapy of Kaposi's Sarcoma in AIDS," *Seminars in Oncology,* March 1984, pp. 60-67.

What Are Clinical Trials All About?, prepared by the Office of Cancer Communications, National Cancer Institute. NIH Publication No. 86-2706.

Young People with Cancer: A Handbook for Parents, prepared by the Office of Cancer Communications, National Cancer Institute. NIH Publication No. 83-2378.

Ziegler, J.L. et al. "Kaposi's Sarcoma: A Comparison of Classical and Endemic Forms," *Seminars in Oncology,* March 1984, pp. 47-52.

The mentioned text is reprinted within this book. See CONTENTS for location.

Chapter 4

Brain Tumor and Brain Cancer

Brain Tumors— Hope Through Research

Editor's Note: The material which follows, describing brain tumors, both benign and malignant, is somewhat different in format from the chapters devoted to other types of tumors and cancers. Unlike those chapters prepared by the National Cancer Institute, this chapter's source was developed by writers at the National Institute of Neurological and Communicative Disorders and Stroke.

She was 20, an attractive English major at a Boston college, engaged to be married. Then she was diagnosed as having a brain tumor of a particularly advanced and malignant type that was invading the right frontal lobe of her brain. Marriage was definitely out, she decided, but she wasn't giving up. The surgeons removed the bulk of the tumor and followed up with radiation and chemotherapy. Now, 7 years later, there is no sign of cancer. She still rules out marriage, but she's back in college.

A 45-year-old minister and biblical scholar recently underwent his fourth operation for a meningioma, a tumor of the outer coverings of the brain. Usually a meningioma is a slow-growing tumor, often completely removable by surgery. In the minister's case, however, the tumor recurred, first after a year or so, then after only months. This time the brain surgeons planned to follow up with a new anticancer drug.

Usually. Slow-growing. Removable. Malignant. Invasive.

Advanced. The words are the common jargon of the cancer expert. The words are familiar to nonexperts as well, for who among us has not been touched by the death of friend or relative who has succumbed to cancer?

When it comes to brain tumors, however, the familiar words take on new meanings. The brain is a special organ, special in the cells that compose it, in its position in the head, and in its relation to the rest of the body. When a tumor grows in the brain, doctors have to consider not only the nature of the tumor, but its relation to the brain's distinctive features.

The Nature of the Brain

First and foremost among those features is that the brain is the organ of thought, emotion, and behavior. The idea that a mass of abnormal tissue could encroach on that domain, undermining the mental faculties that make us human and

41

ultimately threatening life itself, is what terrifies most people when they hear the words *brain tumor.* Yet some brain tumors can be removed completely at surgery leaving no neurological damage. Even advanced cancers growing deep inside the brain are being tackled today by new treatments that have saved or at least prolonged lives, while preserving the integrity of those lives.

Experts can also point to other features of the brain that offer some reason for hope. Tumors are generally classified as benign—if the tumor cells look much like ordinary cells and the tumor is confined to one place—or malignant, if the tumor cells look very disordered and the tumor can spread (metastasize) to other parts of the body. (Strictly speaking, the word *cancer* applies only to malignant growths.) Tumors that' originate in the brain—primary brain tumors—may be either benign or malignant. Surprisingly, while malignant brain tumor cells can spread throughout the brain, only rarely do they spread to other parts of the body. That means that once you destroy a brain cancer, you need not worry that some cells may have escaped to seed tumors elsewhere in the body.

Another fact that startles many people is that brain tumor tissue almost never consists of the fundamental—working cells of the brain—the nerve cells (neurons). Once mature, these complex nerve cells no longer divide and multiply. Instead, it is the surrounding and

supporting cells of the brain that occasionally get out of control. Thus a brain tumor that is diagnosed and treated early may do little or no damage to essential brain matter—the neurons and their circuits that underlie every act of mental life and behavior.

Confusing Symptoms

There are "if's". Brain tumors are not always easy to diagnose. The symptoms can vary widely according to the brain area affected. If a tumor grows in the temporal lobe on the left side of the brain, for example, it may affect speech and memory, or alter mood and emotional state. Such symptoms might suggest mental illness or psychological problems, rather than a brain tumor. If a tumor lies near the cerebellum, an area at the back of the brain important in the control of movement, there may be early symptoms of dizziness and lack of coordination. Tumors growing on or around the major nerves supplying the ears or eyes may lead to symptoms of hearing loss, headaches, or visual problems, diverting attention from the brain as the source of trouble.

On the other hand, some brain tumors may produce few symptoms. Parts of the frontal lobes, for example, are presumed to play a role in thinking and other higher mental activities. Yet tumors can sometimes cause considerable tissue damage in these areas with little effect on a person's behavior.

Once a tumor is found, still another "if" centers on its location in relation to surrounding tissue. The brain is one of the most protected organs in the body. It is wrapped in the tough outer coverings of the meninges, bathed in shock-absorbing and nutrient liquid—the cerebrospinal fluid—and armored by the strong bones of the skull.

If a tumor lies near the skull bones or close to major blood vessels or channels circulating cerebrospinal fluid, it need not grow very large before it blocks blood or cerebrospinal fluid circulation and causes increased pressure inside the skull. Or, if the tumor is discovered deep inside the brain, surgery to remove it may be risky, with too great a chance of damaging vital brain centers. Ironically, the distinction between benign and malignant blurs in such cases. If a benign tumor is inaccessible it can be fatal. On the other hand, the young woman with the malignant tumor invading her frontal lobe had a major portion of the lobe removed and is alive and well today.

Neurosurgeons who treat brain tumor patients are well aware of the ironies of the condition. They can all tell stories of exceptional survivals as well as tragic deaths. Scientists who have made research on brain tumors their specialty are particularly concerned that the public understand the complex problems posed by brain tumors as well as the growing efforts to solve those problems.

Those investigators include scientists supported by the National Institute of Neurological and

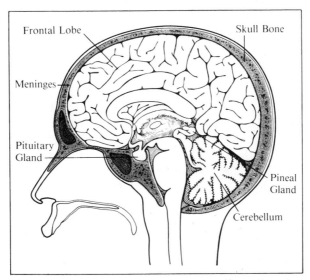

The brain, wrapped in its meningeal coverings, fits snugly against the bones of the skull.

Communicative Disorders and Stroke (NINCDS)—the leading Federal agency supporting research on the brain—the National Cancer Institute, and other Federal health agencies. One major group effort is the clinical research program carried out by NINCDS neurosurgeons working at the Clinical Center, the research hospital of the National Institutes of Health in Bethesda, Md.

11,000 Cases a Year

The chances of developing a primary malignant brain tumor are relatively rare—about 1 in 22,000. Such cancers account for less than 2 percent of all cancers diagnosed in the United States every year. That is still an impressively large number—11,000 brain cancers annually. At least twice as many patients have secondary brain cancers, the result of cancer metastasizing to the brain from other sites in the body, principally the breast, lung, or kidney.

Brain tumors affect children as well as adults. Indeed, primary tumors of the brain or spinal cord (the central nervous system) are the most common tumors of childhood after the leukemias. The peak for brain tumors in children is between the ages of 6 and 9. Childhood brain tumors generally differ in location and cellular makeup from adult tumors, differences thought to reflect a still growing and developing nervous system. Adult brain tumors are most common between the ages of 40 and 60, with men affected slightly more than women.

Why primary brain tumors occur remains a mystery. Tumor sleuths have considered the vast array of environmental and genetic factors that have been linked to cancers in other parts of the body, but in the case of brain tumors there are no clearcut associations. The recent finding of a slightly higher than normal occurrence of brain tumors in workers at certain petrochemical plants is interesting, but the cases are too few for scientists to come to firm conclusions. There are also a few families in the United States where cancer, including brain cancer, occurs frequently. Some genetic factor could possibly account for these families' high cancer prevalence—perhaps some defect in the body's immune system. Again, more detailed genetic and biochemical studies are needed.

Diagnosing Brain Tumors Today

Clearly not every headache, dizzy spell, or visual disturbance is a sign of brain tumor. And while symptoms can vary widely, specialists pay particular attention to certain signs:

■ *Progressive unrelenting symptoms.* Whatever they may be, the symptoms never let up and they get worse over time.

■ *Headache.* Given the tight confines of the head, a growing tumor sooner or later will create pressure or swelling that affects tissues in the head, producing severe headache. Often the patient reports that the headache is worse upon first waking in the morning. Interestingly, brain tissue itself is normally insensitive to pain. But the meningeal layers, blood vessel walls, and the tissues lining the cavities of the brain and skull are rich in nerve endings sensitive to pain.

■ *Visual complaints.* Double vision, blurring or other visual symptoms may occur as a result of increased pressure on the optic nerve or the blood vessels supplying the retina.

■ *Motor signs.* Some patients report weakness or numbness in their arms and legs. Sometimes reflexes (like the familiar knee jerk reflex) are very strong. In the case of spinal cord tumors, patients may experience a growing loss of sensation below a certain level in the trunk, or increasing difficulty in moving limbs.

■ *Seizures.* The onset of seizures or convulsions in a patient who has not been in an accident, been ill with fever, or suffered some other injury or illness is "presumptive evidence of a brain tumor until proven otherwise," says one leading authority.

To confirm the diagnosis, neurologists and neurosurgeons can conduct a battery of tests including simple X-rays of the head, standard brainwave recordings (the electroencephalogram or EEG),

analysis of cerebrospinal fluid, and so on. Their principal diagnostic aid today, however, is the CT scan, the technique that produces a computerized three-dimensional X-ray image of the brain. The CT scan is highly accurate, detecting the presence of a tumor mass in 90 to 95 percent of cases—even when that mass is no larger than half an inch across.

The CT scan can not only indicate the presence of a tumor, but will pin down its location in the brain. At this point the specialist may call for an arteriogram: an X-ray that will outline the arteries supplying blood to the tumor. Some tumors are richly endowed with blood vessels; others are less so. Thus the arteriogram provides another clue to the kind of brain tumor.

The Next Step

Surgery is the first line of attack against brain tumors. How extensive the operation will be depends on the tumor size and location and whether the tumor cells are concentrated in a mass or spread throughout the brain. "Each patient's tumor is different," notes the chief of the NINCDS Surgical Neurology Branch in the NIH Clinical Center. "It is different pathologically, it behaves differently, and it grows differently."

For that reason some of the tissue removed at brain surgery is always reserved for pathological analysis. Studies of this "biopsy" material

45

indicate whether the tumor is benign or malignant. Malignant tumor tissue removed at surgery is also being used in promising research studies aimed at improving treatment—even predicting which treatments will be successful.

Observers examining samples of brain tissue microscopically can tell what kinds of cells make up a tumor, and whether the cells are benign or malignant. Benign cells resemble normal cells of the tissue in question. Malignant cells lose more and more of their distinctive trademarks and acquire the classic characteristics of cancer: large or multiple nuclei, abnormal numbers of chromosomes, and changes in the cell's surface membrane. These changes seem to help very malignant cells to invade and take root in other tissues more easily. The extent of these changes permits classifying tumor cells by degree of malignancy

from Grade I, benign, to Grade IV, the most advanced stage of malignancy.

Tumor Varieties

Most brain tumors are *gliomas*, derived from the glial cells that support the neurons of the brain. Gliomas can be either benign or malignant. Unfortunately, one of the most malignant gliomas—the *glioblastoma multiforme*—is also the most common brain tumor. In all, gliomas account for 43 percent of primary brain cancers. Glial tumors are further described in terms of the type of glial cell they contain:

■ *Astrocytomas.* Star-shaped cells called astrocytes are the cells affected in a large subgroup of gliomas. Benign cerebellar astrocytomas are common childhood tumors. With

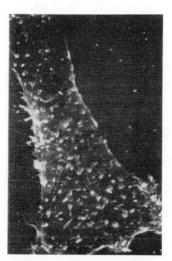

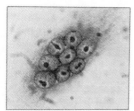

The small finger-like projections dotting the surface of this brain tumor cell are signs of malignancy.

Those bull's-eyes in the center are multiple nuclei in a single glial cell: a sign of malignancy.

46

today's tools and techniques, these tumors are often completely removable surgically. They are one of the recent success stories in tumor treatment. On the other hand, the young woman college student's frontal lobe tumor was a malignant astrocytoma. What makes her story so impressive is that it was a Grade IV malignancy—an aggressive rapidly growing tumor that is usually fatal in a year or so.

■ *Medulloblastomas.* The root "blast" refers to a cell in an early stage of development. Medulloblasts are immature cells that may develop into either neurons or glial cells. Medulloblastomas are malignant tumors found in the rear of the brain. They typically occur in youngsters under 12 and account for a small percentage of all brain tumors.

■ *Ependymomas.* The cells lining

the hollow cavities of the brain—ependymal cells—also give riseto a small percentage of brain tumors. These "ependymomas" tend to be benign.

Other gliomas are composed of other varieties of glial cells, such as those that produce the fatty insulating material (myelin) that surrounds many nerve fibers in the brain.

The second major group of primary brain tumors are those made up of covering cells:

■ *Meningiomas.* Tumors of the meninges (the membrane coverings of the brain and spinal cord) are usually benign, and account for some 15 percent of all brain tumors.

■ *Schwannomas.* These tumors arise from the Schwann cells that form the fatty sheath that envelops

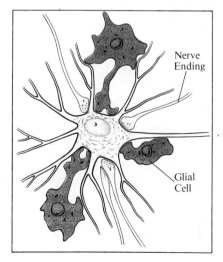

A typical nerve cell in the brain surrounded by glial cells and nerve endings.

Nerve Ending

Glial Cell

nerve fibers in the body. One such tumor develops in relation to the nerve of hearing, the acoustic nerve. Acoustic nerve tumors, called *acoustic neuromas*, are benign tumors which, if detected early, can be completely removed without loss of hearing or other nervous system damage.

The successful removal of acoustic neuromas is a good illustration of how far neurosurgeons have advanced in techniques. During the first decade of this century the mortality rate for acoustic neuroma surgery was close to 80 percent. The tumor was deep-seated and difficult to remove because of its close relation to the brain stem, a core of brain tissue that contains vital nerve centers such as those controlling breathing. By 1917, however, the doctor considered to be the father of neurosurgery, Harvey Cushing, demonstrated a new technique for acoustic neuroma removal which reduced mortality to 20 percent. With more experience Cushing was able to reduce mortality to below 10 percent. Today the mortality rate

for acoustic neuroma is down to 1 percent.

Other kinds of tumor may involve cells in or near the pituitary gland at the base of the brain, or the pineal gland, deep in the center of the brain. In rare instances a brain tumor will develop from types of nerve cells.

Surgery Plus...

In the case of a benign accessible brain tumor, surgery may be the beginning and end of treatment: The tumor is completely removed and the patient resumes activities with little likelihood of recurrence. If the tumor is malignant, it may not be possible to remove it completely. In that case, or if a tumor is large or difficult to reach, treatment will include radiation and chemotherapy. Radiation is sometimes used before surgery in the hope of reducing tumor size.

Today, an increasing number of tumors formerly considered

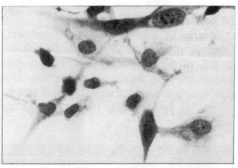

These benign cells from an acoustic neuroma were grown in tissue culture. If diagnosed early, acoustic neuromas can be removed completely with no neurological damage.

inoperable can be tackled surgically. Microsurgery—the use of an operating microscope—has played an important role in that development. But often it is a combination of great technical skill and an ingenious strategy for getting at the tumor that has led to surgical success.

A few neurosurgeons are currently using high frequency sound waves (ultrasound) and laser beams to destroy brain tumors. In one laser technique, for example, the surgeon uses an operating microscope and aims the laser beam at the center of the tumor, using the high intensity rays to burn out the tissue. The exact position of the tumor is calculated by a computer that translates CT scan images into a set of coordinates referable to a framework set up 'around the patient's head. Time will tell whether such techniques will improve the success rate for tumor treatment.

Radiation usually begins within a week or two after surgery and continues for 6 weeks. Among recent refinements in radiation therapy are the use of drugs that make tumor tissue more sensitive to radioactive bombardment, and new radioactive sources that provide more powerful rays or charged particles that can be sharply focused on the tumor.

Chemotherapy, the other major weapon in the attack on brain tumors, has also benefited from refinements and advances. The principal brain tumor-killing drugs in use today go by the initials BCNU and CCNU, both chemically known

as nitrosoureas. These drugs pass readily into the brain when given by mouth or injected into the bloodstream. Many drugs are prevented from reaching brain cells by an elaborate meshwork of fine blood vessels and cells—the blood-brain barrier—that filters blood reaching the brain.

The combined treatment of brain cancers with better drugs and radiotherapy, along with surgical techniques aimed at removing as much tumor tissue as possible, has meant longer survival times and richer lives for brain cancer patients. Further improvements in these traditional forms of treatment can be expected in the years ahead. In addition, scientists are developing new therapies based on promising laboratory studies.

The New Research

If a single word could describe the aim of much current research on malignant brain tumors it might be the word *fingerprint*. Scientists want to characterize tumor tissue in ways that make the tissue as unique to the patient as his or her fingerprints. Armed with that information, the hope is that doctors can design more effective treatments—with added confidence that those treatments will work.

The impetus for this research comes first from the need to determine what kinds of cells are found in the tumor and their degree of malignancy. Second, there is a strong suspicion that the reason that those tumor cells are there to begin with is that the body's immune system is deficient in some way.

Normally, the immune system seeks out and destroys invading organisms or foreign tissue. These defense mechanisms are called into play because foreign tissue is studded with telltale surface proteins—antigens—that differ from the surface antigens normally found on body cells. The immune system recognizes the foreign tissue and is stimulated to make a variety of cells—scavengers, "killer" cells, and others—as well as the protein compounds called antibodies—all specifically designed to fight that particular foreign invader. When the body's *own* cells become cancerous, their surface antigens also change. They, too, should appear foreign. By rights, a person's immune system ought to attack the cancer and destroy it.

There is evidence that the immune system tries to do just that. Investigators have been able to take samples of brain tumor tissue removed during surgery and grow the cells in tissue culture. When the scientists later expose the cultured cells to blood serum from the patient who provided the cells, they find that the serum contains antibodies that attack the tumor cells. The ammunition is there; it is just not powerful enough.

Scientists at NINCDS and elsewhere are exploring ways to boost patients' immune responses so that they can successfully fight their brain tumors or any remnants of tumor tissue not removed during surgery. One way is through immune *stimulation*. The idea is to use the patient's own tumor cells as the stimulating material. The cells are grown in tissue culture and then irradiated to prevent them from reproducing. The cells still contain their surface antigens, however, and so when injected back into the patient's body, they should provoke a strong response—both cells and antibodies—from the immune system. Currently NINCDS investigators are conducting such experimental treatments in selected patients with highly malignant astrocytomas.

The ability to grow human brain cancer cells in tissue culture has paid off in other ways as well. Tumor samples from a patient can be grown on separate culture plates and subjected to a variety of tests. Some tests are used to determine the degree of malignancy of tumor cells, a necessary step in planning treatment. One way to measure malignancy is to observe how rapidly the cells multiply and fill the culture plate. Investigators can also expose the cells to a fine-holed filter and see how aggressively the cells try to penetrate the openings.

Scientists can also transplant human brain tumor cells to laboratory animals to see if the human tumor will take root in the animal's body. The animals used are mice with a hereditary defect that renders them hairless as well as lacking the thymus, an organ important in the immune system. The immune system defect makes these "nude mice" less likely than normal animals to reject foreign tissue. The ability to grow a human cancer in a living animal is in itself of great importance: Scientists can observe how the tumor behaves at all stages of growth, as well as experiment with new therapies.

Tailor-made Treatments

Provided with samples of a patient's tumor cells in tissue culture, investigators can also test the effectiveness of antitumor drugs. There appears to be a correlation between the way tumor cells respond to drugs in the laboratory dish and the way they respond in the brain. Thus if the lab studies show that BCNU and CCNU have little or no effect on cells grown in culture, there is little likelihood that these drugs will benefit the patient. For these "nonresponders," investigators may try other tactics, such as the use of new antitumor drugs still in the experimental stage. (The biblical scholar will receive such an experimental drug.)

With continued experience and refinements in culturing techniques, it may be possible to custom design brain tumor treatment programs, selecting the right drug at the right dosage and initiating treatment quickly, without having to go through a lengthy trial and error period. Such tactics not only save

precious time, they also spare the patient the futility of ineffective treatments and may also reduce side effects.

Tissue culture techniques may also make it easier to diagnose a brain tumor early—when physicians may suspect that a tumor is present, but nothing is detectable on a CT scan. NINCDS scientists and others have taken blood samples from patients with suspected malignancies and added the serum to established laboratory cultures of human brain tumor cells. If the patient has a brain tumor, there is a high probability that the blood serum will contain antitumor antibodies that will react with the tumor cells on the laboratory plate.

Alternative Treatments

The tissue culture and immunotherapy techniques are among the most promising and exciting lines of investigation being explored in brain tumor research today. There are others as well. Radiologists continue to seek out more effective methods of irradiating tumor tissue in the brain without jeopardizing surrounding tissue. Likewise, pharmacologists search for better antitumor drugs and ways of delivering those drugs to the brain. The use of a type of sugar called mannitol, for example, can disrupt the blood-brain barrier for a brief period of time and allow chemicals access to brain tissue. However, specialists have noted that the blood-brain barrier does not appear to be as intact around tumor tissue, so the need to circumvent it may not be so crucial.

Scientists are also exploring the use of agents that can cause malignant cells to become more like normal cells again. Such a transformation may be effective in halting tumor growth or in enhancing sensitivity to other forms of treatment. The advantage of this technique—called *biological modification*—is that the substances used are nontoxic compounds that are normally produced in the body.

Professional journals as well as popular magazines and newspapers report a steady stream of promising new treatments for cancer. One reads, for example, of heat produced by microwaves being used to kill brain tumors. Some investigators are also experimenting with raising body temperature on the theory that an artificial fever will provoke the immune system into action. Another well-publicized potential cure for cancer is interferon, the substance body cells produce naturally to fight infection. These new therapies may prove to be important, but as yet there is not enough evidence to establish their roles as therapeutic agents. All new approaches to treating brain tumors must stand the test of well-designed, carefully controlled clinical tests and long-term followup before any conclusions can be drawn about the safety or the effectiveness of treatments.

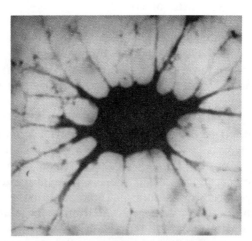

This normal-looking astrocyte is a malignant cell. Experimental treatment with a nontoxic chemical normally found in the body caused the cell to assume a more normal appearance.

Watching The Brain In Action

Aiding and abetting followup of new treatments for brain tumors, as well as providing a versatile research tool in many basic and clinical studies, is a new form of brain scanning called positron emission tomography (PET). PET scans of the brain show which brain cells are most active metabolically. An aggressively growing tumor, for example, might show up on a PET scan as an area lighter or brighter than surrounding tissue, indicating higher metabolic activity. A tumor that is dying, however, might be correspondingly lower in activity, and, over time, shrink in size.

The PET technique depends on the fact that metabolically active cells absorb nutrients at a high rate. The bloodstream of a patient or an experimental animal is injected with a nutrient like sugar that is labeled with a radioactive compound. As the blood circulates in the brain, the most active cells will take up more of the labeled sugar and then broadcast their location by virtue of their radioactivity. Detectors placed around the head pick up the radioactivity, and with the aid of a computer, translate the readings into a brain image. PET scans can be color-coded to make the differences in cell uptake of nutrient stand out better. PET studies are being used to compare the healthy brain with the tumorous brain, and to observe changes in brain metabolism at all stages of disease.

When Brain Tumor Strikes

It is especially important to have a clear idea of the facts, should you or someone close to you be diagnosed as having a brain tumor. The news inevitably comes as a shock, so much so that much of what the specialist may say by way of explanation may be lost in the immediate emotional reaction to the news. Most patients and their families are caught up in a turmoil of feelings which may range from disbelief to paralyzing grief at the thought of impending death. Yet it is precisely at this point that hard decisions have to be made about the course of treatment and about family affairs. During this time you may find it helpful to turn to the larger family, friends, and outside resources such as clergymen or hospital counselors. Such people may assist you with many of the practical arrangements that may have to be made, as well as provide psychological and moral support.

What you should also do is inform yourself about the tried and true treatments as well as the highly regarded clinical research and treatment programs available in major medical centers in the United States. You should also seek treatment by physicians who are experienced in tumor therapy. Because brain tumors are relatively rare, many physicians see only a few brain tumor patients a year. There are others, however, who have made brain tumors their specialty.

53

Psychologically, the brain tumor patient and the family need to adapt to the situation. No one says that this is easy, and it is expected that there may be stages of anger or indignation (Why me?), denial, frustration, sadness, and depression. Some parents have seen a child die from a brain tumor and have written books about their experience, as John Gunther did in *Death Be Not Proud*. Knowing that others experience grief and tragedy, reading their stories, or sharing accounts can help in working through the emotional upheaval. In this regard the Association for Brain Tumor Research, a voluntary health organization formed by individuals concerned about brain tumors—usually because of personal experience—can be a valuable source of information and help. NINCDS, the National Cancer Institute, groups like the American Cancer Society, and major treatment centers like New York's Memorial Sloan-Kettering Center for Cancer Research and Houston's M.D. Anderson Hospital and Tumor Institute are other useful sources of information.

Probably one of the most unsettling aspects of the diagnosis and treatment of brain tumors is the uncertainty with which you have to live. In some cases of secondary brain tumors or advanced primary malignancies, death may be imminent. As we have seen, however, the combination of new and improved therapies have added months or even years to life, while preserving its quality.

As more and more brain tumors come to treatment earlier, and the treatments themselves prove more effective, there will still be worrisome wait-and-see problems. Will the tumor recur? Is a minor memory lapse or mood change an omen of cancer's return? Those questions and fears are not helped when brain tumor patients experience episodes of brain swelling, fever, or headache as a result of treatment. Needless to say checkups can allay such fears, and there are medications that can relieve brain swelling or other side effects of treatment.

In the end, how well patients, friends, and family members adapt to the experience of a brain tumor depends on their understanding of the problem and the inner resources and personality traits they bring to bear on it. For a 27-year-old college student in Boston, it has paid to be an optimist.

Volunteer Health Organizations

The Association for Brain Tumor Research supports research on brain tumors and provides information to the general public through brochures and newsletters.

Association for Brain Tumor Research
6232 N. Pulaski Road, Suite 200
Chicago, Ill. 60646
(312)286-5571

54

The Acoustic Neuroma Association is a new organization for patients, families, and medical personnel concerned with tumors of the acoustic nerve as well as other cranial nerves.

Acoustic Neuroma Association
240 Mooreland Avenue
Carlisle, Pa. 17013
(717) 249-2973

The Candlelighters is an organization for parents of children with cancer. The group publishes a newsletter and promotes the establishment of self-help chapters throughout the country.

The Candlelighters Foundation
2025 I Street, N.W.
Washington, D.C. 20006
(202) 659-5136

The American Cancer Society is a source of information on all varieties of cancer. The society has divisions in many cities in the United States and headquarters in New York.

American Cancer Society
777 3rd Avenue
New York, N.Y. 10017
(212) 371-2900

National Institutes of Health

For additional information on brain tumor research and clinical treatment programs contact:

Office of Scientific and Health Reports
National Institute of Neurological and Communicative Disorders and Stroke
Building 31, Room 8A06
National Institutes of Health
Bethesda, Md. 20205
(301) 496-5751

Office of Cancer Communications
National Cancer Institute
Building 31, Room 10A29
National Institutes of Health
Bethesda, Md. 20205
(301) 496-6631

Chapter 5

Breast Cancer: Biopsy

What You Should Know

Breast Biopsy: What You Should Know

You have a lump or other change in your breast. After you've had an examination, you're told that a biopsy must be performed to find out whether the lump is benign (noncancerous) or malignant (cancerous).

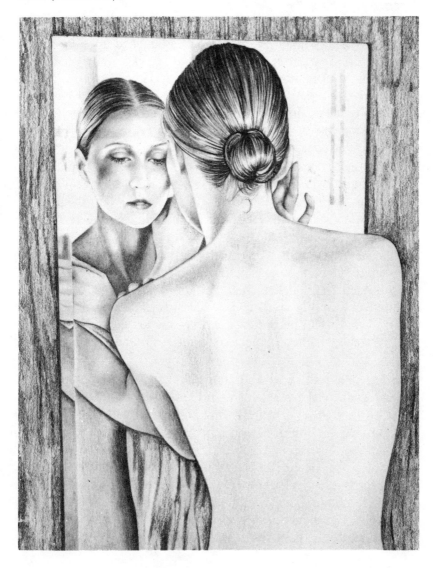

A *biopsy* is a test that establishes the precise diagnosis of your breast problem. It is a simple procedure in which tissue is removed and examined under a microscope by a specially trained doctor called a pathologist. A biopsy can be performed either by inserting a needle to withdraw fluid or by taking tissue from the lump, or by surgically removing the entire lump or a portion or it. The tissue is then analyzed in a laboratory.

Before the Biopsy

When a surgical biopsy is necessary, you have a choice of two procedures that should be discussed and agreed upon by you and your doctor. You can have a biopsy on one day and schedule treatment, if necessary, for a later date. This is called a *two-step procedure*. The biopsy is usually done in a hospital, on either an inpatient or outpatient basis, with local or general anesthesia. The size and location of your lump will help the doctor decide which type of anesthesia is better for you.

Or you can choose to have a *one-step procedure*. Your biopsy will be done in the hospital under general anesthesia. While you are asleep, the suspicious tissue will be removed and analyzed. If cancer is found, your surgeon will immediately perform a mastectomy, the surgical removal of a breast.

This **material** will help you in making the decision between the one-step and two-step procedures. It will also provide information on what to expect during the biopsy procedure. However, it is only a starting point. You will want to discuss this information in more detail with your doctor, a nurse, your family, a close friend, or perhaps another woman who has had a biopsy. You may also want to seek a second medical opinion.

You do not have to rush to make this decision. A short delay will not reduce your chances of successful treatment.

Before the biopsy, it is important to discuss with your doctor the estrogen and progesterone receptor assay tests. If your lump is cancer, these laboratory tests will determine if hormone treatment will benefit you now or in the future. If these tests are not performed at the time of the biopsy, this information may be very difficult to obtain later. Whether you choose a one-step or two-step procedure, you should ask your doctor if arrangements have been made to perform these tests.

Any woman facing breast surgery who thinks she may be interested in breast reconstruction should discuss the options with her surgeon and a plastic surgeon before having her mastectomy. Breast reconstruction, a type of plastic surgery that rebuilds the breast, is growing in popularity, and the techniques of breast reconstruction have improved greatly over the past few years. Some women plan for reconstruction during the same surgery as their mastectomy; others decide on reconstruction several months or even years after mastectomy. For more information, contact the National Cancer Institute for a copy of *Breast Reconstruction: A Matter of Choice.**

The One-Step Procedure

Although a biopsy is the only sure way to determine whether a lump is cancer, your doctor may be able to predict if a mastectomy will be likely. Under such circumstances, many women choose a one-step procedure. If you decide to have the one-step procedure, you will probably enter the hospital the evening before your biopsy. Some routine blood and urine tests will be performed and you will be asked to sign a consent form authorizing your doctor to remove all or part of your breast if the biopsy shows that the tissue is cancer. Shortly before your surgery you will be given some medication to help you relax, and then you will be taken to the operating room where the anesthesiologist will put you to sleep.

The surgeon will remove the suspicious tissue and send it to the pathology department where it will be analyzed. Thin slices of frozen tissue will be mounted on a slide for examination under a microscope. Analysis of this "frozen section" can be completed in just minutes. If the pathologist finds that the tissue contains cancer cells, your surgeon will perform a mastectomy. Surgery will take several hours and you will remain in the hospital for approximately a week to 10 days to recover from the breast surgery.

If the lump is not cancer, the surgeon will close the incision and bandage it; your surgery will be completed in about an hour. You may be discharged within a few hours or you may

---

* *The mentioned text is reprinted within this book. See CONTENTS for location.*

spend the night in the hospital. You should be able to resume your normal activities within a few days. However, for the next week or so your breast may be sore and slightly bruised, and your incision may feel firm for 3 or 4 months.

If there is any question about whether the tissue is cancer, the surgeon will close the incision and wait for a "permanent section" to be done which takes several days.

The one-step procedure requires a doctor to explain the full details of a mastectomy to you before biopsy, even though the lump may not be cancer. If the lump is benign, this may cause unnecessary concern. However, some women who choose the one-step procedure, and who turn out to have cancer, are relieved to know when they wake up from surgery that the cancer has already been removed.

The Two-Step Procedure

When the two-step procedure is chosen, you have a biopsy with local or general anesthesia—usually as an outpatient in a hospital—and then schedule treatment, if necessary, for a later date. You can use the time between biopsy and treatment to have additional tests to find out the extent of the disease, to look into the kind of treatment you want to have, to seek another medical opinion, to prepare yourself emotionally, and to make home and work arrangements for the time you will be in the hospital.

The tissue removed during a two-step procedure is analyzed by both a frozen section and a permanent section. Once the biopsy is complete, the incision is closed and bandaged. After the results of the biopsy are learned, treatment decisions are made. Treatment usually is scheduled within a few weeks. Studies have shown that a short delay between biopsy and treatment will not affect the spread of the disease or reduce the chances for successful treatment.

Outpatient Hospital Procedure for a Biopsy

If you are having a biopsy as an outpatient, you will be admitted to the hospital on the same day that you have your biopsy and go home later that day. Before you go to the hospital, your doctor or nurse will tell you when and where to check in and if there are any restrictions on what you should eat or drink before the biopsy. As a general rule, it is a good idea to leave your money and jewelry at home, but be sure to take your insurance card and Social Security number. Also, if you wear fingernail polish, remove it before going to the hospital. Your doctor will be checking your circulation during the recovery period by pinching the tip of the nail until it turns white and then watching how quickly the color returns to normal.

You will probably have some routine tests performed before your surgery such as urine and blood tests, a chest x-ray, and an EKG (electrocardiogram, which electrically records the activity of your heart). Sometimes the laboratory tests can be done several days before the surgery.

When it is time for your surgery, you will be taken to the operating room where you will be given local or general anesthesia. It usually takes about 30 minutes to an hour to remove the suspicious tissue.

After surgery you will be taken to the outpatient care area. Most women have very little discomfort following a biopsy, but if you had general anesthesia, you will probably be sleepy and want to rest. Your doctor may see you and tell you the results of the frozen section. If the tissue is also being analyzed by permanent section, it may be a few days before your doctor can let you know the diagnosis. Before you leave the hospital, you will be given instructions for taking care of the incision. If you have any questions, ask your doctor or nurse.

Depending on how you feel, you will probably be ready to go home 2 or 3 hours after the biopsy. Most doctors will suggest that a family member or friend meet you at the hospital to take you home. You've been under stress and you may feel weak or tired. Once you are at home, you will return to your usual activities within a day or two. Usually about a week after the biopsy your doctor will want to see you to remove the stitches and discuss further treatment, if needed.

Learn the Facts

Your doctor can answer your questions to help you decide between a one-step and a two-step procedure. The two-step procedure was recommended for most women at a meeting of breast cancer specialists held at the National Institutes of Health in 1979. However, once you know the treatment options available to you, you may prefer the one-step procedure. Don't hesitate to ask questions and learn the facts. Then you will be sure that the decision you make is the right one for you.

Whichever biopsy procedure you select, you will probably want to learn more about the options for treatment—what's involved, what to expect, and how to prepare yourself in the event your breast lump is cancer.

Breast Cancer Treatment

Today's treatments for breast cancer are less disfiguring than ever before. Knowing the options for breast cancer treatment will help you play an active role in your health care.

Mastectomy

Mastectomy, the surgical removal of the breast, remains the most common treatment for breast cancer. There are several types of mastectomy, but *total mastectomy with axillary dissection* is the standard treatment for most breast cancers today. This operation removes the breast and the lymph nodes under the arm, but leaves the chest muscles.

Radiation Therapy

Radiation therapy as a primary treatment for breast cancer is a promising technique for some women who have early stage breast cancer. This procedure allows a woman to keep her breast. Only the breast lump and some or all of the underarm lymph nodes are removed. The remaining breast tissue is then treated with radiation. In some cases, iridium implants are temporarily placed in the breast to supplement the external radiation therapy.

Research is currently under way comparing the effectiveness of radiation therapy with the traditional surgical approach, mastectomy. Preliminary study results are encouraging. Researchers are hoping that over time the survival rates for women who are treated with radiation therapy will remain comparable to those of women treated by mastectomy.

Chemotherapy and Hormone Therapy

Chemotherapy, the use of drugs to destroy cancer cells, is often used in addition to surgery or radiation therapy if the cancer has spread beyond the breast. Finally, depending on the results of the estrogen and progesterone receptor assays, hormone therapy may also be used. Hormone therapy is a way of changing the balance of a woman's hormones to discourage the growth of certain tumors.

Awaiting the Diagnosis

Many women have said that bringing their suspicions of breast cancer to their physician was one of the most difficult and trying experiences of their lives. Waiting for the appointment to discuss your symptoms can heighten fear. When you visit the doctor there are tests, then additional waiting time for test results, and perhaps an appointment with another physician for a second opinion or referral. While waiting, you bear the stress of not knowing what you may have to cope with or how to plan for the future. These emotional concerns are common to women facing the possibility of breast cancer. You may not face all of the problems discussed below, and you may find other ways of dealing with the stressful situations you have to face. Throughout this waiting period, seek support from friends and loved ones, who usually want to help out in stressful times.

Uncertainty

An unpredictable situation frequently causes a great deal of stress. This is especially true for a woman about to undergo a breast biopsy. You may feel better if you:

- Talk over your fears and concerns with someone close to

you. It is very important for you to be open about your feelings with those people who are important to you. Also, expressing healthy anger can give you some vitality and the energy to cope with the unknown. Openness can set the tone for continued sharing. This is a good time to find ways of talking frankly. Don't hide your hurt or pain—share it. You are under a great deal of stress. Don't hesitate to seek professional help to deal with your anxiety or anger.

- Think through how you would deal with a diagnosis of cancer and what sorts of plans you'd make. Spend time learning about treatment options and considering what your needs are—someone to care for your children, who can fill in for you at work, etc. Look into the best medical facility and kind of care that are available to you. Find out what others in your situation have done and learn from their experiences.

Fear of Cancer

Cancer is frightening; however, it can be treated successfully, and it is not necessarily fatal. More than 5 million Americans who have been treated for cancer are considered cured. If you need to have treatment, you may have to adjust your daily activities temporarily, but most cancer patients can expect to return to their usual lifestyle. Many women who have been treated for breast cancer say that they discovered new sources of strength within themselves to cope with the emotional demands they faced.

Fear of Loss

If you think you may have breast cancer, you are naturally concerned about the possibility of losing a breast. The emotions and concerns about sex and intimacy related to that loss are another difficult aspect of the disease. If a mastectomy is necessary, you (and your partner) may experience depression and grief similar to those associated the other losses. Coping with loss is different for each woman, but recognizing and talking about your feelings—which may include anger, frustration, sadness, and fear—can help. These feelings lessen with time, and you may even find that your relationships with loved ones are stronger than before.

Chapter 6

Breast Cancer

Understanding Treatment Options

Breast Cancer: Understanding Treatment Options

As recently as a decade ago, most doctors considered removal of the breast the only treatment for breast cancer. The most common procedure was a radical **mastectomy***, the removal of the entire breast, the chest muscles under the breast, and the underarm lymph nodes. Breast cancer treatment almost always caused women serious physical and emotional trauma. Many women feared the treatment as much as the disease.

Today, radical mastectomies are rarely done. There has been much progress in the early identification and treatment of breast cancer. Beginning with the time a breast lump is found, women have a number of treatment options. As developments occur, doctors are continuing to learn about the advantages and disadvantages of these different treatments. Because of the different stages at which breast cancer is diagnosed, there is no one treatment that is best for all women.

If you discover a lump in your breast or if your doctor suspects you have breast cancer, now is the time to learn about the various treatments available, as well as their risks and benefits. This information will help you get started.

The options available to you will depend on a number of factors, including the type of tumor, the extent of the disease at the time of diagnosis, your age, and your medical history. But your personal feelings about the treatment, your self-image, and your lifestyle will also be important considerations in your doctor's assessment and recommendations. You and your doctor should discuss these treatment methods and how they apply to your situation.

Right now, you may be asking yourself, "Why me?" Cancer has suddenly intruded on your life and threatened your health and well-being. You don't have to lose control of your personal health, however. You can continue to take care of yourself by working in partnership with the health care professionals

---

* *Boldface words are defined in Glossary on page 163.*

69

responsible for your treatment and safe recovery. By becoming informed, asking questions, and participating in treatment decisions, you can have a positive influence on your own well-being.

Biopsy: Learning If You Have Breast Cancer

If you have noticed a lump or other change in your breast, your doctor may recommend several tests to determine if you have cancer. After taking your medical history and performing a manual breast exam, your doctor may recommend a breast x-ray or mammogram. If the lump is suspected to be a cyst, your doctor may use a needle to drain fluid from the lump. Another test is a **biopsy**, in which tissue is removed and examined under a microscope by a pathologist. Part or all of the lump is removed under local or general **anesthesia**. Biopsy is the only certain way to diagnose breast cancer.

During the biopsy procedure, the surgeon removes the suspicious tissue and sends it to the pathology department to be analyzed. The pathologist will examine the tissue to see if it is **benign** or malignant. If it is malignant, the pathologist will try to identify the type of cancer cells present, how fast they reproduce, if the blood vessels or lymph system contains cancer cells, and if the cancer's growth is affected by hormones. All of this information allows your doctor to determine the best treatment for you.

There are two ways that a pathologist prepares the tissue for examination—a "frozen section," which is a quick procedure that takes about 30 minutes, and a "permanent section," which takes a day or two. The frozen section is a quick way of determining whether or not cancer is present. The permanent section is the most accurate method.

The Frozen Section

The frozen section is done while the patient is in the operating room; the surgeon does not continue the operation until the pathologist reports the results from the frozen section.

In the frozen section, the pathologist cuts thin slices of tissue and fast-freezes them to be able to look quickly at the tissue. The disadvantage of the frozen section is that the freezing process distorts the cells and the method is not always accurate.

70

The Permanent Section

The permanent section takes longer than a frozen section—usually a day or two. In this process, the tissue is treated by a series of chemical solutions that give a high-quality slide. The advantage of this process is that it is more accurate and allows the pathologist to make a more correct diagnosis. Permanent sections are always performed, even if a frozen section is done too.

If your lump is cancer, estrogen and progesterone receptor assay tests may be performed. These tests will determine if hormone treatment may benefit you.

Other diagnostic procedures may be performed including special blood tests, additional x-rays, radioisotope scans, and/or computerized body scans.

There are two basic options for having a biopsy: the one-step and the two-step procedures.

One-Step Procedure

In this procedure, biopsy, diagnosis of cancer, and breast removal are completed in a single operation. With this procedure, you and your doctor must agree before surgery that your breast will be removed if the lump is cancerous. Your doctor will explain the full details of a mastectomy (surgical removal of the breast) before biopsy—even though the lump may not be cancerous. In the past, the one-step procedure was thought to be the best way to treat breast cancer. However, recent studies have shown that treatment can safely follow a biopsy by a week or two—even if the lump is cancerous.

Two-Step Procedure

This method involves biopsy on one day; then, if the lump is cancerous, the treatment takes place within a couple of weeks. In many cases, the biopsy can be done on an outpatient basis, and it may be possible to perform the biopsy under local, rather than general, anesthesia. The short time between biopsy and treatment (which will not reduce the chances for success) allows time to examine the permanent section slides, to perform additional tests to determine the extent of the disease, to discuss treatment options, to gain another medical opinion, to make home and work arrangements, and to prepare emotionally for the treatment.

If you are going to have a biopsy, discuss these procedures with your doctor. The two of you can decide which option is best for

71

you. Additional information about biopsy can be found in *Breast Biopsy: What You Should Know*, a National Cancer Institute booklet.

Breast Surgery

Mastectomy is the medical term for surgical removal of the breast. It refers to a number of different operations, ranging from those that remove the breast, chest muscles, and underarm **lymph nodes**, to those that remove only the breast. Other kinds of surgery remove only the breast lump.

The different types of breast surgery are described below. Based on the size and location of the lump, your doctor will recommend the type of surgery that offers you the best chance of successful treatment.

Most medical and surgical procedures carry some risk. The risk may be small or serious, frequent or rare. Because there is such a wide range of potential risks and benefits from the various treatments for the different stages and kinds of breast cancer, you should discuss with your doctor the particular benefits and risks of the treatment methods suitable for you.

Radical Mastectomy

This type of surgery removes the breast, the chest muscles, all of the underarm lymph nodes, and some additional fat and skin. It is also called a "Halsted radical" (after the surgeon who developed the procedure). A radical mastectomy was the standard treatment for breast cancer for more than 70 years and is still used today for some women.

- *Advantages*—Cancer can be completely removed if it has not spread beyond the breast or nearby tissue. Examination of the lymph nodes provides information that is important in planning future treatment.

- *Disadvantages*—Removes the entire breast and chest muscles, and leaves a long scar and a hollow chest area. May cause **lymphedema** (swelling of the arm), some loss of muscle power in the arm, restricted shoulder motion, and some numbness and discomfort. Breast reconstruction is also more difficult.

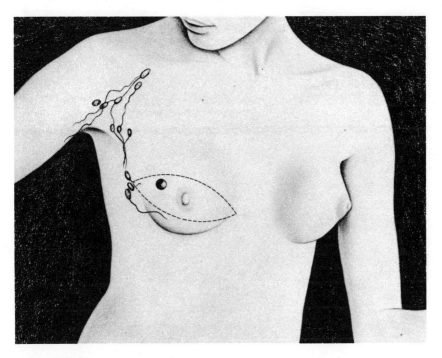

Modified Radical Mastectomy

This procedure removes the breast, the underarm lymph nodes, and the lining over the chest muscles. Sometimes the smaller of the two chest muscles is also removed. This procedure is also called "total mastectomy with axillary (or underarm) dissection" and today is the most common treatment of early stage breast cancer.

- *Advantages*—Keeps the chest muscle and the muscle strength of the arm. Swelling is less likely, and when it occurs it is milder than the swelling that can occur after a radical mastectomy. Leaves a better appearance than the radical. Survival rates are the same as for the radical mastectomy when cancer is treated in its early stages. Breast reconstruction is easier and can be planned before surgery.

- *Disadvantages*—The breast is removed. In some cases, there may be swelling of the arm because of the removal of the lymph nodes.

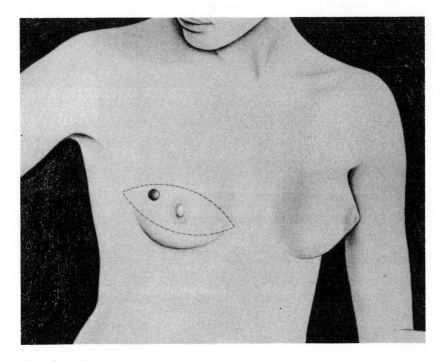

Total or Simple Mastectomy

This type of surgery removes only the breast. Sometimes a few of the underarm lymph nodes closest to the breast are removed to see if the cancer has spread beyond the breast. It may be followed by radiation therapy.

- *Advantages*—Chest muscles are not removed and arm strength is not diminished. Most or all of the underarm lymph nodes remain, so the risk of swelling of the arm is greatly reduced. Breast reconstruction is easier.

- *Disadvantages*—The breast is removed. If cancer has spread to the underarm lymph nodes, it may remain undiscovered.

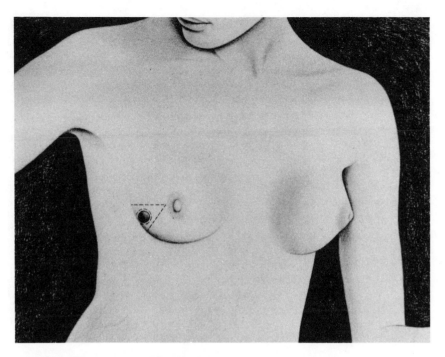

Partial or Segmented Mastectomy

This procedure removes the tumor plus a wedge of normal tissue surrounding it, including some skin and the lining of the chest muscle below the tumor. It is followed by radiation therapy. Many surgeons also remove some or all of the underarm lymph nodes to check for possible spread of cancer.

- *Advantages*—If a woman is large-breasted, most of the breast is preserved. There is little possibility of loss of muscle strength or arm swelling.

- *Disadvantages*—If a woman has small- or medium-sized breasts, this procedure will noticeably change the breast's shape. There is a possibility of arm swelling.

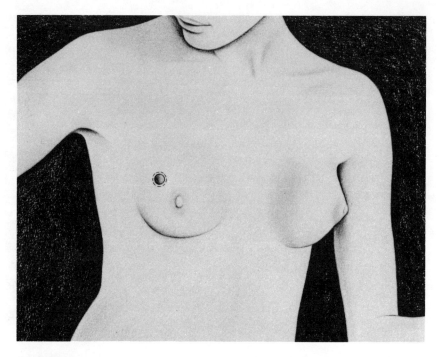

Lumpectomy

Lumpectomy removes only the breast lump and is followed by radiation therapy. Many surgeons also remove and test some of the underarm lymph nodes for possible spread of cancer. Although results of this treatment in patients with early stage breast cancer seem to be equal to those of mastectomy, this has not been scientifically proven. The National Cancer Institute is sponsoring clinical trials to answer this question.

- *Advantages*—The breast is not removed.

- *Disadvantages*—Small-breasted women with large lumps may have a significant change in breast shape. Scar tissue from the treatment may make it more difficult to examine the breast later. There is a possibility of arm swelling.

For more information, contact the National Cancer Institute for a copy of *Mastectomy: A Treatment for Breast Cancer*.*

---

* *The mentioned text is reprinted within this book. See CONTENTS for location.*

A Word About
Breast Reconstruction

As you consider mastectomy as a treatment option, you should be aware of breast reconstruction, a way to recreate the breast's shape after a natural breast has been removed. This procedure is gaining in popularity, although many women are still unaware of it.

Today, almost any woman who has had a mastectomy can have her breast reconstructed. Successful reconstruction is no longer hampered by radiation-damaged, thin, or tight skin, or the absence of chest muscles.

Reconstruction is not for everyone, however. And it may not be right for you. After mastectomy, many women prefer to wear artificial breast forms inside their brassieres.

Both a general surgeon and a plastic surgeon may help you decide whether to have breast reconstruction. If possible, you should discuss breast reconstruction before your surgery because the position of the incision may affect the reconstruction procedure. However, many women consider the option of reconstruction only after surgery.

For more information on breast reconstruction, contact the National Cancer Institute for a copy of *Breast Reconstruction: A Matter of Choice*.*

Radiation Therapy

Radiation therapy*as primary treatment is a promising technique for women who have early stage breast cancer. This procedure allows a woman to keep her breast and involves lumpectomy followed by radiation (x-ray) treatment.

Once a biopsy has been done and breast cancer has been diagnosed, radiation treatment usually involves the following steps:

* Surgery to remove some or all of the underarm lymph nodes to see if the cancer has spread beyond the breast;
* External radiation therapy to the breast and surrounding area; and
* "Booster" radiation therapy to the biopsy site.

For external radiation therapy, a machine beams x-rays to the

---

* See chapters, *Breast Reconstruction,* page 125, and *Radiation Therapy and You,* page 83.

breast and possibly the underarm lymph nodes. The usual schedule for radiation therapy is 5 days a week for about 5 weeks. In some instances, a "booster" or concentrated dose of radiation may be given to the area where the cancer was located. This can be done with an electron beam or internally with an implant of radioactive materials.

If you are having radiation therapy as primary treatment for early stage breast cancer, it should be done by a qualified, board-certified radiation therapist who is experienced in this form of treatment.

- *Advantages*—The breast is not removed. Lumpectomy with radiation therapy as a primary treatment for breast cancer currently appears to be as effective as mastectomy for treating early stage breast cancer. Because this is a new treatment procedure, researchers are continuing to collect information on long-term results. Usually there is not much deformity of surrounding tissues. The skin usually regains a normal appearance after treatment is completed.

- *Disadvantages*—A full course of treatment requires short daily visits to the hospital as an outpatient for about 5 weeks, as well as hospitalization for a few days if implant radiation therapy is used. Treatment may produce a skin reaction like a sunburn, and may cause tiredness. Itching or peeling of the skin may also occur. Radiation therapy can sometimes cause a temporary decrease in white blood cell count, which may increase the risk of infection.

For detailed information about radiation therapy, contact the National Cancer Institute for a copy of *Radiation Therapy: A Treatment for Early Stage Breast Cancer*.

The Breast Cancer Treatment Team

During your treatment you are likely to meet several health professionals who will perform the various tests and treatments your doctor recommends. It may be difficult at first to talk with them about your illness and your feelings about treatment. But

---

* *See chapters, **Breast Cancer: Radiation Therapy**, page 83, and **Radiation Therapy**, page 429.*

each of them can offer information to help you feel more at ease. By talking with the professionals who care for you, you will come to understand more about cancer and its treatment and be better able to cope.

These are some of the specialists you may meet or hear about:

- *Anesthesiologist*—A doctor who administers drugs or gases to put you to sleep before surgery.

- *Clinical nurse specialist*—A nurse with special knowledge in a particular area, such as postoperative care or radiation therapy.

- *Medical oncologist*—A doctor who administers anticancer drugs or chemotherapy.

- *Pathologist*—A doctor who examines tissue removed by biopsy to see if the tissue is cancer.

- *Personal physician*—Your doctor, who will be responsible for coordinating your treatment and working with you to ensure that treatment is satisfactory. Your personal physician may be a surgeon, radiation oncologist, medical oncologist, or family physician.

- *Physical therapist*—A specialist who helps in rehabilitation after surgery by using exercise, heat, light, and massage.

- *Plastic surgeon*—A doctor who specializes in rehabilitative and cosmetic surgery. Plastic surgeons perform breast reconstruction.

- *Radiation oncologist*—A doctor who supervises radiation therapy.

- *Radiation therapy technologist*—A specially trained technician who helps the radiation oncologist give external radiation treatments.

- *Surgeon*—A doctor who performs surgery, such as biopsy and mastectomy.

Informed Consent:
When Surgery Is Recommended

When surgery is recommended, most health care facilities require patients to sign a form stating their willingness to permit diagnosis and medical treatment. This certifies that you understand what procedures will be done and that you have consented to have them performed.

Before consenting to any course of treatment, ask your doctor for information on:

- The recommended procedure;

- Its purpose;

- Risks and side effects associated with it;

- Likely consequences with and without treatment;

- Other available alternatives; and

- Advantages and disadvantages of one treatment over another.

You are likely to discover that your anxiety over treatment decreases as your understanding of breast cancer and its treatment increases.

Making Decisions About Treatment

Important decisions are always hard to make, particularly when they concern your health.

However, there are a number of things you can do to make decisions about breast cancer treatment easier. One is gathering information. You can:

- *Talk with your doctor.* There are a number of treatments that may be used for breast cancer. To make sure you will be comfortable with your decision to have a particular treatment, you may want to get another medical opinion.

- *Gather additional information from published reports.* Many articles and books have been written about breast cancer for patients and professionals. There is also much information available about cancer in general. Some recommended reading materials are listed at the back of this booklet. Others are available at local libraries and may

80

be available through local chapters of the American Cancer Society.

- *Call the Cancer Information Service (CIS).* This program, sponsored by the National Cancer Institute, is available to answer questions about cancer from the public, cancer patients and their families, and health professionals. Call this toll-free number and you will automatically be connected to the CIS office serving your area:

1-800-4-CANCER

In Alaska call 1-800-638-6070; in Hawaii, on Oahu call 524-1234 (call collect from neighboring islands). Spanish-speaking staff members are available to callers from the following areas (daytime hours only): California, Florida, Georgia, Illinois, New Jersey (area code 201), New York, and Texas.

- *Ask your doctor to consult PDQ.* The National Cancer Institute has developed PDQ (Physician Data Query), a computerized database designed to give doctors quick and easy access to the latest treatment information for most types of cancer; descriptions of clinical trials that are open for patient entry; and names of organizations and physicians involved in cancer care. To access PDQ, a doctor may use an office computer with a telephone hookup and a PDQ access code or the services of a medical library with online searching capability. Most Cancer Information Service offices provide a physician with one free PDQ search and can tell doctors how to get regular access. Patients may ask their doctor to use PDQ or may call 1-800-4-CANCER themselves.

Some of the other things you might want to do before making a final decision about various treatments are:

- *Discuss them with friends or relatives.* Although you and your doctor are in the best position to evaluate treatment options, it sometimes helps to discuss your feelings with others whose judgment you respect. Often, close friends and relatives can provide insights that can help your own thinking.

- *Talk with other women who have had breast cancer.* Many women who have been treated for breast cancer are willing to share their experiences. Your local American Cancer Society chapter may be able to direct you to such women through its Reach to Recovery program. This program, which works through volunteers who have had breast cancer, helps women meet the physical, emotional, and cosmetic needs of their disease and its treatment. Some chapters have volunteer visitors who have had a mastectomy, breast reconstruction, radiation, or **chemotherapy.** Sometimes they are able to meet with women before surgery. Contact your local ACS chapter for more information.

Remember that you have time to consider options. Except in rare cases, breast cancer patients do not need to be rushed to the hospital for treatment as soon as the disease is diagnosed. Most women have time to learn more about available options, make arrangements at medical facilities where treatments will be given, and organize home and work lives before beginning treatment. A long delay, however, is not advisable because it may interfere with the success of your treatment.

Chapter 7

Breast Cancer: Radiation Therapy

*A Treatment Option
For Early Stage
Breast Cancer*

Radiation Therapy:
A Treatment for
Early Stage Breast Cancer

Radiation therapy as primary treatment for breast cancer is a promising technique for women who have early stage breast cancer. This procedure, which allows a woman to keep her breast, involves removing the lump or cancerous tissue from the breast (**lumpectomy**)* and some or all of the underarm **lymph nodes**. The breast is then treated with radiation (x-ray).

During the last 20 years, considerable experience has been gained with this form of treatment. Research comparing this treatment with the traditional surgical approach, **mastectomy**, is continuing. Preliminary research results are encouraging, though data on the long-term effects are still being collected. At present, the survival rates for women with early stage breast cancer who are treated with radiation therapy seem to be equal to those for women treated by mastectomy.

This information describes the procedures used in radiation therapy and tells you what to expect—from the beginning of your treatment to your recovery at home. After reading this chapter and discussing it with your doctor, you may want to talk with another woman who has had radiation therapy to treat her breast cancer. She may have some practical advice and be able to answer some of your questions.

---

* *Boldface words are defined in Glossary on page 163.*

Informed Consent: When Treatment Is Recommended

When treatment is recommended, most health care facilities now require patients to sign a form stating their willingness to proceed. This is to certify that you understand what procedures will be done and have consented to have them performed.

Consent to treatment is only meaningful if given by a patient who has had an opportunity to learn about recommended alternatives and to evaluate them. Before consenting to any course of treatment, be sure your doctor lets you know:

- The recommended procedure;
- Its purpose;
- Risks and side effects associated with it;
- Likely consequences with and without treatment;
- Other available alternatives; and
- Advantages and disadvantages of one treatment over another.

Even if you want your doctor to assume full responsibility for all decisionmaking, you are likely to discover that your concerns about treatment decrease as your understanding of breast cancer and its treatment increases.

Questions To Ask Your Doctor
Before Radiation Therapy

- What kind of procedure are you recommending?
- What are the potential risks and benefits?
- Am I a candidate for any other type of procedure?
- What are the risks and benefits of those alternatives?
- How should I expect to look after the treatment?
- How should I expect to feel?

After Radiation Therapy

- When will I be able to get back into my normal routine?
- What can I do to ensure a safe recovery?
- What problems, if any, should I report to you?

- What type of exercises should I do?
- How frequently should I see you for a checkup?

Treatment Steps

Once the lump has been removed and breast cancer has been diagnosed, radiation treatment usually involves the following steps:

- Surgery to remove some or all of the underarm lymph nodes;
- External radiation therapy to the breast and surrounding area; and
- "Booster" radiation therapy to the biopsy site.

Lymph Node Surgery

Before radiation therapy begins, some or all of the underarm lymph nodes are usually removed to determine if the cancer has spread beyond the breast. If all of the lymph nodes are removed, the surgery is called **axillary dissection**; if only some of the lymph nodes are removed, it is called **axillary sampling.** Other tests such as bone and liver scans may also be done to provide your doctor with valuable information needed to plan further treatment. This process is known as "staging" the disease.

Hospital procedures and policies vary, but there are a number of things you can probably expect to have happen when you check in for lymph node surgery.

In the Hospital You will probably be admitted the afternoon before your surgery so that some routine tests, such as blood and urine tests and a chest x-ray, can be performed. Shortly before the operation, the surgical area (underarm) will be shaved, and you may be given some medication to help you relax.

When it is time for your surgery, you will be taken to the operating room and an **anesthesiologist** will put you to sleep. Electrocardiogram sensors will be attached to your arms and legs with adhesive pads to monitor your heart rate during surgery. The surgical area will be cleaned, and sterile sheets will be draped over your body, except for the area around the operation. An axillary dissection usually takes several hours; an axillary sampling, about an hour.

When you awaken from surgery, you will be in the recovery room. Your underarm area will be bandaged, and a tube may be in place at the surgical site to drain any fluid that may accumulate. Your throat may be sore from the tube that was placed in it to carry air to your lungs during surgery. You may also feel a little nauseated and have a dry mouth—these are common side effects of anesthesia.

You will spend an hour or so in the recovery room. Oxygen will be available in case you need it to ease your breathing. Wires may be taped to your chest to measure your heartbeat. An intravenous (IV) tube will be in a vein in your arm to give fluid, nourishment, or medication after surgery. The IV tube will probably be removed after you begin to drink and eat.

It's common to feel drowsy for several hours after surgery. You may feel some discomfort under your arm; some women experience numbness, tingling, or pain in the chest, shoulder area, and upper arm. Your doctor will prescribe medication to relieve any discomfort you may have following your surgery. The numbness under your arm will decrease gradually, but total feeling may not return for a long time.

After you return to your room, a nurse will check your temperature, pulse, blood pressure, and bandage. She will ask you to turn, cough, and breathe deeply to keep your lungs clear after the anesthesia. You may also be encouraged to move your feet and legs to improve your blood circulation. Although each woman reacts to surgery differently, you will probably discover that by the next day you will be able to sit up in bed and walk from your bed to a chair in your room. Your doctor will probably encourage you to walk around and eat solid food as soon as possible.

After Surgery   At first you will have to be careful not to move your arm too much. But by the second or third day, you may be ready to begin exercises to ease the tension in your arm and shoulder. Women who have axillary sampling usually recover their arm motion fairly quickly because their surgery is not as extensive as axillary dissection.

You will be taking sponge baths for a few days after surgery until your incision starts to heal. Before you leave the hospital, ask the doctor or nurse for instructions on taking care of your incision. When you have permission to bathe or shower, do so gently and pat, don't rub, the area of your incision.

The average stay in the hospital for an axillary dissection is 7 to 10 days, and 2 to 4 days for an axillary sampling. Before you leave, the tube that drains fluid from your incision will be removed. Your stitches will be taken out in 1 to 3 weeks at the doctor's office or clinic.

Once you are home, you should continue to exercise until you have regained the full use of your arm. As you increase your exercise and begin to renew your daily activities, you must be careful not to overexert yourself. Take clues from your body; rest before you become tired.

To keep your skin soft and to promote healing, you may want to massage your incision gently with cocoa butter or vitamin E cream. As time goes by, the redness, bruising, and swelling will disappear. But you should watch for any signs of infection such as inflammation, tenderness, or drainage. If you develop any of these signs or a fever, call your doctor. Although each woman recovers from surgery at her own rate, most women are ready for the next part of their treatment, radiation therapy, about 1 or 2 weeks after their lymph node surgery.

Exercising After Surgery   Exercising will help you ease the tension in your arm and shoulder and will hasten your recovery. It is especially important for women who have had an axillary dissection. You will probably be able to begin exercising within a few days of your operation. Your doctor, nurse, or physical therapist can show you what exercises to do.

Ask your doctor if you might begin with these few simple movements:

- Lie in bed with your arm at your side. Raise your arm straight up and back, trying to touch the headboard behind you.
- Raise your shoulders. Rotate them forward, down, and back in a circular motion to loosen your chest, shoulder, and upper back muscles.

- Lying in bed, clasp your hands behind your head and push your elbows into the mattress.
- With your elbow bent and your arm at a 90 degree angle to your body, rotate your shoulder forward until the forearm is down and then backward until it is up.
- With your arm raised, clench and unclench your fist.
- Breathe deeply.
- Rotate your chin to the left and right. Cock your head sideways.

The key is to exercise only to the point of pulling or pain—don't push yourself.

External Radiation Therapy *

During this procedure, high-energy x-rays are aimed at the breast and sometimes at nearby areas that still contain some lymph nodes, such as under the arm (if only a "sampling" was done), above the collarbone, and along the breastbone. The goal of radiation therapy is to destroy any cancer cells that may still remain in the breast or surrounding lymph node areas.

These high-energy x-rays are delivered by a linear accelerator or a cobalt machine. The difference between the two machines is simply that the beams are produced by different energy sources.

Often, a patient's first visit to the radiation department takes 1 to 2 hours and doesn't involve any treatments. You will probably talk with the radiation therapist, a physician with special training in the use of radiation, who will reveiw your records and decide the best way to proceed with your treatment.

You will probably also meet the technician who delivers the treatment, and the radiation therapy nurse, who works closely with the doctor and can answer any questions you have about treatment, potential side effects, and what you can do about them.

During the first visit, ink lines or small tattoo marks will be drawn on your skin around the treatment area to mark exactly where to aim the radiation. The marks are generally made with

---

* *See chapter entitled, **Radiation Therapy and You**. Consult CONTENTS for page location.*

permanent ink, and you should not attempt to wash them off until treatment is completed. These marks ensure that the area treated is the same every day. Many women wear old underclothes during treatment because the marking may stain clothing.

The radiation therapist will consult with the dosimetrist, who computes the dosages of radiation. The standard treatment for early stage breast cancer is almost always 4,400 to 5,000 **rads** (radiation absorbed dose). A rad refers to the amount of radiation that is absorbed by the breast tissue.

Your actual number of treatments will depend on the total dose you need. Usually, treatments are given 5 days a week, Monday through Friday, for about 5 weeks. To protect normal tissue, it is better to give a little radiation each day than to give a lot of radiation all at once. A single treatment takes about 20 to 25 minutes. Only a few minutes of this time are of exposure to radiation; most of the time is spent putting the patient in position. Most people continue to work or pursue other activities throughout the treatment period.

It is very important to have all your treatments. However, if you have to miss a treatment, it can be made up. If you do not finish the full course, you may not have gotten enough radiation to destroy the cancer cells.

For more information about what to expect during radiation therapy, contact the National Cancer Institute for a copy of *Radiation Therapy and You: A Guide to Self-Help During Treatment.**

"Booster" Radiation Therapy

About 1 or 2 weeks after the external radiation therapy has been completed, nearly all women will receive a concentrated "booster" dose of radiation to the area where the breast lump was located.

This treatment may be done either externally, using an electron beam, or internally, using an implant of radioactive material. The electron beam "booster" is delivered by a type of linear accelerator machine similar to the one used in external radiation therapy. The treatment procedure is also similar to that of ex-

---

* The mentioned text is reprinted within this book. See CONTENTS for location.

ternal radiation therapy, with the patient coming to the hospital daily for 5 to 10 days. If you have this type of booster treatment, you may notice an increase in skin redness at the site of the electron beam treatments—this is normal.

The implant procedure requires a short hospital stay of 2 to 3 days. Thin plastic tubes are threaded through the breast tissue where the original lump was removed. This may be done using either a local or general anesthesia. The number and location of the tubes depend on the size and location of the tumor that was removed. The doctor may take an x-ray of your breast after inserting the tubes to make sure they are in the correct position.

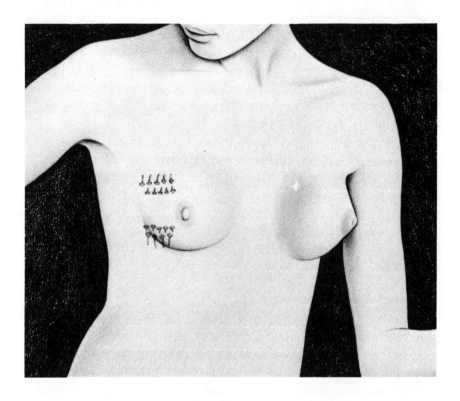

When you return to your hospital room, radioactive seeds (usually iridium) will be inserted into the tubes. The implant will remain in your breast for 2 to 3 days, during which time it will deliver approximately 2,000 rads to the surrounding tissue.

While the implant is in place, you will stay in a private room because the implant emits small amounts of radiation, which may be a possible risk to those who come in close contact with you. For that reason, visitors and the nursing staff will have to limit their time with you.

You may notice some breast sensitivity around the area of the implant, especially if you move around a lot, but you should not have much pain or other discomfort. If you are uncomfortable, ask your nurse for some pain medication. You'll be free to move around your room, sit and read, do needlework or write letters.

The implant will be removed in your room, without anesthesia. The process feels very much like having stitches taken out. Once it is removed there is no risk of radiation exposure to others and you can usually go home.

Side Effects of Radiation Therapy

During Treatment

Many women feel mildly to moderately tired during radiation therapy, especially as treatments progress. Treatment for cancer can be stressful and the daily trips to the hospital take a lot of energy. Try to rest as much as you can and plan your activities at levels that are comfortable for you. Don't push yourself. It is especially important to eat properly while you are having radiation treatments, because your body needs wholesome food to restore its strength and to repair injured cells. It's also important for you to maintain your weight. Even if you are overweight, do not try to lose weight until you have finished all of your treatments.

The skin around the treated area may begin to look reddened, irritated, tanned, or sunburned. In some women the skin becomes quite dry; in others it becomes very moist, especially under the breast fold. These side effects are most likely to occur toward the end of treatment.

Be gentle with your skin. Try not to irritate it. Don't use perfumed or deodorant soaps, ointments, or anything besides lukewarm water and plain soap (such as Ivory) on your breast. Some women wear soft cotton bras, without wiring, or go braless whenever possible. Some like to wear a soft T-shirt or other loose clothing.

Your doctor and nurse will be watching you closely as treatment progresses. Be sure to mention any side effects you may have.

After Treatment

You may notice other changes in your breast due to the radiation therapy and changes may continue for 6 to 12 months after treatment. As the redness goes away, you will notice a slight darkening of the skin—as when a sunburn fades to a suntan. The pores may be enlarged and more noticeable.

You may have some change in skin sensitivity—some women report increased sensation, others have decreased feeling. The skin and the fatty tissue of the breast may feel thicker, and you may notice that your breast is firmer than it was before your radiation treatment. Some older women have said that their breast feels and looks as it did when they were in their twenties. Others report a change in the size of the treated breast—it may become larger because of fluid buildup or smaller because of development of fibrous tissue, but many women have little or no change at all.

After 10 to 12 months, you should notice few additional changes caused by the radiation therapy. If changes in size, shape, appearance, or texture occur after this time, report them to your doctor at once.

Precautions

A problem that may arise after treatment for breast cancer is swelling of the arm on the side of the treatment. This condition, called **lymphedema,** is caused by the loss or damage of underarm lymph nodes and their connecting vessels. It occurs because circulation of lymph fluid is slowed in the arm, making it harder to fight infection. You should take special care of your arm to prevent infection.

Follow these simple rules:

● Avoid burns while cooking or smoking;

- Avoid sunburns;

- Have all injections, vaccinations, blood samples, and blood pressure tests done on the other arm whenever possible;

- Use an electric razor with a narrow head for underarm shaving to reduce the risk of nicks or scratches;

- Carry heavy packages or handbags on the other arm;

- Wash cuts promptly, treat them with antibacterial medication, and cover them with a sterile dressing; check often for redness, soreness, or other signs of infection;

- Never cut cuticles; use hand cream or lotion;

- Wear watches or jewelry loosely, if at all, on the operated arm;

- Wear protective gloves when gardening and when using strong detergents, etc.;

- Use a thimble when sewing;

- Avoid harsh chemicals and abrasive compounds;

- Use insect repellent to avoid bites and stings; and

- Avoid elastic cuffs on blouses and nightgowns.

Call your doctor at once if your arm becomes red, swollen, or feels hot. In the meantime, put your arm over your head and alternately squeeze and relax your fist.

Though you should be cautious, it's also important to use your arm normally—don't favor it or keep it dependent.

Common Questions About Radiation Therapy

Q. Will radiation affect my normal cells?

A. Radiation is a strong treatment for cancer and can sometimes affect normal cells. However, normal cells are not as sensitive to radiation and will usually recover when treatment is finished.

Q. Will anything be done to protect me from excess radiation?

A. The x-ray machine with which you'll be treated has special protections built in to limit your radiation to the specific area outlined. If needed, other areas of your body will be covered by special lead shields.

Q. What will radiation feel like during the treatment?

A. Radiation treatment is like having a regular x-ray; most patients feel no sensation. You may feel warmth or a tingling, but you're not likely to feel any pain or discomfort.

Q. Will I be radioactive after treatments?

A. No. The treatment beam is the only thing that is radioactive when you receive external radiation therapy. Neither your normal tissues nor the cancerous tissues are radioactive during or after treatment. If you have a radiation implant, small amounts of radiation will be emitted. However, once the implant is removed, you are no longer radioactive.

Q. What will my breast look like after treatment?

A. There is no way to predict the cosmetic outcome of this type of treatment for a particular woman. The extent of the initial surgery, the size of the breast, the type of incision, and the effects of radiation on the skin are all factors. However, the breast usually looks quite normal and most women are pleased that they chose this breast-saving treatment.

Q. What is **chemotherapy** *and when is it used?*

A. Chemotherapy is the use of drugs to destroy cancer cells. It may be used in addition to radiation therapy in cases where cancer cells are found in the underarm lymph nodes, suggesting that other cancer cells may be circulating elsewhere in the body. Anticancer drugs are used to reach areas of the body where cancer cells may be hiding, and to eliminate them before they multiply and hurt the normal cells and organs. More information on this supplementary treatment can be found in *Chemotherapy and You: A Guide to Self-Help During Treatment* and *Adjuvant Therapy: Facts for Women With Breast Cancer,* both of which are available from the National Cancer Institute.

Q. How frequently should I plan to see a doctor after radiation therapy treatment?

A. Your doctor will tell you when to schedule your first post-treatment exam. The two of you will then decide whether you should continue to make regular visits to him or her or to a medical oncologist, an internist, a gynecologist, or a family practitioner. Most doctors believe that women treated for breast cancer should have professional exams every 3 to 6 months for the first 3 years after surgery. More information on followup exams, possible signs of recurrence, and taking care of yourself can be found in the chapter, *Breast Cancer: Afterward / A Guide to Followup Care*, which begins on page 153.

Adjusting Emotionally

After you have completed treatment, you'll have a lot of things on your mind. You may think about the fact that you've just been treated for a serious disease and hope this treatment will control your cancer forever. Breast cancer often has a dramatic emotional impact and you may be wondering how it will affect your lifestyle and your personal relationships. You might even be unsure how to act toward your family and friends.

Although every woman reacts to breast cancer differently, these types of concerns are common. Just as you will be taking action to help yourself physically recover from treatment, you can take steps to ease your emotional adjustment as well.

Expressing your feelings to your doctor and the people you love can be important emotional medicine. If you try to handle your problems alone, everyone will lose: you will lose chances to express yourself, your family and friends will lose opportunities to share your difficulties and help you work through them, and your doctor may not understand what you need to fully recover.

Remember, your family and close friends can be your strongest supporters. But chances are, they aren't quite sure how they can show their support. You can help them by being open and honest about the way you feel.

If informal approaches to dealing with your feelings don't work, consider professional help. Psychiatrists, psychologists, social workers, nurses, and religious counselors can help your emotional adjustment.

Others Are Willing To Help

You may also want to talk with other women who have had similar experiences. Reach to Recovery is an American Cancer Society program designed to help breast cancer patients meet the physical, emotional, and cosmetic needs related to cancer and its treatment. Women who have had radiation therapy to treat their breast cancer volunteer to participate in the program by providing practical information and sharing their experiences with others. All volunteers are carefully selected and trained.

Programs vary from city to city. Call your local American Cancer Society unit for more information or contact departments of radiation therapy at major medical centers.

Intimacy

Whether you are single or married, you are likely to wonder how your treatment for breast cancer will affect your intimate relationships. Your partner will also have concerns. You can help each other by expressing them.

Intimate relationships are built on mutual love, trust, attraction, shared interests, common experiences, and a host of other feelings. Breast cancer treatment will not necessarily change these feelings. What it may change is some of the physical aspects of lovemaking—what's pleasurable to you and what's not. It may also temporarily affect your partner's and your attitudes toward intimacy.

Because fatigue often is associated with radiation treatment, you may need additional rest. You can continue to enjoy an intimate relationship by planning special time to spend alone with your partner.

Sometimes a partner is afraid that touching the treated breast will hurt you. Let your partner know what's comfortable to you and what's not. You can bring new closeness to your relationship by talking about your treatment and the way you feel.

Helping Children Cope

Children react to illness in a variety of ways. Some feel angry at their mothers for becoming ill. Others are frightened. Still others worry that they might have caused the illness.

Although you may be tempted to protect your children by not telling them about your disease and its treatment, it's usually better to be honest. Even young children sense when something is wrong. Preschool children often feel deserted when their mother goes to the hospital. And if she returns feeling weak or depressed, they may become frightened. Teenagers sometimes suddenly change their behavior because they fear their mother's illness will keep them from maintaining the independence they have begun to enjoy. If you can avoid imposing too much responsibility on your teenage children, and if you share some of your feelings with them, you may be able to keep their problems to a minimum.

It is a good idea to tell your children the truth as simply and positively as possible. Be careful not to burden them with any more information than is necessary. Encourage their questions, and answer those questions honestly. You will probably find that talking helps your children to accept your illness and the temporary disruption it causes.

Breast Self-Examination

After radiation therapy, breast self-examination (BSE) should continue to be part of your routine. You will want to examine your breasts and your scar (if you had the lymph nodes removed) once a month to note any changes in the way they look or feel. Though you may have been doing BSE before your treatment, you will have to relearn what's considered "normal" for you now.

If you menstruate, the best time to do BSE is 2 or 3 days after your period ends, when your breasts are least likely to be tender or swollen. If you no longer menstruate, pick a day, such as the first day of the month, to do BSE. Here is how to do BSE:

1. Stand before a mirror. Inspect your breast for anything un-

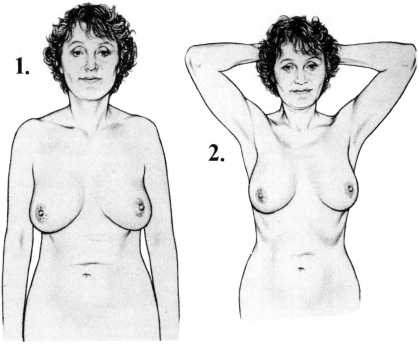

usual, such as any discharge from the nipples, or puckering, dimpling, or scaling of the skin.

In front of the mirror, inspect the scar for swelling, lumps, redness, or color change.

The next two steps are designed to emphasize any change in the shape or contour of your breasts. As you do them, you should be able to feel your chest muscles tighten.

2. Watching closely in the mirror, clasp your hands behind your head and press your hands forward.

3. Next, press your hands firmly on your hips and bow slightly toward your mirror as you pull your shoulders and elbows forward.

The next part of the exam is done while standing. Some women do it in the shower because fingers glide over soapy skin, making it easy to concentrate on the texture underneath.

4. Raise your arm on the untreated side. Using three or four fingers of your other hand, explore your breast firmly, carefully, and thoroughly.

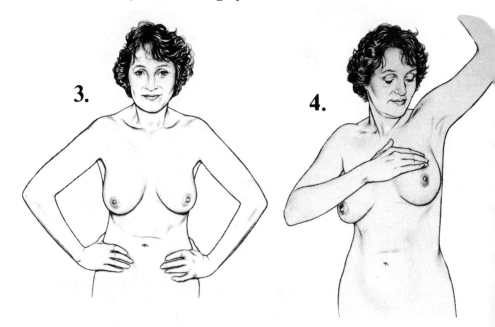

Beginning at the outer edge, press the flat part of your fingers in small circles, moving the circles slowly around the breast. Gradually work toward the nipple. Be sure to cover the entire breast. Pay special attention to the area between the breast and the armpit, including the armpit itself. Feel for any unusual lump or mass under the skin.

5. Gently squeeze the nipple and look for a discharge. Repeat the exam on the treated breast. Raise your arm on the treated side. Use three or four fingers of your other hand and examine your scar from the lymph node surgery. Begin at the top of the scar. Press gently, using small circular motions, and feel the entire length of the scar. Look for thickenings, lumps, or hard places. As with your breasts, familiarity with your scar makes it easier to notice any changes.

6. Steps 4 and 5 should be repeated lying down. Lie flat on your back, raise your arm on the unoperated side over your head and place a pillow or folded towel under your shoulder. This position flattens the breast and makes it easier to examine. Use the same circular motion described earlier.

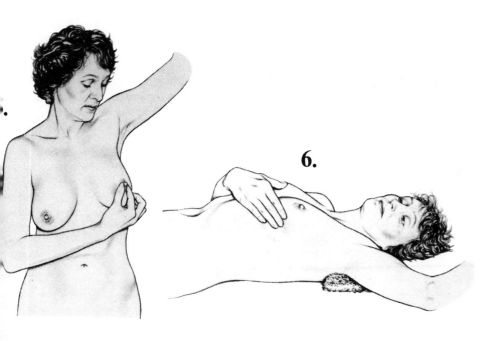

6.

Chapter 8

Breast Cancer: Mastectomy

Mastectomy:
A Treatment for
Breast Cancer

You've been diagnosed as having breast cancer and your doctor has recommended a **mastectomy***. If you're like most women, you probably have many concerns about this treatment for breast cancer.

Surgery of any kind is a frightening experience, but surgery for breast cancer raises special concerns. You may be wondering if the surgery will cure your cancer, how you'll feel after surgery—and how you're going to look.

It's not unusual to think about these things. More than 100,000 women in the United States will have mastectomies this year. Each of them will have personal concerns about the impact of the surgery on her life.

This information is designed to ease some of your fears by letting you know what to expect—from the time you enter the hospital to your recovery at home. It may also help the special people in your life who are concerned about your well-being.

Over the years, mastectomy has proven to be an effective treatment for breast cancer. Today, doctors may choose from a range of procedures depending on the extent of the disease at the time of diagnosis, the patient's medical history, her age, the type of tumor, and other factors. You can feel confident that your doctor is taking steps to see that you can continue to lead an active and full life.

Though breast surgery and recovery will cause you to take time out from your normal routine, it need not cause a permanent change in your lifestyle. Like hundreds of other women who have had mastectomies, you can plan to continue doing the things you enjoy—whether it's working, raising a family, maintaining your home and personal relationships, or pursuing other interests.

---

* Boldface words are defined in Glossary on page 163.

Informed Consent: When Surgery Is Recommended

When surgery is recommended, most health care facilities now require patients to sign a form stating their willingness to permit diagnosis and medical treatment. This is to certify that you understand what procedures will be done and have consented to have them performed.

Consent to surgical or other treatment is only meaningful if given by a patient who has had an opportunity to learn about recommended alternatives and to evaluate them. Before consenting to any course of treatment, be sure your doctor lets you know:

- The recommended procedure;
- Its purpose;
- Risks and side effects associated with it;
- Likely consequences with and without treatment;
- Other available alternatives; and
- Advantages and disadvantages of one treatment over another.

Even if you want your doctor to assume full responsibility for all decisionmaking, you are likely to discover that your concerns about treatment decrease as your understanding of breast cancer and its treatment increases.

Types of Surgery

Mastectomy is the most common treatment for breast cancer today. As recently as 15 years ago, many doctors considered radical mastectomy the only procedure. It removed the entire breast, the chest muscles under the breast, and all underarm lymph nodes, leaving a hollow chest area. Many women feared the treatment as much as the disease.

Thanks to medical advances, there is now a wide range of effective procedures that may be used, depending on the individual case. In addition to the radical mastectomy, also called a "Halsted radical," surgical options include:

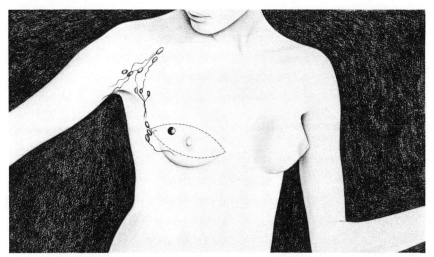

- *Modified radical mastectomy*—Removes the breast and the underarm **lymph nodes**, and the lining over the chest muscles. Sometimes the smaller of the two chest muscles is also removed. This procedure is also called a "total mastectomy with axillary (or underarm) dissection" and today is the most common treatment of early stage breast cancer.

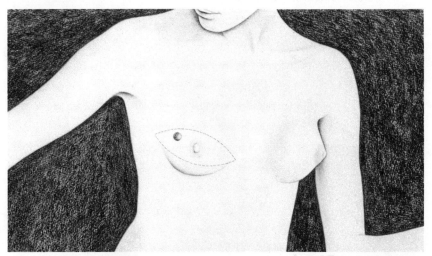

- *Total or simple mastectomy*—Removes only the breast. Sometimes a few of the underarm lymph nodes closest to the breast are removed to see if the cancer has spread beyond the breast. May be followed by radiation therapy.

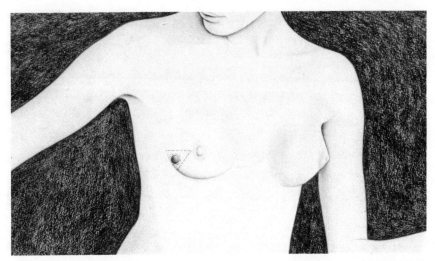

- *Partial or segmental mastectomy*—Removes the tumor plus a wedge of normal tissue surrounding it, including some skin and the lining of the chest muscle below the tumor. It is followed by radiation therapy. Many surgeons also remove some or all of the underarm lymph nodes to check for possible spread of cancer.

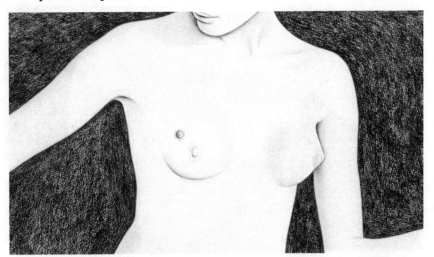

- *Lumpectomy*—Removes the breast lump and is followed by radiation therapy. Many surgeons also remove and test some of the underarm lymph nodes.

A Word About Breast Reconstruction

Since you are about to have breast surgery, you should be aware of breast reconstruction, a way to recreate a breast shape after a natural breast has been removed. Though this procedure is gaining in popularity, many women are still unaware of it. Some women have reconstruction at the same time as their mastectomies; others have it done several months or even years later.

Today, though, almost any woman who has had a mastectomy can have her breast reconstructed. Successful reconstruction is no longer hampered by radiation-damaged, thin, or tight skin, or the absence of chest muscles.

Reconstruction isn't for everyone, however. And it may not be right for you. After mastectomy, many women prefer to wear an artificial breast form, called a **prosthesis**, inside their brassieres.

Both a general surgeon and a plastic surgeon can help you decide whether to have breast reconstruction. If possible, this should be discussed before your surgery because the position of the incision may affect the reconstruction procedure. However, many women consider breast reconstruction only after surgery.

For more information on breast reconstruction, contact the National Cancer Institute for a copy of *Breast Reconstruction:** *A Matter of Choice.*

Questions To Ask Your Doctor

Before Surgery

- What kind of procedure are you recommending?
- What are the potential risks and benefits?
- Am I a candidate for any other type of procedure?
- What are the risks and benefits of those alternatives?
- How should I expect to look after the operation?
- How should I expect to feel?

---

* *The mentioned text is reprinted as the next chapter in this book. See page 125*

After Surgery

- When will I be able to get back into my normal routine?

- What can I do to ensure a safe recovery?

- What problems, if any, should I report to you?

- What type of exercises should I do?

- How frequently should I see you for a checkup?

In the Hospital

Hospital procedures and policies vary, but there are a number of things you probably can expect to have happen when you check in for surgery.

You will probably be admitted the afternoon before your operation so that some routine tests, such as blood and urine tests and a chest x-ray, can be performed. Shortly before the operation, the surgical area (breast and underarm) will be shaved, and you may be given some medicine to help you relax.

When it is time for surgery, you will be taken to the operating room and an anesthesiologist will put you to sleep. Electrocardiogram sensors will be attached to your arms and legs with adhesive pads to check your heart rate during surgery. The surgical area will be cleaned and sterile sheets will be draped over your body, except for the area around the operation. Depending on the procedure, surgery will take between 2 and 4 hours.

Recovery

When you awaken from surgery, you will be in the recovery room. Your breast area will be bandaged and a tube will be in place at the surgical site to drain away any fluid that may accumulate. Your throat may be sore from the tube that was placed in it to carry air to your lungs during surgery. You may also feel a little nauseated and have a dry mouth—common side effects of **anesthesia**.

You will spend an hour or so in the recovery room. Oxygen will be available in case you need it to ease your breathing. Wires may be taped to your chest to measure your heartbeat. An **intravenous** (IV) tube will be inserted into a vein in your arm to give fluid, nourishment, or medication after surgery. The IV will probably be removed after you begin to drink and eat.

It's common to feel drowsy for several hours after surgery. You may also feel some discomfort in your breast area. Some women experience numbness, tingling, or pain in the chest, shoulder area, upper arm, or armpit. Others feel pain in the breast that was removed. Doctors are not sure why this "phantom pain" occurs, but it does exist; it's not imaginary. If you are in pain, ask for medication to relieve it.

After Surgery

After you return to your room, a nurse will frequently check your temperature, pulse, blood pressure, and bandage. The nurse will ask you to turn, cough, and breathe deeply to keep your lungs clear after the anesthesia. You may also be encouraged to move your feet and legs to improve your blood circulation. Although each woman reacts to surgery differently, you will probably discover that by the next day you will be able to drink some juice or broth and, with help, to sit up in bed and walk from your bed to a chair in your room. Your doctor will probably encourage you to walk around and eat solid food as soon as possible.

You will be taking sponge baths for a few days after surgery until your incision starts to heal. Before you leave the hospital, ask the doctor or nurse for instructions on taking care of your incision. When you have permission to bathe or shower, do so gently and pat, don't rub, the area of your incision.

The average stay in the hospital is 7 to 10 days. Before you leave, the tube that drains fluid from your incision will be removed. Some of your stitches may also be removed before you leave the hospital. The remaining stitches will be taken out within 1 to 3 weeks at the doctor's office or clinic.

With your doctor's permission, a Reach to Recovery volunteer may visit you in the hospital. Reach to Recovery is an American Cancer Society program that brings volunteers who have had mastectomies together with breast cancer patients. A volunteer will be able to discuss with you any concerns you may have about coping with your mastectomy. She may also give you a lightweight, fiber-filled or cotton breast form to fasten inside your bra, robe, or nightgown while you are recuperating.

Exercising After Mastectomy

Exercising will help you ease the tension in your arm and shoulder and will hasten your recovery. You will probably be able to begin exercising within a few days of your operation. Your doctor, nurse, or physical therapist can show you what exercises to do. The key is to exercise only to the point of pulling or pain—don't push yourself.

Ask your doctor if you might begin with these few simple movements:

- Lie in bed with your arm at your side. Raise your arm straight up and back trying to touch the headboard.

- Raise your shoulders. Rotate them forward, down, and back in a circular motion to loosen your chest, shoulders, and upper back muscles.

- Lying in bed, clasp your hands behind your head and push your elbows into the mattress.

- With your elbow bent and your arm at a 90 degree angle to your body, rotate your shoulder forward until the forearm is down and then backward until it is up.

- With your arm raised, clench and unclench your fist.

- Breathe deeply.

- Rotate your chin to the left and right. Cock your head sideways.

In addition to exercises such as these, many communities offer swimming, exercise, and dance classes specifically for breast cancer patients.

Precautions

A problem that may arise after treatment is swelling of the arm on the side of the mastectomy. Called **lymphedema**, this condition is caused by the loss of underarm lymph nodes and their connecting vessels. Because the lymph nodes have been removed, circulation of lymph fluid is slowed, making it harder for your body to fight infection. You should take special care of your arm to prevent infection. (If you have had breasts removed, ask your doctor about any special precautions.)

Follow these simple rules:

- Avoid burns while cooking or smoking;

- Avoid sunburns;

- Have all injections, vaccinations, blood samples, and blood pressure tests done on the other arm whenever possible;

- Use an electric razor with a narrow head for underarm shaving to reduce the risk of nicks or scratches;

- Carry heavy packages or handbags on the other arm;

- Wash cuts promptly, treat them with antibacterial medication, and cover them with a sterile dressing; check often for redness, soreness, or other signs of infection;

- Never cut cuticles; use hand cream or lotion;

- Wear watches or jewelry loosely, if at all, on the operated arm;

- Wear protective gloves when gardening and when using strong detergents, etc.;

- Use a thimble when sewing;

- Avoid harsh chemicals and abrasive compounds;

- Use insect repellent to avoid bites and stings; and

- Avoid elastic cuffs on blouses and nightgowns.

Call your doctor at once if your arm becomes red, swollen, or feels hot. In the meantime, try to keep your arm over your head and periodically pump your fist.

Though you should be cautious, it's also important to use your arm normally—don't favor it or keep it dependent.

Recovering at Home

After breast surgery, there are a number of steps you can take to ensure a safe physical recovery. Your physical health will not be your only concern, however. A mastectomy often has a dramatic emotional impact as well.

Taking Care of Yourself

Once you are home, you should continue to exercise until you have regained the full use of your arm. As you increase your exercise and daily activities, be careful not to overdo. Take clues from your body; rest before you become overly tired.

To keep your skin soft and to promote healing, you may want to massage your incision gently with cocoa butter or vitamin E cream. As time goes by and the incision begins to heal, the redness, bruising, and swelling will disappear. As you are healing, be sure to watch for any signs of infection such as swelling, inflammation, tenderness, or drainage. If you see any of these signs or develop a fever, call your doctor.

Although each woman recovers from a mastectomy at her own rate, you will probably discover that within 2 to 3 weeks after surgery you will be doing most of the things you have always done. Within about 6 weeks you will be able to resume your normal activities. Over time the numbness under your arm will decrease, but total feeling may not return for a long time.

Adjusting Emotionally

After you've had a mastectomy, you'll have a lot of things on your mind. You may think about the fact that you've just been treated for a serious disease. You've had an operation that has changed your appearance, perhaps your self-image. You might wonder how the mastectomy will affect your lifestyle and your personal relationships. You might even be unsure how to act toward your family and friends.

Though every woman reacts to mastectomy differently, these types of concerns are common. Just as you will be taking action to help yourself physically recover from treatment, you can take steps to ease your emotional adjustment as well.

Expressing your feelings to your doctor and the people you love can be important emotional medicine. If you try to handle your problems alone, everyone will lose: you will lose chances to express yourself, your family and friends will lose opportunities to share your difficulties and help you work through them, and your doctor may not understand what you need to fully recover.

Remember, your family and close friends can be your strongest supporters. But chances are, they aren't quite sure how they can show their support. You can help them by being open and honest about the way you feel.

Others Are Willing to Help

In addition to talking with your doctor, your nurse, and the people closest to you, you may also want to talk with other women who have had similar experiences.

As described earlier, Reach to Recovery is an American Cancer Society program designed to help patients meet the physical, emotional, and cosmetic needs related to breast cancer and its treatment. Women who have had mastectomies volunteer to participate in the program by sharing their experiences with others. All volunteers are carefully selected and trained.

If your doctor authorizes a visit from a Reach to Recovery volunteer, she will contact you about an appointment while you are in the hospital or shortly after you go home. When you get together, she'll bring a kit containing a temporary breast form and information for husbands, children, other loved ones, and friends. She'll be prepared to discuss all aspects of mastectomy, including your personal concerns. Programs vary from city to city, so contact your local American Cancer Society chapter for more information.

ENCORE is a national YWCA discussion and exercise program for women who have had breast cancer. This once-a-week 90-minute program consists of floor and swimming pool exercise sessions and group discussions. Contact your local YWCA for more information about ENCORE.

If informal approaches to dealing with your feelings don't work, consider professional help. Psychiatrists, psychologists, social workers, nurses, and religious counselors can help you adjust.

Intimacy

Whether you are single or married, you are likely to wonder how your mastectomy will affect your intimate relationships. Your partner will also have concerns. You can help each other by expressing them.

Intimate relationships are built on mutual love, trust, attraction, shared interests, common experiences, and a host of other feelings. A mastectomy will not necessarily change these feelings. What it may change is some of the physical aspects of love-making—what's pleasurable to you and what's not. It may also temporarily affect your partner's and your attitude toward intimacy.

After mastectomy you will still be the person your partner has come to love and enjoy. You can bring new closeness to your relationship by talking about the changes in your body, accepting them, and reaffirming your joy of being alive and being together.

At first, there may be some awkward moments. It may be helpful to let your partner see your body soon after surgery to decrease the anxiety both of you may feel. Sometimes a partner is afraid that touching a mastectomy incision will hurt you. Let your partner know what's comfortable to you and what's not.

Sometimes a partner assumes that you will not be ready for sex for some time after surgery. Women often interpret this waiting as rejection. You may prevent this potential problem by letting your partner know when you feel ready for sex, that you still need your partner, and that it is important for you to know that your partner still finds you attractive and desirable.

Helping Children Cope

Children react to illness in a variety of ways. Some feel angry at their mothers for becoming ill. Others are frightened. Still others worry that they might have caused the illness.

Although you may be tempted to protect your children by not telling them about your operation or the disease that caused it, it's usually better to be honest. Even young children sense when something is wrong. Preschool children often feel deserted when their mother goes to the hospital. And if she returns feeling weak or depressed, they may become frightened. Adolescents sometimes suddenly change their behavior because they fear their mother's illness will keep them from maintaining the independence they have begun to enjoy. If you can avoid imposing too much responsibility on your teenage children, and if you share some of your feelings with them, you may be able to keep their problems to a minimum.

It is a good idea to tell your children the truth as simply and positively as possible. Be careful not to burden them with any more information than is necessary. Encourage their questions, and answer those questions honestly. You will probably find that talking helps your children to accept your illness and the temporary disruption it causes. A booklet that may be helpful to you is called *When Someone In Your Family Has Cancer.* It is written for young people who have a parent or sibling with cancer and is available*from the National Cancer Institute.

---

* *The mentioned text is reprinted within this book. See CONTENTS for location.*

Common Questions
About Breast Surgery

Q. *Is breast surgery dangerous?*

A. Doctors have been performing mastectomies for many years and are continuing to improve their techniques. There are risks associated with any kind of surgery, however. Risk depends on a lot of things, including your age, your medical history, your response to anesthesia, and your general health. After considering these factors, your doctor will recommend the type of surgery that will offer you the most benefit with the least amount of risk.

Q. *How frequently should I plan to see a doctor after a mastectomy?*

A. Your surgeon will tell you when to schedule your first postoperative exam. The two of you will then decide whether you should continue to make regular visits to the surgeon, or to a medical oncologist, an internist, a gynecologist, or a family practitioner. Most doctors believe that women treated for breast cancer should have professional exams every 3 to 6 months for the first 3 years after surgery. More information on followup exams, possible signs of recurrence, and taking care of yourself can be found in *After Breast Cancer: A Guide to Followup Care,** another booklet available from the National Cancer Institute.

Q. *What is chemotherapy and when is it used?*

A. Chemotherapy is the use of drugs to treat cancer. It may be used in addition to surgery in cases where cancer cells are found in the underarm lymph nodes, suggesting that other cancer cells may be circulating elsewhere in the body. (Remember, a mastectomy treats only the cancer in the breast.) Anticancer drugs are used to reach areas of the body where cancer cells may be hiding, and to destroy them before they multiply and hurt the normal cells and organs. More information on this supplementary treatment can be found in *Chemotherapy and You:* A Guide to Self-Help During Treatment* and *Adjuvant Therapy:* Facts for Women With Breast Cancer,* both of which are available from the National Cancer Institute.

---

* *The mentioned text is reprinted within this book. See CONTENTS for location.*

Breast Self-Examination

After a mastectomy, breast self-examination (BSE) should be part of your routine. You will want to examine your natural breast and the surgical site once a month to note any changes in the way they look or feel. Though you may have been doing self-exams before your surgery, you will have to relearn what's considered "normal" for you now. About half the women who have mastectomies report that their remaining breast becomes larger.

If you menstruate, the best time to do BSE is 2 or 3 days after your period ends, when your breast is least likely to be tender or swollen. If you no longer menstruate, pick a day, such as the first day of the month, to do BSE.

Here is how to do BSE:

1. Stand before a mirror. Inspect your breast for anything unusual, such as any discharge from the nipple, or puckering, dimpling, or scaling of the skin.

    Inspect the scar for new swelling, lumps, redness, or color change. Although redness can be a result of irritation from your bra or prosthesis, report it to your physician.

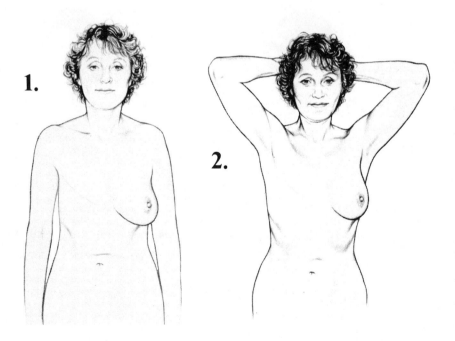

1.

2.

119

The next two steps are designed to emphasize any change in the shape or contour of your breast. As you do them, you should be able to feel your chest muscles tighten.

2. Watching closely in the mirror, clasp your hands behind your head and press your hands forward.

3. Next, press your hands firmly on your hips and bow slightly toward your mirror as you pull your shoulders and elbows forward.

The next part of the exam is done while standing. Some women do it in the shower because fingers glide over soapy skin, making it easy to concentrate on the texture underneath.

4. Raise your arm on the unoperated side. Using three or four fingers of your other hand, explore your breast firmly, carefully and thoroughly.

   Beginning at the outer edge, press the flat part of your fingers in small circles, moving the circles slowly around the

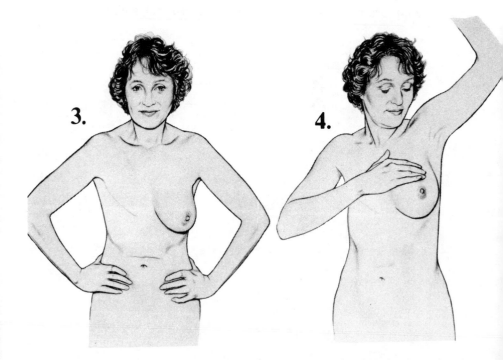

breast. Gradually work toward the nipple. Be sure to cover the entire breast. Pay special attention to the area between the breast and the underarm, including the underarm itself. Feel for any unusual lump or mass under the skin.

5. Gently squeeze the nipple and look for a discharge. Raise your arm on the operated side. Use three or four fingers of your opposite hand and begin at the top of the scar. Press gently, using small circular motions, and feel the entire length of the scar. Look for thickenings, lumps, and hard places. As with your breast, familiarity with your scar makes it easier to notice any changes. Lumps, thickening, and inflammation are among changes you should bring to the attention of your doctor.

6. Steps 4 and 5 should be repeated lying down. Lie flat on your back, raise your arm on the unoperated side over your head and place a pillow or folded towel under your shoulder. This position flattens the breast and makes it easier to examine. Use the same circular motion described earlier.

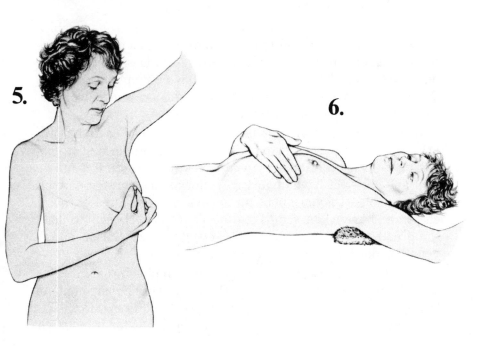

5.

6.

Shopping for a
Permanent Prosthesis

Ask your doctor when it's appropriate for you to shop for a permanent breast form. You can probably begin shopping as soon as you're feeling strong and the swelling and tenderness are gone from the incision. If you are planning to have breast reconstruction, you may want a prosthesis before it's time for your surgery.

Breast forms are available in many shapes and sizes. Some prostheses feel like plastic bags, some are rubbery, some feel very much like skin. They may be covered with a soft fabric, polyurethane, or a silicone envelope, and they may be filled with foam rubber, water, air, chemical gel, polyethylene materials, polyurethane foam, silicon gel, or ceramic particles. Like natural breasts, prostheses vary in weight, and their consistency varies from very soft and pliable to relatively firm. Some brands have models specifically for the right or left side; some are made with a modified nipple and can be worn with or without a bra. Custom-made forms, which adhere to the chest wall and closely match the remaining breast, are also available.

Small prostheses, sometimes called equalizers, are available for women who have had lumpectomies or segmental mastectomies. Women whose reconstructive surgery does not replace the nipple or whose breast form does not have a nipple may choose a nipple prosthesis. Extremely lightweight forms are available to wear in a nightgown or with leisure clothes.

When selecting your prosthesis you'll also need to find a properly fitting bra that will hold the breast form in place. You may be able to wear the same bra you have always worn if it fits well and does not have underwires. Special postmastectomy bras are available—they are built up to cover a larger area of the chest and have wider straps and pockets inside the cup to hold the prosthesis. You can sew a pocket into your swimsuit and your standard bras to keep the breast form in place.

Breast prostheses are sold in surgical supply stores, in lingerie and corset shops, and in the underwear departments of large department stores. Many stores that sell breast forms also carry lingerie and sportswear specially designed for women who

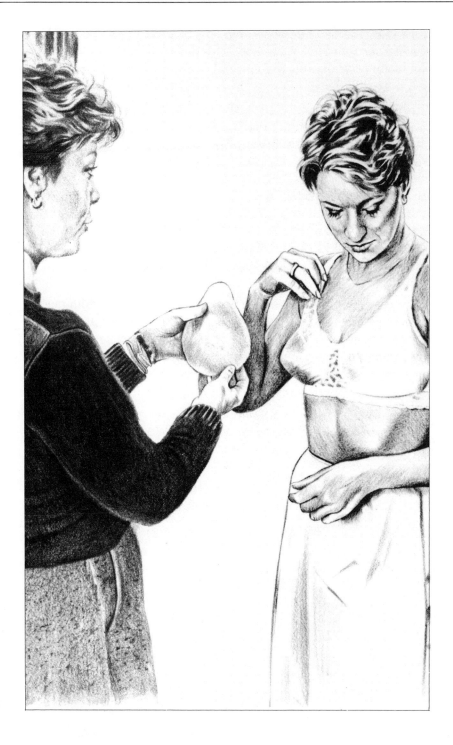

have had mastectomies. Look in the *Yellow Pages* under "Brassieres" or "Surgical Appliances." Reach to Recovery volunteers can often provide information on types of permanent prostheses and a list of where they are available locally.

Before you go out to try various breast forms, you should call ahead and see if the supplier has a professional fitter to meet with you. More than a dozen different breast forms are on the market, and the only way to find the best one for you is to try them on. Your breast form should feel comfortable, have a natural contour and consistency, and remain in place when you move. It may feel heavy at first, but you will get used to the extra weight. Ask the fitter if the form absorbs perspiration or other chemicals from the skin and how to clean and care for your prosthesis. Most prostheses are guaranteed for 1 to 5 years.

Prices for breast forms range from $7 to $265. Custom-made forms are more expensive. The expense is covered, at least partly, by most medical insurance policies. A written prescription from your doctor will help ensure payment. If your insurance does not cover a prosthesis, you may be able to deduct the cost as a medical expense on your income tax.

If you want some emotional support when you shop, ask your partner or a good friend to go with you. Wear a form-fitting blouse or sweater so you can see how the form will make you look.

The most important thing to do is shop around. It's worth your time to find a prosthesis that feels comfortable and keeps you looking your best.

Chapter 9

Breast Cancer: Reconstructive Surgery

A Matter of Choice

Breast Reconstruction: A Matter of Choice

Thanks to recent advances in plastic surgery techniques, a mastectomy need not have the same physical and emotional consequences it did in the past. Women of all ages who have had all or part of a breast removed are finding that breast reconstruction can be a step toward restoring their bodies and their former lifestyles.

Whether you are about to have a mastectomy or have already had your surgery, the information given in this chapter may answer some of your questions about breast reconstruction and ease your concerns. The section headed "Glossary," (beginning on page 163) explains many of the medical terms you may hear in discussions of breast cancer and reconstructive surgery.

Although the procedure is gaining in popularity, many women still are unaware that a breast can be reconstructed after surgery. The fact is that today virtually any woman who has had a mastectomy for breast cancer can have her breast reconstructed. Radiation-damaged skin, grafted, thin, or tight skin, and the absence of chest muscles are no longer obstacles to successful reconstruction.

Reconstruction isn't for everyone, however. And it may not be right for you. Many women prefer to wear breast forms rather than having additional surgery. The important thing is that most breast cancer patients have a choice. This booklet is designed to help you decide whether breast reconstruction is for you.

Its Your Choice

The decision to have plastic surgery is a personal one. It depends on a lot of things, including your self-image, but the issue goes beyond simple vanity. Breast reconstruction can help promote a sense of wellness. It can also help your family or others close to you to resolve their feelings about your having had cancer.

You may be thinking about breast reconstruction because you believe it will help you feel "whole" again. Or it may make it

127

easier for you to get back to a normal routine after a period of illness.

Here's what some women have to say about breast reconstruction:

"I decided to have reconstruction because . . .

. . . I wanted to be able to wear all my favorite clothes— including bathing suits and low-cut dresses."

. . . I felt it would help me regain my sense of femininity; make me feel more attractive."

. . . I tried wearing a breast form and found it uncomfortable and inconvenient."

"Reconstruction was not the best choice for me because . . .

. . . I was perfectly comfortable with a breast form."

. . . the idea of having additional surgery was too frightening. I wasn't willing to take the risk."

. . . I wasn't satisfied with the results my doctor told me I could expect."

You may agree with any of these women—or have your own ideas about whether or not to have breast reconstruction. The first step in deciding is to get additional information about all aspects of the surgery.

Reconstructive Surgery

Plastic surgeons have been developing methods of breast reconstruction since the late 19th century. Until the late 1960's, however, the standard surgical procedure was very complex and the results were often disappointing. Few women chose to have the operation.

Two medical advances have made reconstruction more popular in recent years:

• Creation of **silicone gel*** implants and

• Development of ways to transfer skin and muscle to the chest area from other areas of the body.

These advances have helped make breast reconstruction an option for many women who have had surgery for breast cancer, including those who have had **radical mastectomies**.

Reconstruction of the entire breast, including the nipple and **areola** (the dark-colored skin around the nipple), is a procedure

---

* *Boldface words are defined in Glossary on page 163.*

that may require two or more operations over 6 to 12 months' time. A hospital stay of several days to a week is usual for each operation in the process.

Several types of **breast implants** are used in reconstruction. Generally, they are soft, fluid-filled sacs, available in various sizes. The surgeon chooses the size and shape that will best match the patient's opposite breast.

The simplest type of implant is a sac made of tough, elastic silicone rubber and filled with silicone gel or other fluids. Silicone implants are an improvement over liquid silicone injections, which were once used for **breast enlargements** but have now been banned by the Food and Drug Administration. There is no evidence that silicone gel implants cause cancer.

Common Procedures

Like any other type of plastic surgery, breast reconstruction is a personalized procedure. There are three major types: simple implant placement, tissue expansion, and tissue transfer. Your doctor will recommend the best one for you after considering the type of mastectomy performed, your postsurgery treatment, your skin and muscle conditions, your breast size, and other factors.

- *"Simple" implant placement*—This procedure, which may be done as outpatient surgery, is used when the patient has a healthy chest muscle and enough good-quality skin to cover the implant. In this procedure, the surgeon makes a small incision, usually through the mastectomy scar, and inserts the implant in a pocket created under the chest muscle. A drain may be inserted to remove fluid that may accumulate during the next few days, and the incision is then closed. The operation takes 1 to 2 hours. It is usually done while the patient is under general **anesthesia**, but local anesthesia is sometimes used. The appearance of the mastectomy scar can be improved during the reconstruction, but the scar cannot be eliminated. If the surgeon makes the incision in the original mastectomy scar, there will be no additional scarring.

"Simple" Implant Placement

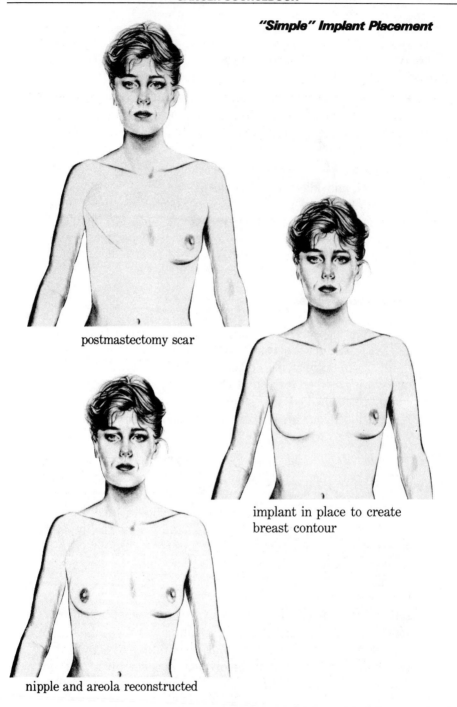

postmastectomy scar

implant in place to create
breast contour

nipple and areola reconstructed

- *Tissue expansion*—A temporary tissue expander may be used when there is good-quality skin and muscle but the quantity is not enough to cover an implant that matches the size of the opposite breast. In this procedure, the remaining tissue is gradually stretched so that an implant that matches the opposite breast can be inserted. While the women is under local or general anesthesia, the surgeon makes an incision in the mastectomy scar and inserts the deflated tissue expander under the skin and muscle. (In some instances, the expander may be inserted at the time of the mastectomy.) After the tissue expander is in place, it is filled with a small amount of sterile fluid. The operation takes 1 to 1½ hours. During the next 8 to 12 weeks, the patient visits her doctor's office on the average of once a week where the doctor injects additional fluid, gradually enlarging the expander and stretching the tissue over it. While this expansion is taking place, the patient can keep up her normal activities, with little or no discomfort. Then, when the tissue has stretched enough to hold an implant of the desired size, the surgeon removes the tissue expander and inserts the permanent implant. This last step can be done on an outpatient basis, usually with local anesthesia.

- *Tissue transfer*—There are three kinds of breast reconstruction that involve the moving, or transfer, of tissue from one part of the body to another.

— *"Latissimus dorsi" reconstruction*—This procedure may be used when more radical surgery has removed more of the chest muscles and a large amount of skin, leaving too little soft tissue to hold and cover an implant. During this operation, the surgeon transfers skin and muscle from the patient's back to the mastectomy site. To create a new muscle on the front of the chest, the surgeon uses the latissimus dorsi, a broad, flat muscle on the back below the shoulder blade. An implant is then placed under the new chest muscle. Drains may be inserted and kept in place for several days after surgery to remove fluid. The operation takes several hours and patients stay in the hospital for about a week. This procedure leaves a scar on the back in addition to the mastectomy scar on the chest.

"Latissimus Dorsi" Reconstruction

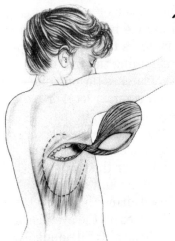

latissimus dorsi muscle and
skin flap raised

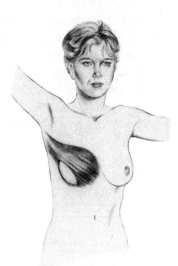

flap tunneled under skin from
back to front of chest

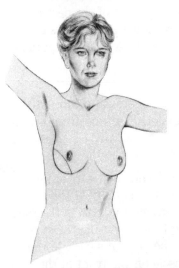

flap in place recreating breast contour with
reconstructed nipple and areola

— *Abdominal advancement reconstruction*—This procedure is
often used for women who are large breasted. During this
operation, the surgeon advances skin and fat from the chest
and abdomen below the mastectomy site to the breast area. The
advantages of this procedure are the good match of skin color
and texture, less scarring to other areas of the body, and
relative ease of performance.

— *"Rectus abdominus" reconstruction*—This procedure is also
used for women whose mastectomy has removed a lot of skin
and muscle. To move tissue to the chest, the surgeon transfers
one of the two parallel vertical abdominal muscles (the rectus
abdominus muscles) to the breast area along with skin and fat
from the abdomen. The surgeon shapes this flap of muscle, skin,

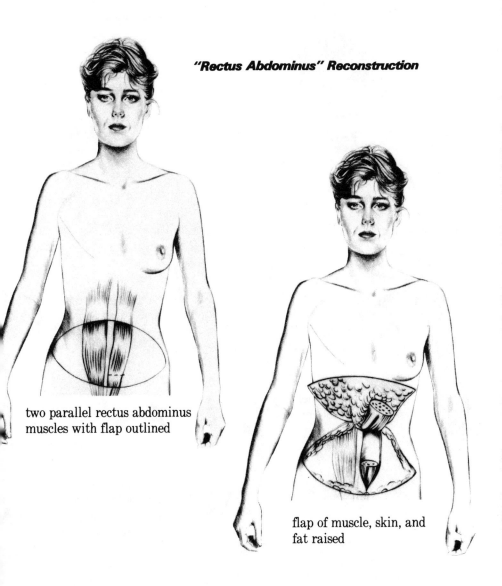

"Rectus Abdominus" Reconstruction

two parallel rectus abdominus
muscles with flap outlined

flap of muscle, skin, and
fat raised

and fat into the contour of a breast. If there is enough abdominal tissue available, no implant is needed. Transferring tissue from the abdomen to the chest also results in tightening of the stomach, called a "tummy tuck." This procedure leaves a horizontal scar across the lower abdomen in addition to the mastectomy scar on the chest.

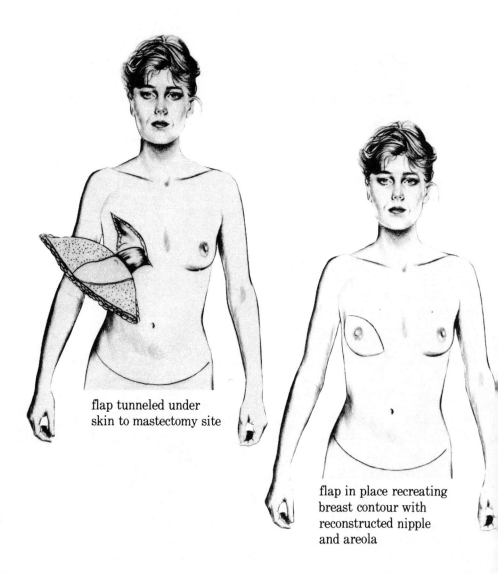

flap tunneled under
skin to mastectomy site

flap in place recreating
breast contour with
reconstructed nipple
and areola

Recreating the Nipple and Areola

After the breast shape has been reconstructed, most doctors prefer to wait several weeks or months before doing surgery to construct the nipple and areola. This is done to allow the new breast tissue to settle in place so minor adjustments in size and position can be carried out when the nipple and areola are reconstructed. Women who are primarily concerned with improving their appearance in clothing may be satisfied with reconstruction of the contour alone and choose not to have the nipple and areola reconstructed.

Reconstruction of the nipple and areola can be accomplished in a variety of ways. The operation usually takes between 1 and 2 hours.

The most common technique for reconstructing the areola is to use the skin from the upper inner thigh or skin from behind the ear. The nipple is usually reconstructed by using tissue from the newly created breast mound or by grafting a piece from the opposite nipple. In another technique, skin from the vaginal lips can be used to reconstruct the nipple and areola. If the reconstructed areola is not dark enough, ultraviolet light may be used to improve the color match.

Possible Complications

As with all surgical procedures, there are certain risks associated with breast reconstruction. You should discuss possible complications and side effects with your doctor before having any operation.

In breast reconstruction, complications may arise if a woman's body reacts unfavorably to a foreign substance—the implant. In about 20 percent of patients, the body's response causes a problem known as "capsular contracture" where the body creates a firm, fibrous capsule around the implant to protect itself. The capsule may become very thick, creating a spherical "baseball" appearance and possibly causing discomfort. Sometimes a contracture softens, as it is absorbed by the body, and improves. Frequently, the surgeon can manipulate it by hand to split the capsule, and the implant then assumes its normal size and shape. Contractures may need to be released surgically.

There are a number of other possible complications. If an infection occurs at the breast site, the implant may have to be removed until the infection heals; it can usually then be replaced. The implant may also have to be temporarily removed if large areas of skin die. Sometimes all or part of a transferred muscle may fail to survive. If the abdominal tissue is used, there is a small chance of an abdominal hernia developing.

Women who are considering reconstructive breast surgery should be aware that mastectomy and reconstruction scars are permanent, although the degree of scarring varies among individuals. As with any other type of plastic surgery, it is difficult to predict the overall result. Also, you should not expect that reconstruction will restore the sensation lost through mastectomy. Any surgery on the breast can damage the sensitive nerves in that area.

Common Questions About Breast Reconstruction

Q. *What does a reconstructed breast look like?*

A. The breast created by inserting an implant under the chest wall muscle does not look like a natural breast, but small differences won't be noticeable in clothing. The new breast will probably look more flattened than tapered. It may have a more youthful appearance than the natural breast, in that it may not droop as much. Plastic surgeons may be able to show you photographs of reconstructed breasts, but you should not expect your reconstructed breast to look like any other woman's.

Q. *Does a reconstructed breast feel different?*

A. Breast implants are designed to be much like a natural breast in weight and density, so you should feel a balance between the reconstructed breast and its partner. The fluid-filled sacs are soft and pliable, like natural breast tissue. In place, the implant can move about to some extent, so the reconstructed breast may have some "bounce" to it. The skin over the breast will, of course, feel natural to the touch because it's your own skin; but sensations in the surgical area will probably be diminished. If abdominal tissue is used, the texture will be more like that of a normal breast.

Q. *Can a plastic surgeon "match" my natural breast?*

A. While plastic surgeons make every attempt to match the opposite breast, a reconstructed breast is rarely an exact duplicate of its partner in size, shape, or contour. This is true of a reconstructed nipple and areola as well. Often, surgeons will suggest modifying the natural breast to give a more balanced appearance. Operations on the natural breast may be done at the time of the reconstruction or in a second operation. The most common types of modifications to the natural breast are reduction, enlargement, or lifting. If a woman is at high risk of developing cancer in the remaining breast, a surgeon may recommend a **prophylactic mastectomy**. With one technique that is sometimes used, the procedure removes most underlying tissue from the natural breast but leaves the skin and nipple. The operation could be followed by immediate reconstruction.

Q. *What if I'm not pleased with the results?*

A. Your level of satisfaction with the reconstruction will depend in large part on your expectations before the operation. Be sure to discuss them with your doctor before you decide to proceed. If an implant is used, after the operation you will be instructed to massage and exercise the muscles surrounding your implant. If you are dissatisfied with the results, after waiting a few months for the skin and muscle to stretch and for the reconstructed breast to take on a more natural appearance, discuss your concerns with your plastic surgeon. Often, the position or the size of the breast mound can be adjusted under local anesthesia.

Q. *How long must I wait after surgery before having my breast reconstructed?*

A. Surgeons have different opinions about the most desirable waiting period. Most believe that the mastectomy incision should be well healed and the skin easily movable and elastic before reconstruction. This generally takes from 3 to 6 months. Some surgeons feel that no delay is necessary; they may create a new breast at the same time the natural breast is removed. Most recommend that reconstruction be delayed until **chemotherapy** and/or **radiation therapy** are completed.

Your feelings also play an important role in the timing of reconstructive surgery. You should be comfortable with your decision before giving the signal to proceed. In most cases, reconstruction can be successfully performed even years after a mastectomy.

Q. *How much will breast reconstruction cost?*

A. Plastic surgeon's fees vary with the complexity of the procedure. For example, simple insertion of an implant costs less than other procedures; creation of a nipple increases the cost. Fees also vary considerably in different parts of the United States. Hospital costs are extra. Most health insurance plans now cover part of the cost of breast reconstruction, because it is considered corrective surgery for postmastectomy rehabilitation, not cosmetic surgery. Some insurance companies, however, do not cover rehabilitation of any kind. Ask your insurance company representative if reconstruction is covered under your policy.

Q. *How long is the recovery period?*

A. Depending on the extent of the operation, most women are able to resume normal activities in 2 to 3 weeks. It may be several more weeks before they can do strenuous exercise, however.

Q. *Do I continue breast self-examination after reconstruction?*

A. By all means. Breast reconstruction does not cause cancer to come back, nor does it prevent recurrence. After reconstruction, you will continue to have periodic physical and laboratory exams. In addition, you should examine both of your breasts monthly, following your doctor's instructions.

Q. *Could a breast implant hide a new cancer?*

A. Plastic surgeons and radiologists believe there is little or no difficulty in promptly detecting a recurrence of cancer, either beneath or around an implant, using examination by hand or mammography (x-rays of the breast). If cancer were to recur in the reconstructed breast, it would most likely be located just under the skin and be easy to find.

Making Decisions About Reconstruction

After a mastectomy, you may decide to have your breast reconstructed, to use an artificial breast form, or to make no attempt to alter your appearance. It's a choice that can have a significant impact on your lifestyle. And it is a choice that you need not make immediately or without help.

In considering reconstruction, you should:

• Talk with your doctor about the benefits and risks;

• Consult one or more plastic surgeons about the best procedure for your particular situation;

• Talk with women who have had reconstructive surgery and those who have chosen not to have it; and

• Discuss your concerns with family members and friends.

Choosing a Plastic Surgeon

Both a general surgeon and a plastic surgeon may help you decide whether to have reconstructive surgery. If possible, you should discuss reconstruction with the doctor before you have surgery for breast cancer because the position of the mastectomy incision may affect the reconstruction procedure. However, many women consider the option of reconstruction only after surgery. A time lag, even if it's years, between mastectomy and reconstructive surgery need not be an obstacle to the success of the procedure.

In choosing a plastic surgeon, you will want someone who is technically competent and well-experienced in this procedure. Your surgeon should also be someone who is sensitive to the emotional issues associated with breast reconstruction. You may want to talk with a number of doctors. Discussing your feelings openly will help you decide if you are comfortable with a particular doctor.

Most mastectomies performed today are the **modified radical** type in which the breast and the underarm lymph nodes are removed but the chest muscles remain. After a modified radical mastectomy, the reconstruction procedures are relatively straightforward and can be performed successfully by nearly all plastic surgeons. Women who have had radical mastectomies might seek a surgeon with exceptional expertise in breast reconstruction.

Your doctor may be able to recommend a plastic surgeon. In addition, you can contact the following organizations:

- *American Society of Plastic and Reconstructive Surgeons*— This professional society may give you names of board-certified members in your area. Write to the ASPRS (Suite 1900, 233 N. Michigan Avenue, Chicago, IL 60601) or call its 24-hour patient referral service (312-856-1818).

- *The Amercian Cancer Society (ACS)*—Call your state or local unit (listed under American Cancer Society in the telephone book) to see if it has names of surgeons who perform reconstruction.

- *Medical societies*—Your local medical society also may recommend qualified surgeons who perform breast reconstruction.

Sharing Experiences With Other Women

Your surgeon and plastic surgeon may be able to refer you to other breast cancer patients they have treated. Other women who have made a decision about having reconstruction can provide insight that may help you decide what's best for you.

Many women who have had reconstructive surgery are happy to meet with others considering the procedure. The American Cancer Society's Reach to Recovery Program is one means to meet such volunteers. Another is the YWCA's ENCORE program for postoperative breast cancer patients. For more information, contact your local units of ACS and YWCA.

Questions To Ask A Plastic Surgeon

The list of questions below can help you in getting the information you need to consider before you decide to have breast reconstruction. You may have other questions that are not listed here. If so, write them in at the end of the list; then take this booklet with you when you consult a plastic surgeon.

- What type of surgery would you recommend for me? Why?
- What are the risks and benefits associated with it?
- What is your experience with operations of this type?
- May I see photographs of other patients who have had breast reconstruction?
- May I talk with other patients about the operation?
- What can I expect my reconstructed breast to look and feel like? Right after the surgery? In 6 months? In a year?
- How long will I be in the hospital?
- How long is the recovery period after surgery?
- What will I have to do to ensure a safe recovery?
- How much will it cost?
- When can I have the operation?
- What else should I consider in determining whether to have reconstructive surgery?
- Others?

_____

_____

_____

_____

_____

When you visit the plastic surgeon, be prepared for a candid discussion of your expectations for breast reconstruction and your understanding of the impact it will have on you and those close to you. Your motivation for considering breast reconstruction is another area that the surgeon will want to know about.

Breast Self-Examination

After reconstruction, breast self-examination (BSE) should be part of your routine. You will want to examine your natural breast and the reconstructed breast once a month to note any changes in the way they look or feel. Although you may have been doing self-exams before your surgery, you will have to relearn what's considered "normal" for you now. About half the women who have mastectomies report that their remaining breast becomes larger.

If you menstruate, the best time to do BSE is 2 or 3 days after your period ends, when your breast is least likely to be tender or swollen. If you no longer menstruate, pick a day, such as the first day of the month, to do BSE.

Here is how to do BSE:

1. Stand before a mirrow. Inspect your breast for anything unusual, such as any discharge from the nipple, or puckering, dimpling, or scaling of the skin.

   Inspect the scar for new swelling, lumps, redness, or color change. Although redness can be a result of irritation from your bra or prosthesis, report it to your physician.

   The next two steps are designed to emphasize any change in the shape or contour of your breast. As you do them, you should be able to feel your chest muscles tighten.

2. Watching closely in the mirror, clasp your hands behind your head and press your hands forward.

3. Next, press your hands firmly on your hips and bow slightly toward your mirror as you pull your shoulders and elbows forward.

(See page 99 for illustrations of self-examination method)

The next part of the exam is done while standing. Some women do it in the shower because fingers glide over soapy skin, making it easy to concentrate on the texture underneath.

4. Raise your arm on the unoperated side. Using three or four fingers of your other hand, explore your breast firmly, carefully and thoroughly.

   Beginning at the other edge, press the flat part of the your fingers in small circles, moving the circles slowly around the breast. Gradually work toward the nipple. Be sure to cover the entire breast. Pay special attention to the area between the breast and the underarm, including the underarm itself. Feel for any unusual lump or mass under the skin.

5. Gently squeeze the nipple and look for a discharge. Raise your arm on the operated side. Use three or four-fingers of your opposite hand and begin at the top of the scar. Press gently, using small circular motions, and feel the entire length of the scar. Look for thickenings, lumps, and hard places. As with your breast, familiarity with your scar makes it easier to notice any changes. Lumps, thickening, and inflammation are among changes you should bring to the attention of your doctor.

6. Steps 4 and 5 should be repeated lying down. Lie flat on your back, raise your arm on the unoperated side over your head and place a pillow or folded towel under your shoulder. This position flattens the breast and makes it easier to examine. Use the same circular motion described earlier.

Chapter 10

Breast Cancer: Adjuvant Therapy

Adjuvant Therapy
Facts for Women With Breast Cancer

Early in its development, breast cancer may begin to spread beyond the breast to other parts of a woman's body by way of the bloodstream and the lymph system. To control this spread, a form of cancer treatment called adjuvant therapy is sometimes used following primary treatment with either surgery or surgery combined with radiation therapy. In breast cancer, adjuvant therapy involves the use of drugs that either kill cancer cells (chemotherapy) or deprive them of hormones needed for growth (hormone therapy). Adjuvant therapy is being used with increasing success for breast cancer patients who are at risk of having their cancer recur after primary treatment.

Planning Treatment

In deciding if a woman needs adjuvant therapy and what type of treatment would help her the most, doctors must consider several factors. First they must find out if the cancer has spread beyond the breast.

One of the first places breast cancer may spread is to the lymph nodes under the arm. Lymph nodes are bean-shaped structures that filter impurities from the lymph fluid that circulates through the breast and all other parts of the body. During surgery, some or all of the underarm lymph nodes are removed and are examined later under a microscope. Lymph nodes with cancer cells are said to be "positive." Nodes are described as "negative" when there is no evidence that cancer cells have spread to them. If cancer cells are found in the lymph nodes, there is a strong possibility that other cancer cells are circulating in the body. At the present time, adjuvant therapy is recommended for women with positive underarm lymph nodes and should be considered for other women at high risk of having their cancer recur.

Doctors also know that some types of breast cancer depend partly on the female hormones (estrogen and progesterone) for growth. By using certain drugs that block the effects of hormones or lower their levels in the blood, doctors can extend the survival of women whose breast cancer is hormone-dependent.

In addition to examining the lymph nodes when planning treatment, doctors also try to identify women who are most likely to respond to hormone therapy. To do this, they perform tests on a sample of the tumor that was removed during the biopsy. These tests, called hormone receptor assays, show that about two-thirds of all women with breast cancer have tumors that contain estrogen receptors (ER). Women who are ER positive are more likely to respond to hormone therapy than are women who are ER negative (no estrogen receptors). A further way to tell if hormone treatment will be effective is a second test, for progesterone receptors (PR). A woman whose tumor is both ER and PR positive has an 80 percent chance of responding to hormone therapy.

Another factor that is important in planning for adjuvant therapy is a woman's menopausal status. Studies have shown that the effectiveness of different types of adjuvant therapy for breast cancer depends on whether a woman is pre- or postmenopausal. Women who are premenopausal generally respond better to adjuvant chemotherapy. Women who are postmenopausal and ER-positive generally respond to adjuvant hormone therapy. As discussed below, other factors may be considered in deciding treatment for an individual patient.

Options for Treatment

Adjuvant chemotherapy and hormone therapy are both effective treatments for breast cancer patients. While significant advances in treatment research have been made, there is no single best therapy for any group of patients.

Menopausal Women

- For premenopausal breast cancer patients with positive underarm lymph nodes, adjuvant chemotherapy has been shown to be of much benefit, regardless of hormone receptor status. Adjuvant chemotherapy with a combination of drugs is recommended.

- For premenopausal patients with negative lymph nodes, adjuvant therapy is generally not recommended. However, it should be considered for certain high-risk patients. Patients at high risk include those women who have large or aggressive tumors, those who have negative hormone receptors, those who develop breast cancer during pregnancy, or patients who are under age 40. These women have a higher risk of recurrence and may be helped by adjuvant chemotherapy.

Postmenopausal Women

- For postmenopausal patients with positive nodes and positive hormone receptor levels, hormone therapy with a drug called tamoxifen is recommended.

- For postmenopausal patients with positive nodes and negative hormone receptor levels, chemotherapy may be considered.

- For postmenopausal patients with negative nodes, there is no indication for routine adjuvant therapy. For certain high-risk patients, however, adjuvant chemotherapy should be considered.

At this time, scientists are conducting clinical trials*(research with patients) using adjuvant therapy. They are evaluating the possible benefits of this type of treatment in women with negative lymph nodes. Other studies are designed to find the most effective adjuvant therapy for women with positive nodes. Breast cancer patients and their doctors are encouraged to participate in such clinical trials. Patients who take part in research make an important contribution to medical science and have the first chance to benefit from improved treatment methods.

At many hospitals throughout the country, the National Cancer Institute supports studies of new treatments for breast cancer. To learn about these clinical trials, your doctor may use PDQ (Physician Data Query), a new computer information system. PDQ can give your doctor the latest information on clinical trials for each type and stage of cancer. Doctors have access to PDQ through their personal computers or a library.

---

*For in-depth discussion of clinical trials see chapter entitled, *Clinical Trials: What Are They All About?* See CONTENTS for location.

Course of Treatment

Drugs commonly used to treat breast cancer include cyclophosphamide (Cytoxan), methotrexate, 5-fluorouracil (5-FU), doxorubicin (Adriamycin), vincristine (Oncovin), L-PAM (also known as melphalan or L-phenylalanine mustard), and prednisone, given in combinations of two to five drugs. Research indicates that combinations of drugs are generally more effective than single drugs, but no one combination has proved best. Tamoxifen, an antiestrogen drug, is given to postmenopausal women who are ER-positive.

Chemotherapy is given by mouth or by injection into a vein or muscle on a daily, weekly, or monthly schedule. Therapy generally starts shortly after surgery or radiation therapy and may last from 6 months to a year, Tamoxifen, which is taken orally appears to be more effective when given for a longer period (at least 2 years). However, exactly how long adjuvant therapy should be given for best results has not been determined.

Side Effects

The powerful drugs used in chemotherapy destroy constantly dividing cancer cells. Unfortunately, they also affect healthy dividing cells, causing side effects such as nausea and vomiting, loss of appetite, weakness, mouth ulcers, fatigue, hair loss, weight gain, menstrual changes, and lowered resistance to infections.

Whether a woman will have side effects depends on the drugs she is taking and her own response to them. However, most side effects are temporary and gradually go away once treatment is stopped, although some side effects can be permanent. For example, certain drugs may cause sterility or, in the case of Adriamycin, injury to the heart. There is even the remote chance that some drugs may cause a second cancer to develop in the future.

Tamoxifen is tolerated well by most patients. However, it does cause short-term side effects related to lowered levels of estrogen such as hot flashes. Long-term side effects of tamoxifen are unknown at present but appear to be minimal.

Side effects can sometimes be prevented and often they can be treated or minimized. Cancer researchers are working to make chemotherapy more effective and to lessen its side effects. Most doctors believe that the overall benefits achieved by adjuvant therapy for breast cancer outweigh the risk of serious side effects. Each woman and her doctor need to evaluate the known and potential side effects of adjuvant therapy when making decisions about treatment. More information on side effects and other aspects of chemotherapy can be found in the National Cancer Institute publication, Chemotherapy and You:*A Guide to Self-Help During Treatment.

Emotional Concerns

Concerns about breast cancer and its treatment may have a dramatic emotional impact on a woman. The need for chemotherapy and its effect on a woman's life can cause a range of feelings. Fear, anxiety, and depression are common to many breast cancer patients undergoing adjuvant therapy.

When a woman starts chemotherapy, her lifestyle may change. She may have to adjust her routine to fit treatment schedules. And, her overall health may suffer from treatment side effects. These kind of changes are not pleasant, but they can be handled. It is important for all women who are undergoing treatment for breast cancer to remember that they are not alone. Many other cancer patients have successfully dealt with similar feelings and problems.

During treatment, a woman may wonder what is happening to her, whether the drugs are working, and how she can deal with her stress and anxiety. If a woman doesn't understand what is happening, she should ask questions. If she doesn't understand the way it is explained, she should keep asking until she does. A woman should also be aware of her emotional well-being, and remember that it is just as important as her physical health. If a woman feels frightened or discouraged, she should seek out help.

Talking with an understanding friend or family member or with another patient may be helpful. She may wish to talk things over with a member of the clergy or a health professional with whom she feels comfortable. She can talk with her doctor, nurse, or

---

* The mentioned text is reprinted within this book. See CONTENTS for location.

social worker, or ask about seeing a mental health professional. Many hospitals have support groups for people undergoing chemotherapy. Everyone needs some support during difficult times, and she should not hesitate to ask for help while she's being treated for breast cancer.

Followup Care

Any woman who has had cancer in one breast is at an increased risk of developing cancer in her other breast, so breast self-examination (BSE) is very important. No matter what kind of treatment a woman has had, she needs to do BSE once a month. Her doctor can tell her how to do BSE if she doesn't already know. Nurses are also trained to teach BSE.

Most doctors believe that women treated for breast cancer should have regular exams every 3 to 6 months for the first 3 years after treatment, and once or twice a year thereafter. During some visits the doctor will perform a physical exam of the breast tissue, chest area, underarms, and neck. Other visits may include a mammogram of the breast, X-rays, blood tests, and bone scans.

These tests will help the doctor to check for reappearance of cancer cells in the original site and elsewhere in the body. After 3 years, these exams may be done once or twice a year. However, a woman should always remain under a doctor's care for her breast disease. More information about followup care can be found in the National Cancer Institute booklet, After Breast Cancer:* A Guide to Followup Care.

---

* *The mentioned text is reprinted as the next chapter in this book.*

Chapter 11

Breast Cancer: Afterward

A Guide to Followup Care

After Breast Cancer: A Guide to Followup Care

The majority of women with early stage breast cancer are successfully treated by surgery and/or radiation therapy, sometimes combined with chemotherapy. Now that you have completed your treatment, you've gone through a number of physical and emotional changes and are probably ready to get on with the rest of your life. However, you should be aware of your continuing need for followup care. It is important for you to return to your doctor for scheduled examinations, continue to practice breast self-examination, and know about the signs of possible recurrence.

This **text** provides some helpful suggestions for taking care of yourself after breast cancer: how to cope with emotional needs, what to expect during your followup examinations, and how to spot possible signs of recurrence. A short glossary near the end of the **material** explains some of the medical terms you might hear, and the "Resources" section can direct you to additional information and assistance.

Adjusting Emotionally

Dealing with the physical aspects of breast cancer treatment

155

is only one part of the healing process. Understanding and managing the emotional side is another. While the treatment you've had may control your cancer forever, the threatening nature of the disease can make you feel upset, depressed, angry, afraid, bitter, or frustrated. Your family and others who are close to you may share some of these feelings as well.

During treatment you had frequent, perhaps daily, contact with health professionals. Many women report that when their treatment ends, they feel they have lost the support of those most concerned with their physical needs and well-being. Some say they feel abandoned. If you feel this way, it may be a good idea to talk over your feelings with those on your health care team that you have been close to during treatment. Busy health professionals can sometimes use a reminder that the patients they are no longer treating continue to need personal support.

Coping with treatment has consumed much of your physical and mental energy. Yet, some women find that the demands of treatment were somehow reassuring: at least they were *doing something* to treat the cancer. Some women report feeling anxious when they no longer have to deal with the side effects of a specific therapy because suddenly they feel that they are no longer taking any action against their disease. If you feel this way, remind yourself that you have followed the recommendations of medical professionals and that you and your doctor are continuing to monitor your health.

If you feel comfortable talking about your feelings, do so. Expressing your feelings to your doctor and the people you love can be important emotional medicine. Think about how you have solved other problems in your life, and apply those techniques now. Here are some suggestions for handling this period of readjustment:

○ There will be days that your spirits will be low—not only because you must deal with uncertainty but also because you have been through a difficult time. Pretending you're always happy, without mentioning times when you do feel upset, can cut off channels for communication. Discuss your experience and fears openly with family and friends, and ask for their support. Tackling the situation together can give those close to you the feeling that they are doing something to help.

o Whatever was important to you before your cancer treatment can remain part of your life now. Remember that the qualities that make a good friend, a valuable worker, a loving mate, and a caring mother are still there in you.

o If informal approaches to dealing with your feelings do not seem to be working, don't hesitate to ask for help from professionals. Psychiatrists, psychologists, social workers, nurses, and religious counselors can help you.

o Some women do find that having breast cancer restores their sense of values, sharpens their appreciation of life, brings them closer to people they love, and leads to insights about the meaning of their lives. You may wish to seek out other women who have had breast cancer to find out how they coped with the disease.

Above all, remember that you, as the patient, can set the tone and pace of communication with your doctor, and you *should* have input in decisions regarding your health. Assume your rightful share of the responsibility for your followup care.

Continuing Health Care
Breast Self-Examination

Any woman who has had cancer in one breast is at an increased risk of developing cancer in her other breast, so breast self-examination (BSE) continues to be important. Whether you have had a mastectomy or had radiation therapy as the primary treatment for breast cancer, you need to do BSE*once a month.

As you do BSE, you will become familiar with the usual appearance and consistency of your breast tissue, chest area, and any scar tissue. Breast tissue usually feels different after radia-

(See page 99 for illustration on self-examination method)

157

tion therapy, and you may need a few BSE sessions to learn what is now the "usual" for you. Likewise, if you've had a breast removed, you will need practice to know what is usual for the scar and surrounding area. Early discovery of a change from "normal" is the main idea behind BSE. By practicing BSE regularly, you should soon be able to detect any change that requires your doctor's attention.

The doctor who will be handling your followup care can tell you how to do BSE if you don't already know. Most nurses are also trained to teach BSE. If you haven't received BSE instructions, ask them about it.

If you menstruate, the best time to examine yourself is 2 or 3 days after your period ends. If you no longer menstruate, pick a regular date, such as the first of each month, to do BSE. In any case, be sure to follow all the prescribed steps, both standing and lying down.

Written materials can help you while you're practicing BSE at home. Detailed guidelines for BSE after mastectomy can be found in *Mastectomy:*A Treatment for Breast Cancer*. Detailed guidelines for BSE after radiation therapy can be found in *Radiation Therapy:*A Treatment for Early Stage Breast Cancer*. Contact the National Cancer Institute if you need a copy*of either booklet.

Followup Examination

Your doctor will tell you when to schedule your first post-treatment examination. After that, regular visits to a physician are important, and you and your surgeon or radiation therapist should decide which doctor will be responsible for your followup care. Many surgeons and radiation therapists continue to monitor their patients after treatment. Others refer their patients to a medical oncologist, an internist, a gynecologist, or a family physician.

During the first 3 years after breast cancer treatment, you should have periodic professional examinations. Check with your doctor to see when you should return for an examination; often doctors recommend followup visits about every 3 to 6 months.

The mentioned text is reprinted within this book. See CONTENTS for location.

If you have a mastectomy and are considering surgery for breast reconstruction, you may need to see your regular doctor more often, in addition to visits with a plastic surgeon. Your doctor can also advise you about when you can start to wear a breast prosthesis if you wish to.

During some visits, your doctor will simply perform a physical exam that includes breast tissue, any incisions, the chest area, underarms, and neck. Other visits, however, may include all or some of the following procedures:

○ A mammographic breast examination;

○ A complete physical examination;

○ Blood tests for liver function and/or liver scans, if indicated;

○ Other blood tests and urine analysis; and

○ X-rays and/or scans of the chest, spine, and pelvis.

These tests will help the doctor to check for reappearance of cancer at the original site and in other parts of the body. In cases where breast cancer metastasizes (spreads to other organs), it most often shows up in the bones, lungs, liver, or brain.

After 3 years, the above examinations may be done at less frequent intervals, probably once or twice a year. However, you should always remain under continuing followup care for your breast disease.

A Possible Complication

Some women, after treatment for breast cancer, develop a condition known as lymphedema, which is caused by the loss of or damage to the underarm lymph nodes and their connecting vessels. Because of surgical or radiation treatment to the lymph nodes, circulation of lymph fluid from the affected arm may be slowed and the ability to fight infection impaired. Not all women develop this complication, but if swelling should occur, the doctor will advise you on the proper steps to take, for example, doing special exercises and wearing an elastic sleeve to stimulate circulation.

Women who have had the underarm lymph nodes removed or who have been treated by X-ray need to take special care of the affected arm and try to *prevent* infection in it. Some simple rules to help prevent infection are:

o Avoid burns while cooking or smoking;

o Avoid sunburns;

o Have all injections, vaccinations, blood samples, and blood pressure tests done on the other arm whenever possible;

o Use an electric razor with a narrow head for underarm shaving to reduce the risk of nicks or scratches;

o Carry heavy packages or handbags on the other arm;

o Wash cuts promptly, treat them with antibacterial medication, and cover them with a sterile dressing; check often for redness, soreness, or other signs of infection;

o Never cut cuticles; use hand cream or lotion;

o Wear watches or jewelry loosely, if at all, on the treated arm;

o Wear protective gloves when gardening and when using strong detergents, etc.;

o Use a thimble when sewing;

o Avoid harsh chemicals and abrasive compounds;

o Use insect repellent to avoid bites and stings; and

o Avoid elastic cuffs on blouses and nightgowns.

Call your doctor at once if your treated arm swells or becomes red, or if it feels hot. In the meantime, put your arm over your head and pump your fist. Though you should be cautious, it's also important to use your arm normally—don't favor it or keep it dependent.

Possibility of Recurrence

Recurrent breast cancer can be successfully treated if it is detected and treated early. Sixty percent of all recurrences appear within the first 3 years after initial treatment, 20 percent within the next 2 years, and 20 percent in later years. As a result, you should be examined frequently during the first 5 years after your treatment, and you should continue to be checked by your doctor as often as recommended in the years afterward.

While you should be careful to observe and to report any symptoms of recurrent disease to your doctor, do not let yourself become obsessed with watching for a new cancer. Remember that the symptoms listed below can also be caused by arthritis, influenza, menopause, or even the common cold.

Between professional examinations, you should report to your doctor the following:

o Changes you detect in a breast or in your scar during breast self-examination, especially lumps, thickenings, or inflammation;

o Persistent pain in the breast, shoulder, hip, lower back, or pelvis;

o Persistent coughing or hoarseness;

o Digestive disturbances such as nausea, vomiting, diarrhea, or heartburn that persist for several days;

o Loss of appetite or unexplained weight changes;

o Changes in your menstrual cycle or flow; and

o Persistent dizziness, blurred vision, severe and frequent headaches, or difficulties in walking.

None of these symptoms is a clear indication that the cancer has recurred, so you should not let them frighten you. But do report any such changes to your doctor immediately so that an accurate diagnosis can be made.

Questions To Ask Your Doctor

o How often should I return for an examination? For lab tests?

o What tests will be performed at those times?

o What will the tests tell us?

o When I do a breast exam, what am I looking for?

o Should I watch for any particular signs of recurrence?

Resources

The National Cancer Institute sponsors a toll-free *Cancer Information Service* (CIS), open 7 days a week to help you. By dialing 1-800-4-CANCER (1-800-422-6237), you will be connected to a CIS office, where a trained staff member can answer your questions and listen to your concerns.

In Alaska, call 1-800-638-6070; in Hawaii, on Oahu call 524-1234 (on neighboring islands, call collect).

Spanish-speaking staff members are available to callers from the following areas (daytime hours only): California, Florida, Georgia, Illinois, northern New Jersey, New York, and Texas.

The American Cancer Society's *Reach to Recovery* program offers support to breast cancer patients as they adjust to their disease and treatment. The volunteers' goals are to let the patient know that many women share her problems and to provide a positive role model for the patient. Reach to Recovery also provides the husband and family members with a letter to help them understand some of the problems the patients might be experiencing. For further information, contact the local unit of the American Cancer Society listed in your telephone book.

ENCORE (Encouragement, Normalcy, Counseling, Opportunity, Reaching Out, Energies Revived) is a national YWCA program for postoperative breast cancer patients. ENCORE meetings include exercise to music, water exercises, and a discussion period. Many ENCORE programs are ongoing, and a woman may join a group as early as 3 weeks after surgery for breast cancer. For further information, contact your local YWCA.

Glossary

Anesthesia—loss of feeling or sensation resulting from the administration of drugs or gases.

Anesthesiologist—a doctor who administers drugs or gases to put a patient to sleep before surgery.

Areola—the circular field of dark-colored skin surrounding the nipple.

Aspiration—withdrawal of fluid from a cyst with a hypodermic needle.

Assay, estrogen receptor and progesterone receptor—a laboratory test conducted on cancerous tissue to determine if the cells need the female hormones estrogen and progesterone for their growth.

Axillary dissection—removal of all the underarm lymph nodes.

Axillary sampling—removal of some of the underarm lymph nodes.

Benign—not cancerous.

Biopsy—removal of a sample of tissue to see if cancer cells are present.

Breast enlargement—an operation in which an implant is inserted under normal breast tissues to make the breast larger.

Breast implant—a round or teardrop-shaped sac inserted in the body to restore a breast form.

Breast prosthesis—an artificial breast form that can be worn under clothing after a mastectomy.

Breast reduction—an operation in which breast skin and tissue are removed and the nipple is moved up onto the newly contoured breast to make the breast smaller.

Chemotherapy—treatment with drugs to destroy cancer cells. Most often used to supplement surgery and/or radiation therapy.

Frozen section—a part of the biopsy tissue frozen immediately. A thin slice is then mounted on microscope slides and examined by a pathologist. The analysis can be completed in just a few minutes.

Intravenous (IV)—being within or entering by way of the veins.

Lump—any kind of mass in the breast or elsewhere in the body.

Lumpectomy—surgical removal of the lump or cancerous tissue from the breast, usually followed by radiation therapy.

Lymph nodes—part of the lymphatic system that removes wastes from body tissue and carries fluids that help the body fight infection.

Lymphedema—swelling in the arm caused by excess fluid that collects when the lymph nodes and vessels are removed during surgery or damaged by radiation therapy.

Mammography—the process of X-raying the breast to detect tumors before they can be felt.

Mastectomy—surgical removal of the breast as treatment for breast cancer.

Mastectomy, modified radical—the most common mastectomy performed today. Also called "total mastectomy with axillary dissection." The breast, breast skin, nipple, areola, and underarm lymph nodes are removed, while the chest muscles are saved.

Mastectomy, prophylactic—a procedure sometimes recommended for patients at very high risk of developing cancer in one or both breasts. One type, called a "subcutaneous" mastectomy, removes the breast tissue but leaves muscle, skin, and nipple.

Mastectomy, radical—the surgical removal of the breast, breast skin, nipple, areola, chest muscles, and underarm lymph nodes. This operation leaves a hollow area in the chest wall under the collarbone and in front of the armpit. Also call a "Halsted radical."

Oncologist—a doctor who is a specialist in the treatment of cancers.

One-step procedure—biopsy performed under general anesthesia; if cancer is found, the surgeon immediately performs a mastectomy.

Palliative therapy—a treatment that may relieve symptoms without curing the disease.

Pathologist—a doctor with special training in diagnosing disease from samples of tissue.

Pectoral muscles—muscles that overlay the chest wall and help to support the breasts.

Permanent section—a thin slice of the biopsy tissue mounted on slides to be examined under a microscope by a pathologist. Permanent sections require long preparation time and are not used for diagnosis with the one-step procedure.

Prosthesis—an artificial breast form (or any artificial replacement for a body part).

Rad—stands for "radiation absorbed dose." A unit of measurement for radiation therapy.

Radiologist—a physician with special training in the diagnostic and/or therapeutic use of X-rays and other forms of radiant energy.

Radiation oncologist—a doctor who specializes in using radiation to treat cancer.

Radiation therapy—the use of high-energy penetrating rays to treat disease; sources of radiation include X-ray, cobalt, and radium.

Recurrence—reappearance of cancer at the same site (local), near the initial site (regional), or in other areas of the body (metastatic).

Silicone gel—medical-grade silicone rubber gel that has fluid qualities similar to the normal breast.

Tumor—an abnormal mass of tissue that results from excessive cell division and performs no useful body function; tumors are either *benign* or *malignant*.

Two-step procedure—biopsy and treatment performed in two stages.

Chapter 12

Cancer of the Colon and Rectum

Introduction

This text describes current knowledge of the incidence, possible causes and prevention, detection and diagnosis, and treatment of cancer of the colon and rectum. The information presented here was gathered from medical textbooks, recent articles in the periodical literature, National Cancer Institute (NCI) researchers, and other scientists.

Knowledge about cancer of the colon and rectum is increasing rapidly. For up-to-date information on this and other cancer-related subjects, you may call the toll-free Cancer Information Service at 1-800-4-CANCER.

Description and Function of the Colon and Rectum

The chief function of the digestive system, also called the gastrointestinal (GI) tract, is to convert food into substances that can be absorbed into the bloodstream and transported throughout the body. It thus supplies the body with essential nutrients, fluids, and electrolytes (such as sodium and potassium). Another function of the GI tract is to store and dispose of waste.

The large bowel, or large intestine, is the last part of the

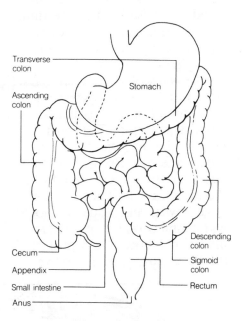

digestive tract. About 5 feet long and 1 to 3 inches in diameter, the large bowel is a tubular organ composed of the cecum, the colon, and the rectum.

The cecum, a pouch in the lower right part of the abdomen, is the first part of the large bowel. It connects the small intestine with the colon. (Attached to the cecum is the appendix, a 3-inch-long organ whose function, if any, is not understood.)

The colon, the middle section of the large bowel, extends from the cecum to the rectum in the shape of an inverted "U." The four parts of the colon—beginning on the right side and extending upward, across the body, and down the left side—are the ascending, transverse, descending, and sigmoid sections. The sigmoid colon leads to the rectum, and the final inch or so of the rectum, the anal region, leads to the opening called the anus.

The walls of the digestive tract have four layers of tissue: mucosa, submucosa, muscularis externa, and serosa. The innermost layer is the mucosa, a mucous membrane that forms a continuous lining of the GI tract from the mouth to the anus. In the large bowel, this tissue is smooth and contains cells that produce mucus to lubricate and protect the inner surface of the bowel

wall. Connective tissue and muscle separate the mucosa from the second layer, the submucosa, which contains blood vessels, lymph vessels, and nerves. Next to the submucosa is the muscularis externa, consisting of two layers of muscle fibers—one that runs lengthwise and one that encircles the bowel. The fourth layer, the serosa, is a thin membrane that produces fluid to lubricate the outer surface of the bowel so that it can slide against adjacent organs.

The main functions of the large bowel are to absorb water and to store and eliminate waste. Semiliquid waste, composed

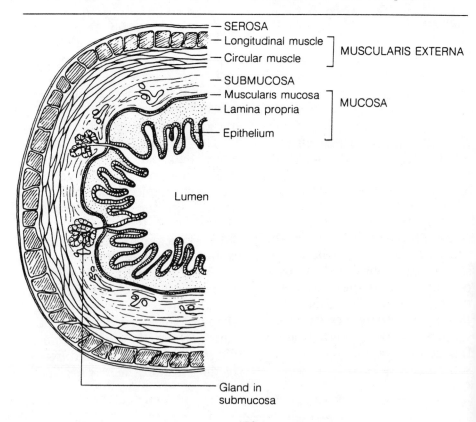

— SEROSA
— Longitudinal muscle ⎤
— Circular muscle ⎦ MUSCULARIS EXTERNA

— SUBMUCOSA
— Muscularis mucosa ⎤
— Lamina propria ⎥ MUCOSA
— Epithelium ⎦

Lumen

Gland in submucosa

mainly of water and partly digested food, enters the large bowel from the small bowel. Fluids and electrolytes that reach the large bowel are absorbed, mainly in the cecum and the ascending colon. Bacteria that normally live in the colon break down remaining carbohydrates and proteins and convert food components into vitamin K and some of the B vitamins. Muscle contractions, called peristalsis, move fecal matter (waste) through the transverse colon into the descending colon and then into the sigmoid colon. Depending on the amount and the type of food in the diet, about 5 ounces of fecal matter are produced each day. The anus is kept closed by the action of several muscles, including the sphincter muscle surrounding the anal opening. These muscles relax to allow the stool to pass.

Like other tissues and organs of the body, the large bowel is composed of individual cells. To repair worn-out or injured tissues and to allow for growth, cells normally divide and replace themselves in an orderly, controlled way. When cell division becomes disorderly and uncontrolled, too many cells are produced, abnormal growth takes place, and masses of tissue known as tumors are formed.

Tumors may be benign (noncancerous) or malignant (cancerous). Benign tumors that grow from the wall into the interior space (lumen) of the large bowel are called polyps. Polyps may interfere with normal functions, but they do not spread to other parts of the body, and generally they are not life threatening. However, some types of intestinal polyps have the potential to become cancerous as they grow larger.

Cancers that develop in the cecum, colon, and rectum are known as colorectal cancers. Like other types of cancer, they can invade and destroy normal tissues and extend into surrounding structures. Also, cancer cells can break away from a primary tumor and metastasize, or spread, to other parts of the body through the lymphatic system or the bloodstream. When colorectal cancer cells spread, they most often travel to the liver. Cells that migrate to the liver or other organs can continue to divide abnormally and form secondary (metastatic) tumors. The cancer cells that form metastatic tumors in the liver, lungs, or elsewhere in the body have the same characteristics as the cells of the primary tumor. Although another organ is affected, the disease is still called colon cancer or rectal cancer. Methods used to treat the metastatic disease depend on the site and type of the primary (original) cancer and on the location and extent of the secondary tumors.

Most colorectal cancers are adenocarcinomas, which arise in the epithelial tissue, or lining, of the large bowel. Cancers that begin in connective tissue (sarcomas) or lymphatic tissue (lymphomas) and other uncommon cancers (such as carcinoid tumors) in the colon and rectum are not discussed in this *Research Report*.

Incidence and Mortality

The incidence of colorectal cancer in the United States is among the highest in the world. Cancers of the colon and rectum affect roughly 5 percent of Americans at some time in their lives. These cancers account for about 15 percent of all cancers diagnosed in this country. Only cancer of the lung and common skin cancers occur more frequently, and only lung cancer causes more deaths. It is estimated that 147,000 new cases of colorectal cancer (76,000 in women and 71,000 in men) were diagnosed in this country in 1988, with colon cancer affecting more than twice as many people as rectal cancer.

Data collected and analyzed by the Surveillance, Epidemiology, and End Results (SEER)

Program of the NCI show that the incidence rate of colorectal cancer (the annual number of new cases per 100,000 population) in this country increased 9.6 percent from 1973 to 1985. During that period, the incidence of colon cancer remained relatively constant among white females, rose slightly among white males, and increased sharply for blacks of both sexes. For rectal cancer, the incidence remained about the same for all groups.

Colorectal cancer is rare in young people. Fewer than 6 percent of cases occur before the age of 50. Incidence increases markedly after age 50, continues to rise until age 75, and then tapers off. The average age at the time of diagnosis is 60.

Certain patterns are apparent in the worldwide variation in the incidence of colorectal cancer. These cancers are more common in densely populated, industrialized regions than in rural areas. High rates are observed in North America and northern and western Europe. People in less developed areas—Africa, Latin America, and most of Asia— seldom develop colorectal cancer. In eastern and southern Europe,

Japan, and urban areas of some South American countries, the rates are between the low rate of rural Africa and the high rates of Europe and North America. Although it is still relatively low, the rate in Japan is rising. Some studies of incidence patterns within the United States have shown a higher-than-average risk among Americans of Irish, Czech, and German ancestry and a low risk among Mormons and Seventh-Day Adventists.

Geographic differences in death rates from colorectal cancer also exist within the United States. For both sexes and both races, the rates are highest in New Jersey, Massachusetts, parts of New York State, and urban areas in the Great Lakes region. Large areas in the South and Southwest have significantly lower colorectal cancer mortality rates than the average for the rest of the country.

The national mortality rate (the annual number of deaths per 100,000 population) from colorectal cancer declined 5.5 percent from 1973 to 1985. This decrease probably indicates that the disease is being detected at an earlier, more treatable stage and that treatment and patient management are becoming more effective. Nevertheless, these cancers cause roughly 60,000 deaths each year—about 12 percent of all cancer deaths in the United States.

Causes and Prevention

Scientists believe that cancers of the colon and rectum develop over a period of many years as the result of gradual changes in cells. Although both heredity and environment seem to be involved, the causes of the disease are not well understood. Doctors can seldom explain why an individual develops colorectal cancer. In most cases, the onset of colorectal cancer is probably triggered by the complex interactions of several different factors.

Lifestyle

Although many investigators have observed that colon and rectal cancers occur more often in urban, industrialized regions, they have not been able to identify the underlying cancer-causing factors. In studies of ethnic groups with unusually high or unusually low rates, it has been difficult to separate genetic factors from lifestyle and environment. However, studies of migrant populations point to the importance of lifestyle as a risk factor. Groups that have migrated from areas with low rates of colorectal cancer to areas with higher rates begin to exhibit the rates of the population in the new area, often within one generation. In Hawaii, for example, the colorectal cancer rate among Japanese immigrants has risen to equal that of the Caucasians in that State. Furthermore, when Americans move from high-risk to low-risk parts of the country—as from the urban North to the rural South—the incidence in the new area does not seem to rise. Rather, the migrants apparently take on the lower risk of their new neighbors.

Diet

Numerous animal experiments and population studies suggest that the development of colorectal cancers is linked to low intake of dietary fiber and that increased dietary fiber has a protective effect. Fiber, often referred to as "roughage" or "bulk," is the indigestible part of plants. Scientists do not yet understand exactly how dietary fiber reduces the risk of colorectal cancer, but several possible mechanisms have been suggested. We know that increased fiber results in greater stool bulk and more rapid movement through the colon. Thus, high-fiber diets may reduce both the concentra-

tion of carcinogens (cancer-causing substances) in the stool and the amount of time during which carcinogens come in contact with the bowel wall. In addition, increased fiber may change the chemical composition of the stool by altering the nature and behavior of the bacteria in the colon.

Animal and population studies also indicate that colon cancer risk is related to the amount of dietary fat. Considerable evidence links a high-fat diet to a high incidence of colon cancer. Scientists theorize that dietary fat increases the amount of bile acids in the colon. These substances may act directly to damage the bowel lining, or they may be converted to secondary bile acids, which are known to produce tumors in animals. A high-fat diet may also affect colon cancer incidence by increasing the amount of damaging chemicals (lipid peroxides) in the bowel, by causing changes in cell membrane, and/or by affecting hormone (prostaglandin) regulation.

The NCI suggests that Americans increase fiber from a variety of sources and reduce fat as part of a balanced diet that includes the recommended daily allowances (RDAs) of vitamins, minerals, and protein. The amount of fiber in the American diet, which currently averages 8 to 12 grams per day, should be increased to 20 to 30 grams, but should not exceed 35 grams. (Fiber comes chiefly from vegetables, fruits, and whole-grain breads and cereals.) The portion of calories supplied by fats should be reduced from the current average of nearly 40 percent to 30 percent or less. (The major sources of fat in the American diet are meat, eggs, dairy products, and oils used in cooking and in salad dressings.) Although precise predictions are impossible, some scientists estimate that by the year 2000, more than 20,000 cases of large bowel cancer might be prevented annually by these simple dietary modifications.

Other dietary factors are under study. Several with a possible, though still unproven, link to colorectal cancer include compounds produced in the body's metabolism of protein; chemicals produced by frying, smoking, or grilling meat and fish; and certain nitrogen-containing compounds.

Scientists are trying to learn more about the cancer-causing potential of substances known as mutagens that are present in our food. They know that mutagens damage the genetic makeup (DNA) of cells, but they have not determined whether such changes are related to the development of cancer. Certain groups of people who consume a high-fat/low-fiber diet have higher levels of mutagens in their stools and also have an increased risk of colon cancer, but a cause-and-effect relationship has not been proven. One such mutagen currently under study is known as fecapentaene-12 (fec-12). While researchers have shown that fec-12 damages human cells grown in the laboratory, they have not demonstrated that it causes cancer in humans.

Researchers are also trying to determine whether specific dietary factors can inhibit the development of cancer in humans. They have shown that increased levels of certain vitamins and minerals can reduce the number of colon cancers in animals. But whether increased amounts of these nutrients can reduce the risk of large bowel cancer in humans has not been determined. Currently, the NCI is conducting two types of cancer prevention studies related to diet: chemoprevention (using natural and/or synthetic agents as dietary supplements) and dietary intervention (changing the diet to alter the intake of specific nutrients, food groups, or non-nutritive food components).

Some of this work is looking at the actions and effects of selenium, vitamins A, C, and E, beta-carotene (a precursor to vitamin A), minerals such as calcium, and certain enzymes that inhibit protein breakdown. This research is in the early stages. The role that these dietary factors may have in the prevention of colorectal cancer has not been defined, and at this time, NCI scientists do not recommend dietary supplements. Instead, they advise a well-balanced diet that includes a wide variety of foods high in fiber and low in fat.

Occupation

Most scientists believe that occupational risks account for a very small fraction of the total number of cases of colorectal cancer. A Canadian study suggests that workers exposed to certain substances in the manufacture of synthetic fibers have an increased incidence of colorectal cancer. More study is needed to explore possible risks associated with on-the-job exposure to asbestos, dyes, fuel oil, solvents, aromatic hydrocarbons, and abrasives.

Heredity

The role of heredity in the development of large bowel cancer is not fully understood. Some geneticists believe that, overall, an inherited tendency toward colorectal cancer is a contributing factor in roughly 5 to 7 percent of all cases. Among family members of patients with colorectal cancer, the risk of developing the same disease is 3 to 4 times greater than the risk in the general population. Some families prone to colon cancer have an increased risk of developing cancer in other organs, particularly the uterus. For most of these families, the importance of heredity as compared with environment and lifestyle has not been determined. In certain families, however, chiefly those in which colon cancer occurs at an unusually early age, a dominant inheritance pattern has been identified. For the offspring of colorectal cancer patients in these families, the chance of developing the disease is close to 50 percent.

Various genetic conditions involving colon polyps are known to lead to cancer. One example is familial polyposis, a rare inherited disease in which multiple polyps (often several hundred) develop throughout the colon during adolescence and early adulthood. As many as one-half to two-thirds of patients with this disorder develop cancer during their thirties and forties; by the age of 55, the probability of their having bowel cancer is nearly 100 percent.

A similar condition is Gardner's syndrome, which involves multiple polyps of the colon along with other noncancerous growths, usually in the skin and the bones of the jaw and skull. The colon polyps generally appear at a later age than in familial polyposis, but the risk of cancer is the same. These and other forms of inherited polyposis—including Turcot's syndrome and Oldfield's syndrome—are uncommon conditions. Familial polyposis, for example, affects 1 person in about 8,000; Gardner's syndrome affects only 1 in roughly 14,000. In all, fewer than 1 percent of all colorectal cancers occur in persons with genetic polyps.

At the present time, most doctors agree that surgery is the best way to prevent bowel cancer in patients with inherited polyposis. Generally, the surgeon removes the entire colon and rectum and creates an ostomy, an opening in the abdominal wall for the elimination of waste. In some cases, when the polyps are located above the rectum, it may be possible to remove just the colon and attach the ileum, the lower part of the small intestine, to the anus. Also, physicians are evaluating a new procedure, removing the colon and rectal mucosa, but not removing the rectum or the sphincter muscle. The ileum is pulled through the rectum and attached to the anus, thus preserving muscle control.

Polyps

Sporadic (not inherited) intestinal polyps, or adenomas, are another risk factor. These polyps—chiefly those classified as adenomatous (or tubular), villous, and intermediate (or tubulovillous)— may become cancerous, particularly if they grow larger than an inch in diameter. These growths, which arise most often in the rectum and sigmoid colon, are different in their appearance, texture, microscopic characteristics, and potential for cancerous change. Adenomatous polyps are believed to occur in up to 15 percent of the adult population in the United States. Although these polyps usually do not cause symptoms, they can cause intermittent bleeding and, if they are large, can obstruct the passage of waste material. Invasive cancer develops in roughly 5 percent of adenomatous polyps. Villous polyps are less common,

177

affecting fewer than 3 or 4 percent of the population. These growths bleed easily and may cause the passage of mucus with bowel movements. An estimated 40 percent become cancerous. Intermediate polyps are somewhat more common than the villous type; cancer develops in about 23 percent. The most common colorectal polyps, called hyperplastic polyps or hyperplastic mucosal tags, are harmless.

Scientists now believe that many—perhaps most—cancers of the large bowel arise from adenomatous, villous, and intermediate polyps. Removing these growths (polypectomy), often through a sigmoidoscope or colonoscope (described on pages 12 and 14), is one way to prevent colorectal cancer. Also, because new polyps develop in nearly half of all patients who have had such growths removed, careful followup is necessary. An ongoing study is testing the possibility that vitamins C and E may reduce the recurrence rate of colorectal polyps. Thus far, however, research does not suggest that people should take vitamin supplements to try to prevent the growth of colorectal polyps.

Inflammatory Bowel Diseases

A history of ulcerative colitis or granulomatous colitis (Crohn's disease) increases the risk of bowel cancer. These diseases cause inflammation of the lining and wall of the bowel. Scientists believe that cancer arises in an overgrowth of epithelium as new cells are generated to replace diseased tissue. For patients with ulcerative colitis, the risk of eventually developing colon cancer appears to be 5 to 11 times higher than that of the general population. The probability of cancer is especially high when the disease develops during childhood, persists for more than 10 years, involves the entire colon, and is continuous rather than intermittent. Crohn's disease increases the risk of cancer of both the large and small bowel, but the degree of risk is smaller than with ulcerative colitis.

For many years, doctors advocated surgery (removing the colon or both the colon and rectum) to prevent patients with inflammatory bowel disease from developing colorectal cancer. Recently, new techniques that allow doctors to view the entire colon have made it possible to monitor ulcerative colitis patients closely and postpone surgery until precancerous tissue or early cancer is found.

178

Other Cancers

For an individual with a history of colorectal cancer, the risk of developing a new primary cancer of the large bowel is roughly three times that of the general population. In women, a history of cancer of the breast and/or reproductive tract also increases the risk of colorectal cancer.

Detection

Early detection is one of the best ways to reduce the number of deaths from colorectal cancer. Researchers are seeking safe, reliable, cost-effective ways to detect these cancers at an early stage, when they are most treatable. It is estimated that cure rates of 75 percent or higher can be achieved if colorectal tumors are found and treated before they cause symptoms.

Screening and Early Detection

Only 2 percent or less of colorectal cancers develop in people known to be at high risk because of conditions that require frequent monitoring.

Therefore, to reduce the overall mortality from these cancers, screening and early detection practices need to focus on the general population.

Screening is the attempt to detect cancer in persons who have *no symptoms* of the disease. To encourage screening for colorectal cancer in the general population, the NCI has worked with representatives of other medical organizations to formulate early detection guidelines for use by physicians. These guidelines are based on current statistical and clinical information, and they are subject to change as new scientific data become available. At present, based only on age as a risk factor, recommended screening techniques include digital rectal examination, sigmoidoscopy, and fecal occult blood testing.

- The *rectal examination* is recommended for all adults seen in the physician's office for a periodic health examination. This exam is easy to perform and not uncomfortable for the patient. Inserting a lubricated, gloved finger into the rectum, the doctor checks the surface of the rectal wall for irregular or abnormally firm areas. Roughly 12 to 15 percent of all colorectal cancers arise in tissues that can be felt by a doctor performing a routine digital rectal examination.

• *Sigmoidoscopy* (sometimes called proctosigmoidoscopy) should be performed every 3 to 5 years, beginning at age 50. The sigmoidoscope is a lighted, tubular instrument that is inserted into the large bowel through the anus. It enables the physician to visually examine the walls of the rectum and the sigmoid portion of the colon, where more than half of all large bowel cancers occur. This procedure may be somewhat uncomfortable but is seldom painful.

• The *fecal occult blood test* should be done every year, beginning at age 50. This is a safe, relatively simple, inexpensive chemical test for hidden blood in a stool sample. However, it is only a test for blood, *not* a specific test for cancer. A positive test result can be caused by bleeding from a cancerous growth, as well as from hemorrhoids, ulcers, polyps, or other non-cancerous conditions. In fact, in a number of screening programs, fewer than 10 percent of all positive occult blood tests were the result of cancer.

In addition, the occult blood test is negative in many patients with proven large bowel cancer—perhaps because some tumors bleed intermittently, some bleed too little to be detected, and some do not bleed at all. Also, the outcome of an occult blood test can be affected by a variety of other factors, including how a patient prepares for the test and how the stool specimen is processed.

Studies are in progress to determine whether the death rate from colorectal cancer can be reduced by mass screening with an occult blood test. These studies will look at the benefits of using this test to screen very large numbers of people who have no signs or symptoms of the disease.

In addition to these procedures, physicians should continue to identify high-risk patients—including those with a strong family history of colon cancer and those with a personal history of colorectal polyps, colon cancer, or inflammatory bowel disease—for special attention. The three detection techniques described above and various others may be recommended for these individuals.

Scientists are trying to learn whether the likelihood of developing colorectal cancer is signaled by any chemical or biological changes in the body prior to tumor growth. Such markers could then be used to help identify individuals at high risk. These people might benefit from special prevention and detection efforts. Similar research may lead to the identification of colorectal tumor markers (substances produced by the tumor) that would signal the presence of cancer and make detection possible at a very early stage.

Symptoms

At present, most colorectal cancers are detected only after symptoms have appeared. Changes in bowel habits (such as constipation or diarrhea); very dark, mahogany red, or bright red blood in or on the stool; and abdominal discomfort are the most common warning signs. Other signals are persistent narrowing of the stools, tenesmus (an urgent, painful need to defecate), and the feeling of incomplete emptying following bowel movements. Symptoms may also include unexplained weight loss, anemia, unusual paleness, and fatigue. Certain symptoms depend on the location and size of the tumor.

On the right side, colon tumors sometimes grow large before causing discomfort because the contents of the ascending colon are fluid and can pass through a constricted area. If discomfort is caused by a tumor on the right side, it is usually dull and vague. A tumor on the left side, where fecal matter is more solid, is likely to cause intermittent gas pains, cramps, or obstruction.

Because of the importance of early diagnosis and treatment, any symptom that lasts for 2 weeks or more should be reported to a physician. The warning signs of colorectal cancer can also be signs of other ailments, and only a physician can determine what is causing the problem.

Diagnosis

If colon or rectal cancer is suspected, the patient undergoes a series of tests to diagnose the condition. The doctor takes the patient's medical history and performs a general physical examination, which includes a rectal exam. Certain laboratory tests also may be performed, including a fecal occult blood test and exfoliative cytology (microscopic examination of stool samples to look for cancer cells). An important step in diagnosis is direct visual inspection by sigmoidoscopy or colonoscopy and/or x-ray examination of the large bowel.

Sigmoidoscopy is described on page 180. Fiberoptic colonoscopy is carried out with a lighted tube (colonoscope) that bends around the curves of the colon; in most patients, the physician can see the entire length of the large bowel—from the anus to the cecum. The sigmoidoscope and the colonoscope can be used to collect small samples of tissue (biopsy) for microscopic examination by a pathologist. These instruments also have a wire loop that makes it possible to grasp polyps and remove them.

X-rays of the lower gastrointestinal tract are called a "lower GI series," or barium enema. For this test, an enema fills the bowel with barium, a chalky substance that appears white on x-ray film. The barium coats the inside of the large intestine, and x-rays reveal abnormal growths, as well as constricted or displaced areas. Air may be pumped into the colon during the test to expand the bowel and make small tumors easier to see. This technique is called an air-contrast or double-contrast barium enema.

Another diagnostic test is the measurement of blood levels of a protein known as carcinoembryonic antigen (CEA). This substance is present in the human embryo but is normally found only in minute amounts in healthy adults. Many patients with colorectal cancer have increased blood levels of CEA, but measuring CEA is not a conclusive test for colorectal cancer because CEA values are not elevated in all persons with the disease. Moreover, the level of this antigen can be abnormally high in the blood of individuals who do *not* have cancer, including smokers and persons with noncancerous growths or inflammation of the gastrointestinal tract. The CEA assay can, however, signal the need for further diagnostic tests. (See the discussion of CEA under Followup.)

Staging

Once cancer has been diagnosed, other tests help determine the extent of the disease (staging), so that appropriate treatment can be planned. These staging procedures may include further blood tests, including tests to measure liver function; x-rays of the chest and, in some cases, the kidneys; and computed tomographic (CT) scans of the abdomen. (The CT scan gives a three-dimensional x-ray image of the area examined.)

Several staging systems have been used for colorectal cancer. The Dukes system, developed over 40 years ago and later modified, is widely used by both clinicians and researchers. It divides colorectal cancers into several stages.

- Stage A refers to carcinoma *in situ,* a small cancer in the mucosa that has not spread; the cancer cells have not reached the submucosa, where lymph and blood vessels are located;

- Stage B1 tumors extend through the submucosa into the muscularis externa;

- Stage B2 describes tumors that penetrate through the bowel wall;

- Stage C means that regional lymph nodes are involved; and

- Stage D indicates that the disease has spread to other organs.

Recently, the American Joint Committee on Cancer developed a staging system that takes into account some major factors that influence prognosis. The proposed system is based on coded descriptions of *t*umor size (T), lymph *n*ode involvement (N), and degree of *m*etastasis (M). In the TNM system, the extent of the tumor is designated TX (if it cannot be assessed), T*is* (car-

cinoma *in situ*), or T with a number from 0 to 5 to describe the extent of the tumor's growth through the layers of bowel wall or into nearby tissue. The site and degree of spread to lymph nodes are indicated by NX or N with a number from 0 to 3. Finally, M with X, 0, or 1 indicates whether the cancer has spread to distant parts of the body.

Using TNM designations, physicians divide colorectal cancers into five stages. The following is a simplified description of these stages:

Stage 0: Means carcinoma *in situ;* the cancer does not extend beyond the smooth muscle (muscularis mucosa) that separates the mucosa from the submucosa (T*is*, N0, M0);

Stage I: Refers to cancer confined to the mucosa, submucosa, or muscularis externa; the cancer does not extend through the bowel wall (T1 or T2, N0, M0);

Stage II: Describes cancer that penetrates all layers of the bowel wall, with or without invasion of adjacent tissues (T3, N0, M0);

Stage III: Means that the cancer involves regional lymph nodes, or it extends into nearby tissues or organs without spread to lymph nodes (any T, N1-N3, M0; or T4, N0, M0); and

Stage IV: Cancer has spread to distant sites, usually the liver or lungs (any T, any N, M1).

Treatment

Combining all races, both sexes, and all stages of disease, the 5-year relative survival rate (a measure that takes normal life expectancy into account) for patients diagnosed between 1979 and 1984 is 54 percent for colon cancer and 50 percent for rectal cancer. These figures compare with 50 percent and 48 percent respectively for patients diagnosed from 1974 to 1976. Until recently, improvements in survival statistics appeared to be related primarily to refinements in surgical techniques and supportive care, including better preoperative preparation, antibiotics, anesthesia, and blood banking. Patients in the 1980s are also benefiting from the results of clinical trials, which have led to important improvements in other methods of treating colorectal cancer. (Information about clinical trials is found on page 190.

Many factors affect the outlook of an individual colorectal cancer patient, including the location of the primary tumor, the stage of the cancer, certain features of the cancer cells, and the person's age and general health. Patients have the best chance of survival if the disease is found and treated at an early stage, as it is in more than 40 percent of all cases. Included below are separate discussions of the treatment of colon and rectal cancers.

Colon Cancer Treatment

Surgery is the primary treatment for most colon cancers and leads to cure in about half of all cases. Often *in situ* cancers (stage 0) are removable through the colonoscope. Standard primary treatment for colon cancer at stages I, II, and III is abdominal surgery (bowel resection). The type of operation depends mainly on the location and size of the tumor. Usually, the surgeon removes the tumor and some normal bowel tissue on each side of the tumor. This operation is called a partial colectomy, or hemicolectomy. In some colon cancer patients, the whole colon must be removed in an operation called complete or total colectomy. In both types of surgery, the abdominal lymph nodes that drain the area also are removed because the lymph system is a major route of spread.

Most often, the surgeon can immediately reconnect the healthy segments of the bowel, and the patient experiences little or no change in bowel function. If infection, obstruction, or other problems make immediate reconnection (anastomosis) impossible, the surgeon may perform a colostomy, creating an opening called a stoma in the abdominal wall for the elimination of waste. The colostomy is usually temporary to allow time for healing. In a small number of cases, anastomosis cannot be performed, and the stoma is permanent.

For some patients with stage IV colon cancer, surgery may be recommended to bypass the tumor or to remove all or part of it. In such cases, the goal of surgery may be palliative (to relieve symptoms), rather than curative. In certain patients, surgery to remove secondary tumors in the liver significantly improves the prognosis.

Radiation therapy in the treatment of colon cancer is still under investigation. In some cases, preoperative radiotherapy to shrink the tumor may improve the results of surgery or even make it possible to remove an otherwise inoperable tumor. Radiation therapy also can arrest the growth of cancer cells that remain in the area after the tumor is removed and, thus, reduce the risk of recurrence in some patients.

In addition, radiotherapy may have value for patients with inoperable or metastatic tumors. Although it is seldom curative under these circumstances, radiation can sometimes offer significant relief from symptoms, such as pain and bleeding.

Further study is needed to clarify the value of radiotherapy in specific groups of patients. Research is in progress to define the role of preoperative, postoperative, and a combination of pre- and postoperative ("sandwich technique") radiation treatment. Researchers are conducting clinical trials to compare the effectiveness of surgery alone vs. surgery preceded by low-dose irradiation for patients with stage I cancer at specific sites in the colon. Other studies are comparing the effectiveness—as well as the side effects and the complications—of sandwich vs. postoperative radiotherapy in patients with more advanced disease (stages II and III).

Chemotherapy has been used for some time to treat patients with colon cancer. Of the many drugs that have been tried, the most active and most commonly used is 5-fluorouracil (5-FU).

About half of all colon cancers are diagnosed and treated after the tumor has penetrated the bowel wall but apparently has not spread to other organs of the body. In a significant number of these patients, the disease reappears later on, even though the initial surgery seemed to be curative. To improve the outlook for this group of patients, researchers have been looking at the effectiveness of using chemotherapy to kill undetectable cancer cells that remain in the body after surgery. Recently, this approach—called adjuvant chemotherapy—has improved both disease-free survival time and overall survival time, especially for stage II and certain stage III patients. Researchers will need to work with large numbers of patients in carefully designed clinical trials to test the merits of various adjuvant drug combinations and also to identify subgroups of patients for whom this approach will be most

beneficial. These very important studies offer patients treatment under the care of doctors expert in the evaluation of new types of therapy.

About 20 percent of patients with metastatic colon cancer respond to intravenous or oral 5-FU. Recent studies suggest that combinations of 5-FU and other anticancer agents may be more active against colon cancer than 5-FU alone. Patients with advanced disease may experience partial remission or relief of symptoms, but in most cases the improvement lasts only a few months. At present, scientists are working to develop and evaluate new anticancer agents, treatment schedules, dosages, and drug combinations, as well as innovative methods of drug administration. One treatment method under study uses a thin tube called a catheter to infuse anticancer drugs—usually 5-FU or a related compound called FUDR (floxuridine)—directly into the liver to treat metastatic tumors. Researchers hope this method will improve the effectiveness of chemotherapy by exposing the liver to a high concentration of the drug without increasing the amount that circulates throughout the body. In some studies using this technique, preliminary results have been encouraging, but so far, direct infusion has not proven superior to systemic chemotherapy. In addition to the studies of this mode of treatment for metastatic disease, clinical trials are being carried out to see whether adjuvant infusion chemotherapy can prevent liver metastasis in patients at high risk of recurrence.

Immunotherapy (sometimes called biotherapy) is another important area of research. Scientists have identified a number of natural and synthetic substances called biological response modifiers (BRMs), which may boost, direct, or restore the body's normal defenses (immune response). Clinical trials are exploring the potential of various BRMs, both alone and in combination with chemotherapy, for colon cancer.

Researchers are looking at the role that BRMs may have in the adjuvant treatment of colon cancer. Preliminary results have encouraged them to persist in their search for ways to use the immune system to delay or prevent recurrence after surgery. Researchers are using a BRM called interleukin-2 (IL-2) to stimulate the growth of lymphocytes (white blood cells produced by the immune system) in the body and in blood that has been removed from the body.

The patient is treated with the stimulated cells—called lymphokine-activated killer (LAK) cells—and additional doses of IL-2. The IL-2 and LAK cells may be injected into the bloodstream, or they may be infused directly into the lower abdomen (peritoneum) if the disease is confined to that area.

Other BRMs under investigation as adjuvant treatment include several types of interferon and an immune system stimulator called levamisole. Researchers are also working with monoclonal antibodies (substances that can locate and bind to tumor cells in the body). To eliminate tumors, these antibodies can be used alone, or they can be linked to various cell-killing substances. Thus, monoclonal antibodies can be used to deliver drugs, toxins, or radioactive material directly to the cancer cells.

Rectal Cancer Treatment

Surgery is the primary treatment for most rectal cancers. The type of operation depends largely on the size and site of the tumor. Whenever possible, doctors attempt to preserve the anal sphincter muscle; only about 15 percent of rectal cancer patients require a permanent ostomy.

In situ rectal cancer (stage 0) is nearly always curable with conservative surgery. The surgeon removes only the tumor itself or a wedge that encompasses the tumor and some surrounding tissue. Similar treatment also may be feasible in some stage I patients. Another technique under study for early stage rectal cancers is electrocoagulation, which uses a high-frequency electric current to destroy the tumor.

Surgery and anastomosis (reattachment of healthy sections of the large bowel) is possible for most patients with stage I, II, and III rectal cancers if the tumor is located in the upper third of the rectum. When the tumor is low in the rectum, however, the anal sphincter usually cannot be saved. The surgeon removes the tumor, the rectum, and the sigmoid colon, closing the anus and connecting the remaining section of the bowel to a stoma in the abdominal wall. For patients with tumors arising in the middle third of the rectum, the type of operation depends on the size and position of the tumor, the sex of the patient, and other factors.

Radiation therapy may be used instead of surgery to treat some rectal cancer patients. In a procedure called endocavitary irradiation, an x-ray tube is fitted into a special proctoscope, allowing the physician to see inside the rectum and aim the rays directly at the tumor. Radiation therapists with the necessary special equipment and experience may use endocavitary irradiation to cure early (stage I) rectal cancer or to control pain and bleeding in patients with inoperable tumors.

More often, radiotherapy is used in addition to surgery, not as an alternative to it. Because rectal cancers tend to recur at their original site, many doctors now recommend radiation as a precaution. Recent research indicates that irradiation given before and/or after surgery reduces the risk of local recurrence, but patients in most studies have not been followed long enough to show whether irradiation also improves survival. Still, reduction of painful local recurrence is itself an important benefit for rectal cancer patients.

Intraoperative radiation therapy for rectal cancer is a new technique currently being evaluated in clinical trials. The radiation is given at the time of surgery, when the tumor is exposed and the surrounding normal tissues can be shielded.

Chemotherapy for metastatic (stage IV) rectal cancer does not improve survival time, but may offer some patients temporary relief of symptoms. However, the results of recent clinical trials indicate that patients with stage II and stage III rectal cancer do benefit from adjuvant chemotherapy (given after surgery to reduce the chance of recurrence). In these trials, researchers have observed fewer local recurrences and better overall survival in patients treated with a combination of radiotherapy and chemotherapy compared with those treated with surgery alone.

Immunotherapy, whether for early stage or advanced disease, is considered investigational at this time. The studies for colon cancer, described on page 187, generally include rectal cancer patients as well.

Followup

Colorectal cancer can recur at or near the site of the original tumor, and it can spread to organs in other parts of the body. Also, patients treated for large bowel cancer have a 2 to 10 percent chance of developing a *new* cancer in the colon or rectum, one that is not a recurrence of the original tumor. It is important for patients to be followed carefully, so that if these problems occur, they can be found and treated as early as possible.

Followup studies may include periodic physical examination, fecal occult blood testing, sigmoidoscopy and/or colonoscopy, double-contrast barium enema, blood tests, x-rays, and scans. The CEA assay (described on page 14) is commonly used with other tests to follow colorectal cancer patients. Often the CEA level in a patient's blood is high before surgery and returns to normal within several weeks after the tumor has been removed. If the amount of CEA rises again, it may be an indication that the cancer has recurred—sometimes before there are any other signs. However, the CEA assay is not always reliable, and the CEA level sometimes remains normal even when the cancer has recurred or may go up for other reasons.

Another tumor marker under study for colorectal cancer is known as carbohydrate antigen 19-9 (CA 19-9). Although this substance is not a dependable signal of recurrence when used alone, CA 19-9 may be helpful when used along with the CEA assay and other tests.

Clinical Trials and PDQ

To improve the outcome of treatment for patients with cancers of the colon and rectum, the NCI supports clinical studies at many hospitals throughout the United States. Patients who take part in this research make an important contribution to medical science and may have the first chance to benefit from improved treatment methods. Physicians are encouraged to inform their patients about the option of participating in such trials. To help patients and doctors learn about current trials, the NCI has developed PDQ (Physician Data Query), a computerized database to give doctors quick and easy access to:

- descriptions of current clinical trials that are accepting patients, including information about the objectives of the study, medical eligibility requirements, details of the treatment program, and the names and addresses of physicians and facilities conducting the study;

- the latest treatment information for most types of cancer; and

- names of physicians and organizations involved in cancer care.

To access PDQ, doctors may use an office computer with a telephone hookup and a PDQ access code or the services of a medical library with online searching capability. Most Cancer Information Service offices (1-800-4-CANCER) provide physicians with free PDQ searches and can explain how to obtain regular access to the database. Patients may ask their doctor to use PDQ or may call 1-800-4-CANCER to request a search themselves. Information specialists at this toll-free number use a variety of sources, including PDQ, to answer questions about cancer prevention, diagnosis, treatment, and research.

Selected References

The materials marked with an * are distributed free of charge by the NCI. The other items can be found in medical libraries, many college and university libraries, and some public libraries.

Bates, S.E. and Longo, D.L. "Use of Serum Tumor Markers in Cancer Diagnosis and Management," *Seminars in Oncology,* Vol. 14(2), June 1987, pp. 85-88.

Calabresi, P. et al., eds. *Medical Oncology: Basic Principles and Clinical Management of Cancer.* New York: Macmillan Publishing Co., 1985.

*"Cancer Prevention Research: Chemoprevention and Diet." Prepared by the Office of Cancer Communications, National Cancer Institute. February 1987.

Cancer Rates and Risks. Prepared by the Office of Cancer Communications, National Cancer Institute. NIH Publication No. 85-691.

Chemotherapy and You: A Guide to Self-Help During Treatment. Prepared by the Office of Cancer Communications, National Cancer Institute. NIH Publication No. 86-1136.

Daly, J.M. and Kemeny, N. "Therapy of Colorectal Hepatic Metastases." In *Important Advances in Oncology, 1986* (DeVita, V.T., et al., eds.). Philadelphia: J.B. Lippincott Co., 1986.

DeVita, V.T. et al., eds. *Cancer: Principles and Practice of Oncology.* 2nd ed. Philadelphia: J.B. Lippincott Co., 1985.

Diet, Nutrition and Cancer Prevention: The Good News. Prepared by the Office of Cancer Communications, National Cancer Institute. NIH Publication No. 87-2878.

Fenoglio-Preisler, C.M. and Hutter, R.V.P. "Colorectal Polyps: Pathologic Diagnosis and Clinical Significance," *Ca-A Cancer Journal for Clinicians,* Vol. 35(6), November/December 1985, pp. 322-344.

Greenwald, P., Lanza, E., and Eddy, G. "Dietary Fiber in the Reduction of Colon Cancer Risk," *Journal of the American Dietetic Association,* Vol. 87(9), September 1986, pp. 1178-1188.

Greenwald, P. and Lanza, E. "Role of Dietary Fiber in the Prevention of Cancer." In *Important Advances in Oncology, 1986* (DeVita, V.T. et al., eds.). Philadelphia: J.B. Lippincott Co., 1986.

Haskell, C.M., ed. *Cancer Treatment.* 2nd ed. Philadelphia: W.B. Saunders Co., 1985.

Holland, J. and Frei, E., III, eds. *Cancer Medicine.* 2nd ed. Philadelphia: Lea and Febiger, 1982.

Radiation Therapy and You: A Guide to Self-Help During Treatment. Prepared by the Office of Cancer Communications, National Cancer Institute, NIH Publication No. 86-2227.

Simon, J.B. "Occult Blood Screening for Colorectal Carcinoma: A Critical Review," *Gastroenterology,* Vol. 88(3), March 1985, pp. 820-837.

✴ *The mentioned text is reprinted within this book. See CONTENTS for location.*

Chapter 13

Hodgkin's Disease and the Non-Hodgkin's Lymphomas

Introduction

This Report: *Hodgkin's Disease and the Non-Hodgkin's Lymphomas* describes current research on the causes, incidence, symptoms, diagnosis, and treatment of Hodgkin's disease and the non-Hodgkin's lymphomas. The information presented here came from medical textbooks, recent articles in the scientific literature, discussions with National Cancer Institute (NCI) scientists and other researchers, and various scientific meetings.

The Immune System

Lymphomas are cancers of the immune system, the complex network of specialized organs and cells that defends the body against infection. The organs of the immune system are often referred to as "lymphatic" organs because they are concerned with the growth, development, and deployment of lymphocytes, the white blood cells that are the key operatives of the immune system. Lymphatic organs include the bone marrow, thymus, spleen, and lymph nodes, as well as the tonsils, appendix, and clumps of lymphatic tissue in the small intestine known as Peyer's patches. Some nonlymphatic organs, like the skin, liver, and lungs, also contain circulating lymphocytes and play a major role in immunity.

Blood cell growth begins with the formation of immature stem cells in the bone marrow, the spongy interior of the long bones. Some of these young cells mature in the thymus, a multi-lobed organ that lies behind the breastbone. There they multiply and mature into cells capable of mounting an immune response. Stem cells that develop in the thymus are called "T-cells." Other lymphocytes, which appear to mature either in the bone marrow itself or in lymphatic organs other than the thymus, are called "B-cells." Most lymphomas arise from B-cells.

B-cells secrete substances called antibodies. A given antibody exactly matches a specific invading antigen, or foreign substance, much like a key matches a lock. When an antibody interlocks with its matching antigen, it can inactivate the antigen. The body is capable of making antibody to about a million antigens.

T-cells do not secrete antibodies, but their help is essential for antibody production. Some

T-cells become "helper" cells that turn on B-cells or other T-cells, while others become "suppressor" cells that turn these cells off. T-cells also secrete a variety of potent chemicals that can call into play many other cells and substances. Both B-cells and T-cells can be divided into a number of subsets, all with different functions. Besides the lymphocytes, other white blood cells, like macrophages and monocytes, also contribute to the immune response.

Much like the blood circulatory system, lymphatic vessels carry lymph, a fluid containing white blood cells, to all parts of the body. Situated along the vessels are bean-shaped glands, called lymph nodes, that trap and help destroy foreign particles and disease-causing agents. As the lymph passes through lymph nodes, foreign substances are filtered out and more lymphocytes are picked up.

During their travels, circulating lymphocytes may spend several hours in the spleen, an organ located near the stomach. The spleen is the only organ capable of mounting an immune response to blood-borne antigens. It is also involved with the final destruction of aging blood cells and various stages in the production of lymphocytes.

Types of Lymphoma

In all forms of lymphoma, the cells in the lymph tissue begin growing abnormally and, if left untreated, spread to other organs. There are a number of different forms of lymphoma, whose symptoms, rate and pattern of spread, as well as treatment vary, depending on the type. For this reason, the disease should be diagnosed by a pathologist who is experienced in recognizing the cellular features of these cancers.

Hodgkin's disease, the most common lymphoma, has special characteristics that distinguish it from the others. Often it is identified by the presence of a unique cell, called the Reed-Sternberg cell, in lymphatic tissue that has been surgically removed for biopsy. Hodgkin's disease tends to follow a more predictable pattern of spread, and its spread is generally more limited than that of the non-Hodgkin's lymphomas. By contrast, the non-Hodgkin's lymphomas are more likely to begin in extra-nodal sites (organs other than the lymph nodes, like the liver and bones).

Pathologists around the world use six different systems to classify the non-Hodgkin's lymphomas. Some of the systems place major emphasis on structure of the cell that becomes cancerous; others on the arrangement of the cells when examined under the microscope. In 1981 meetings sponsored by the National Cancer Institute, an international panel of expert pathologists developed a new classification system for the non-Hodgkin's lymphomas, called the International Working Formulation, to help standardize terms and apply new knowledge gained from the science of immunology. In the Working Formulation, lymphomas are classified as low grade, intermediate grade, or high grade depending on the type of cell found in the cancer and the arrangement of the cells.

Although many doctors have begun using the Working Formulation, the most commonly used classification is still the Rappaport system. In this system, a non-Hodgkin's lymphoma is described as either nodular or diffuse, based on the growth pattern of the cancer cells as seen through the microscope. The disease is further classified by cell type as lymphocytic—if the cancer cells are small and resemble lymphocytes; histiocytic—if the

cancer cells are large and resemble macrophages or histiocytes; or mixed—if the cells have both features. Pathologists using the Rappaport system also describe lymphoma cells as either poorly differentiated or well differentiated. The term differentiated is used to describe the microscopic appearance of cells. Poorly differentiated cancer cells are irregular in structure and size and have poorly defined borders. Cancer cells that are more normal in their microscopic appearance are referred to as well differentiated.

The unique features of each lymphoma arise from the structure and growth pattern, or histology, of the cancer cells involved. Most nodular lymphomas are called "indolent" or "favorable histology" lymphomas because they spread slowly, often taking years to develop into aggressive disease. However, the "aggressive" or "unfavorable" histologies, which include most of the diffuse types, tend to progress quickly. Without treatment, these rapidly growing lymphomas are quickly fatal.

Aggressive and indolent lymphomas occur at about the same rate in the population. In the

Rappaport classification, the most common subtypes are nodular poorly differentiated lymphocytic lymphoma and diffuse histiocytic lymphoma. Most non-Hodgkin's lymphomas appear to develop from B-cells.

Certain kinds of non-Hodgkin's lymphomas have unique cellular and clinical features that distinguish them from other non-Hodgkin's lymphomas. Among these are mycosis fungoides (a T-cell lymphoma first appearing in the skin), Burkitt's lymphoma (a childhood B-cell lymphoma generally found in tropical Africa), and lymphoblastic lymphoma (a childhood lymphoma most often of T-cell origin).

Causes and Prevention

About 37,000 new cases of lymphoma—or 12 new cases per every 100,000 people—are diagnosed yearly in the United States. Hodgkin's disease is the most common, accounting for nearly one-fourth of all lymphomas. Unlike most cancers, Hodgkin's disease is often found in relatively young people, with peak incidence between the ages of 15 and 34. Lymphoblastic and Burkitt's lymphomas are also more common in young people, but the other lymphomas occur in all age groups.

The causes of lymphomas are not fully understood. Research has shown an increase in the rate of certain of these cancers among survivors of the atomic bomb in Hiroshima. It is also known that persons with damaged immune systems, caused either by immune disorders or immunosuppressive drugs, are more susceptible to this group of diseases. Kidney transplant patients, whose immune systems are suppressed with medications, develop non-Hodgkin's lymphomas 40 to 100 times more often than the general population. The short latent period—onset is often within one year of the organ transplant—and the fact that transplant patients are more prone to infection with certain viruses linked with cancer suggest that viral infection may play a role in non-Hodgkin's lymphoma, perhaps in combination with other factors.

Viruses

Scientists think that, in some cases, a viral infection may be one step in a complex series of events leading to the development of a lymphoma. However, researchers have not been able to identify any virus as a cause of the more common lymphomas, including Hodgkin's disease. Only two rare types of lymphoma have been clearly linked with a viral infection: adult T-cell leukemia-lymphoma (ATLL), a cancer of mature T-cells that is rare in the United States, and African Burkitt's lymphoma, a childhood lymphoma that is common in tropical regions of Africa. Burkitt's lymphoma that occurs in the United States does not appear to be associated with a virus.

The virus associated with adult T-cell leukemia-lymphoma is called "HTLV-1." It was isolated and described by NCI researcher Dr. Robert Gallo and his co-workers in 1978. Studies are under way to determine the worldwide incidence of ATLL and exposure to the HTLV-1 virus, which is thought to be most common in Caribbean countries, parts of South America, and in southern Japan, where in some areas over 50 percent of adult lymphomas are related to HTLV-1. Scientists believe the virus is transmitted primarily through sexual contact or exposure to contaminated blood and that ATLL is not contagious like influenza or other common viral diseases.

ATLL is unlike the more common, well-known types of lymphoma and leukemia. In patients with ATLL, the disease tends to progress rapidly, often with enlarged liver, spleen, and lymph nodes. High levels of calcium are found in the blood and skin eruptions may also occur. In some ways ATLL resembles other rare T-cell cancers that begin in the skin, such as mycosis fungoides and Sezary syndrome, but the unique features of adult T-cell leukemia-lymphoma lead scientists to believe that it is distinct from other T-cell cancers.

Burkitt's lymphoma has been associated with a common, herpes-like virus known as Epstein-Barr virus (EBV). EBV is known to cause infectious mononucleosis, an illness of young people that produces fever and swelling of the lymph glands. By adulthood, most people have been exposed to and have developed antibodies to EBV. Scientists think that EBV plays a role in the development of Burkitt's lymphoma in African children, although other genetic and environmental factors, such as malaria infection, may also contribute to the onset of this cancer. The association between EBV and Hodgkin's disease is less certain. According to several studies, people who have had infectious mononucleosis run a higher, but still very small, risk of developing Hodgkin's disease.

Various studies have found a higher rate of Hodgkin's disease among the brothers and sisters of Hodgkin's patients and among people in certain occupations, such as woodworkers and chemists. According to this research, young Hodgkin's patients are more likely to come from small, high-income families, and have well-educated parents. Studies on the incidence of Hodgkin's disease have found little evidence of "clustering"— unusually high concentrations of cases in one area at the same time.

Herbicides

In occupational studies, workers exposed to the herbicides phenoxyacetic acid or chlorophenol have a higher than expected incidence of lymphoma. A recent study by the National Cancer Institute and the University of Kansas found that Kansas farmers who used herbicides had a higher risk for non-Hodgkin's lymphoma than nonfarmers.

The above-normal rates were associated with the use of phenoxy herbicides, especially 2,4-D. These herbicides are commonly used on pastureland and in growing wheat, corn, sorghum, and rice.

Detection and Diagnosis

Symptoms

The symptoms of lymphatic cancer vary from person to person and may easily be confused with noncancerous conditions. In most cases, the first sign of lymphoma is a painless swelling in the neck, armpit, or groin caused by enlarged lymph glands. In non-Hodgkin's lymphoma, the swelling may arise in the abdomen. Some lymphoma patients complain of persistent or recurrent fever, night sweats, fatigue, and weight loss. Sometimes, itching of the skin (pruritus) marks the early stages of Hodgkin's disease and other lymphomas.

Although all of these symptoms can be present in other illnesses, they may suggest lymphoma, particularly when lymph node swelling lasts more than 6 weeks and does not respond to antibiotics. Still, the only sure way to determine whether lymphoma is present is by examination of lymph tissue surgically removed by biopsy.

Staging

Once a diagnosis of lymphoma has been confirmed by a pathologist, other clinical and laboratory tests are used to determine how far the cancer cells have spread. This step, known as staging, helps the physician select the best treatment for each patient.

Staging usually includes laboratory blood tests, chest x-rays, a needle biopsy of the bone marrow, and lymphangiograms (x-ray studies of the lymph system after injection of a dye). Computerized tomography (CT) scans, ultrasound tests, liver biopsy, and abdominal exploratory surgery with spleen removal may also be necessary for some patients.

Hodgkin's disease begins in a lymph node, often in the neck, and spreads through the lymphatic system to nearby nodes. In advanced Hodgkin's disease, the lungs, spleen, liver, and bone marrow may also be affected. However, by the time non-Hodgkin's lymphoma is diagnosed, cancer cells often have already spread throughout the body, involving abdominal lymph nodes, liver, bone marrow, and the gastrointestinal tract.

Stage I   Disease is limited to one lymph node area or a single extranodal organ

Stage II   Disease has spread to more than one node area or is present in one extranodal organ and adjacent groups of lymph nodes on the same side of the diaphragm

Stage III   Disease has spread to nodes above and below the diaphragm with or without spread to the spleen or extranodal organs

Stage IV   Disease has spread to extranodal sites such as liver, bone marrow, and lungs

An additional subclassification system is used in staging to indicate further extent of the disease:

A   No systemic (generalized) symptoms

B   Systemic symptoms, such as fever, night sweats, or weight loss greater than 10 percent of body weight

E   Extension into adjacent organs

Treatment

Hodgkin's Disease

Before 1970, few patients with advanced Hodgkin's disease recovered from their illness. Most died within 2 years. This grim prognosis has given way to a far brighter outlook, thanks to major strides in drug treatment as well as improved staging techniques. Now, more than half of all patients with advanced Hodgkin's disease are disease-free after followup of more than 10 years. For early stage Hodgkin's patients, the cure rate has risen to nearly 90 percent in some treatment centers, due mainly to advances in radiotherapy.

The usual treatment for most patients with early stage Hodgkin's disease is high-energy radiation of the lymph nodes. Research has shown that radiation therapy to large areas at high doses (3,500 to 4,500 rads) is more effective in preventing relapse than radiation of the diseased nodes alone.

Modern radiotherapy equipment, like the linear accelerator, can sharply focus high-intensity radiation to the targeted area. Doctors use treatment planning devices to tailor the radiation exactly to the patient's body along with special shields that protect normal tissue.

Combination chemotherapy also is effective in the treatment of early stage Hodgkin's disease. In addition, chemotherapy is the treatment of choice for advanced (stages III and IV) Hodgkin's disease and for patients who have relapsed after radiotherapy. Drugs and radiation are sometimes given together, mainly in treating patients with tumors in the chest or abdomen.

The first effective chemotherapy regimen for advanced Hodgkin's disease, known as the MOPP program, was developed by researchers at the National Cancer Institute and is considered one standard therapy. MOPP consists of four anticancer drugs in combination: mechlorethamine (nitrogen mustard), vincristine (Oncovin), procarbazine, and prednisone. Since the development of MOPP, other combinations have proven to be equally effective and are now also considered standard options when chemotherapy is indicated.

One such drug combination, ABVD (doxorubicin, bleomycin, vinblastine, and DTIC), has shown strong anticancer activity in NCI-supported studies of Hodgkin's disease at the National Cancer Institute in Milan, Italy. An advantage of the ABVD regimen is that it does not appear to produce infertility as frequently as MOPP. One study found that by giving MOPP and ABVD in alternating cycles, fewer patients relapsed.

In spite of their effectiveness, some cancer treatments are suspected to be cancer-causing themselves. For example, several studies have shown an association between certain therapies and the development of leukemia many years later. The risk of leukemia, estimated at around 5 percent at 10 years by most studies, seems highest in patients aged 40 years and older who have been treated with both intensive radiotherapy and intensive chemotherapy. Recent NCI research indicates that the risk of leukemia seems to decline after 10 years.

Scientists are continuing their search for safer and more effective drugs to combat Hodgkin's disease. In addition to new drugs that may play an important role in the treatment of this cancer, studies are under way using biological response modifiers, such as interleukin-2/LAK and monoclonal antibodies. Biological response modifiers are substances that boost, direct, or restore many of the normal defenses of the body. Carefully controlled studies comparing established treatments with new and promising approaches using drugs, immunotherapy (sometimes called biological therapy), and radiation are yielding steady progress in the treatment of Hodgkin's

disease and other forms of lymphatic cancer. Information about these studies may be obtained from NCI's computer database, PDQ (Physician Data Query), which is described in more detail at the end of this text.

Aggressive Non-Hodgkin's Lymphomas

Several forms of non-Hodgkin's lymphoma are aggressive cancers that, if left untreated, spread rapidly and become fatal. Approximately half of all patients with non-Hodgkin's lymphoma have these aggressive types. In the Rappaport system, they include:

- Nodular histiocytic lymphoma

- Diffuse histiocytic lymphoma

- Diffuse mixed lymphocytic histiocytic lymphoma

- Diffuse undifferentiated lymphoma

- Diffuse lymphoblastic lymphoma.

Intensive combination chemotherapy is the mainstay of treatment for patients with these lymphomas, since most already have systemic or advanced disease at the time of diagnosis. Sometimes localized radiotherapy is also used.

Researchers have made immense strides in treating aggressive lymphomas with anticancer drugs. One of the first therapies to produce long-term, disease-free survival was C-MOPP, a combination of cyclophosphamide (Cytoxan), vincristine, procarbazine, and prednisone. Although C-MOPP is still used to treat these lymphomas, investigators from NCI and other cancer centers have almost doubled the survival rate of this early drug program by developing regimens with cure rates of 60 to 70 percent, according to more recent clinical trials. Based on the results of these studies, some of the combinations now considered most effective are:

- ProMACE-MOPP (cyclophosphamide, doxorubicin, etoposide, prednisone, and high-dose methotrexate with leucovorin rescue in alternating cycles with mechlorethamine, vincristine, procarbazine, and prednisone);

- ProMACE-CytaBOM (cyclophosphamide, doxorubicin, etoposide, prednisone, cytarabine, bleomycin, vincristine, methotrexate, and cotrimoxazole antibiotic prophylaxis);

- M-BACOD (high-dose methotrexate, bleomycin, doxorubicin, cyclophosphamide, vincristine, and dexamethasone);

- MACOP-B (methotrexate with leucovorin rescue, doxorubicin, cyclophosphamide, vincristine, prednisone, bleomycin, and cotrimoxazole antibiotic prophylaxis);

- COP-BLAM (cyclophosphamide, vincristine, prednisone, bleomycin, doxorubicin, and procarbazine).

Patients with bone marrow involvement run a high risk of relapse in the brain. To prevent this, some specialists advise using radiation to the brain or anticancer drugs injected into the cerebrospinal fluid (intrathecal chemotherapy).

Aggressive lymphomas are the most common forms of lymphoma in children. The most promising results for treating advanced disease are coming from intensive combination chemotherapy. Intrathecal chemotherapy with or without cranial radiotherapy is usually added to prevent a relapse of lymphoma in the brain.

Before 1960, lymphoblastic lymphoma, which usually arises in the chest, was an invariably fatal cancer of adolescents. Now, combination chemotherapy for young patients with advanced disease is yielding 45 to 65 percent long-term survival in various studies.

Most patients with aggressive lymphomas who achieve complete remission can look forward to long-term, disease-free survival. Scientists have observed that most patients with these lymphomas who survive the first 2 years without a relapse (instead of the usual 5-year standard) are permanently cured.

One promising area of research is bone marrow transplantation (BMT)—an experimental and highly technical procedure that has been used successfully in some types of leukemia. Researchers from various cancer centers are reporting encouraging results using bone marrow transplantation in patients with different types of B-cell non-Hodgkin's lymphoma that had become resistant to drug therapy. However, some scientists think that BMT may work best in patients whose disease has not become resistant to drug therapy, for example, those in first remission.

To prepare a patient for a bone marrow transplant, specialists administer intensive chemotherapy, whole body irradiation, or the two in combination in an effort to destroy all cancer cells in the body. The dosages must be so high that the healthy marrow is also destroyed, leaving the patient wholly dependent on supportive care for defense against infection and hemorrhage. In allogeneic bone marrow transplantation, a small amount of the marrow from a matched donor is then infused into the patient's bloodstream. The donated cells travel from the blood to the bones and in time grow into functioning marrow.

Autologous ("self") bone marrow transplantation is an experimental approach that may play a role in the future treatment of lymphoma because it sidesteps the need for a matched donor and the problem of graft-versus-host disease, a potentially fatal reaction in which the donated marrow rejects the tissue of the patient. In autologous transplantation, some of the patient's own marrow is removed during remission, frozen, and reinfused later when the disease becomes resistant to established therapies. Investigators are now focusing on ways to remove any cancer cells from the withdrawn marrow with monoclonal antibodies and chemotherapeutic agents and to improve therapy immediately before transplantation in order to reduce the chances of recurrence. The major clinical use of bone marrow transplantation at this time is in patients with aggressive forms of lymphoma who have relapsed from complete remission.

Indolent Non-Hodgkin's Lymphomas

Another group of non-Hodgkin's lymphomas, called the indolent lymphomas, are slow-growing cancers affecting mainly adults over age 40. Patients with nodular or diffuse poorly differentiated lymphocytic, nodular mixed, diffuse well differentiated lymphocytic lymphoma, or diffuse intermediate differentiated lymphocytic lymphoma usually have no symptoms other than painless enlargement of the lymph nodes in the neck, armpit, or groin. Although most patients with indolent lymphomas are found to have stage III or IV disease at diagnosis, those with early stage disease are often curable with radiation therapy. Several years after onset, the cancer can become aggressive, causing fever, night sweats, and weight loss. At this time, an indolent lymphoma may change to one of the aggressive forms.

There are two schools of thought regarding treatment of the indolent forms of lymphomas when detected in stages III and IV. One approach, based on a Stanford University study of 83 patients seen over a 15-year period, is to "watch and wait," deferring treatment for an indefinite time in patients who are relatively symptom-free. The patient is closely monitored and begins to receive treatment only if the disease shows symptoms of progression.

Another approach is to begin treatment at the time of diagnosis in an effort to achieve and maintain complete remission. The patient may be treated with chemotherapy, radiation, or the two therapies used together. In a review of low-grade lymphoma cases treated at the NCI from 1953 to 1975, researchers found that chemotherapy or chemotherapy plus radiation produced complete responses in approximately 75 percent of patients with stages III and IV disease. Treatment with total body irradiation yielded about the same results. Still, despite the initial success in achieving remission, most patients with indolent lymphoma eventually relapse. Long-term studies comparing various approaches are helping scientists identify the safest, most effective therapy for these diseases. Meanwhile, investigators are continuing their search for new ways to prevent recurrence and to bolster the body's natural defenses against cancer. One substance under active study is interferon, which has shown activity against the indolent lymphomas in early clinical trials.

Mycosis Fungoides

Mycosis fungoides is a T-cell

lymphoma of the skin that, scientists believe, is caused by the uncontrolled growth of helper T-cells, a class of white blood cells that regulates antibody production by B-cells. Its appearance is often preceded by a long history of skin disorders, such as chronic eczema and psoriasis. Even after a diagnosis of mycosis fungoides is confirmed, the cancer may progress very slowly.

Staging of disease, with special attention to lungs and liver for possible spread, is as important a step in treating mycosis fungoides as it is in other lymphomas. Topical approaches using nitrogen mustard (mechlorethamine) and electron beam radiation have been very successful in controlling mycosis fungoides limited to the skin. Electron beams, which have a limited range of penetration, can be used to irradiate the entire body surface without penetrating and damaging deeper tissues. This form of radiation therapy has few side effects and has achieved a 93 percent rate of complete remission in patients with limited disease. Many stay in remission for extended periods after one course of electron beam therapy.

PUVA therapy (8-methoxy-psoralen followed by long-wave ultraviolet exposure) often clears the skin of superficial growths but is less useful in eradicating deeper eruptions. When treat-ment is stopped, the cancerous growths reappear. However, investigators from Yale University recently reported encouraging results from a different application of 8-methoxypsoralen in patients with advanced cutaneous T-cell lymphoma. In this study, patients took the light-activated drug orally. Blood was removed from one arm, and the white cells, separated from the rest of the blood, were exposed to ultraviolet light, thus activating the drug and damaging the white blood cells. The patient's blood, along with the injured white cells, was then reinfused. The Yale researchers, who reported that 27 of 37 patients improved after this treatment, believe that the therapy somehow stimulates the immune system to suppress cancerous T-cells.

Researchers are also testing various other approaches for their possible role in treating mycosis fungoides. For patients with advanced disease, early study results suggest that systemic chemotherapy and high-energy x-rays may be beneficial. Preliminary research with interferon shows that it may also have therapeutic value for the treatment of this lymphoma. Studies are also under way exploring the benefits of 2'-deoxycoformycin (an antimetabolite that may target T-cells), retinoids, and combination chemotherapy.

Burkitt's Lymphoma

Burkitt's lymphoma, one of the fastest growing human cancers, can be cured with chemotherapy alone. Although rare in the United States, it is a common childhood cancer in tropical Africa. In African children, Burkitt's lymphoma most often originates in the jaw, ovaries, and kidneys. However, in Americans the lymph nodes of the neck and digestive system are the most common locations. Because it is such an aggressive cancer, Burkitt's lymphoma patients may need surgery to remove intestinal obstruction. Surgery also helps to reduce tumor size in some patients, either before or after chemotherapy begins. When surgery is not feasible, radiation has been used to reduce tumor bulk. High doses of drug combinations, such as COMP (cyclophosphamide, methotrexate, vincristine, and prednisone) have been found highly effective in treating Burkitt's lymphoma.

PDQ

The National Cancer Institute has developed PDQ (Physician Data Query), a computerized database designed to give doctors quick and easy access to:

• the latest treatment information for most types of cancer;

• descriptions of clinical trials that are open for patient entry; and

• names of organizations and physicians involved in cancer care.

To get access to PDQ, a doctor may use an office computer with a telephone hookup and a PDQ access code, or the services of a medical library with on-line searching capability. Most Cancer Information Service offices (1-800-4-CANCER) provide a physician with one free PDQ search, and can tell doctors how to get regular access to the database. Patients may ask their doctor to use PDQ or may call 1-800-4-CANCER themselves. Information specialists at this toll-free number use a variety of sources, including PDQ, to answer questions about cancer prevention, diagnosis, and treatment.

Additional Information

For additional information on this subject and for other NCI publications, write to the Office of Cancer Communications, National Cancer Institute, Bethesda, MD 20892, or call the Cancer Information Service toll-free at

1-800-4-CANCER

208

Selected References

Materials marked with an asterisk (*) are available from the National Cancer Institute (NCI). Other items can be found in medical libraries, many college and university libraries, and some public libraries.

Bonadonna, G. "Chemotherapy Strategies to Improve the Control of Hodgkin's Disease," The Richard and Hinda Rosenthal Foundation Award Lecture, *Cancer Research*, Vol. 42(11), Nov. 1982, pp. 4309-4319.

Cancer Rates and Risks. Prepared by the Office of Cancer Communications, National Cancer Institute. NIH Publication No. 85-691.

Chemotherapy and You: A Guide to Self-Help During Treatment. Prepared by the Office of Cancer Communications, National Cancer Institute. NIH Publication No. 86-1136.

DeVita, V.T., Jr., et al., eds. *Cancer: Principles and Practice of Oncology.* 2nd ed. Philadelphia: J.B. Lippincott Co., 1985.

DeVita, V.T., Jr., "Hematologic Malignancies: Non-Hodgkin's Lymphomas," *Hospital Practice*, Vol. 21(9), Sept. 15, 1986, pp. 103-118.

Edelson, R.E. et al. "Treatment of Cutaneous T-cell Lymphoma by Extracorporeal Photochemotherapy: Preliminary Results," *The New England Journal of Medicine*, Vol. 316(6), Feb. 5, 1987, pp. 297-303.

"Farming and Cancer." Prepared by the Office of Cancer Communications, National Cancer Institute. Sept. 1986.

Holland, J. and Frei, E. III, eds. *Cancer Medicine.* Philadelphia: Lea and Febiger, 1982, pp. 1478-1537.

Horning, S.J. and Rosenberg, S.A. "The Natural History of Initially Untreated Low-Grade Non-Hodgkin's Lymphomas," *The New England Journal of Medicine*, Vol. 311(23), Dec. 6, 1984, pp. 1471-1475.

Kinsella, T.J. "Role of Combined-Modality Therapy in the Curative Management of Advanced-Stage 'Favorable' Non-Hodgkin's Lymphomas," *Cancer Treatment Reports*, Vol. 66(3), March 1982, pp. 421-425.

Radiation Therapy and You: A Guide to Self-Help During Treatment. Prepared by the Office of Cancer Communications, National Cancer Institute. NIH Publication No. 86-2227.

Research Report: Bone Marrow Transplantation. Prepared by the Office of Cancer Communications, National Cancer Institute. NIH Publication No. 87-1178.

Rosenberg, S.A. et al. "National Cancer Institute Sponsored Study of Classification of Non-Hodgkin's Lymphomas," *Cancer*, May 15, 1982, pp. 2112-2135.

Rosenberg, S.A. "The Low-Grade Non-Hodgkin's Lymphomas: Challenges and Opportunities," Karnofsky Memorial Lecture, *Journal of Clinical Oncology*, Vol. 3(3), March 1985, pp. 299-310.

Schottenfeld, D. and Fraumeni, J., eds. *Cancer Epidemiology and Prevention.* Philadelphia: W.B. Saunders, 1982, pp. 739-794.

Understanding the Immune System. Prepared by the Office of Research Reporting and Public Response, National Institute of Allergy and Infectious Diseases. NIH Publication No. 85-529.

What Are Clinical Trials All About? Prepared by the Office of Cancer Communications, National Cancer Institute. NIH Publication No. 86-2706.

★ *The mentioned text is reprinted within this book. See CONTENTS for location.*

Chapter 14

Adult Kidney Cancer and Wilms' Tumor

Introduction

This *Research Report* describes current research on the causes and prevention, symptoms, diagnosis, and treatment of kidney cancers in adults and children. The information presented here was obtained from medical text-books and recent articles in the medical literature, discussions with National Cancer Institute (NCI) scientists and other researchers, and various scientific meetings.

Description and Function of the Kidneys

The kidneys are a pair of purplish-brown organs located behind the abdominal cavity on each side of the spine, just above the waist. Enclosed by a capsule of fibrous connective tissue called Gerota's fascia, each kidney is cushioned by layers of fatty tissue. The kidney of a 3-year-old child is about 2 inches long, 1 inch wide, and weighs about 4 ounces. The adult kidney is 4 to 5 inches long, 2 to 3 inches wide, and weighs 6 to 8 ounces.

The firm outer region of the kidney, the cortex, makes up about a third of the kidney tissue. The inner portion, called the medulla, has a hollow center, known as the renal pelvis. An indentation in the side of each kidney, the renal hilum, is the passageway for nerves and the vessels that carry blood into and away from the kidney. These vessels—the renal artery and the renal vein—connect directly with the aorta and the vena cava, which are the major vessels that carry blood leaving and entering the heart.

The kidneys are highly complex organs whose main function is to remove waste products from the bloodstream and produce urine to excrete these wastes. These organs also produce the hormone erythropoietin, which regulates the formation of red blood cells.

To help maintain the correct balance of water, salts, and acids in body fluids, the kidneys filter some of these substances out of the blood via approximately 2 million filtration units. Blood coming from the heart via the aorta enters the kidneys through the right and left renal arteries. Inside the kidneys, the renal arteries branch into smaller and smaller arterioles. Arteriole branching ends in microscopic glomeruli, which are masses of tiny, intertwined capillaries. Control of the chemical makeup of the blood and production of urine actually begin here. The thin walls of the glomeruli filter water, salts, sugar, and nitrogen-containing wastes (products of protein metabolism in the body) out of the blood. For the glomeruli to function well, blood-flow through the vessels of the kidneys must be maintained at a proper level. Should flow in the arterioles drop, the kidneys secrete renin, an enzyme that restores blood pressure by constricting the walls of these small vessels.

A cuplike structure surrounding each glomerulus collects the filtered substances and conveys them into the long, twisted renal tubule. Leading from the glomeruli to the renal pelvis, the tubule passes through another network of capillaries. Here, just the right amount of water, salts, and sugar are returned to the bloodstream. What remains is urine, containing excess water and a variety of waste products such as urea, creatinine, and uric acid. Every day a healthy adult produces about one to two quarts of urine, which leaves the renal pelvis via the ureter. This muscular tube extends out of the kidney at the hilum and transports urine to the bladder. Following temporary storage in the bladder, urine is excreted through another tube called the urethra.

Like other organs, the kidneys are composed of individual cells. Normally, growth and repair of tissues take place through the orderly division and reproduction of cells. When cell division is disordered, abnormal growth causes masses of tissue known as tumors to build up. These tumors may be benign or cancerous. Benign tumors may block normal organ function and may crowd adjacent organs, but they do not spread to other parts of the body and generally are not life threatening. Usually, benign tumors can be removed by surgery, and they are not likely to recur. Many scientists feel that certain small, benign tumors in the kidney, called adenomas, are precursors to cancer; that is, they have the potential to become cancerous as they grow larger.

Cancers of the kidney can invade and destroy normal tissues and can extend into surrounding structures. Cancer cells also can break away from the primary tumor and metastasize, or spread, to other parts of the body through the lymphatic system or the bloodstream. When kidney cancers spread, the cells often migrate to the bones, lungs, liver, and brain, where they can continue to divide abnormally and form secondary tumors. Cancer cells that make up these secondary tumors are usually identical to those of the primary cancer, and although another organ of the body is affected, the disease is still kidney cancer.

Certain kinds of cancer have a tendency to spread to the kidneys. In fact, metastatic tumors in the kidneys are more common than cancers that actually begin there.

Several different types of cancer can arise in the kidney. Renal cell carcinoma of the cortex and transitional cell carcinoma of the renal pelvis almost always occur in adults. A different type of kidney cancer, called Wilms' tumor, develops only in children.

Kidney Cancer in Adults

Renal cell carcinoma, the most common type of kidney cancer in adults, arises in the lining of the renal tubules. Also known as renal adenocarcinoma, hypernephroma, and Grawitz' tumor, it accounts for more than 85 percent of all adult kidney cancers. The next most common form is transitional cell carcinoma of the renal pelvis, which, in many ways, resembles bladder cancer. (Other cancers that originate in the kidney, mainly soft tissue sarcomas, are quite rare and are not discussed in this *Research Report*.)

Incidence

Cancer of the kidney accounts for about 2 to 3 percent of all cancers in American adults. Data collected and analyzed by the Surveillance, Epidemiology, and End Results (SEER) Program of the National Cancer Institute show the following average incidence (the number of cases per year per 100,000 population) in the United States for cancers of the kidney and renal pelvis for the years 1978 to 1981: 10.0 for white males, 9.2 for black males, 4.4 for white females, and 4.5 for black females. An estimated 20,000 cases of kidney cancer will be diagnosed in the United States in 1986.

Renal cell carcinoma affects twice as many men as women and is slightly more common among white men than black. It occurs most often between the ages of 50 and 70. Transitional cell carcinoma affects three times as many men as women, is twice as common among white males as black, and develops mainly after the age of 65.

Adult kidney cancers are more common in urban, industrialized areas, but there is little variation among different racial and ethnic groups. Worldwide, the incidence of renal cell carcinoma is higher in Northern Europe and North America and lower in Africa, Asia, and South America. For transitional cell carcinomas, rates are higher in the United States and Western Europe and lower in Japan and Scandinavian countries. Researchers have not found a satisfactory explanation for these geographic differences.

Cause and Prevention

The causes of kidney cancer are not fully understood, although scientists have identified some factors that increase risk for the disease. One such risk factor is tobacco use. Overall, smokers are twice as likely to develop kidney cancer as nonsmokers. Some researchers estimate that cigarette smoking is linked to 30 percent of kidney cancers in men and 24 percent in women. This link appears to be considerably stronger for transitional cell carcinoma than for renal cell carcinoma; in fact, recent studies implicate cigarette smoking as the major cause of cancer of the renal pelvis. For smokers, the risk of developing this type of cancer may be six to seven times higher than for nonsmokers, and the risk is apparently dose-related; that is, the more a person smokes, the higher the risk. One researcher calculates that more than 80 percent of renal pelvis cancers in men and more than 60 percent in women would be avoided if people stopped smoking.

Because they filter waste, the kidneys are exposed to many chemical substances, some produced by the body and others inhaled or ingested. A number of chemicals—such as nitrosamines, aflatoxins, lead acetate, and potassium bromate—do cause renal cell carcinoma in laboratory animals. However, the same effect has not been observed in humans.

Scientists have known for some time that an increased risk of renal pelvis cancer is associated with heavy, long-term use of non-narcotic analgesic drugs. In recent studies, researchers isolated phenacetin as the particular analgesic that raised the risk of cancer of the renal pelvis. Furthermore, phenacetin and tobacco appear to act together in causing this disease. The risk for people who both smoke and use large amounts of phenacetin is 19 times that of the general public. It appears likely that phenacetin also may be implicated in some cases of renal cell carcinoma. (The Food and Drug Administration withdrew its approval for marketing phenacetin-containing products in 1983.)

As is true of several other forms of cancer, there is evidence that obesity may increase one's risk of developing cancer of the kidney. In several studies, obesity has been associated with increased risk in women, and one recent report suggests that being overweight may be a risk factor for men, too. The reasons for this are not clear. One hypothesis is that the increased risk in women may be related to an excess of the hormone estrogen produced in their fatty tissue.

The synthetic estrogen diethylstilbestrol (DES) can cause kidney cancers to develop in hamsters especially bred for use in research. However, researchers have not seen a greater-than-average risk of renal cell carcinoma in people treated with DES or other estrogens. One study did suggest a slightly increased risk of renal pelvis cancer in females using estrogen-containing drugs, but it was not proven that the drugs actually caused the disease.

In the laboratory, animals that have had one kidney surgically removed and are later exposed to ionizing radiation develop cancerous tumors in the second kidney. However, animals subjected to either the surgery or the radiation, but not both, do not have an unusual incidence of cancer in the remaining kidney. In humans, women treated with radiotherapy, mainly for certain disorders of the uterus, may have a slightly increased risk of developing cancer of the bladder and, possibly, the renal pelvis. Patients who were exposed to thorium dioxide, a radioactive substance used in the 1920's with certain diagnostic X-rays, have an increased rate of renal cell carcinoma. However, this substance is no longer in use, and scientists think that ionizing radiation plays a minor role in the total number of kidney cancers.

A very small number of adult kidney cancers are familial. Certain inherited disorders (including von Hippel-Lindau's disease, tuberous sclerosis, Sturge-Weber syndrome, neurofibromatosis, and ataxia telangiectasia) put patients at increased risk for kidney tumors. A few familial cases not associated with one of these inherited conditions have been reported, but they are extremely rare.

Viruses cause kidney cancer in certain species of frogs, but there is no evidence that viruses contribute to the development of kidney cancer in humans. Kidney cancer is not transmissible from one person to another. Moreover, it is uncommon in people with immune disorders, who are susceptible to viral infections.

Recently, a number of studies have examined occupational exposures to see whether they raise workers' chances of developing kidney cancer. Some studies suggest that coke oven workers and insulation workers have above-average rates of kidney cancer, but suspect chemicals have not been identified. Among cadmium workers, a fourfold risk of renal cell carcinoma is seen in smokers, perhaps due to a synergistic effect similar to that seen for phenacetin and tobacco.

Researchers also have investigated several types of workplace exposure already linked with a higher incidence of bladder cancer. Reports now show that workers in the rubber, leather, petroleum, dye, textile, and plastics industries have an increased risk of transitional cell carcinoma of the renal pelvis. The rates of both types of kidney cancer in other occupations are under study.

Another concern is the recent observation that patients on long-term dialysis to treat chronic kidney failure have an increased risk of developing renal cysts and renal cancers. Further study is needed to determine how this finding may affect the care of patients with kidney failure.

Detection and Diagnosis

Detection

In its early stages, kidney cancer usually presents no obvious signs or troublesome symptoms. However, it is sometimes detected at an early stage during an examination for another condition or in the course of a routine checkup.

As a kidney tumor grows, it may cause symptoms that resemble those of other kidney diseases. The most common symptom is visible blood in the urine. Sometimes there is a lump or mass that can be felt in the kidney region and/or pain (a constant, dull ache) in the side, abdomen, or back. Other symptoms (known collectively as "paraneoplastic syndromes") occur less often but may lead the doctor to suspect cancer of the kidney. These include high blood pressure, intermittent fever, weight loss, fatigue, anemia, liver dysfunction, hypercalcemia (excess calcium in the blood), and erythrocytosis (an increase in red blood cells). These problems can be symptoms of cancer or a variety of other diseases.

Most cases of kidney cancer in adults (about 60 percent) are found only after the cancer has begun to spread. One goal of current research is to find ways of detecting the disease early. Researchers are working to identify a "biological marker," a measurable substance in the blood that could signal onset of the disease before symptoms appear, but at present, there are no reliable markers for kidney cancer. Some patients have elevated levels of renin, erythropoietin, or other chemicals in the bloodstream, but none of these is a consistent warning sign.

Researchers have developed a new animal model for both adult and childhood kidney cancers. A specially bred strain of mouse provides a much closer parallel to human kidney cancer than animal models used in the past. Scientists working with the mouse model have identified a number of hormones that are synthesized and secreted by adult kidney cancers and Wilms' tumor in humans. They hope that one or more of these hormones can form the basis for a simple blood test to screen individuals who are at above-average risk for kidney cancer.

Diagnosis

Renal cell carcinoma is often difficult to diagnose. Clues come from the physical examination, the patient's pattern of symptoms, and various laboratory tests. Improved imaging techniques now help to distinguish solid tumors (usually cancerous) from noncancerous, fluid-filled cysts. The diagnostic workup relies principally on X-ray examinations and may also include ultrasonography and blood and urine tests.

One of the first procedures used to diagnose a kidney problem is the excretory urogram, or intravenous pyelogram (IVP). This X-ray examination, performed with a contrast medium that usually contains iodine, provides a silhouette of the kidney, revealing any changes in the shape of the kidney, the ureter, or the neighboring lymph nodes.

If the IVP reveals a mass in the kidney, it is often followed by another series of X-ray studies called nephrotomography. This test, which gives a three-dimensional image of the kidney, can often distinguish a tumor from a cyst. In addition, computerized tomographic (CT) scans provide information about the size, density, extent, and other characteristics of the growth. CT scans also show in-volvement of the vena cava, renal vein, or regional lymph nodes.

Another test physicians sometimes use in the diagnostic process is ultrasonography. An ultrasound examination provides pictures from the echo patterns of soundwaves bounced back from internal organs. This technique may also help distinguish fluid-filled growths from solid ones.

Selective renal arteriography, which gives an X-ray image of renal blood vessels, is usually the final step in the diagnosis of kidney cancer. A substance opaque to X-rays is injected into the bloodstream, permitting doctors to see the veins and arteries that serve the kidneys. This test helps show the extent of a mass and is 95 to 98 percent accurate in diagnosing renal cell carcinoma. To confirm the diagnosis, doctors sometimes insert a needle into the tumor to withdraw sample cells for microscopic examination. This procedure is known as a fine-needle biopsy.

Doctors use additional tests to diagnose transitional cell carcinoma of the renal pelvis. The retrograde pyelogram is an X-ray picture taken after a contrast substance is injected into the kidney through the ureter.

With cystoscopy, a doctor can inspect the bladder through a lighted tube passed through the urethra. Urine and/or tissue can be analyzed for the presence of cancer cells. Also, researchers recently have developed a new device called a ureteropyeloscope, a lighted instrument that gives the doctor access to the ureter and renal pelvis without major surgery. It may even be possible to remove small tumors through the ureteropyeloscope, although the effectiveness of this technique remains to be tested.

A sensitive new diagnostic tool known as magnetic resonance imaging (MRI) can produce cross-sectional images of the kidney similar to those produced by computerized tomography. MRI, which employs only magnetic fields, does not expose the patient to ionizing radiation. Many researchers are enthusiastic about the potential of this new device, but its value in diagnosing kidney cancers must be defined by clinical studies.

Staging

Once kidney cancer has been found, other clinical and laboratory tests are used to establish the stage, or extent, of the disease. These tests usually include chest X-ray films, radioisotope bone and liver scans, abdominal CT scans, and blood tests. Additional X-ray studies of the renal blood vessels, the aorta, and the vena cava are sometimes needed to stage the disease and provide information the physician needs to plan the patient's treatment.

Stage I: The tumor appears to be confined to the kidney.

Stage II: The cancer involves the tissues that lie close to the kidney but has not spread beyond Gerota's fascia; cancer cells have not invaded regional lymph nodes or blood vessels.

Stage III: The cancer has invaded the renal vein, other blood vessels, and/or nearby lymph nodes.

Stage IV: The cancer has invaded neighboring organs or has spread to the opposite kidney or to distant sites in the body.

Treatment

Kidney cancer can often be cured if found and treated at an early stage, as it is in about 40 percent of all patients with the disease. Over the past three decades, progress has also been made against more advanced disease. Data from the NCI's SEER Program indicate that the overall 5-year relative survival rate for adult kidney cancer (combining patients of all races, both sexes, and all stages of disease) is 50 percent for those diagnosed between 1976 and 1981.

Improvements in survival appear to be due mainly to advances in surgical procedures, including better techniques in anesthesia and blood banking. Besides surgery, treatment may include radiation therapy, hormonal therapy, chemotherapy, and immunotherapy, depending on the stage and the specific needs of the patient. Integrated treatment, aggressive surgery in some cases for secondary tumors, intensive followup, and better supportive care have led to increases in the number of patients surviving 5, 10, and even 15 years. These are noteworthy achievements, particularly for a population in whom the average age at diagnosis is 55 to 60.

Surgery

Nephrectomy—the surgical removal of the kidney—was first used to treat adult kidney cancer in 1871. The remaining kidney generally is able to perform the work of both kidneys, and for more than a century this procedure has continued as the mainstay of treatment for adults with this disease. Experts generally agree that the more extensive "radical" nephrectomy, introduced in the 1950's, should replace "simple" nephrectomy as the standard surgical technique for most patients.

Simple nephrectomy is the surgical removal of just the kidney. In radical nephrectomy, the surgeon ties off the renal artery and vein and removes the kidney, as well as the adrenal gland (which lies just above the kidney) and some of the surrounding tissue. In addition, the surgeon usually removes the lymph nodes near the kidney, in case cancer cells have migrated there. Though some physicians question the therapeutic benefit of removing lymph nodes, they generally agree that this step can contribute to accurate staging.

Nephrectomy can cure most patients with localized kidney cancer (stage I); many in whom cancer cells have begun to spread from the kidney (stage II); and some with locally advanced tumors (stage III).

Nephrectomy is sometimes recommended for advanced or metastatic disease (stage IV) to control symptoms, such as excessive bleeding or abnormal hormone production, or to alleviate pain. For the 10 percent of stage IV patients who have a single metastatic tumor, further surgery to remove the secondary tumor has sometimes led to long-term survival.

Another technique—radical nephrectomy preceded by arterial embolization—is used to treat some patients diagnosed with large, locally advanced, or metastatic renal cancer. Small particles of a special substance such as gelatin sponge (Gelfoam) are injected into the renal artery through a very narrow tube called a catheter. This material blocks the small vessels that supply the tumor and thus deprives the cancer cells of nourishment. In some cases, preoperative arterial embolization may simplify later nephrectomy.

For certain patients—primarily those with small, less aggressive tumors and those with only one kidney—some physicians prefer to use a more conservative procedure, the partial nephrectomy. This method of treatment removes the tumor while preserving normal kidney tissue and, thus, kidney function.

Radiation Therapy

Clinical trials comparing the effectiveness of radiation before surgery with nephrectomy alone for stages I and II kidney cancer have not produced consistent results. Preliminary data from some recent research suggest that survival may be better among patients in the irradiated group. Other studies suggest that although survival time may not be improved, local recurrences may be decreased with preoperative radiation. Definitive answers will come from long-term followup of patients in studies like these.

Reports on the benefits of postoperative radiation have not produced clear-cut results yet, either. Some authorities think this mode of therapy may reduce local recurrence in patients with early stage disease and may also contribute to control of tumors that extend outside the kidney.

The importance of radiation therapy in alleviating problems caused by secondary tumors in the bone, lung, and abdominal wall is well established. It may also be useful in the care of certain patients with very large tumors or those who, for various reasons, cannot have surgery.

Hormonal Therapy

In clinical trials, hormonal treatment (usually synthetic forms of progesterone) has not been effective. However, doctors sometimes believe that trying this type of treatment is justified because some responses have been reported (especially in male patients with lung metastases).

Chemotherapy

At this time, anticancer drugs, successful in controlling many other forms of cancer, have not made important contributions in the treatment of kidney cancer in adults. Identifying effective drugs for patients with advanced disease remains a major challenge.

In early efforts to treat this disease with drugs, vinblastine (also known as Velban) appeared to hold promise, particularly if it could be given in high doses. However, more recent work has failed to demonstrate that vinblastine is effective in controlling cancer of the kidney in more than a small number of patients. Many other agents have been studied—both alone and in various combinations—with generally disappointing results. Nonetheless, researchers are continuing to look for new drugs, new drug combinations,

and innovative ways of using existing ones.

Some of the new agents now under study for renal cell carcinoma include gallium nitrate, N-methylformamide, carboplatin, and 4'-deoxydoxorubicin. Antitumor drugs being evaluated for their effectiveness in treating transitional cell cancers of the urinary tract include methotrexate, dichloromethotrexate, and cisplatin.

Methotrexate, a drug used successfully for years in other cancers, is being given to patients with no evidence of metastasis following surgery for cancer of the renal pelvis in an attempt to determine whether chemotherapy can prevent or delay recurrences. In other clinical trials, investigators are trying to learn whether inoperable kidney tumors can be treated effectively by chemoinfusion, delivering anticancer drugs to the tumor directly through the renal blood supply, rather than through the general circulation. This approach might allow the use of larger and potentially more effective doses of the drugs, but it is a complex procedure that has not been studied adequately.

Some investigators believe that it may be possible to identify useful antitumor drugs by growing human renal cancer cells in the laboratory and testing them for sensitivity to various agents. In addition, a new animal screening model may help accelerate studies of potentially useful therapies.

Immunotherapy

For the past several years, researchers have been actively exploring ways to enlist the body's immune system in fighting cancer. In both laboratory and clinical studies, scientists are evaluating a number of biological response modifiers (BRMs), natural and synthetic substances that may boost or strengthen the body's natural defenses against the disease. The results of recent studies with interferon, the best known of these agents, have been encouraging. Clinical trials suggest that interferon may be active against metastatic renal cell carcinoma, and further studies will test whether patients' responses can be improved by altering the doses and types of interferon.

In addition, in 1985, a team of NCI researchers reported the development of a new form of immunotherapy. Their approach uses a BRM called interleukin-2 (IL-2) to activate killer cells (a type of white blood cell) removed from the patient's blood. The result is a unique population of cells called lymphokine activated killer (LAK) cells. The patient is treated with the LAK cells and additional IL-2. In preliminary trials with a small number of patients, renal cell carcinoma appeared to respond to this type of immunotherapy. Clinical studies of this new approach are in progress at a number of institutions throughout the United States.

Physicians have observed long-term stabilization of secondary tumors in a few cases following embolization and nephrectomy. They theorize that interrupting the blood supply to renal tumors may cause the release of certain substances into the bloodstream and, through a series of complex steps, improve the body's natural antitumor response. However, this possibility has not been confirmed in controlled clinical trials.

Wilms' Tumor

Incidence

The most common kidney cancer in children, nephroblastoma, has been called Wilms' tumor since 1899 when Dr. Max Wilms published his detailed paper describing the disease. About 500 new cases of Wilms' tumor occur in the United States each year. It accounts for 6 to 8 percent of childhood cancers. This disease affects 1 child in about 10,000 in this country, and the worldwide incidence is similar. Wilms' tumor occurs mainly in children under the age of 7, with most cases developing between the ages of 1 and 4. Boys and girls are affected equally.

Cause

The causes of Wilms' tumor are not known. The disease seems to be unrelated to race, climate, or environment, and it is apparently not linked to birth order, birth weight, maternal age, or maternal history of previous stillbirths.

About 10 percent of children with Wilms' tumor have certain congenital abnormalities. Aniridia (absence of the iris, the colored part of the eye) is seen in about 1 percent of children with Wilms' tumor, hemihypertrophy (abnormal, asymmetrical enlargement of one half or one part of the body) in about 3 percent, and various genitourinary defects in about 5 percent. Although the exact relationship of these conditions to kidney cancer is not understood, physicians who are aware of the occasional association can diagnose and treat Wilms' tumor at an early stage.

Scientists believe that there are both hereditary and nonhereditary forms of the disease. The hereditary type often arises at an earlier age and is likely to affect both kidneys or several sites in one kidney. Scientists suspect that a defective gene causes abnormalities in the fetal kidney, and chromosome studies point to a small region on the short arm of chromosome number 11 as the location of the defective gene(s). The proportion of Wilms' tumor patients whose families carry a genetic tendency toward the disease is not known. Moreover, researchers do not yet know whether the offspring of recovered Wilms' tumor patients are at higher risk of developing the disease.

Detection and Diagnosis

Detection

A swelling on one side of the upper abdomen is the most common symptom of Wilms' tumor. Other signs may include blood in the urine, low-grade fever, loss of appetite, paleness, weight loss, and lethargy. These problems are most often due to conditions other than cancer, but parents who observe such symptoms should consult a doctor promptly.

Diagnosis

The doctor takes a complete medical history and performs a physical examination. If Wilms' tumor is suspected, readily available diagnostic tests can lead to an accurate diagnosis in most patients. Blood tests to assess kidney and liver function are likely to be part of the initial workup. Production of excess erythropoietin may lead to erythrocytosis (an increase in the red blood cell count). Some patients may have abnormally high blood pressure believed to be caused by secretion of renin. Urinalysis is performed to detect blood in the urine.

The diagnosis of kidney cancer in a child depends primarily on imaging techniques (described on pages 9 and 10). The IVP is usually enough to identify Wilms' tumor. In some cases, ultrasonography and/or computerized tomography can help determine whether the abnormal growth is a solid tumor or a fluid-filled cyst. These tests can also show whether a cancerous growth has spread and can help determine if the opposite kidney is involved. Selective renal arteriography may be used if results of the other tests are inconclusive.

When clinical and laboratory data indicate kidney cancer, surgical exploration generally is the next step in diagnosing the disease. (Needle biopsies are seldom performed.)

Staging

Prognosis depends largely on the stage of the disease, or the extent of spread, at the time of diagnosis, and on certain microscopic features of the cancer cells. The staging system used most widely was developed by the nationwide association of cancer clinics and hospitals cooperating in the National Wilms' Tumor Study. This system takes into account the results of diagnostic tests, as well as the observations of the surgeon and the pathologist.

Stage I: The tumor is confined to the kidney and is completely removed surgically. Nearly half of all children with Wilms' tumor have stage I disease.

Stage II: The tumor extends beyond the kidney but is still completely removed by surgery. Almost one-fourth of patients are in this group.

Stage III: The cancer is found in surrounding tissues, lymph nodes, or blood vessels in the abdomen and cannot be entirely removed by surgery. Nearly one-fifth of children with Wilms' tumor are in stage III.

Stage IV: Cancer cells have spread and formed secondary tumors at distant sites, most commonly the lungs, liver, bone, and brain. About 5 percent of Wilms' tumor cases are described as stage IV.

Stage V: Cancer is bilateral, affecting both kidneys, at the time of diagnosis. The disease is in stage V in about 5 percent of Wilms' tumor cases.

Each tumor is designated "favorable histology" (FH) or "unfavorable histology" (UH), as determined by the pathologist. While all cancer cells lack the orderly arrangement of normal cells, those designated UH are especially primitive and extremely lacking in organized microscopic structure. The vast majority of children diagnosed with kidney cancer (about 90 percent) have cell types described as favorable. (Kidney tumors that contain elements of sarcoma—cancer that arises from supportive or connective tissue rather than from lining tissue—are also designated UH, although most specialists believe that these cancers are a different disease and should not be classified as Wilms' tumor.)

Treatment

In general, children respond better than adults to cancer therapy, and this advantage is especially clear in the treatment of kidney cancer. Wilms' tumor is one of modern medicine's success stories. Treatment plans that combine modern techniques in surgery, radiotherapy, and chemotherapy have brought dramatic progress in treating this disease. How the various treatment methods are combined depends on the extent and cellular characteristics of the cancer, as well as the child's medical history, general health, and age.

Experience has shown that children treated for Wilms' tumor can be considered cured if they survive for 2 years without any sign that the disease has returned. In the early part of this century, Wilms' tumor was almost invariably fatal; only a few children survived as long as 2 years after diagnosis. Statistics now show that nearly 80 percent of children with Wilms' tumor are being cured; in those with favorable histological types, the cure rate approaches 90 percent. The small number of children with aggressive cell types (unfavorable histology) or with widespread disease at the time of diagnosis have a poorer outlook, but many of these patients are curable with intensive therapy.

Surgery

In the 1930's and 1940's, improvements in surgery, anesthesia, and pre- and postoperative care made it possible to perform nephrectomies successfully in very young patients. As a result, about 40 percent of children with Wilms' tumor survived the disease. Radical nephrectomy (described on pages 11 and 12) remains the cornerstone of treatment for Wilms' tumor.

Radiation Therapy

Although the value of radiotherapy for adult kidney cancer is still questionable, it can be important in the treatment for Wilms' tumor. Since 1915, doctors have recognized that Wilms' tumor responds to radiation therapy. By the 1950's, the combination of nephrectomy and postoperative radiation therapy had yielded survival rates of almost 50 percent.

Chemotherapy

The next major advance was the discovery that certain drugs, particularly actinomycin D and vincristine, could reduce the size of Wilms' tumors. These drugs were tested for safety and effectiveness in a series of small-scale clinical studies starting in the 1960's. In one study, investigators found that a 15-month course of repeated treatment with actinomycin D was superior to a single dose of the drug given after surgery. Since then, "maintenance" therapy of varying lengths has been an accepted principle of drug treatment for Wilms' tumor.

After the addition of chemotherapy, treatment centers began adopting a modern team approach in caring for Wilms' patients. With pediatric surgeons, radiotherapists, and oncologists working together, these centers have consistently reported overall 2-year survival rates of 70 to 80 percent.

Side Effects

Although each form of cancer treatment can be accompanied by undesirable effects, all patients do not have the same problems, nor do they experience difficulties to the same degree. Chemotherapy and radiotherapy often cause nausea and vomiting, but these problems are temporary and usually can be curbed with medication. A more serious short-term side effect is the suppression of bone marrow. In killing cancer cells, chemotherapy and radiotherapy also destroy some normal cells in the bone marrow. If the white cells, red cells, and platelets fall too low, patients can become susceptible to bleeding and infection. Such reactions are temporary, and supportive care, such as antibiotic therapy, helps to protect patients from these complications during their treatment.

Pediatric oncologists are particularly concerned with adverse effects that may appear long after successful cancer treatment. For example, radiation therapy can disrupt normal bone growth, especially in very young children. Irradiation can also injure organs, disturb hormonal and reproductive functions, and, in a small percentage of cases, induce new cancers years after therapy. Doctors are also concerned that chemotherapy may cause new primary cancers to develop many years later.

Beginning in the 1960's, as more and more children were being cured of Wilms' tumor, researchers began to examine the accepted treatment programs in an effort to reduce the complications of therapy. Since that time, a series of clinical trials has been designed to identify treatment methods to give Wilms' patients the best chance of being cured while sparing them as many complications as possible. Investigators continue to explore more aggressive approaches to improve the outlook for patients whose tumors are resistant to standard treatment.

National Wilms' Tumor Study

Because Wilms' tumor affects only a small number of children, researchers recognized that pooling resources and data would help speed answers to important questions about improvements in treatment. In 1969, the National Wilms' Tumor Study (NWTS), a national consortium of hospitals and clinics treating children with cancer, was created with National Cancer Institute support to carry out controlled clinical trials. Since then, treatment for Wilms' tumor has been refined in a series of studies enrolling more than 2,300 patients. In the first study (NWTS-1), carried out between 1969 and 1974, the overall 2-year survival rate was 80 percent. The second trial (NWTS-2), which ended in 1978, achieved a 2-year survival rate of 87 percent. The treatment currently received by most Wilms' tumor patients in this country is based on the results of these studies. (NWTS-3 is still in progress.)

NWTS-1 found that stage I patients under 2 years of age given actinomycin D did not require postoperative radiotherapy. The first trial also showed that, for stages II and III, the combination of actinomycin D and vincristine was superior to either drug used alone.

Data gathered in NWTS-2 revealed that combination chemotherapy could replace radiotherapy in the treatment of stage I patients, regardless of the child's age. (At present, postoperative irradiation is generally reserved for patients with unfavorable histology or more advanced disease.)

NWTS-2 also demonstrated that the period of maintenance chemotherapy could be cut from 15 months down to 6 months without changing the cure rate for stage I patients. In addition, the second study showed that treatment of more advanced cases could be improved by adding a third drug, Adriamycin, to the other two. (The three-drug combination also is used for less advanced cases with unfavorable histology.)

When the third study began in 1979, analysis of the NWTS experience showed an overall 2-year survival rate of 89 percent for cases with favorable histology, but only 39 percent for those with unfavorable histology. With this strong evidence of the impact of histologic tumor characteristics on prognosis, NWTS-3 was designed to evaluate the effectiveness of therapy that is more limited for patients in the FH group and more aggressive for those in the UH group.

Preliminary results of this ongoing study, reported in May 1984, suggest that tumors designated FH can be successfully treated with less intensive regimens. For example, NWTS-3 investigators have found that for stage II-FH, results after intensification of the standard two-drug combination (by the addition of either Adriamycin or radiation therapy) apparently are not improved. Also, evidence to date indicates that stage III-FH patients treated wtih three-drug combination chemotherapy and low doses of radiation have done just as well as a similar group treated with more intense radiotherapy.

NWTS-3 has also evaluated the benefits of adding cyclophosphamide to the three drugs in current use for patients with advanced disease (stage IV) and those with unfavorable histology at any stage. The four-drug combination does not appear to offer these children a significant advantage, and researchers now are considering other ways of improving the care of patients with metastatic disease or unfavorable cell types.

PDQ

The National Cancer Institute has developed PDQ (Physician Data Query), a computerized database designed to give doctors quick and easy access to:

- the latest treatment information for most types of cancer;

- descriptions of clinical trials that are open for patient entry; and

- names of organizations and physicians involved in cancer care.

To get access to PDQ, a doctor may use an office computer with a telephone hookup and a PDQ access code or the services of a medical library with online searching capability. Most Cancer Information Service offices (1-800-4-CANCER) provide a physician with one free PDQ search and can tell doctors how to get regular access to the database. Patients may ask their doctor to use PDQ or may call 1-800-4-CANCER themselves. Information specialists at this toll-free number use a variety of sources, including PDQ, to answer questions about cancer prevention, diagnosis, and treatment.

Suggestions for Additional Reading

Except as noted, the following materials are not available from the National Cancer Institute. They can be found in medical libraries, many college and university libraries, and some public libraries.

Brady, Luther W., Jr. "Carcinoma of the Kidney—The Role for Radiation Therapy," *Seminars in Oncology,* Vol 10, December 1983, pp. 417-421.

Cancer Rates and Risks, *prepared by the Office of Cancer Communications, National Cancer Institute. NIH Publication No. 85-691.

Chemotherapy and You: *A Guide to Self-Help During Treatment,* prepared by the Office of Cancer Communications, National Cancer Institute. NIH Publication No. 84-1136.

D'Angio, Giulio J. et al. "The Treatment of Wilms' Tumor: Results of the National Wilms' Tumor Study," *Cancer,* Vol 38, August 1976, pp. 633-646.

D'Angio, Giulio J. et al. "The Treatment of Wilms' Tumor: Results of the Second National Wilms' Tumor Study," *Cancer,* Vol 47, May 1981, pp. 2302-2311.

Dayal, Hari and Kinman, Judith. "Epidemiology of Kidney Cancer," *Seminars in Oncology,* Vol 10, December 1983, pp. 366-377.

DeKernion, Jean B. and Berry, David. "The Diagnosis and Treatment of Renal Cell Carcinoma," *Cancer,* Vol 45, April 1980 (Supplement), pp. 1947-1956.

DeVita, Vincent T., Jr. et al., eds. *Cancer: Principles and Practice of Oncology,* Second Edition. Philadelphia: J.B. Lippincott Co., 1985.

Haskell, Charles M., ed. *Cancer Treatment,* Second Edition. Philadelphia: W.B. Saunders Co., 1985.

Holland, James and Frei, Emil, III, eds. *Cancer Medicine,* Second Edition. Philadelphia: Lea and Febiger, 1982.

Javadpour, Nasser. *Cancer of the Kidney.* New York: Thieme-Stratton, 1985.

McCredie, Margaret et al. "Analgesics and Tobacco as Risk Factors for Cancer of the Ureter and Renal Pelvis," *The Journal of Urology,* Vol 130, July 1983, pp. 28-30.

McCune, Craig S. "Immunologic Therapies of Kidney Carcinoma," *Seminars in Oncology,* Vol 10, December 1983, pp. 431-436.

McDonald, Michael W. "Current Therapy for Renal Cell Carcinoma," *The Journal of Urology,* Vol 127, February 1982, pp. 211-217.

McLaughlin, Joseph K. et al. "Etiology of Cancer of the Renal Pelvis," *Journal of the National Cancer Institute,* Vol 71, August 1983, pp. 287-291.

Meadows, Anna T. and D'Angio, Giulio J. "Late Effects of Cancer Treatment: Methods and Techniques for Detection," *Seminars in Oncology,* Vol 1, March 1974, pp. 87-90.

Meadows, Anna T. et al. "Oncogenesis and Other Late Effects of Cancer Treatment in Children: Report of a Single Hospital Study," *Radiology,* Vol 114, January 1975, pp. 175-180.

Outzen, Henry C. and Maguire, Henry C., Jr. "The Etiology of Renal-Cell Carcinoma," *Seminars in Oncology,* Vol 10, December 1983, pp. 378-384.

---

* *The mentioned text is reprinted within this book. See CONTENTS for location.*

Pochedly, Carl and Baum, Edward, eds. *Wilms' Tumor: Clinical and Biological Manifestations.* New York: Elsevier Science Publishing, 1984.

Quesada, Jorge et al. "Renal Cell Carcinoma: Antitumor Effects of Leukocyte Interferon," *Cancer Research,* Vol 43, February 1983, pp. 940-943.

Radiation Therapy and You: A Guide to Self-Help During Treatment, prepared by the Office of Cancer Communications, National Cancer Institute. NIH Publication No. 85-2227.

Rieselback, R.E. and Garnick, M.B. *Cancer and the Kidney.* Philadelphia: Lea and Febiger, 1982.

Robson, C.J. et al. "The Results of Radical Nephrectomy for Renal Cell Carcinoma," *Transactions of the American Association of Genito-Urinary Surgeons,* Vol 60, 1968, pp. 122-126.

Rosenberg, Steven A. et al. "Observations on the Systemic Administration of Autologous Lymphokine-Activated Killer Cells and Recombinant Interleukin-2 to Patients with Metastatic Cancer," *The New England Journal of Medicine,* Vol 313, No 23, December 5, 1985, pp. 1485-1492.

Sutow, W.W. et al., eds. *Clinical Pediatric Oncology,* Third Edition. St. Louis: Mosby, 1984.

Swanson, David A. et al. "The Role of Embolization and Nephrectomy in the Treatment of Metastatic Renal Cancer," *Urologic Clinics of North America,* Vol 7, October 1980, pp. 719-730.

*What Are Clinical Trials All About?,** prepared by the Office of Cancer Communications, National Cancer Institute. NIH Publication No. 85-2706.

*Young People With Cancer:*A Handbook for Parents,* prepared by the Office of Cancer Communications, National Cancer Institute. NIH Publication No. 83-2378.

This *Research Report* was written by Linda C. Slan under contract with the National Cancer Institute. The scientific content of this publication has been approved by NCI scientists. Please direct questions or comments to the *Research Reports* editor, National Cancer Institute, Office of Cancer Communications, Bethesda, MD 20892.

---

* The mentioned text is reprinted within this book. See CONTENTS for location.

Chapter 15

Leukemia

Introduction

This Research Report describes current research on the causes and prevention, symptoms, diagnosis, and treatment of the various types of leukemia. The information presented here came from recent articles in the scientific literature, discussions with National Cancer Institute scientists and other researchers, and various scientific meetings.

Description and Function of Blood Cells

The term "leukemia" describes a variety of cancers that arise in the blood-forming cells. To understand the various leukemias, their causes, outlook and treatment, it helps to be familiar with the functions of the blood and the different types of cells found in the bloodstream.

The blood is a vital organ that supplies food, oxygen, hormones, and other chemicals to all of the body's cells. It helps remove waste products and assists the lymph system in fighting infection.

Whole blood is composed of red cells, white cells, and clotting cells that circulate in a clear fluid called plasma. Blood cell growth, known as hematopoiesis, begins with the formation of immature stem cells in the bone marrow, the spongy interior of the large bones. (In the fetus, blood cell production takes place in the spleen and liver.) Each stem cell is highly active, producing as many as thousands of cells daily. Stem cells give rise to "committed" cells, which in turn start a series of changes that lead to a distinct type of mature blood cell. When the body is healthy, the numbers of red cells, white cells, and platelets circulating in the blood are kept in balance. Worn-out cells are destroyed and removed from the blood as fast as new cells are produced.

Red Blood Cells (Erythrocytes)

The function of red blood cells (erythrocytes) is to transport oxygen from the lungs to all tissues of the body. Erythrocytes contain hemoglobin, an iron-rich protein that can take up oxygen as the blood passes through the lungs, and release it to the tissues. Too few red blood cells, a condition known as anemia, may cause weakness, dizziness, headaches, and irritability.

Clotting Cells (Platelets)

Platelets help prevent excessive bleeding by forming clots at injured sites. A deficiency of platelets—thrombocytopenia—may cause bleeding of the mucous membranes or other tissues, such as the skin.

White Blood Cells (Leukocytes)

There are three major groups of mature white blood cells, or leukocytes. Each type of white blood cell plays a different role in defending the body against infection:

- *Monocytes* make up 5 to 10 percent of circulating white blood cells and defend the body against bacterial infections.

- *Granulocytes* also help fight infection. Granulocytes are subdivided into eosinophils, basophils, and neutrophils. Neutrophils comprise 60 percent of circulating white blood cells and are capable of pass-

ing through capillary walls to engulf and destroy invading bacteria. Eosinophils and basophils also destroy invading bacteria, but their action is not clearly understood. A deficiency of neutrophils is called neutropenia, which may result in an increased susceptibility to infections and ulcerations of the mucous membranes.

- *Lymphocytes* arise from lymphoblasts and mature in the lymphatic system (thymus gland, spleen, lymph nodes, and Peyer's patches in the intestines). Lymphocytes make up 30 percent of circulating white blood cells. The two types of lymphocytes (T cells and B cells) each provide a different type of immunity. T cells attack and destroy virus-infected cells, foreign tissue, and cancer cells. B cells produce antibodies—proteins that help destroy foreign substances. These two types of white cells interact in complex ways to regulate the immune response. A deficiency of normal lymphocytes, called lymphocytopenia, increases susceptibility to infection.

238

Types of Leukemia

Leukemia is a cancer of the blood-forming tissues. Abnormal white blood cells, unable to perform their infection-fighting roles, fill the bone marrow and bloodstream. Leukemic cells crowd the bone marrow, spill into the circulating blood, and infiltrate vital organs like the liver, lungs, and kidneys. Leukemic cells may even invade the brain and spinal cord by crossing the blood-brain barrier, a system of tightly meshed cells that helps to protect the central nervous system.

Because the bone marrow of leukemia patients cannot maintain normal production of red cells, white cells, and platelets, they are more susceptible to fatigue, bleeding, and infection. The accumulation of uric acid in the blood, caused by the rapid destruction of cells, may inhibit kidney function.

The healthy bone marrow does not contain more than 5 percent blasts, or immature cells, nor are blasts normally present in the bloodstream. In the leukemia patient, though, blasts often constitute more than 5 percent of the cells in the marrow and may be found in the blood stream.

Leukemic cells differ in appearance and function from normal white blood cells:

	Normal White Cells	Leukemic Cells
Appearance:	mature	immature
	no nucleolus visible	prominent nucleoli
	coarse dispersement of chromosomes	fine dispersement of chromosomes
Function:	multiply in response to stimulation	multiply continuously
	defend the body against infection	provide no defense against infection

Leukemia is classified as acute (progressing rapidly) or chronic (progressing slowly). In acute leukemia, there is abnormal growth of immature cells called blasts. Chronic leukemia is characterized by the proliferation of more mature cells, although abnormal immature cells may also be present. Leukemia also is classified according to the type of white cell that predominates.

Acute Lymphocytic Leukemia (ALL)

Patients with acute lymphocytic leukemia have an abnormal increase of immature lymphocytes in their blood and bone marrow. This form of leukemia, also known as acute lymphoblastic leukemia, acute lymphatic leukemia, or childhood leukemia, accounts for 85 percent of leukemia in children, and about 15 percent of leukemia cases in adults. Scientists can classify ALL cells as T-cell; B-cell; or non T-cell, non B-cell types. Most ALL patients have lymphoblasts that exhibit neither T-cell nor B-cell features, when classified by standard immunologic techniques. However, recent studies using more sensitive molecular markers show these cells as originating from a B-cell precursor. T-cell ALL accounts for 15 to 20 percent of all cases of acute lymphocytic leukemia.

Acute Nonlymphocytic Leukemia (ANLL)

Other forms of acute leukemia are grouped under the heading "acute nonlymphocytic leukemia." The most common of these is acute myelocytic leukemia (AML), also called acute granulocytic leukemia or acute myelogenous leukemia. AML involves the neutrophils, a type of granulocyte, and is the most common form of acute leukemia in adults. Other rare forms of acute nonlymphocytic leukemia include monocytic leukemia (monocytes and monoblasts predominate); promyelocytic leukemia (promyelocytes predominate); erythroleukemia

(immature red and white cells predominate); and myelomonocytic leukemia (mixed myelocytes and monocytes). Treatment for these forms of acute leukemia is similar to that for acute myelocytic leukemia.

Smoldering Leukemia and Preleukemia

Several bone marrow disorders, called preleukemia and smoldering leukemia, may, in a small percentage of cases, precede the onset of ANLL by months or years. Patients with preleukemia are generally elderly and have a deficiency of white cells, red cells, and platelets in their blood, with signs of red- and white-cell abnormalities. Smoldering leukemia is a form of acute myelocytic leukemia that begins slowly and, scientists believe, involves abnormal changes in more than one cell line. Generally, chemotherapy for these conditions is not begun until the disease shows signs of becoming aggressive.

Chronic Lymphocytic Leukemia (CLL)

The most common of the chronic leukemias, CLL is characterized by an abnormal increase in lymphocytes. These lymphocytes usually have B-cell features and resemble normal lymphocytes but lack their infection-fighting ability. Scientists think that the lymphocytes of CLL are produced in the lymph nodes and spleen rather than in the bone marrow. The average age of onset for CLL is 60 years.

Besides CLL, several rare forms of chronic leukemia also originate in the lymphocytes. One is called hairy cell leukemia because of the unique, hairy-like appearance of the leukemic cell under the microscope. Scientists believe hairy cell leukemia originates in the B cells. Another rare human leukemia is called adult T-cell leukemia/lymphoma, and is now known to be caused by a virus. This disease, which has a rapid clinical course, has been found in southern Japan, parts of the Caribbean, the southeastern United States, and elsewhere. (See also the discussion of viruses under *Cause and Prevention.*)

Chronic Myelogenous Leukemia (CML)

In chronic myelogenous leukemia, abnormal granulocytes accumulate in the bone marrow and bloodstream. (CML is also known as chronic granulocytic leukemia, chronic myelocytic leukemia, or chronic myelosis.) The average age of CML patients at diagnosis is 40 years.

Causes and Prevention

Together, the leukemias represent about 5 percent of all cancer cases. In 1987, about 26,400 new cases of leukemia—or 10 new cases per 100,000 people—will be diagnosed in the United States. About half of these are acute leukemia, the other half chronic leukemia. Although often thought of as mainly a childhood disease, leukemia strikes many more adults than children (24,600 adult cases compared with 2,000 in children in 1987).

In the United States, leukemia occurs slightly more often among whites than among blacks, and Jews have a somewhat higher incidence than other whites. The male-to-female ratio for all leukemias is about 1.7 to 1. Men have almost two times more chronic lymphocytic leukemia than do women.

The specific forms of leukemia are very different in their age patterns. Acute leukemias account for almost all leukemias in children and young adults and for about two-fifths of those in older adults. In young children, acute lymphocytic leukemia (ALL) is most common. After puberty, however, acute myelocytic leukemia (AML) predominates. CLL is almost never seen before adulthood but is common after age 50.

The causes of leukemia are not fully understood, but certain factors are known to increase the risk of developing leukemia. Among the factors now associated with higher leukemia incidence are certain genetic abnormalities, disorders of the immune system, excessive exposure to ionizing radiation, chemicals that suppress bone marrow function, and a virus recently isolated from a rare type of T-cell leukemia.

Radiation

Statistical evidence strongly suggests that ionizing radiation, either from a single, large dose or repeated small doses, can induce leukemia in humans. Leukemia has been reported to occur at higher-than-average rates among persons exposed to intense radiation: survivors of the atomic bomb explosions in Japan, persons who received large amounts of radiation for treatment of certain medical conditions, and radiologists (in early years of the specialty). Since the potential hazard of excess exposure to medical x-rays has been widely publicized, exposure to this radiation source has declined.

A study of survivors of the atomic bomb explosions in Japan has produced convincing evidence that a single-dose exposure to radiation can increase the likelihood of leukemia in humans. Overall, there was a tenfold to twentyfold increased incidence of leukemia among atomic bomb survivors who were exposed to radiation compared to a control population. Research by the Atomic Bomb Casualty Commission has shown that the frequency of leukemia increases proportionately to doses above about 35 rad. (For comparison, the dose of a breast x-ray exam is typically less than 0.5 rad.) Studies of the time of onset of these cases showed that there may be a delay of up to 20 years before the leukemia develops. In recent years, the rate of chronic myelocytic leukemia in the atomic bomb survivors has returned to normal, but some small increase in the incidence of acute leukemia has persisted.

In general, it is extremely difficult to detect biologic effects either in animals or in people who are exposed to low-level radiation (under 10 rad). If there are effects, they make take years to become apparent, and even then may be difficult to detect. For this reason, scientists are uncertain about whether there is a threshold dose—a "safe" dose below which no leukemia occurs.

The Japanese study also illustrated the fact that susceptibility to radiation-induced leukemia varies from one individual to another. Among persons who survived the largest radiation doses, only 1 in every 40 has developed leukemia.

Genetic Factors

The genetic basis of leukemia is still uncertain. Studies of families and of twins have shown a higher than expected incidence of some forms of leukemia among relatives. It has also been found that leukemia occurs together with certain congenital defects more often than can be attributed to chance. Some of these diseases are characterized by abnormal numbers or shapes of the chromosomes, the cellular materials that carry hereditary information passed from one generation of cells to the next. For example, children with Down* syndrome, a congenital disease characterized by an extra

chromosome, have a risk of developing leukemia about 20 times greater than that for the general population. Still, these findings do not in themselves mean that leukemia is an inherited disease. Scientists think it is more likely that genetic makeup may somehow increase susceptibility to a host of leukemia-causing environmental factors.

Chromosomal abnormalities have been found in the bone marrow cells of a high percentage of patients with acute leukemia who show no congenital defects. The abnormalities disappear during remission—periods when signs and symptoms of the disease vanish in response to treatment. It is not known if these chromosomal abnormalities are a cause or a result of the disease.

Eighty percent of patients with chronic myelogenous leukemia have an abnormality known as the Philadelphia (Ph[1]) chromosome. This abnormal chromosome pattern (characterized by a translocation, or swap, of parts between two chromosomes) has been observed in all phases of the disease and is only rarely affected by treatment. It also has been seen in the acute leukemias

* *Also referred to as Down's syndrome*

243

and other allied diseases, but less commonly.

In animals, chromosomal abnormalities can occur after exposure to radiation, cancer-causing chemicals, or certain viruses. Some scientists think that chromosomal abnormalities, whether inherited or acquired, may be a common factor in the origin of leukemia, but that the disease is triggered by a combination of environmental agents.

Viruses

Scientists have long known that retroviruses (also known as RNA tumor viruses, or type-C viruses) can cause leukemias and lymphomas in certain animal species, but no such virus had been found in human cancer cells. Several years ago, however, National Cancer Institute (NCI) researcher Dr. Robert Gallo and coworkers isolated and described a human T-cell leukemia virus, now called "HTLV-1," from a form of human leukemia that originates in mature T cells. Although unusual in the white U.S. and European populations, this virus-associated leukemia is more common in Caribbean countries, southern Japan, and very likely Africa and South America. Human T-cell leukemia has no association with the more common, well-known types of

leukemia, like childhood leukemias, chronic leukemias, and the majority of adult acute leukemias. Human T-cell leukemia more closely resembles rare T-cell cancers that begin in the skin, such as mycosis fungoides and Sezary syndrome. Even so, the unique features of the leukemia from which HTLV-1 has been isolated lead scientists to believe that it is distinct from other, recognized T-cell cancers.

In human T-cell leukemia patients seen so far, the disease usually progresses rapidly, often with enlarged liver, spleen, and lymph nodes. High calcium levels and skin eruptions occur in more than half of these patients. Scientists have identified antibodies to HTLV-1 in blood samples from a small percentage of the population who live in areas where the virus is more common. It is estimated, however, that only about 1 in every 80 individuals infected by HTLV-1 actually develops cancer. Researchers believe the virus can only be spread by prolonged, intimate contact and is not contagious like influenza or other common viral diseases.

It is known that feline leukemia can be transmitted from one cat to another by a retrovirus.

National Cancer Institute scientists conducted laboratory tests on blood samples of pet owners, veterinarians, research workers who handle these viruses, cancer patients, and people from the general population. In spite of extensive attempts to detect antibodies against the virus or other indications of infection, none of the groups showed evidence of infection. At the present time, therefore, this virus is not considered a causative agent of leukemia in humans.

Chemicals and Drugs

Long-term exposure to certain chemicals and drugs has been linked with a higher risk of various forms of leukemia. One such chemical is benzene, an aromatic hydrocarbon found in petroleum and coal-tar distillates. The risk of acute leukemia is estimated to be 20 times higher for workers heavily exposed to benzene than for the general population. Therapeutic drugs known to cause chromosomal damage or to interfere with bone marrow function, such as chloramphenicol and phenylbutazone, are also associated with a higher incidence of leukemia years after treatment began.

Despite their effectiveness in treating cancer, some anticancer drugs are believed to be cancer-causing agents themselves. A number of studies have shown an association between some drugs used to treat cancer and the development of second cancers years later. A class of anticancer drugs called alkylating agents, for example, has been linked with the later development of acute leukemia in some patients treated for Hodgkin's disease or ovarian cancer. The risk of leukemia, estimated by most studies at around 5 percent 10 years after treatment, seems highest in patients age 40 and over who have been treated with intensive chemotherapy alone or in combination with intensive radiotherapy.

These findings do not suggest that patients treated with alkylating agents (e.g., nitrogen mustard or cyclophosphamide) should stop or avoid their use. The proven benefits of these drugs, which are capable of curing diseases that would otherwise soon be fatal, far exceed their risks. The findings do suggest caution in using them for the treatment of cancer patients at low risk of relapse, and for patients with noncancerous conditions. In these two groups, dose and duration of the use of these drugs should be kept to a minimum.

Symptoms

It is often difficult to make an early diagnosis of leukemia. Some of the first signs of acute leukemia are identical to those of common infectious illnesses. In children, the symptoms may be even less specific, resembling the day-to-day fluctuations in energy, appetite, and temperament also seen in healthy children.

Fever and influenza-like symptoms may be the first signs of acute leukemia. The lymph nodes, spleen, and liver become infiltrated with white blood cells and may be enlarged. Bone or joint pain, paleness, weakness, tendency to bleed or bruise easily, and frequent infections are associated symptoms. The symptoms of acute lymphocytic leukemia may be the same as those for acute myelocytic leukemia.

The symptoms of chronic leukemia, if any, are generally more subtle. In fact, the disease is often discovered when a patient is examined for an unrelated complaint. When symptoms do occur, they may be a general feeling of ill health, fatigue, lack of energy, fever, loss of appetite, or night sweats. Some patients may notice enlarged lymph nodes in the neck or groin. Some may show signs of an enlarged spleen, anemia or infection.

Detection and Diagnosis

Leukemia can only be diagnosed by microscopic examination of the blood and bone marrow. A blood test may show low hemoglobin, low levels of normal white cells, and a low platelet count. Leukemic blast cells may be present. While these findings suggest a diagnosis of leukemia, a bone marrow biopsy (obtained by inserting a needle into the bone and withdrawing a small tissue sample) is needed to confirm the diagnosis and predominant cell type. Several bone marrow samples are taken to assess the extent of disease, since abnormal cell growth may vary from site to site. Using cell markers, researchers are able to identify the major leukemic cell type or types involved. Cell marker studies are especially useful to help distinguish acute B-cell from T-cell leukemia. Following diagnosis, a sample of cerebrospinal fluid from the lumbar region of the spine is examined for signs of leukemic cell infiltration of the central nervous system.

The presence of Auer rods, or rod-shaped granules, in the cellular material outside the nucleus of leukemic cells helps identify acute myelocytic leukemia. Researchers have noted that Auer rods also are a valuable predictor of treatment response. Patients with Auer rod-positive leukemia generally achieve higher rates of remission, and longer periods of remission, than patients with Auer rod-negative leukemia.

These and other advances in immunology and biochemistry are helping scientists identify patients at high risk of recurrence and plan their therapy accordingly.

Treatment

Researchers have made such strides in treating acute childhood leukemia that it is now considered one of the most curable forms of cancer. Thirty years ago a child with acute lymphocytic leukemia—the major childhood cancer—lived only about 3 months after diagnosis. In the past decade alone, the number of children with ALL alive 4 years after diagnosis has increased from 51 percent to 65 percent. In adults, the once grim outlook for acute lymphocytic leukemia has also improved dramatically, with recent studies reporting up to 50 percent 5-year survival for adults with ALL.

Progress in treating acute myelocytic leukemia, although slower in coming, has been steady. Using anticancer drugs, doctors are now able to induce remission—restore normal bone marrow function and eradicate leukemic cells—in about 70 percent of AML patients. Despite this initial remission, most patients with acute myelocytic leukemia eventually relapse. However, new treatment approaches stressing intensive chemotherapy, supportive care during treatment, and, in some cases, bone marrow transplantation, are beginning to achieve prolonged survival—up to 25 percent in some studies.

The slowly progressing chronic leukemias have been less responsive to known therapies than the acute leukemias. Chemotherapy given during the chronic phase of the disease usually destroys enough leukemic cells to keep the patient symptom-free for years. Recently, however, leukemia specialists have begun using intensive chemotherapy and new approaches to supportive care during treatment in an attempt to achieve complete remission, and with it, the hope of prolonged cure.

The goal of leukemia treatment is to achieve and prolong remission—the disappearance of all signs of disease—by ridding the body of all abnormal blood cells and restoring the normal balance of less than 5 percent blasts in the bone marrow. The state of complete remission occurs when symptoms disappear and abnormal cells are no longer found in the bone marrow and bloodstream. Complete remission does not always mean cure, though, since residual leukemic cells may still be present and multiply over time. If leukemic cell growth recurs, the patient is considered to be in a state of relapse.

Acute Leukemia

When acute leukemia is diagnosed, abnormal white blood cells usually make up 50 percent or more of the white cells in the bone marrow. Often, there are signs of leukemic cell infiltration of the spleen, lymph nodes, liver, and other tissues. Blood samples show abnormally low levels of red cells, platelets, and mature white cells. Leukemic cells may be found in the bloodstream, but their numbers do not always correspond to the amount of abnormal blood cell growth in the bone marrow. Left untreated, acute leukemia leaves the body open to infection and bleeding, and is rapidly fatal.

The mainstay of treatment for acute leukemia is combination chemotherapy, although radiation therapy and bone marrow transplantation may also be used. Anticancer drugs may be given orally, intravenously, or intramuscularly.

Treatment begins with induction therapy, which usually lasts 4 to 6 weeks. This is the most intensive stage of treatment since its purpose is to destroy as many abnormal white blood cells as possible. Combinations of the following drugs have proved highly effective in obtaining remission in patients with acute leukemia:

vincristine (Oncovin)
cyclophosphamide (Cytoxan)
prednisone
doxorubicin (Adriamycin)
6-mercaptopurine
cytosine arabinoside (Ara-C)
daunorubicin
methotrexate
thioguanine
asparaginase
rubidazone

Induction treatment for AML differs from that for ALL in the combinations and dosages of drugs used. For childhood acute lymphocytic leukemia, combinations of vincristine and prednisone, together with asparaginase or daunorubicin are standard initial therapy, inducing remission in 95 percent of cases. (More intensive regimens are under study, especially for patients who are at high risk.) Despite this initial success, however, cancer cells often become resistant to even the most effective anticancer drugs. Research has clearly shown that without the second phase of treatment, called consolidation therapy, the leukemia quickly recurs. It is the goal of this second phase to kill any cancer cells that survived the first stage of treatment. Drugs commonly used for consolidation therapy are:

methotrexate
cyclophosphamide
cytosine arabinoside
6-mercaptopurine
asparaginase
daunorubicin
thioguanine
carmustine (BCNU)

During consolidation therapy, specialists often use different anticancer drugs in an effort to overcome possible cancer cell resistance to drugs administered earlier. Another cornerstone of therapy for ALL, which helps reduce the chances of relapse, is to treat the central nervous system directly (see *Central Nervous System Therapy*).

Maintenance chemotherapy, the final stage of treatment for childhood ALL, is given over a longer period of time (2 to 3 years), but its purpose is the same—to destroy all residual cancer cells. In AML, however, the role and duration of maintenance chemotherapy is still under study.

In general, children with acute leukemia respond better to chemotherapy than adults. Scientists think this may be due to biologic differences in the leukemic cells. In addition, children are better able to tolerate intensive chemotherapy.

Acute lymphocytic leukemia is a less common disease in adults, and the prognosis for adult ALL patients tends to be poorer. With new strides in chemotherapy, however, the outlook for adults with ALL has brightened. Initial treatment, which produces remission in 80 to 90 percent of cases, usually consists of high doses of vincristine and prednisone, plus other anticancer drugs like daunorubicin and asparaginase. This is followed by consolidation therapy with a different combination of drugs. Various combinations and schedules have achieved similar results. The patient then receives lower doses of maintenance chemotherapy over a 30-month period in an attempt to kill any remaining cancer cells.

Acute myelocytic leukemia is more resistant to treatment than ALL, so higher doses of chemotherapy may be needed to obtain remission. The need for supportive care, with antibiotics and blood transfusions, is also greater for AML patients, due to the side effects of intensive chemotherapy and the reduced immunity associated with the disease itself.

Daunorubicin is probably the single most effective drug for the treatment of AML. Combining daunorubicin with Ara-C has resulted in complete remission rates of 60 to 80 percent. Some cancer centers are using more intensive induction regimens involving very high doses of Ara-C or the addition of other drugs such as 6-thioguanine.

Investigators are also working on ways to induce second remissions in AML patients whose disease has become resistant to standard therapy. Some of the newer agents that appear from clinical trials to be active in relapsed AML are m-AMSA, mitoxantrone, diaziquone, and homoharringtonine.

Another approach to treating the relapsed leukemia patient is bone marrow transplantation. This procedure is discussed more fully under the heading *Bone Marrow Transplantation.*

Central Nervous System Therapy

The blood-brain barrier is a network of selectively permeable capillary walls that prevent anticancer drugs from reaching the brain and spinal cord, thus creating a natural haven for cancer cells. In the past, patients with ALL often had a relapse of leukemia in the central nervous system (CNS) despite intensive chemotherapy. This discovery led scientists to develop a special approach, called CNS preventive therapy or CNS prophylaxis, to attack hidden cancer cells early in treatment. CNS prophylaxis generally consists of whole brain irradiation combined with the injection of drugs, such as methotrexate, in the cerebrospinal fluid (intrathecal chemotherapy).

CNS prophylaxis plays a crucial role in the treatment of acute lymphocytic leukemia. Without it, ALL patients run a serious risk of relapse. Yet CNS therapy has itself been linked with certain temporary as well as long-term side effects. In one followup study of children who received combined radiation and intrathecal chemotherapy, NCI researchers noted learning problems, such as in the development of mathematical skills, and loss of motor function in treated children when compared to their healthy siblings. These effects were more pronounced in children who received treatment before 5 or 6 years of age.

Intensive research is under way at cancer centers nationwide to find alternative approaches to CNS preventive therapy that provide the same protection but are not associated with long-term side effects. NCI investigators have been studying high-dose infusion of methotrexate into the bloodstream to see if this method is an equally effective, but perhaps less toxic, way of killing cancer cells in the central nervous system. Other studies are attempting to reduce the dose of radiation or eliminate radiotherapy altogether, depending on the patient's risk of relapse.

Scientists are uncertain about the need for CNS prophylaxis in the treatment of acute myelocytic leukemia. CNS involvement is less common in AML than in ALL, but as survival for AML patients increases—and with it the chances of relapse in the central nervous system—CNS therapy may play an increasingly important role.

Supportive Care

Long-term studies of various drug combinations are helping scientists identify the safest, most effective therapy for acute leukemia. Many of the drugs now used to combat leukemia injure normal cells as well as cancer cells, so managing chemotherapy's side effects is an important part of treatment. Both drugs and leukemia interfere with the patient's ability to produce two important blood elements: platelets, which are essential for blood clotting, and white blood cells (granulocytes), which help control infection. In the last few years, great strides have been made in controlling hemorrhage and infection, the two most common causes of death in leukemia patients.

Transfusions of blood platelets have reduced the rate of fatal hemorrhage fourfold during the last decade, making it possible to use effective anticancer drugs even though they may depress platelet production. In some cases, patients become resistant to platelets obtained from persons of different platelet "types." When this occurs, the donated platelets are rapidly destroyed, and the patient is again in danger of hemorrhage. Fortunately, platelets can be typed according to a histocompatibility system (HL-A). Studies at the National Cancer Institute have shown that HL-A-matched platelets often survive normally in patients who have become resistant to nonmatched platelets.

HL-A typing can thus frequently identify a suitable donor. Further research has shown that platelets obtained from the patient in remission can be frozen and reinfused during relapse.

The success achieved with platelet transfusion prompted NCI scientists to attempt granulocyte (white cell) replacement for treatment of infection in acute leukemia patients. Granulocyte transfusions may help an occasional patient with bacterial infections, but it has been difficult to obtain enough of these cells from normal blood donations to justify their routine use.

Another approach to controlling infection in leukemia patients is the use of relatively germ-free environments plus decontamination procedures, to reduce contact with bacteria. Germ-free, laminar air-flow rooms developed by NCI are now used at major cancer centers throughout the country for certain patients at very high risk of infection.

Newly developed antibiotics are very useful in the treatment of bacterial infections. Aggressive antibiotic therapy has greatly aided the treatment of infectious complications in cancer patients. A search is under way for antibiotics that are more effective against certain resistant bacteria, fungi, and viruses.

Bone Marrow Transplantation

Bone marrow transplantation is a highly technical procedure that may help some leukemia patients who have relapsed, are at high risk of relapse, or have failed to respond to chemotherapy. Recently, it has become clear that bone marrow transplantation is more likely to succeed in patients transplanted during remission than in those who undergo the transplant during relapse or partial remission. For this reason, some researchers believe transplantation should be performed during the first remission in AML patients and during the second remission for poor-risk ALL patients who have an immunologically matched donor, usually a brother or sister.

To prepare the patient for a bone marrow transplant, specialists administer intensive chemotherapy and whole body irradiation in an effort to destroy all leukemic cells. The dosages must be so high that the bone marrow is destroyed, leaving the patient wholly dependent on supportive care for defense against infection and hemorrhage. In allogeneic transplantation, a small amount of the marrow from a matched donor is then infused into the patient's bloodstream. The donated cells travel from the blood to the bones and in time grow into functioning marrow.

One major problem with allogeneic bone marrow transplantation is the risk of graft-versus-host disease (GVHD), a potentially fatal reaction in which the donated bone marrow rejects the tissue of the patient. Despite improved matching techniques, GVHD is not uncommon. The high risk of GVHD, recurrent leukemia, and fatal infection following bone marrow transplantation are the main reasons why this procedure is only considered as a last resort.

Autologous, or "self," bone marrow transplantation is an experimental approach that may play a broader role in the treatment of leukemia because it sidesteps the problem of GVHD. Some of the patient's own bone marrow is removed during remission, frozen, and then reinfused if the patient relapses. Research now is focusing on ways to cleanse the withdrawn marrow of cancer cells and to improve therapy immediately before transplantation in order to reduce the chances of recurrence.

Immunotherapy

Research has shown immunotherapy to be of little value against large numbers of leu-

kemia cells. Its use has therefore been limited to patients in remission with the goal of prolonging the disease-free period. Intensive research continues on ways to stimulate the body's natural immune defenses against disease. So far, however, results of studies using immunotherapy in the most common types of leukemia have proved disappointing.

Chronic Lymphocytic Leukemia

Chronic lymphocytic leukemia is a disease of old or middle age in which there is an abnormal increase in lymphocytes. The course of CLL varies a great deal from person to person. Generally, however, the disease begins slowly and progresses to an aggressive stage after a period of years.

Doctors generally favor monitoring the patient and delaying anticancer treatment until symptoms, such as anemia or lymph node enlargment, appear. Most patients respond well to moderate doses of chemotherapy, such as chlorambucil (or another alkylating agent) with or without prednisone. Radiation therapy also produces remission in a large number of patients. A recent study reported good results in obtaining remission by combining low-dose total body irradiation with cyclophosphamide and prednisone.

Initially, chronic lymphocytic leukemia responds well to treatment. Eventually, however, leukemic cells develop resistance to therapy, and most patients relapse. Various studies are using experimental chemotherapies, both as single agents and in combination, to overcome drug resistance. More information about such studies may be obtained from PDQ, NCI's database of clinical trials, which is described on the next page.

Hairy Cell Leukemia

At diagnosis, patients with hairy cell leukemia may have an enlarged spleen and a deficiency of red blood cells, white blood cells, and platelets. Although rarely cured, many patients have prolonged survival with little or no therapy. If the disease shows signs of progressing, most patients respond well to splenectomy, or removal of the spleen. Patients who relapse or fail to improve after splenectomy often benefit from treatment with alpha interferon, which was recently approved by the Food and Drug Administration as an effective therapy for hairy cell leukemia.

Low-dose alklyating agents, like chlorambucil, may be useful in treating persistent leukemia. According to recent studies, an experimental drug called pentostatin (2'-deoxycoformycin) may also have a promising role in the treatment of hairy cell leukemia.

Chronic Myelogenous Leukemia

Chronic myelogenous leukemia is a slowly growing form of leukemia found mainly in adults. CML usually begins with a chronic, treatable stage of low-grade leukemia that may persist for years before progressing to an acute phase of disease. During the chronic phase, practically all CML patients respond well to chemotherapy. Standard therapy consists of oral doses of busulfan (Myleran) or hydroxyurea. Rarely, however, does treatment eradicate the abnormal Philadelphia chromosome often found in the white cells of CML patients.

CML becomes more resistant to treatment once it progresses to the acute phase. Patients with high levels of lymphocytes may respond to vincristine and prednisone, anticancer drugs used in

254

the treatment of acute lympho-cytic leukemia. Other combinations of anticancer drugs are also being studied in an attempt to control the growth of resistant leukemic cells. Younger patients with matched donors should be considered for bone marrow transplantation while they are still in the chronic phase.

PDQ

The National Cancer Institute has developed PDQ (Physician Data Query), a computerized database designed to give doctors quick and easy access to:

- the latest treatment information for most types of cancer;
- descriptions of clinical trials that are open for patient entry; and
- names of organizations and physicians involved in cancer care.

To get access to PDQ, a doctor may use an office computer with a telephone hookup and a PDQ access code or the services of a medical library with on-line searching capability. Most Cancer Information Service offices (1-800-4-CANCER) provide a physician with one free PDQ search and can tell doctors how to get regular access to the database. Patients may ask their doctor to use PDQ or may call 1-800-4-CANCER themselves. Information specialists at this toll-free number use a variety of sources, including PDQ, to answer questions about cancer prevention, diagnosis, and treatment.

Suggestions for Additional Reading

Materials marked with an asterisk (*) are available from the National Cancer Institute (NCI). Other items can be found in medical libraries, many college and university libraries, and some public libraries.

Bone Marrow Transplantation: Questions and Answers. Prepared by the Leukemia Society of America, 733 Third Ave., New York, NY 10017.

Research Report: Bone Marrow Transplantation. Prepared by the Office of Cancer Communications, National Cancer Institute. NIH Publication No. 86-1178.

Bortin, M.M. et al. "Bone Marrow Transplantation for Acute Myelogenous Leukemia: Factors Associated with Early Mortality," *Journal of the American Medical Association,* Vol. 249(9), March 4, 1983, pp. 1166-1175.

Cancer Rates and Risks. Prepared by the Office of Cancer Communications, National Cancer Institute. NIH Publication No. 85-691.

Champlin, R.E. and Golde, D.W. "Chronic Myelogenous Leukemia: Recent Advances," *Blood,* Vol. 65(5), May 1985, pp. 1039-1047.

**The mentioned text is reprinted within this book. See CONTENTS for location.*

Clavell, L.A. et al. "Four-Agent Induction and Intensive Asparaginase Therapy for Treatment of Childhood Acute Lymphoblastic Leukemia," *New England Journal of Medicine,* Vol. 315(11), Sept. 11, 1986, pp. 657-663.

Cohen, H. and Boros, L. "Environmental Exposure: Its Role in Acute Leukemia," *Your Patient and Cancer,* Vol. 3, 1982, pp. 56-62.

DeVita, V.T., Jr. et al., eds. *Cancer: Principles and Practice of Oncology.* 2nd ed. Philadelphia: Lippincott, 1985.

Gunz, F.W. and Henderson, E.S. *Leukemia.* 4th ed. New York: Grune and Stratton, 1983.

Jacobs, A.D. and Gale, R.P. "Recent Advances in the Biology and Treatment of Acute Lymphoblastic Leukemia in Adults," *New England Journal of Medicine,* Vol. 311(19), Nov. 8, 1984, pp. 1219-1231.

Margolies, C.P. and McCredie, K.B. *Understanding Leukemia,* New York: Charles Scribners, 1986.

Moore, I.M. et al. "Late Effects of Central Nervous System Prophylactic Leukemia Therapy on Cognitive Functioning," *Oncology Nursing Forum,* Vol. 13(4), July/Aug. 1986, pp. 45-51.

Owens, M.R. "Chronic Lymphocytic Leukemia: Histopathology, Diagnosis and Staging," *Primary Care and Cancer,* Vol. 6(11), Nov. 1986, pp. 10R-60R.

Owens, M.R. "Chronic Lymphocytic Leukemia: Treatments of Choice," *Primary Care and Cancer,* Vol. 7(1), Jan. 1987, pp. 270R-320R.

Poplack, D.G. "Acute Lymphoblastic Leukemia and Less Frequently Occurring Leukemias in the Young." In *Cancer in the Young* (Levine A.S., ed.). New York: Masson Publishing, 1982, pp. 405-461.

Quesada, J.R. et al. "Alpha Interferon for Induction of Remission in Hairy Cell Leukemia," *New England Journal of*

Medicine, Vol. 310(1), Jan. 5, 1984, pp. 15-18.

Radiation Risks and Radiation Therapy, Medicine for the Layman Series. Prepared by the Clinical Center, Building 31, Room 2B58, National Institutes of Health, Bethesda, MD 20892. NIH Publication No. 83-2367.

Shottenfeld, D. and Fraumeni, J., eds. *Cancer Epidemiology and Prevention.* Philadelphia: W.B. Saunders, 1982, pp. 728-738.

Spiers, A.S.D. et al. "Remissions in Hairy Cell Leukemia with Pentostatin," *New England Journal of Medicine,* Vol. 316(14), Apr. 2, 1987, pp. 825-830.

Talpaz, M. et al. "Hematologic Remission and Cytogenic Improvement Induced by Recombinant Human Interferon Alpha$_A$ in Chronic Myelogenous Leukemia," *New England Journal of Medicine,* Vol. 314(17), Apr. 24, 1986, p. 1065-1069.

Thomas, E.D. et al. "Marrow Transplantation for the Treatment of Chronic Myelogenous Leukemia," *Annals of Internal Medicine,* Vol. 104(2), Feb. 1986, pp. 155-163.

Wiernik, P.H. "Acute Nonlymphocytic Leukemia in Young People." In *Cancer in the Young* (Levine A.S., ed.). New York: Masson Publishing, 1982, pp. 461-472.

Additional Information

The Leukemia Society of America, Inc., is a voluntary health agency that sponsors leukemia research, provides financial aid to patients, and conducts programs in public and professional education about leukemia. For further information, contact your local chapter or the national headquarters, Leukemia Society of America, Inc., 733 Third Avenue, New York, NY 10017 (212/573-8484).

Chapter 16

Cancer of
the Lung

Introduction

Research Report: Lung Cancer describes current research on the causes, prevention, detection, symptoms, diagnosis, and treatment of lung cancer. The information presented here came from medical textbooks, recent articles in the scientific literature, discussions with National Cancer Institute (NCI) scientists, and various scientific meetings.

Description and Function of the Lungs

The lungs, which are part of the respiratory system, are a pair of cone-shaped organs composed of pinkish-gray, spongy tissue that occupy most of the chest cavity, or thorax. They are separated from each other by the mediastinum, containing the heart and its large blood vessels, the trachea (windpipe), esophagus, thymus gland, and lymph nodes. The surface of each lung closest to the mediastinum contains a slit called the hilus, through which the bronchi (air tubes), pulmonary blood vessels, and nerves enter and exit.

The right lung, divided into three sections or lobes, is slightly larger than the left lung, which has two lobes. Although fairly large, the lungs together weigh only about 2 pounds. They are filled with air and are enclosed and protected by a two-layer membrane called the pleura.

The function of the lungs is the continuous exchange of gases between the body and the atmosphere. They alternately exhale carbon dioxide, a waste product of the body's cells, and inhale oxygen, a necessity for cellular function. Oxygen-rich air enters the body through the nose and mouth and travels down the main passageway of the throat, or pharynx. From here it passes through the voice box, or larynx, and then into the chest through the tube-like structures of the tracheobronchial tree, which extend into the lungs.

The tracheobronchial structure looks like a tree placed upside down in the chest, with its trunk extending up into the throat.

Types of Lung Cancer

The World Health Organization classification of lung cancer specifies 13 different types according to the kind of cells that are involved. The four cell types described below make up more than 90 percent of all lung cancer cases. Sometimes, a single lung tumor contains more than one type of cancerous cell.

Small cell lung cancer (SCLC) comprises 20 to 25 percent of all cases of lung cancer. The tumor cells are small; they may be predominantly "oat celled" (cells resembling oats), "fusiform" (spindle shaped), or "polygonal" (many sided). Because of the microscopic appearance of SCLC cells, these cancers were at one time believed to be sarcomas (cancers originating in the bone and connective tissue). SCLC develops in the bronchial submucosa (a layer of tissue beneath the epithelium).

Epidermoid, or *squamous cell,* carcinoma of the lung makes up about 33 percent of all lung cancers. It often begins in the large bronchi and tends to remain localized in the chest for longer periods than other types of lung cancer. Patients with epidermoid carcinoma have a better 5-year survival rate than those with other types of lung cancer.

Adenocarcinoma, which accounts for 25 percent of lung cancers, is composed of cube- or column-shaped cells and often develops along the outer edges of the lungs and under the membranes lining the bronchi. This type of lung cancer has been found around scar tissue, but it is not known whether these scars are a result or a cause of the cancerous growth. Some recent reports indicate that the incidence of adenocarcinoma is increasing, and studies are under way to examine this possibility.

Large cell carcinoma comprises 16 percent of all lung cancer cases. These tumors originate most frequently in the smaller bronchi. The large cells found in this tumor include the two subtypes of giant cells and clear cells. A diagnosis of large cell lung cancer is made when the tumor cells cannot be classified as epidermoid, adenocarcinoma, or SCLC.

Epidermoid carcinoma, adenocarcinoma, and large cell carcinoma are grouped together under the general classification of "nonsmall cell lung cancer" (NSCLC). Their pattern of spread and treatment differ markedly from the other major type, small cell lung cancer.

This trunk (trachea) descends into the chest cavity and divides into the primary bronchi, one leading to the right lung and the other to the left. Each primary bronchus divides to form smaller bronchi—the secondary (lobar) bronchi. The secondary bronchi continue to branch, forming still smaller bronchi, called tertiary (segmental) bronchi, which eventually divide into bronchioles. The bronchioles end in about 300 million tiny air sacs called alveoli. The walls of the alveoli contain a network of capillaries. Through the walls of these tiny blood vessels, red blood cells exchange carbon dioxide for the oxygen in the alveoli. The lungs expel the carbon dioxide, and red blood cells carry the oxygen to all cells of the body.

Like all tissues and organs of the body, the lungs and tracheobronchial tree are composed of individual cells. Several different kinds of cells are found in the lining (epithelium) of the lungs and tracheobronchial tree. For example, some cells produce mucus, which covers the surface of the bronchial tubes and traps foreign particles in the air breathed in and out of the lungs. Other cells have tiny hairlike projections (cilia), which sweep mucus up toward the throat, helping to cleanse the lungs of impurities.

Normal cells divide and reproduce in an orderly manner, replacing worn-out and injured tissue. When cell division becomes disordered, abnormal growth takes place and masses of tissue known as tumors result. These tumors may be benign or cancerous. Benign tumors may interfere with normal organ function and crowd adjacent organs, but they do not spread to other parts of the body and generally are not life threatening. Cancerous growths compress, invade, and destroy normal tissue. In addition, cancer cells may break away from a tumor and spread (metastasize) through the blood and lymph systems to other parts of the body where they can form secondary tumors. Lung cancer cells most commonly travel to the adrenal glands, liver, brain, kidneys, and bones. Cancer cells that comprise these secondary tumors are usually identical to those of the primary cancer, and although another organ is affected, the disease is still lung cancer. Similarly, certain other kinds of cancers, such as breast cancer and a number of childhood cancers, including Wilms' tumor and Ewing's sarcoma, tend to metastasize to the lungs and form secondary tumors there.

NSCLC may be subdivided according to the microscopic appearance of the tumor cells. Cells that are termed "poorly differentiated" are very different in appearance from normal cells, while "well-differentiated" cells look more like normal ones.

A less prevalent type of lung cancer is the *carcinoid tumor,* which accounts for 2 percent of lung cancer cases. Carcinoids are composed of cells arranged in strands. They usually arise from glands near the bronchi.

Another uncommon lung cancer is *bronchioalveolar carcinoma,* a subtype of adenocarcinoma. This cancer develops around scars on the outer edges of the lungs. These cancer cells often produce mucin, a substance containing a complex of protein and polysaccharide—the main component of mucus.

The steps involved when normal cells become cancerous are not clearly understood. However, animal studies and data obtained from autopsies point to the following sequence of events in the case of epidermoid lung cancer. First, damage to the tissue causes a nonspecific inflammatory reaction, which is followed by changes in the mucus-secreting and ciliated cells. Second, the normal cells of the epithelium are replaced with abnormal cells (metaplasia). The metaplastic cells become more and more abnormal. Because these cellular changes have been observed in 93 percent of active smokers, but in only 6 percent of ex-smokers and 1 percent of nonsmokers, scientists believe that the process up to this point may be reversible. The next step in the process is called carcinoma *in situ,* meaning that the cells have become cancerous but have not spread from their site of origin. The events in the transition from carcinoma *in situ* to invasive cancer are not known, although research is under way to determine the steps in the invasion process.

Adenocarcinomas of the lung develop from immature (stem) cells in the epithelium or from the glands found below this tissue. The origin of large cell carcinoma is not known.

Similarly, the origin of SCLC is unknown, but scientists do have some theories about where these tumors develop. One concept is that SCLC arises in certain stem cells, called neuroendocrine cells, found in the lung. A neuroendocrine cell is one that is capable of releasing a hormone in response to stimulation of nerve cells.

Causes

Scientists believe that at least 80 percent of lung cancer is caused by substances that have been identified as carcinogens (capable of causing cancer). Because the tissue lining the lungs and tracheobronchial tree is directly exposed to inhaled air, it is a target for airborne carcinogens and, in fact, most lung cancers develop in the epithelial cells of the bronchial tree. Although several environmental agents are known to cause lung cancer, tobacco smoke is unquestionably the major culprit.

Smoking appears to cause all types of lung cancer, although it is most strongly associated with epidermoid carcinoma and SCLC. Overall, smokers are 10 times more likely to die from lung cancer than are nonsmokers, and it is clear that the risk of developing lung cancer increases with the number of cigarettes smoked. However, this risk gradually begins to level off upon cessation of smoking, and after 15 to 20 years the ex-smoker's risk of dying from lung cancer is similar to that of an individual who has never smoked. Persons who smoke filtered, low-tar cigarettes generally have a lower lung cancer risk than those who smoke nonfiltered, high-tar

cigarettes. However, the cancer risk for such smokers is still far greater than for nonsmokers.

Still, not all heavy smokers develop lung cancer, and not all people with lung cancer are heavy smokers. About 10 to 20 percent of all cases of lung cancer occur in nonsmokers. Occupational hazards, air pollution, and other environmental factors have been implicated.

Workers who are exposed to carcinogens face an even greater chance of developing lung cancer if they smoke cigarettes. For example, epidemiologic studies show that workers in the asbestos industry who have been exposed to large concentrations of asbestos dust have a risk of lung cancer that is three to four times greater than that of workers who are not exposed to asbestos. Furthermore, the risk for asbestos workers who smoke cigarettes is 30 times greater than that of nonsmoking workers, and 90 times greater than workers who neither smoke nor work with asbestos.

Other workers facing an increased risk of lung cancer include uranium and fluorspar miners who inhale radon, a radioactive gas present in these mines. In addition, if these miners smoke, they are roughly 4 to 10 times more likely to develop lung cancer than co-workers who do not smoke. Studies of copper smelter workers in the western United States, Japan, and Sweden show an increased lung cancer risk among workers heavily exposed to arsenic, a byproduct of copper refining. Likewise, NCI scientists report an increased risk of lung cancer associated with employment for 15 years or more in the steel industry in eastern Pennsylvania. The researchers observed that long-term steel workers who were heavy smokers were at the greatest risk.

Several studies indicate that bis-chloromethyl ether (BCME) and chloromethyl methyl ether (CMME) may cause lung cancer. In a 5-year survey of CMME workers at a chemical manufacturing plant in the United States, the incidence of lung cancer was eight times higher than that of a comparable group of men with similar smoking histories in the general population. Similar studies in Germany and Japan have confirmed the high incidence of lung cancer among workers exposed to BCME.

Studies are under way to determine if involuntary smoking, or secondhand exposure to others' cigarette smoke, may be a cause of disability and disease, including cancer. Sidestream smoke (smoke released from a cigarette between active puffs) contains carcinogens similar to those in smoke that is directly inhaled. In a number of these epidemiologic studies it has been shown that there is an increased risk of lung cancer for non-smoking wives of smoking husbands. This growing body of evidence leads scientists to believe that there is a need to recognize and examine further the possible association between involuntary smoking and cancer.

Aside from the general risk of lung cancer from occupational and environmental exposures, some families may have an inherited susceptibility to the carcinogenic effects of these exposures. The exact role of genetic factors in causing lung cancer is still unclear. According to the current theory that the development of cancer is a multistage process, scientists believe that at least two independent events must occur to change a normal cell to a cancerous one. A genetic predisposition may be one such event, but in most instances it is probably not by itself enough to initiate a cancer.

Incidence and Mortality

Primary lung cancer accounts for about 15 percent of all cancer cases and 25 percent of all cancer deaths in the United States. It is the most common cause of cancer death among American men and is expected to surpass breast cancer in 1986 as the number one cause of cancer mortality in American women as well. The age at time of diagnosis is usually greater than 40, with a peak during the seventies.

For many years, lung cancer rates in the United States have increased rapidly. This increase in lung cancer follows by about 20 years a similar increase in cigarette smoking. However, incidence may be leveling off, corresponding to a reduction in cigarette consumption. It seems likely that, when rates are adjusted to take age into account, lung cancer rates will reach a plateau and begin to drop during the next few years.

Lung cancer is also the leading form of cancer in many other countries, particularly in western Europe and other parts of North America. At present, the incidence is comparatively low in China, India, and several Latin American and African countries. Yet, even in these areas of the world lung cancer ranks as one of the three most common types of cancer in men. In large part, the worldwide variation can be attributed to differences in tobacco use.

Lung cancer mortality rates also vary within countries, with a generally higher rate in urban areas and coastal communities. People in cities tend to smoke more than those on farms, but a small excess in deaths from lung cancer in urban areas is still evident after taking smoking behavior into account. NCI scientists have analyzed and mapped U.S. lung cancer mortality rates on a county level. The lung cancer pattern for white males revealed clustering in the Northeast and Midwest, but some of the highest mortality rates were found in coastal areas of the South.

Prevention

Cigarette smoking is responsible for about 85 percent of lung cancer deaths. If the number of smokers were cut by half, thousands of lives could be saved before the end of this century. As part of its prevention efforts, the NCI has established a Smoking, Tobacco, and Cancer Program, with a goal to reduce the incidence and mortality from cancer caused by or related to smoking and the use of tobacco products.

The NCI also has intensified research efforts in the area of chemoprevention of lung cancer. Chemoprevention is the use of natural and synthetic substances to reduce the incidence of cancer. One goal of this research is to find ways to halt or reverse the development of cancer in people already exposed to known or potential cancer-causing agents, such as those found in cigarette smoke. For example, one study will attempt to determine whether people with low dietary levels of selenium, an essential element found in seafoods, organ meats, and grains grown in some geographic areas, are at increased risk of developing lung cancer.

Intervention trials in chemo-prevention also are under way. These studies are attempting to determine the effect dietary sup-plementation and modification may have on lung cancer risk. In one such study, persons at high risk of lung cancer from occupational exposure to asbestos are receiving daily oral beta-carotene and retinol, which are precursors (substances from which other substances are formed) of vitamin A. Another trial involving cigarette smokers and ex-smokers is designed to assess the value of daily oral

vitamin A in preventing cancer. However, since conclusive data are not yet available on the effectiveness of this preventive approach, reducing smoking prevalence is still the NCI's highest prevention priority.

Basic research in lung cancer prevention is designed to identify exactly what causes a normal lung cell to become cancerous. Scientists have found genetic changes in the DNA (genetic material) of some lung cancer cells, which may provide clues in this area. Every cell in the body contains 23 pairs of thin strands of DNA. These strands, or chromosomes, contain regions known as genes, which are responsible for transmitting in-herited characteristics. Research-ers in several laboratories have isolated and cloned what they believe is a lung cancer gene (oncogene). Scientists believe that this research will ultimately be helpful in their efforts to develop more effective therapies for lung cancer.

Detection and Diagnosis

Early Detection

Early detection of lung cancer is not always possible. Present methods, using the most modern equipment, can disclose fewer than 25 percent of lung cancers at a localized stage when they can be effectively treated.

In an attempt to reduce lung cancer mortality, the NCI initiated the Cooperative Early Lung Cancer Detection Program to determine the effectiveness of screening programs for large groups of heavy smokers judged to be at high risk of developing this form of cancer. The Program is composed of three studies being conducted at Johns Hopkins Medical Institutions, Mayo Clinic, and Memorial Sloan-Kettering Cancer Center. The examinations used in the Program combine chest x-rays and sputum cytology (a microscopic examination of cells obtained from deep-cough sputum samples). Some scientists believe that sputum cytology may offer a method for earlier detection of lung cancer. Abnormal cells in the sputum can indicate a cancer too small to be seen in x-rays, but the presence of these cells cannot reveal the tumor's exact location. Consequently, if such cells are detected, further examination to identify the tumor site is necessary.

Results from the Program published to date indicate that some lung cancers can be detected at an earlier stage than was previously possible. However, this technique has not resulted in a reduction in mortality for the participants in the study. Long-term followup of the patients in the Cooperative Program is necessary to determine if earlier detection actually decreases mortality.

Symptoms

The symptoms of lung cancer can result from local tumor growth and invasion of adjacent structures; regional growth, including spread to nearby lymph nodes; spread of the cancer to distant parts of the body; and paraneoplastic syndrome, a variety of symptoms caused by hormones that are produced by lung cancer cells.

Lung cancers that originate and grow in the bronchi can produce a variety of symptoms—pain, cough, shortness of breath, pneumonia, hoarseness caused by pressure on a nerve, difficulty swallowing due to obstruction of the esophagus, and swelling of the neck, face, and upper extremities caused by pressure on blood vessels. Cancer cells that have broken away from the primary tumor and have spread to the brain, distant lymph nodes, bone, liver, or other parts of the body can cause a variety of symptoms. Depending on which organs are affected, these symptoms can include headache, weakness, pain, bone fractures, jaundice, and bleeding.

Paraneoplastic symptoms, which are most frequently associated with SCLC, can be caused by many different hormones. For example, some lung cancer cells produce arginine vasopressin (AVP), which acts on the kidneys to cause a drastic reduction of the concentration of sodium in the body. Sodium deficiency in turn causes severe confusion and may even produce coma. Another paraneoplastic symptom is caused by adrenocorticotropic hormone (ACTH), the hormone normally produced by the pituitary gland to act on the adrenal glands and regulate various body functions. Unrestrained ACTH production by lung cancer cells causes elevated blood sugar levels, diabetes, decreased concentration of potassium in the blood, and an increase in body fat and hair growth. Hypercalcemia (abnor-

mally high concentration of calcium compounds in the circulating blood), caused by production of a parahormonelike substance, occurs in about 5 percent of lung cancer patients. Symptoms produced by hypercalcemia include loss of appetite, nausea, drowsiness, constipation, and mental confusion.

Diagnosis and Staging

If lung cancer is suspected or detected, a patient undergoes a series of diagnostic tests designed not only to confirm the disease (diagnosis), but to determine how widely the cancer has spread (staging). The choice of therapy is based in large part on the type of cancer cell involved and the location and extent of the tumor.

The procedures used to diagnose and stage lung cancer depend on the individual situation. The first step for all patients, however, is a thorough physical examination, followed by chest x-rays. Following these procedures, it is necessary to obtain cells from any suspicious area for microscopic examination. These cells may be obtained by biopsy (removal of cells by needle aspiration or surgery) or by other techniques. For example, if the physician finds lymph glands above the collarbone that feel abnormal, they should be biopsied.

A diagnostic technique called bronchoscopy permits direct visual examination of the breathing tubes through a hollow lighted tube (a bronchoscope) inserted into the airways. This tube may be rigid or flexible, but with the advent of the flexible fiberglass bronchoscope, the use of a rigid bronchoscope is less common. The bronchoscope is inserted into the patient's nose or mouth and threaded into the bronchi. Special instruments can be passed through the bronchoscope to brush cells from the bronchial walls or snip tissue specimens for microscopic study. This procedure generally is done on an outpatient basis; the patient is given a local anesthetic and is awake during the procedure.

An experimental technique currently under study is called diagnostic fluorescence bronchoscopy. In this procedure, hematoporphyrin derivative (HPD), a nontoxic dye that is fluorescent under violet light and is attracted to cancer cells, is injected into the patient's bloodstream. Then, violet light from a krypton laser, a device that produces a powerful, narrow beam of light at one wavelength, is directed into the bronchial tubes by means of a fiberoptic bronchoscope. The dye causes a tumor to fluoresce under the light of the laser. One problem with this technique is that it is sometimes difficult to distinguish between the fluorescence of a very small tumor and the natural fluorescence of surrounding normal tissue.

A new technique that has proved useful for obtaining suspicious cells in areas not accessible to the bronchoscope is called transthoracic fine needle aspiration biopsy under fluoroscopic guidance. In this procedure, a needle is passed through the chest wall and directed to the abnormal tissue using fluoroscopy, an x-ray procedure that transmits an image to a fluorescent screen rather than a photographic plate. Fluoroscopy permits internal organs such as the heart to be observed while in motion.

To determine if the cancer has spread to the lymph nodes in the mediastinum, a procedure similar to bronchoscopy, called mediastinoscopy, may be employed. Because this test involves inserting the mediastinoscope through an incision above the collarbone, it must be conducted under general anesthetic and is not recommended for all patients. Mediastinotomy is a procedure similar to mediastino-scopy, except the incision is made either to the right or left side of the breastbone, rather than above the collarbone.

Using radioactive tracers, physicians may perform scans to locate tumors that have spread to the brain, bone, or liver. In these tests, a radioactive substance is injected into the bloodstream and is taken up by the body. Then a machine scans the patient to measure radiation emission levels, which indicate whether a tumor is present. Computed tomography (CT or CAT scans) also is used to determine if the cancer has spread. In a CT scan, an x-ray, cross-sectional image of a body part is produced with the aid of a computer and displayed on a cathode ray tube.

Other tests sometimes used to stage lung cancer patients include pulmonary angiography (an x-ray study in which dye or material visible on x-ray is injected into the blood vessels leading to the lung) and bron-chography (x-ray filming of the respiratory system after injection of a dye that makes the parts of the system visible on x-ray).

A sensitive new technique known as magnetic resonance imaging (MRI) produces images of the internal organs of the body without exposing the patient to ionizing radiation. Investigators are conducting studies to evaluate the usefulness of this technique in staging lung cancer.

Investigators also are trying to identify cell surface antigens and hormone receptors found on lung cancer cells. Hormone receptors are protein molecules located on the surface of cells to which hormones bind. When these antigens and receptors are identified, it may be possible to prepare monoclonal antibodies, pure antibodies specific against these receptors or antigens, and "tag" them with various radio-active isotopes. When injected into a patient's bloodstream, the antibodies circulate through the body, but bind only to the lung cancer cells, allowing researchers to identify lung cancer cells anywhere in the body.

Staging

Different staging systems are used for NSCLC and SCLC. A complex "TNM" system, pro-posed by the American Joint Committee for Cancer Staging and End Results Reporting, is usually employed for NSCLC. In this classification, T with digits 0, X, *is,* 1, 2, or 3 describe the size and extent of the primary tumor; N with digits X, 0, 1, or 2 tell whether regional lymph nodes have cancer cells in them; and M with digits X, 0, or 1 indicate whether the cancer has metastasized to distant parts of the body.

Doctors use this TNM system to divide NSCLC into four groups. A simplified description of this grouping is as follows:

Occult Stage: Cancer cells are present in lung secretions, but no tumor can be found in the lung.

Stage I: The tumor is smaller than 3 centimeters (cm).

Stage II: The tumor is larger than 3 cm and/or has spread only to lymph nodes located near the hilus or bronchi.

Stage III: The tumor is larger than 3 cm and/or has spread to lymph nodes located in the mediastinum and/or to distant parts of the body.

The detailed TNM system, however, is used less often to stage patients with SCLC. Instead, physicians use a simple two-stage system developed by the Veterans Administration Lung Cancer Study Group. In this system, SCLC is classified into two groups:

Limited Stage: The tumor is confined to the side of the thorax in which it originated, the mediastinum, and lymph nodes immediately above the collarbone.

Extensive Stage: The tumor has spread beyond the sites defined for limited-stage disease.

Treatment

Nonsmall Cell Lung Cancer

Patients with NSCLC generally can be divided into three groups, which reflect the extent of the disease and optimal treatment. The first group consists of patients whose tumors can be removed surgically (usually stages I and II). This operation may include removing a small portion of the affected lung (wedge resection), the entire lobe of the lung (lobectomy), or the entire right or left lung (pneumonectomy). Because patients with adenocarcinoma and large cell carcinoma have a high rate of brain metastases, some physicians also recommend preventive, or prophylactic, cranial irradiation (PCI). This group of patients has the best prognosis, with 30 to 80 percent surviving 5 years or more. Patients in this

271

group who cannot have their cancers removed surgically because of other medical conditions may be treated with radiation therapy. About 20 percent of them survive at least 5 years.

The second group consists of NSCLC patients whose tumors have invaded nearby tissue or have spread to mediastinal lymph nodes. Treatment for these patients usually consists of radiation therapy, sometimes in combination with other forms of treatment, especially surgery. Certain patients can be treated effectively with surgery, depending on the size and location of the tumor and affected nodes. About 10 percent of patients in this group survive 5 years.

The third group includes patients whose cancer has spread to distant parts of the body. Treatment for these patients is intended to shrink the tumor and relieve symptoms (palliative treatment). Radiation may be used to palliate symptoms from the primary tumor or from metastases in locations such as the bone or brain. Chemotherapy also may be employed as palliative treatment.

Because current methods of treatment for NSCLC are generally unsatisfactory, many scientists are conducting intensive research to find more effective therapies. Thus far, many combinations of anticancer drugs have been evaluated, and some look promising, but none has been shown to produce overall survival benefit. Studies with new drugs and new combinations of drugs are continuing. Some investigators are comparing the effectiveness of combination chemotherapy when used alone with the same drugs plus radiation therapy. In addition, scientists at several centers are looking at the usefulness of lasers in treating early-stage lung cancer and in relieving symptoms in advanced NSCLC and SCLC.

Other clinical studies are continuing to examine the effectiveness of whole-brain irradiation in preventing the spread of nonsmall cell cancers to the brain and the usefulness of radiation therapy following surgical removal of tumors that have invaded nearby tissue in the chest wall.

An important area of research centers on the role that biological response modifiers (BRMs) may play in NSCLC treatment. BRMs are substances that boost, direct, or restore many of the normal defenses (immune response) of the body. One such BRM is thymosin, a protein made by the thymus gland, which helps immature immune cells grow and develop. Clinical trials are in progress to determine if thymosin administered after radiation therapy to the primary tumor and mediastinum will improve survival rates for patients with nonmetastatic NSCLC.

Another BRM is bacillus Calmette-Guerin (BCG), a vaccine that has long been used to immunize patients against tuberculosis. Although previous studies with BCG have not shown a benefit in treatment of NSCLC, researchers are continuing to evaluate variations in BCG therapy following surgery. Another experimental approach using BRMs is known as radioimmunoglobulin therapy. In this technique, a radioactive element is coupled to specific monoclonal antibodies, which then bind to tumor cells. Studies are under way at a number of centers to evaluate this therapy for NSCLC patients. A clinical trial designed to test the safety and effectiveness of monoclonal antibodies coupled to anticancer drugs also has been initiated.

Small Cell Lung Cancer

Small cell carcinoma of the lung has a tendency to spread quickly to distant parts of the body, and these secondary tumors often cannot be detected by routine clinical tests. For these reasons, treatment such as surgery and chest radiotherapy are usually ineffective in controlling SCLC, even in patients with tumors that appear to be localized.

Patients with limited-stage disease are commonly treated with combination chemotherapy or chemotherapy plus chest irradiation. The radiotherapy is directed to the primary tumor, while the chemotherapy is intended to control secondary tumors in other parts of the body. Many different combinations of drugs have been used in chemotherapy for SCLC. Most programs employ a three- or four-drug regimen that includes cyclophosphamide plus two or three of the following agents: doxorubicin (Adriamycin), vincristine (Oncovin), methotrexate, CCNU (Lomustine), or etoposide (VP-16). The use of more than three or four drugs has not been shown to be beneficial. Chemotherapy produces a fourfold to fivefold improvement in median survival time and is usually effective in relieving symptoms that are present at the time of diagnosis.

Sometimes prophylactic cranial irradiation also is used for patients who respond to primary treatment. For SCLC patients with extensive disease, adding chest irradiation to chemotherapy does not appear to improve survival rates, although radiotherapy is important in relieving symptoms of metastatic disease. Long-term survival for SCLC patients in both staging groups using these treatments is about 7 percent overall: 10 to 30 percent for those with limited disease and 1 to 2 percent for patients with extensive disease.

Although surgical treatment for SCLC has been ineffective in most cases, the small group of patients whose disease is confirmed to be limited to its original location may benefit from resection. Some investigators believe that patients who respond to an initial course of chemotherapy also may be helped by subsequent surgical resection. Studies to examine this possibility are under way.

As in the case of NSCLC, a major effort is under way to find better forms of treatment for SCLC. One area of study is focusing on more effective ways to administer the anticancer drugs already in use and to identify new drugs that may prove more active against the disease. For example, investigators are trying to determine if very high doses of chemotherapy with and without radiation therapy and autologous bone

marrow transplantation will prove helpful in treating SCLC patients. The bone marrow, the spongy interior of the large bones, produces young blood cells—red cells, white cells and platelets. A bone marrow transplant replaces damaged marrow with healthy marrow. In autologous transplantation, the patient's own marrow is withdrawn before chemotherapy and/or radiotherapy, frozen, and reinfused into the patient after treatment. Bone marrow transplantation allows doctors to use very high doses of anticancer drugs and radiation— doses ordinarily precluded because they cause such severe damage to the bone marrow.

Clinical trials to find chemotherapies active against SCLC have been disappointing. However, recent basic research has yielded new knowledge about how this type of cancer behaves, so it is now possible to grow colonies of SCLC cells outside the body (*in vitro*). Cells obtained by biopsy can be grown in test tube cultures and exposed to various anticancer drugs to see which ones, if any, kill the cancer cells. NCI scientists are investigating the usefulness of this technique in both SCLC and NSCLC.

Other basic research with lung cancer cell cultures seeks to determine what these cells require to grow. After testing various growth factors and hormones, scientists have learned that, among those that stimulate cell growth, some (for example, insulin and transferrin) are produced outside the cells; others, called autocrine factors, are made by the cancer cells themselves (bombesin and arginine vasopressin). Because SCLC cell lines produce a bombesinlike substance, scientists are now attempting to develop ways to block the action of this growth-promoting substance and, thereby, halt tumor growth. One way to accomplish this may be through the use of monoclonal antibodies. Studies have shown that an antibombesin monoclonal antibody stopped tumor growth in mice, although some of these cancers did recur. Clinical trials have yet to determine whether this approach will be effective in humans.

As with NSCLC, scientists are examining the role that biological response modifiers may play in treating SCLC. Research is under way to evaluate the usefulness of thymosin when it is combined with radiation therapy and chemotherapy for patients with inoperable small cell lung cancer.

Suggestions for Additional Reading

Except as noted, the following materials are not available from the NCI. They can be found in medical libraries, many college and university libraries, and some public libraries.

*Cancer Rates and Risks.** Prepared by the National Cancer Institute. NIH Publication No. 85-691.

Clearing the Air: A Guide to Quitting Smoking. Prepared by the Office of Cancer Communications, National Cancer Institute. NIH Publication No. 84-1647.

DeVita, Vincent T., Jr. et al., eds. *Cancer: Principles and Practice of Oncology,* Second Edition. Philadelphia: J.B. Lippincott Company, 1985.

The Health Consequences of Smoking: Cancer, A Report of the Surgeon General. Office on Smoking and Health, U.S. Department of Health and Human Services. PHS Publication No. 82-50179.

Holland, James F. and Frei, Emil, III, eds. *Cancer Medicine,* Second Edition. Philadelphia; Lea and Febiger, 1982.

Ihde, Daniel. "Current Status of Therapy for Small Cell Carcinoma of the Lung," *Cancer,* Vol. 54, December 1984, pp. 2722-2728.

Shottenfeld, Daniel and Fraumeni, Joseph, eds. *Cancer Epidemiology and Prevention.* Philadelphia: W.B. Saunders, 1982.

Smoking and Health: A Report of the Surgeon General. Office on Smoking and Health, U.S. Department of Health, Education, and Welfare. PHS Publication No. 79-50066.

*What Are Clinical Trials All About?** Prepared by the Office of Cancer Communications, National Cancer Institute. NIH Publication No. 86-2706.

---

* *The mentioned text is reprinted within this book. See CONTENTS for location.*

Chapter 17

Melanoma

Introduction

This material describes current research on incidence, possible causes, prevention, detection, diagnosis, and treatment of melanoma. When this tumor develops in the skin, it is called melanoma, or malignant melanoma. When it affects the eye, it is called ocular melanoma. These two cancers are discussed separately.

This information was gathered from medical textbooks, recent articles in the medical literature, and discussions with researchers at the National Cancer Institute (NCI) and other scientists.

Knowledge about melanoma is increasing steadily. The most up-to-date information on this and other cancer-related subjects is available from the toll-free Cancer Information Service at 1–800–4–CANCER.

Cutaneous Melanoma

Description and Function of the Skin

As the body's outer covering, the skin offers protection from extreme temperatures, light, injury, infection, and many chemicals. The largest organ of the body, the skin

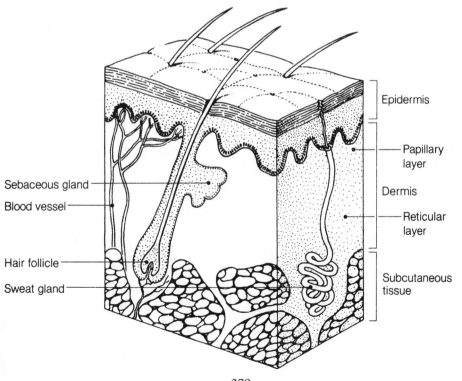

Sebaceous gland
Blood vessel
Hair follicle
Sweat gland

Epidermis
Papillary layer
Dermis
Reticular layer
Subcutaneous tissue

also regulates body temperature, stores water and fat, and helps to make vitamin D. By sending information to the brain about temperature, pressure, vibration, pain, and touch, the skin also senses the environment.

The skin has two main layers—the inner dermis and the outer epidermis. The dermis, in turn, is divided into an upper part called the papillary dermis and a lower portion named the recticular dermis. The dermis contains cells, fibrous tissue, blood and lymph vessels, sweat and sebaceous glands, and the follicles (hair shafts) through which hair grows. Blood vessels in the dermis supply the skin with nutrients. When sweat evaporates, it cools the skin and regulates body temperature. The sebaceous glands produce sebum, an oily substance that keeps the skin from drying out. Sweat and sebum reach the skin's surface through tiny openings called pores.

The epidermis, the outermost layer of the skin, is made up mostly of flat, scalelike cells called squamous cells. Less common are the round basal cells, found mainly in the lower part of the epidermis. This part of the epidermis also contains melanocytes, the cells that produce the pigment called melanin. The amount of melanin in the skin accounts for the variations in skin color found among different races and individuals.

Types of Skin Cancer

Skin cell growth begins at the base of the epidermis. New cells push older cells to the skin's surface, where they eventually die and flake off. In this way, the skin constantly repairs itself as new cells grow and multiply in an orderly way to replace dying ones.

Sometimes, though, cell growth becomes disordered, abnormal growth takes place, and a mass of tissue known as a tumor develops. Tumors can be either benign or malignant. Benign tumors are not cancer. They do not spread to other parts of the body and generally do not threaten life. Benign growths can usually be removed and seldom return. Malignant tumors are cancerous. They can invade and destroy healthy tissue and extend into nearby healthy tissues and organs. Cancer cells can also break away from the original (primary) tumor and spread, or metastasize, through the bloodstream or lymphatic system to form metastatic (secondary) tumors in distant organs. Cancer cells that make up secondary tumors are usually identical to those found in the primary cancer. Thus, although another part of the body is affected, the new tumor is still the same type of cancer.

280

Melanoma, the subject of this Research Report, is a serious type of cancer that develops in the melanocytes. This disease is diagnosed and treated differently from other (nonmelanoma) skin cancers. Melanoma spreads both by extension into neighboring tissues and to other parts of the body through the lymphatic system and bloodstream. Metastatic melanomas may involve any organ.

The two most common types of skin cancer are basal cell carcinoma, which arises in the basal cells, and squamous cell carcinoma, which begins in the squamous cells of the epidermis. These cancers are often diagnosed and treated in the same way and are almost always curable. They are discussed in *Research Report: Nonmelanoma Skin Cancers—Basal and Squamous Cell Carcinomas.** In addition to melanoma, other, much less common types of cancer that can affect the skin include Kaposi's sarcoma and cutaneous T-cell lymphoma (also called mycosis fungoides). These cancers are not discussed in this Research Report.

Incidence

Approximately 27,000 new cases of cutaneous melanoma and 5,800 deaths from this disease were estimated for the United States in 1988. The incidence of melanoma in this country has increased steadily over the past 40 years. The lifetime risk is now estimated to be about 0.8 percent. Whites develop melanoma much more frequently than blacks or Asians and, therefore, suffer many more deaths from the disease as well. In the United States, the annual incidence among whites approaches 10 per 100,000 individuals; in blacks, the rate is about 1 per 100,000.

Causes and Prevention

Causes

As with other forms of skin cancer, the development of cutaneous melanoma is related to exposure to ultraviolet (UV) radiation from the sun. UV radiation covers wavelengths between 0 and 400 nanometers (nm). The group of wavelengths between 290 and 330 nm, called UV-B, reaches the earth's surface and causes most of the sun damage to the skin. People who live close to the equator receive more direct sun and, if not protected by darker skin, are more susceptible to developing melanoma. For example, Australia, which receives a high level of UV-B radiation, has an annual incidence of more than 17 cases per 100,000 people—one of the highest rates in the world. In addition, the rate of new cases of melanoma in the southwestern United States is now equal to or greater than the rate in Australia.

---

* The mentioned text is reprinted within this book. See CONTENTS for location.

The rising incidence of melanoma may be due, in part, to changes in lifestyle and leisure activities. More people are exposing themselves to intense sunlight. In addition, concern is increasing that the atmosphere's ozone layer, which protects us from UV-B radiation, is being depleted by manmade products called chlorofluorocarbons, such as Freon. These products serve as propellants in aerosol sprays and as cooling agents in refrigerators and air conditioners. As the ozone layer thins, more UV-B radiation reaches the earth, increasing the likelihood that more cases of melanoma will be seen in the next decade.

Melanoma usually occurs in different areas of the body in light-skinned women and men. It develops most often on the arms and lower legs in women and on the head and neck in men. These sites are commonly exposed to light. However, another common site for melanoma to occur in men is the trunk. Because this site is not normally exposed to light, the relationship between UV-B exposure and melanoma location is not as clearcut as is the relationship of UV-B to the development of nonmelanoma skin cancers. It appears likely that other risk factors play a role in the development of melanoma.

There is evidence that certain types of moles known as dysplastic nevi may give rise to cutaneous melanomas. (Nevus is the medical term for mole.) These nevi, which are different from common moles, can be inherited (familial dysplastic nevi), or they may occur sporadically in people who have no family history of dysplastic nevi.

Individuals with dysplastic nevi should be monitored by a doctor to detect and remove abnormal moles that are likely to lead to melanoma. Photographs of nevi are often helpful for followup examinations. Dysplastic nevi are generally larger than ordinary moles and have irregular borders that fade into the surrounding skin. They may be flat or raised above the skin surface. Their color—usually not uniform—may be dark brown, sometimes with pink or red areas. While the average adult has 10 to 40 moles, persons with dysplastic nevi often have more than 100 unusual moles on their skin. More information about this condition is given in the NCI publication titled *About Dysplastic Nevi*.

People with dysplastic nevi may have an increased risk of developing melanoma during their lifetime. Melanoma usually develops in the dysplastic nevi but may also develop in normal skin. The risk of developing melanoma is increased more than a hundredfold for persons with dysplastic nevi who are also from melanoma-prone families (i.e., people with two or more first-degree relatives—parents, children, brothers, sisters—with melanoma). Adult family members who do not have dysplastic nevi appear to have a nearly normal risk of developing melanoma.

Melanoma is also related to other noncancerous conditions. People who sunburn easily and tan poorly or who have blue eyes, red hair, or many moles have a greater risk of developing melanoma than do people who do not have these characteristics. Individuals with very large moles (20 centimeters, or 7.8 inches, in diameter) that are present from birth have a 5 to 20 percent risk of developing melanoma. Also, people with xeroderma pigmentosum, a rare hereditary disease in which the skin and eyes are extremely sensitive to light, are 1,000 times more likely to develop melanoma than the general population.

Prevention

Reducing sun exposure is one of the easiest ways to decrease the risk of developing melanoma, particularly for those individuals in sun-sensitive high-risk groups. Ultraviolet radiation exposure can be reduced 50 percent by avoiding the sun between 11 a.m. and 1 p.m. (12 p.m. and 2 p.m., daylight saving time). During spring and summer months, exposure to sunlight should be gradual. During winter vacations to tropical areas, intense exposure to the sun should be limited. Wearing protective clothing (such as hats and long sleeves) and using an effective sunscreen are also important. Sunscreens that block UV radiation usually contain para-aminobenzoic acid (PABA) or related compounds; they are rated in strength from 2 to 15 or higher. This sun protection factor (SPF) must be printed on the container. The higher the SPF rating, the greater the blockage of UV radiation.

To prevent melanoma, a person with dysplastic nevi is best advised to avoid excessive sunlight and have changing moles (as described on pages 284-5) surgically removed. Dysplastic nevi on the scalp should be removed because it is difficult to see changes in growths covered by hair. Individuals with dysplastic nevi from families with multiple cases of melanoma should be examined on a regular basis.

Detection and Diagnosis

Melanoma can begin in an existing mole or as a new, mole-like growth. If detected early, it can be effectively treated and cured. The first warning signs of melanoma should be promptly brought to the attention of a physician:

- *Large size.* If there is an increase (gradual or sudden) in the size of a mole, it may be a melanoma. Melanomas generally are at least 5 millimeters (mm) across (about ¼ inch).

• *Multiple colors.* Melanomas tend to have a variety of colors—red, white, blue, and sometimes black or dark brown—within a single mole.

• *Irregular border.* Melanomas often have uneven or notched borders.

• *Abnormal surface.* A mole may be a melanoma if it is scaly, flaky, oozing, bleeding, or has an open sore that does not heal.

• *Unusual texture.* If a mole feels hard or lumpy, it may be a melanoma.

• *Abnormal skin around a mole.* If pigment, or color, from a mole has spread to surrounding skin or if nearby skin is red or swollen or has lost its pigmentation (becomes white or gray), a melanoma may be present.

• *Unusual sensation.* A mole may be a melanoma if it itches or is painful and tender.

• *Change in appearance of the skin.* Melanomas may develop as new pigmented spots in a skin area that had been normal.

While experienced physicians, especially dermatologists, can often identify a melanoma on sight, a biopsy is the only sure way to make a diagnosis. The biopsy—surgical removal of the mole—can usually be done using local anesthesia in a doctor's office. Suspicious-looking areas should never be burned off. By examining the tissue under a microscope, a pathologist can determine whether the growth is benign (a mole) or cancerous (a basal or squamous cell carcinoma or a melanoma).

Staging

Once melanoma has been diagnosed, other tests help determine the extent (stage) of the disease. Staging procedures generally include a thorough physical examination and various x-rays. The stage of the melanoma, which is an important factor in selecting treatment, is determined by the thickness of the growth, the depth of skin penetration, and whether the cancer has spread to nearby lymph nodes or distant parts of the body.

Microstaging

Various researchers have studied the relationship between prognosis (outcome of the disease) and either the level of skin invaded or the thickness of the melanoma. Dr. Alexander Breslow, at the George Washington University, suggested measuring the thickness of the tumor. When he grouped melanoma by thickness, he found that the thicker the growth, the more likely that metastasis had occurred. He also found that survival ranged from almost 100 percent for patients with growths equal to or thinner than 0.75 mm, about $\frac{1}{32}$ inch, to no greater than 20 percent for those with melanomas equal to or thicker than 4.0 mm (slightly greater than $\frac{1}{8}$ inch).

Dr. Wallace Clark, Jr., at the University of Pennsylvania, found that a deeper level of invasion was associated with a poorer prognosis. Clark's classification system groups melanomas into five levels:

Level I: A cancer involving only the epidermis (the outer skin layer). Characterized by the abnormal growth of cells (atypical melano-cytic hyperplasia), it is sometimes called melanoma *in situ* and may be regarded as nonmalignant.

Level II: Melanoma reaches into the papillary dermis (upper portion of the dermis).

Level III: Cancer extends to the bottom of the papillary dermis.

Level IV: Melanoma invades the reticular dermis (lower part of the dermis).

Level V: Cancer penetrates through the layers of the skin into the underlying tissue.

Stage of the Disease

The American Joint Committee on Cancer has developed a staging system based on coded descriptions of tumor size (T), lymph node involvement (N), and degree of metastasis (M). The amount of skin invasion determines the extent of the primary tumor. Cutaneous melanoma is classified TX when there is no evidence of primary tumor or this factor has not been or cannot be assessed; T0 when there is abnormal, but not cancerous, growth; or T with a number from 1 to 4, depending on the degree of skin invasion. Lymph nodes are classified NX if they cannot be assessed; N0 if no cancer cells are found in the node(s); or N with the number 1 or 2, depending on the location of the node(s) containing cancer cells. Distant metastases are classified as MX when metastases cannot be assessed; M0 when no distant disease is found; M1 when distant metastases are present in the skin or tissues underneath it; or M2 when the disease affects distant organs.

The following staging system takes into account microstaging (Breslow's classification and Clark's levels) and the extent of spread to lymph nodes or distant organs.

Stage 0:   Sometimes called *in situ;* Clark's level I.

Stage IA: Melanomas thinner than 0.75 mm ($\frac{1}{32}$ inch); Clark's level II. (T1, N0, M0)

Stage IB: Melanomas 0.76 mm to 1.5 mm ($\frac{1}{32}$ to $\frac{1}{16}$ inch) in thickness; Clark's level III. (T2, N0, M0)

Stage IIA: Melanomas 1.51 mm to 4.0 mm ($\frac{1}{16}$ to $\frac{1}{8}$ inch) in thickness; Clark's level IV. (T3, N0, M0)

Stage IIB: Melanomas 4.1 mm ($\frac{1}{8}$ inch) thick or greater; Clark's level V. (T4, N0, M0)

Stage III: Melanomas that have spread to only one group of nearby lymph nodes. (any T, N1, M0)

Stage IV: Melanomas that involve one enlarged and fixed lymph node group, more than one lymph node group, or another organ or area of skin. (any T, N2, M0; or any T, any N, M1 or M2)

Treatment

Treatment of melanomas that have not spread beyond the original area of growth (especially if they are thin and have not invaded the papillary dermis) is highly effective, and most of these cancers can be cured. Some melanomas that have spread to nearby lymph nodes also can be treated effectively. At present, however, current methods of therapy for melanomas that have spread to distant parts of the body are unsatisfactory, and many scientists are conducting basic research and clinical trials to find better forms of treatment.

Surgery

About 95 percent of all patients with melanoma are treated with surgery. When the tumor is thin and has not spread beyond the initial area of growth (stage I), it is usually curable with surgery alone. Generally, the doctor removes the growth and a border of normal tissue around it to eliminate any cancer cells that may have spread from the tumor. Researchers have found that the removal of tissue surrounding the cancer is necessary to prevent recurrence. Wide excision, the removal of a large margin of tissue around a melanoma, is used to treat stage II and stage III disease. For this procedure, a skin graft may be necessary. At this time, a clinical trial is being conducted to determine whether wide excision is equivalent to or better than removing a smaller border of tissue during treatment for stage I melanoma.

This trial will also determine

whether there is any benefit in taking out regional lymph nodes at the time a stage I melanoma is removed. Currently, lymph node removal is optional for treatment of stage I and stage II melanoma; removal may eliminate undetected cancer cells that have spread from the original cancer to the lymph nodes. Regional lymph nodes, or those affected by disease, are removed during a wide excision for stage III melanoma. For very advanced disease (stage IV), surgical removal of metastatic tumors and lymph nodes may help relieve symptoms and provide pain relief.

Chemotherapy
Patients with stage II and stage III melanoma face a high risk of disease recurrence. To improve the outlook for these patients, researchers are evaluating the use of chemotherapy to kill undetectable cancer cells that remain in the body after surgery (adjuvant chemotherapy). Drugs under investigation for the adjuvant treatment of stage II and stage III disease include carmustine (BCNU), cisplatin (Platinol), dacarbazine (DTIC), dactinomycin (Cosmegan), vinblastine (Velban), and vincristine (Oncovin).

An innovative method of administering chemotherapy is under investigation for patients with stage II or stage III melanoma in an arm or leg. Known as limb, or isolation, perfusion, this method enables patients to receive high doses of anticancer drugs in the affected area so that side effects are not experienced throughout the body. This technique is based on the heart-lung machine developed in the early 1950's for heart surgery. In isolation perfusion, blood is withdrawn from the patient and pumped through a special machine that adds oxygen and the anticancer drugs. The blood is then pumped back into the major artery supplying the limb being treated. Often, the blood is heated to enhance the effects of the drugs. Drugs commonly used for perfusion are melphalan (Alkeran), mechlorethamine (Mustargen), and DTIC.

Because current methods of treatment for advanced melanoma are generally ineffective, researchers are looking for new anticancer drugs and combinations of drugs that may prove useful. Although many drugs and drug combinations have been evaluated, none has improved long-term survival for patients with widespread disease. Thus, clinical trials with chemotherapeutic agents are continuing, and patients with advanced disease should consider participating in these trials to evaluate new treatments. Drugs under investigation for stage IV or recurrent melanoma include vincristine, cisplatin, carmustine, and dacarbazine.

Biological Therapy

Biological therapy, also called immunotherapy, is another important area of research. Scientists have identified a number of naturally occurring and synthetic substances called biological response modifiers (BRMs), which can boost, direct, or restore the body's normal defenses (immune system). Clinical trials are exploring the potential of various types of biological therapy, both alone and in combination with other forms of treatment such as chemotherapy.

Researchers are studying the usefulness of certain BRMs in the adjuvant treatment of melanoma. One such BRM is interferon, a protein formed in small amounts by the body's cells; it can now be produced in the laboratory using recombinant interferon technology. Clinical trials are under way to determine whether the addition of recombinant interferon to initial surgical treatment will prevent recurrence of melanoma.

Studies are also under way to evaluate treatment of metastatic melanoma (stages III and IV) with recombinant interleukin-2 (IL-2), a biological response modifier that activates the patient's white blood cells to form a unique type of killer cell. These cells, called lymphokine-activated killer (LAK) cells, destroy cancer cells. A patient may receive IL-2 alone or combined with LAK cells produced by treating the patient's white blood cells with IL-2. Thus far, results of studies with IL-2 and IL-2/LAK cell therapy have been promising. In other trials, monoclonal antibodies are combined with IL-2 or used alone for metastatic disease. Monoclonal antibodies are proteins produced in the laboratory. These special antibodies seek out specific cancer cells or parts of cancer cells; they can be bound to dyes, radioactive compounds, or poisons to locate and/or destroy the targeted cancer cells.

Radiation Therapy

Radiation therapy is of limited value in treating melanoma. However, in cases where the disease has spread (stage IV) to the lung, gastrointestinal tract, bone, or brain, radiation may provide relief from such symptoms as pain.

Recurrent Disease

Treatment for recurrent melanoma depends on prior therapy, the location and extent of recurrence, the patient's age and general health, and other factors. Investigational treatment, including chemotherapy and biological therapy, should be considered in patients with recurrent disease.

Followup Care

Because melanoma patients are at high risk for recurrence and for the development of new melanomas, they should be examined by a physician on a regular basis. Depending on the stage of the original growth, followup exams may include x-rays. Patients should also regularly examine their own skin.

Ocular Melanoma

Description and Function of the Eye

The eye is composed of three tissue regions and two inner cavities. The tissue regions are the outer group (the fibrous tunic) consisting of the sclera in the back of the eye and the cornea in the front; the middle group (the vascular tunic) consisting of the choroid, ciliary body, and the iris; and the inner retina, or nervous tunic. The anterior cavity located at the front of the eye and the posterior cavity at the back help give the eye its shape.

Sometimes, as described on page 280, normal pigmented cells grow in a disordered and abnormal way, giving rise to a cancerous tumor or

melanoma. Ocular melanoma develops in the pigmented vascular tunic. Also called the uvea, this area includes the iris, the ciliary body, and choroid. The iris is a circular group of muscles that contract or relax to control the amount of light entering the pupil. The ciliary body is located at the edges of the iris, to which it is attached. It contains a muscle that alters the shape of the lens, which sits behind the iris and focuses light. The lens also separates the two eye cavities. At the back of the eye, the ciliary body connects with the choroid layer. The choroid layer nourishes the layer above it, called the retina. Ocular melanoma may develop in any of these three structures (iris, ciliary body, or choroid).

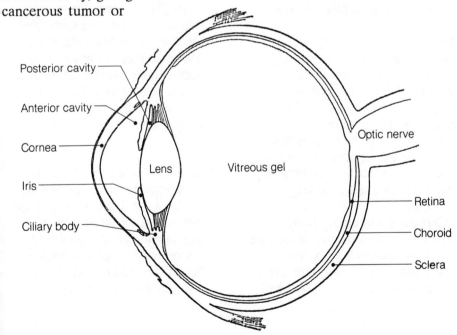

Incidence and Causes of Ocular Melanoma

Although ocular melanoma is the most common primary eye cancer in white adults, it is still very rare, with fewer than 6 new cases in every million people diagnosed each year. This form of melanoma is even rarer in blacks and Asians.

The causes of ocular melanoma are not well understood. One study suggests that sunlight plays a role in the development of this disease. Another study on the relationship of sunlight to this form of melanoma is in progress. Based on animal studies, some scientists believe that viruses and certain chemicals may be involved in the formation of ocular melanoma.

Symptoms and Diagnosis

Symptoms
Signs of this disease depend on where in the eye the cancer develops. Melanoma that develops in the iris may produce a pigmented spot, often noticed by the patient. Other signs include distortion of the pupil, presence of new blood vessels, curling of the iris near the pupil, and cataract formation.

Choroidal and ciliary body melanomas often reach a large size before symptoms are observed. These may include loss or deterioration of vision and the presence of floating spots. Cataracts, secondary glaucoma, and inflammation also may occur. Tumors in the choroid and ciliary body may not produce any symptoms and are often diagnosed during a routine eye examination.

Diagnosis
Diagnostic procedures for ocular melanoma depend upon where the disease begins. Melanoma that starts in the iris is easy to detect by the presence of a changing spot that varies in color from velvety brown to translucent or pink. Several diagnostic procedures for this tumor include:

- *Slit lamp examination,* in which light is projected into the eye through a slit, allowing the doctor to use a microscope to study the inside of the eye, lens, iris, cornea, and the surface of the eye. Sometimes the doctor may take pictures at successive appointments to see whether the tumor is growing. This procedure is called serial slit lamp photography.

- *Gonioscopy,* a procedure in which the doctor examines the angle of the front portion of the eye with a slit lamp or another instrument called a gonioscope. An obstruction of this angle may signal the presence of glaucoma and possibly melanoma.

- *Ophthalmoscopy,* the visual examination of the eye's interior, in which the doctor uses drops to dilate the pupil and a special instrument called an ophthalmoscope to view the inner eye, including the retina. Fundus photography, or pictures taken using an ophthalmoscope, is helpful in locating and characterizing an ocular melanoma.

Diagnosis of melanomas that begin in the choroid and ciliary body (grayish to brown tumors) usually include the examination techniques mentioned above, in addition to several others:

- *Fluorescein angiography,* in which the eye's blood vessels, including those that supply a tumor, are highlighted with a dye. This procedure can help distinguish an ocular melanoma from other types of tumors that may begin in the eye.

- *Ultrasonography,* a procedure in which high-frequency sound waves are projected into the eye and the echoes converted by a computer into a picture showing the shape, location, and tissue characteristics of a tumor inside the eye.

- *Computed tomography* (CT), in which a computer is used to produce a detailed x-ray picture of a cross-section of the eye. This test helps the doctor determine whether the tumor extends to the back of the eye.

When a diagnosis of ocular melanoma is made, a patient undergoes a full medical examination, which may include blood tests, x-rays, and scans of different organs to determine if the cancer has spread to other parts of the body. In 1 to 3 percent of patients with ocular melanoma, metastases to other areas are detected at the time of initial diagnosis. When melanoma spreads outside the eye, it most often appears in the liver. It can also spread to the lungs and areas directly under the skin. Other sites are less common.

Classification and Staging

Melanomas are classified by where they begin in the eye (iris, ciliary body, or choroid) and by their size. Small melanomas have a diameter of less than 10 mm ($^5/_{12}$ inch), medium-size melanomas are between 10 and 15 mm ($^5/_{12}$ to $^5/_8$ inch), and large melanomas exceed 15 mm (over $^5/_8$ inch) in diameter. In addition, ocular melanomas are classified by the microscopic appearance of the cells. Most melanomas of the iris and some melanomas in the choroid and ciliary body are made of spindle cells. Spindle cell tumors are less likely to metastasize than nonspindle cell types. More aggressive melanomas include those composed of several nonspindle cell types and tumors in which spindle cells are mixed with nonspindle types.

Treatment

When ocular melanoma is detected and treated at an early stage, it may be curable, and vision can be preserved in some cases. The selection of treatment depends, in part, on tumor size, location, site of origin (whether it began in the iris, ciliary body, or choroid), and growth rate. Other factors affecting the choice of treatment are the degree of tumor invasion into the eye cavity and spread to nearby tissues, the presence of distant metastases, the patient's age and general health, eyesight in the affected and unaffected eye, and the patient's preference.

Iris

Melanomas of the iris are generally smaller, slower growing, and less aggressive than melanomas in the choroid and ciliary body. A doctor may recommend only careful monitoring of a melanoma in the iris if it appears to grow slowly and doesn't interfere with vision. For faster-growing tumors, surgical removal of the tumor may be suggested. If the tumor has grown over a large portion of the iris, impaired vision, or is too large to be excised, the whole eye may be removed in a procedure called enucleation. On the rare occasions that the tumor spreads beyond the eye, exenteration (removal of the eye plus the surrounding tissues) may be necessary.

Choroid and Ciliary Body

Until fairly recently, enucleation was the usual treatment for choroidal and ciliary melanomas. However, patients with melanomas in these areas of the eye now have more treatment options. Patients may simply be observed by a doctor, especially if the tumor is small and appears slow-growing or inactive. Alternatively, the doctor may decide to use external radiation to shrink or destroy the tumor.

A new study is under way to develop a standard treatment for choroidal melanomas. One portion of this Collaborative Ocular Melanoma Study (COMS), sponsored by the National Eye Institute, will determine whether radiation therapy is better than enucleation in treating medium-size tumors. Half the patients receive radiation and half undergo enucleation. Radiation is given in the form of a radioactive plaque, made by placing radioactive pellets in a plastic disc covered on one side with a gold plate. The disc is sewn to the eye over the tumor. Radiation is directed to the tumor, while the gold plate protects the rest of the eye and surrounding tissues. This study will compare the effectiveness of each treatment, the relative risk of developing distant metastases, and the long-term survival of patients.

The amount of radiation needed to destroy a large melanoma, whether given by plaque or by other means, is often so great that the eye itself is severely injured or destroyed. Therefore, enucleation (or exenteration in the case of extraocular tumor extension) is still the recommended treatment for large tumors of the ciliary body and choroid. It is not known, however, whether external radiation given to shrink a tumor prior to enucleation improves the effectiveness of surgery. To help answer this question, patients in the COMS study with large melanomas will undergo either external radiation followed by enucleation or enucleation alone.

Side effects accompany each form of treatment. After enucleation, the eye area may be temporarily painful. Serious problems following radiation therapy may include bleeding within the eye (hemorrhage), cataract formation, glaucoma, inflammation, and other conditions. For this reason, patients should discuss treatment options and possible side effects with their doctor before beginning treatment. Several doctors, including an ophthalmologist (eye specialist) and an oncologist (cancer specialist), may need to be consulted to develop the best treatment plan.

The NCI is supporting an investigational study comparing external radiation using charged helium particles with radioactive iodine radiation implants in the treatment of localized ocular melanoma. This study will compare the effectiveness of each treatment, long-term effects of treatment on vision, the relative risk of developing distant metastases, and long-term patient survival.

Doctors are looking at several investigational techniques to treat certain patients with ocular melanoma. Small melanomas of the choroid and ciliary body may be removed by surgical resection, in which the tumor plus underlying tissue is removed. One experimental procedure that reduces the amount of radiation necessary for treatment combines external radiation with hyperthermia, a technique in which the tumor is heated. However, hyperthermia may result in complications, including pain, inflammation, retinal detachment, loss of vision, and blindness.

Photocoagulation is a procedure being studied in the treatment of small tumors. In this process, the blood vessels entering the tumor are heated by a light beam and destroyed, thereby depriving the tumor of nutrients. Photocoagulation may be used in combination with radiation to treat small (under 10 mm) and medium-size (10–15 mm) tumors. In addition, photodynamic therapy with hematoporphyrin derivative (HPD) may be useful in treating these melanomas. Photodynamic therapy uses an interaction between light and a substance that makes cells more sensitive to light (photosensitizing agent) to destroy tumor tissue. When injected into the body, the HPD travels to and enters the tumor cells, sensitizing them to light. The tumor is destroyed when a beam of light is then directed at it.

Rehabilitation and Followup

Treatment results, side effects, and evidence of metastatic disease may not appear for several months to years following the initial therapy. Therefore, it is important that patients have regular followup examinations. Patients may also undergo some type of reconstructive surgery after treatment. For a patient who undergoes enucleation, a silicone ball is sewn inside the eye socket; this implant usually heals within 4 to 8 weeks. The patient is then fitted with an artificial eye, or prosthesis, which fits over the front of the silicone ball. The artificial eye looks and moves much like a real eye. Patients should discuss this and other reconstructive options with their doctor prior to therapy.

Selected References

The materials marked with an * are distributed free of charge by the NCI. The other items are not available from the NCI; they can be found in medical libraries, many college and university libraries, and some public libraries.

*About Dysplastic Nevi. Single copies available from the National Cancer Institute; multiple copies available from Modern Talking Picture Service, 5000 Park Street N., St. Petersburg, Florida 33709-2254.

Balch, C. M. "The Role of Elective Lymph Node Dissection in Melanoma: Rationale, Results, and Controversies," Journal of Clinical Oncology, Vol. 6(1), January 1988, pp. 163–172.

*Chemotherapy and You: A Guide to Self-Help During Treatment. Office of Cancer Communications, National Cancer Institute. NIH Publication No. 86-1136.

Coleman, D. J., et al. "Ultrasonic Hyperthermia and Radiation in the Management of Intraocular Melanoma," American Journal of Ophthalmology, Vol. 101(6), June 1986, pp. 635–642.

*"Consensus Conference—Precursors to Malignant Melanoma," Journal of the American Medical Association, Vol. 251(14), April 13, 1984, pp. 1864–1866.

DeVita, V. T., et al., eds. Cancer: Principles and Practice of Oncology, 2nd Ed. Philadelphia: J. B. Lippincott Co., 1985.

*Eating Hints. Office of Cancer Communications, National Cancer Institute, NIH Publication No. 86-2079.

Fairchild, R. G. "New Radiotherapeutic Techniques in Nuclear Ophthalmology," Seminars in Nuclear Medicine, Vol. 14(1), January 1984, pp. 35–45.

Friedman, Robert J., et al. "Early Detection of Malignant Melanoma: The Role of Physician Examination and Self-Examination of the Skin," Ca—A Cancer Journal for Clinicians, Vol. 35(3), May/June 1985, pp. 130–151.

Garretson, B. R., et al. "Choroidal Melanoma Treatment with Iodine 125 Brachytherapy," Archives of Ophthalmology, Vol. 105, October 1987, pp. 1394–1397.

Gragoudas, E. S., et al. "Long-Term Results of Proton Beam Irradiated Uveal Melanomas," Ophthalmology, Vol. 94(4), April 1987, pp. 349–353.

*Greene, M. H., et al. "Acquired Precursors of Cutaneous Malignant Melanoma—The Familial Dysplastic Nevus Syndrome," The New England Journal of Medicine, Vol. 312(2), January 10, 1985, pp. 91–97.

*"Identifying Melanoma-Prone Individuals: The Familial Dysplastic Nevus Syndrome." Office of Cancer Communications, National Cancer Institute, January 1985.

Manschot, W. A. and Van Strik, R. "Is Irradiation a Justifiable Treatment of Choroidal Melanoma? Analysis of Published Results," British Journal of Ophthalmology, Vol. 71, 1987, pp. 348–352.

*Radiation Therapy and You: A Guide to Self-Help During Treatment. Office of Cancer Communications, National Cancer Institute. NIH Publication No. 86-2227.

Scotto, J., et al. "Biologically Effective Ultraviolet Radiation: Surface Measurements in the United States, 1974-1985," Science, Vol. 239, February 1988, pp. 762-764.

Scotto, J. and Fears, T. R. "The Association of Solar Ultraviolet and Skin Melanoma Incidence Among Caucasians in the United States," Cancer Investigation, Vol. 5(4), 1987, pp. 275–283.

*What Are Clinical Trials All About? Office of Cancer Communications, National Cancer Institute. NIH Publication No. 86-2706.

Van Peperzeal, H. A. "Treatment of Retinoblastoma and Choroidal Melanoma: A Multidisciplinary Approach," International Ophthalmology, Vol. 7, 1985, pp. 255–258.

★ The mentioned text is reprinted within this book. See CONTENTS for location.

Veronesi, U., et al. "Thin Stage I Primary Cutaneous Malignant Melanoma: Comparison of Excision with Margins of 1 or 3 Cm," *The New England Journal of Medicine,* Vol. 318(18), May 5, 1988, pp. 1159–1162.

This Research Report was written by Lauren E. Dickie and its scientific content has been approved by National Institutes of Health scientists.

Chapter 18

Mesothelioma

Introduction

This *Research Report* describes current research on the causes and prevention, symptoms, diagnosis, and treatment of mesothelioma. The information presented here came from recent articles in the scientific literature, discussions with National Cancer Institute (NCI) scientists and other researchers, and various scientific meetings.

Description and Function of the Mesothelium

The lungs, heart, digestive organs and parts of the reproductive system are surrounded by a single layer of flat cells called the visceral membrane. This is connected to another layer of flat cells, the parietal membrane. The two membranes form an envelope, the mesothelium, which contains and protects the internal organs of the body. The mesothelium produces a fluid that lubricates moving organs such as the beating heart and the expanding and contracting lungs.

The mesothelium around the lungs is the pleural mesothelium. The peritoneal mesothelium encases the digestive organs, and the pericardial mesothelium surrounds the heart.

Normally, growth and repair of tissues take place through the orderly division and reproduction of cells. When cell division is disordered, masses of tissue known as tumors begin to grow. These tumors may be benign or cancerous. Most mesotheliomas—tumors that arise in mesothelial tissue—are cancerous, but benign tumors do occur. (Benign growths may block normal organ function and crowd adjacent organs, but they do not spread to other parts of the body and generally are not life-threatening. Usually, benign tumors can be removed by surgery, and they are not likely to recur.)

Malignant, or cancerous, cells invade and destroy normal tissues and extend into surrounding structures. Cancer cells also can break away from the primary tumor and metastasize, or spread, to other parts of the body through the lymphatic system or bloodstream.

About 81 percent of all reported mesotheliomas are pleural mesotheliomas and 15 percent are peritoneal. The remaining 4 percent include pericardial mesotheliomas and those that arise from the mesothelium of the ovaries, uterus, fallopian tubes, genital tract, and testes.

Incidence

Mesothelioma is relatively rare. The National Cancer Institute's SEER (Surveillance, Epidemiology, and End Results) Program estimates that about 1,000 to 1,500 new cases of mesothelioma are diagnosed yearly. The disease occurs at a rate of 1.1 cases per 100,000 population a year among men, while among women the incidence is 0.3 cases. Mesothelioma occurs most often in white men between the ages of 40 and 60, but can appear at any age; cases of mesothelioma have been reported in children as young as 2 years old.

Although it accounts for only a small percentage of all cancer deaths, mesothelioma is usually fatal.

Cause and Prevention

The major risk factor for mesothelioma is airborne exposure to asbestos, a mineral composed of silicate fibers. It is strong, durable, flexible, and fire-resistant, making it useful in a variety of industrial products such as asbestos cement and plastics, insulation, and fabrics.

The term "asbestos" refers to fibrous minerals of the serpentine or amphibole types. Chryso-tile asbestos is the only serpentine of commercial importance. Amphiboles have straight, rod-shaped fibers. All forms of asbestos are composed of large fibers that can be broken down into bundles of minute, finer fibrils, microscopic or submicroscopic in size.

Asbestos exposure had been suspected as a risk factor for mesothelioma since 1943, but it wasn't until 1960 that a study of asbestos miners and neighborhood residents in South Africa firmly established the association. Forty-seven cases of mesothelioma were observed among this population in 5 years. Since then, additional studies have supported the connection between asbestos exposure and mesothelioma, and animal studies have shown asbestos to be cancer-causing.

One of the most studied groups at risk for mesothelioma is shipyard workers. Asbestos was a primary component in the insulation of ships. A large increase in incidence of mesothelioma has been found among shipyard workers who were exposed to asbestos.

Increased risk has also been noted among workers in asbestos mines, asbestos mills and factories, and among workers who manufacture and install asbestos insulation.

Nonoccupational exposure to asbestos also increases risk. Household contacts of employees who work with asbestos have higher-than-normal rates of asbestosis, lung cancer, and mesothelioma.

Zeolite, a family of mineral fibers of volcanic origin found in Cappadocia, Turkey, and elsewhere has also been associated with mesothelioma. This finding has led to further questions about the cancer-causing ability of other natural and man-made fibrous materials. Recent studies have also suggested that heavy exposure to ionizing radiation may also increase the risk of mesothelioma.

Cigarette smoking increases the risk of lung cancer by about 90-fold for those exposed to asbestos, compared to people who neither smoke nor have asbestos exposure. Smoking alone is not known to increase risk of mesothelioma.

Although asbestos has been recognized as a potential health hazard since the turn of the century, it was not until 1960 that legal standards for asbestos exposure were set in the United States. Under the Walsh-Healy Act, exposure levels were set at 5 million particles per cubic foot

(mppcf), but these restrictions applied only to companies doing more than $10,000 worth of business with the U.S. Government. In 1972, the Occupational Safety and Health Act established national emission standards of 2 fibers per cubic centimeter for all industries.

The Environmental Protection Agency (EPA) restriction is "no visible emissions." This standard, which is now being revised by EPA, does not take into account the very small asbestos fibers, invisible to the naked eye, that are associated with mesothelioma.

A number of consumer products, ranging from toasters to pipe insulation, contain asbestos. Before 1978, certain types of hand-held hair dryers were made with asbestos to protect the heat cone casing. Air forced across the heating coil could become contaminated with asbestos fibers. Questions about these appliances may be directed to the U.S. Consumer Product Safety Commission (CPSC).

Little doubt exists that asbestos exposure can cause mesothelioma. Estimations from epidemiological studies show that about 70 to 80 percent of all patients with mesothelioma have had some documented exposure, occupational or environmental, to asbestos fibers.

Because it is commercially valuable, asbestos is present in many manufactured products and has a history of widespread use. By the end of World War II, for example, 1,722,500 people had worked in the building, repair, renovation, maintenance, and/or demolition of ships. Between 1960 and 1969, over 40,000 tons of fireproofing material containing 10 to 20 percent asbestos were sprayed each year in high-rise and office buildings during construction. Individuals exposed to asbestos from such sources may be at increased risk of developing mesothelioma or other asbestos-related illnesses. However, the magnitude of the increase is difficult to estimate because of uncertainties regarding the extent of exposure as well as precise dose-response relationships between exposure and risk of cancer onset.

Detection and Diagnosis

Symptoms

Chest pain and fluid in the chest cavity are the most common signs of pleural mesothelioma. Other symptoms are shortness of breath, cough, loss of ap-

petite, fever, hoarseness, low blood sugar, weakness and weight loss. If cancer cells have spread to underlying organs such as the heart or lungs, rib destruction and soft tissue masses may occur.

Pain and swelling in the abdomen are the most common symptoms of peritoneal mesothelioma. Others are nausea, vomiting, bowel and urinary obstruction, soft tissue masses, swelling of the lower extremities, fever, and hernia.

Diagnosis

Diagnosing mesothelioma is difficult because the disease resembles other cancers that have spread to the mesothelium from a primary tumor located elsewhere in the body. Treatment may be delayed because of this confusion despite improvements in diagnostic tools and procedures.

About 50 percent of mesotheliomas appear to originate in epithelial cells. Twenty percent are predominantly fibrous in appearance under the microscope. Fibrosarcomas often form a pseudocapsule which contains invasive prongs of malignant tissue. This feature makes sarcomas extremely difficult to cure.

Because of the symptoms of pleural mesothelioma, chest X-rays are commonly used in detecting the disease. An abnormal X-ray may alert the physician to the possibility of mesothelioma, although a tissue biopsy is needed to confirm the diagnosis.

Sample tissue may be obtained through surgical incision into the chest (thoracotomy) for pleural mesothelioma, or surgical incision into the peritoneum (laparotomy or peritoneoscopy) for peritoneal mesothelioma.

Screening/Detection

The Mayo Clinic in Rochester, Minnesota; the Johns Hopkins Hospital in Baltimore, Maryland; and Memorial Sloan-Kettering Cancer Center in New York City have screening programs for detecting early-stage lung cancer in people who are at high risk for the disease. However, no such program exists for the early detection of mesothelioma.

In 1978 the National Cancer Institute conducted a large-scale program to inform people about the health risks associated with asbestos. As part of this campaign, NCI sent mailings to 400,000 U.S. physicians explaining the relationship of asbestos to health problems, disseminated materials on the risk of asbestos, and sponsored public announcements in the media. Trade unions, asbestos companies, and other groups have also conducted local information campaigns.

Treatment

Patients with solitary benign pleural mesothelioma may be cured with surgery, but there is no standard, effective therapy for malignant mesothelioma. Because of the rarity of this cancer and the consequent problems of evaluating treatment, the National Cancer Institute suggests that newly diagnosed patients be considered for clinical research applying new approaches to treatment. Investigational therapy may consist of radical surgery, radiation, chemotherapy, or combinations of these approaches.

Surgical procedures used to treat mesothelioma include incisional biopsy, excisional biopsy, wide excision, and radical local resection. Incisional and excisional biopsy—the removal of part or all of the tumor for examination under the microscope—may be used in diagnosis.

Wide excision is removal of the tumor and a margin of normal surrounding tissue. Because of the location and size of the tumor, surgeons often find it impossible to perform a sufficiently wide excision.

Radiation therapy is more useful in controlling pain and pleural effusions than as a cure. The standard dose of 6,000 rads of radiation has little curative value in mesothelioma. Limited studies with aggressive, high-dose radiotherapy have shown some benefit, but further information is needed.

Instillation of radioactive compounds into diseased tissue has been used to treat some patients. Radioactive colloidal gold (Au[198]) placed in the space between the two pleural membranes has been associated with longer survival (over 2 years) in a small number of patients, but its effectiveness is limited to patients with early-stage mesothelioma.

Radioactive chromic phosphate, p[32], may have value for patients with peritoneal mesothelioma. Investigators have not fully evaluated this approach, because of the small numbers of patients studied.

Information about the effectiveness of chemotherapy is also incomplete due to the rarity of the disease. Some responses have been noted with Adriamycin (doxorubicin), Cytoxan (cyclophosphamide), 5-fluorouracil, and 5 azacytidine. Doxorubicin and cyclophosphamide are considered the most active drugs; response rates have ranged from 0 to 35 percent among patients in limited studies. Other drugs that have shown some effect are cisplatin, high-dose methotrexate, interferon, anthracycline analogues, and vinblastine. Further studies on the effectiveness of these and other drugs are being conducted in various clinical centers across the country, supported with funding from the NCI.

Combination chemotherapy yields mixed results; response rates for the combinations are often similar to the response rate of the single agents doxorubicin or cyclophosphamide.

Surgery supplemented with radiation and/or chemotherapy has shown some good results in animal studies. More information is needed about the effectiveness of such treatment in humans.

Side Effects

Although each form of cancer treatment can be accompanied by undesirable side effects, all patients do not have the same problems, nor do they experience difficulties to the same degree. Chemotherapy and radiotherapy often cause nausea and vomiting, but these problems are temporary and usually can be curbed with medication. A more serious short-term side effect is the suppression of bone marrow. In killing cancer cells, chemotherapy and radiotherapy also destroy some normal cells in the bone marrow. If the white cells, red cells, and platelets fall too low, patients can become susceptible to bleeding and infection. Such reactions are temporary, and supportive care, such as antibiotic therapy, helps protect patients from these complications during treatment.

PDQ

The National Cancer Institute has developed PDQ (Physician Data Query), a computerized database designed to give doctors quick and easy access to:
- the latest treatment information for most types of cancer;
- descriptions of clinical trials that are open for patient entry; and
- names of organizations and physicians involved in cancer care.

To get access to PDQ, a doctor may use an office computer with a telephone hookup and a PDQ access code or the services of a medical library with online searching capability. Most Cancer Information Service offices (1-800-4-CANCER) provide a physician with one free PDQ search, and can tell doctors how to get regular access to the database. Patients may ask their doctor to use PDQ or may call 1-800-4-CANCER themselves. Information specialists at this toll-free number use a variety of sources, including PDQ, to answer questions about cancer prevention, diagnosis, and treatment.

Suggestions for Additional Reading

Except as noted, the following materials are not available from the National Cancer Institute. They can be found in medical libraries, many college and university libraries, and some public libraries.

Aisner, J. and Wiernik, P.H. "Malignant mesothelioma: Current status and future prospects," *Chest,* vol. 74 (4), 1978, pp. 438-444.

Antman, K.H. "Clinical presentation and natural history of benign and malignant mesothelioma," *Seminars in Oncology,* vol. 3, 1981, pp. 313-320.

Antman, K.H. "Malignant mesotheliomas," *New England Journal of Medicine,* vol. 303 (4), 1980, pp. 200-202.

Antman, K.H. et al. "Malignant mesothelioma following radiation exposure," *Journal of Clinical Oncology,* (11), 1983, pp. 695-700.

Brenner, J. et al. "Malignant mesothelioma of the pleura: Review of 123 patients," *Cancer,* vol. 49, 1982, pp. 2431-2435.

Chahinian, A.P. "Malignant mesothelioma," In *Cancer Medicine,* 2nd Ed. (Holland J.F., Frei E. III, eds). Philadelphia: Lea & Febiger, 1982, pp. 1744-1751.

Craighead J.E. and Mossman, B.T. "The pathogenesis of asbestos-associated diseases," *New England Journal of Medicine,* vol. 306 (24), 1982, pp. 1446-1455.

Dimitrov, N.V., McMahon S.M., and Carr D.T. "Multidisciplinary approach to management of patients with mesothelioma (The international workshop on multidisciplinary approach to treatment of mesothelioma)," *Cancer Research* vol. 43, August 1983, pp. 3974-3976.

Fraumeni J.F. and Blot W.J. "Lung and pleura," *In Cancer Epidemiology and Prevention* (Schottenfeld D. and Fraumeni J.F., Jr., eds). Philadelphia: W.B. Saunders, 1982, pp. 576-582.

Harington J.S. "Fiber carcinogenesis: Epidemiologic observations and the Stanton hypothesis," *Journal of the National Cancer Institute,* vol. 67 (5), 1981, pp. 977-988.

McDonald, A.D. and McDonald J.X. "Malignant mesothelioma in North America," *Cancer* vol. 46, 1980, 1650-1656.

Miller, A.B. "Asbestos fibre dust and gastro-intestinal malignancies. Review of literature with regard to a cause/effect relationship," *Journal of Chronic Disease* vol. 31, 1978, pp. 23-33.

Rom, W.N. and Lockey, J.E. "Diffuse malignant mesothelioma: A review," *Western Journal of Medicine,* 137 (6), 1982, pp. 548-554.

Selikoff, I.J. "Occupational respiratory diseases: Asbestos-associated disease," *In Public Health and Preventive Medicine,* 11th Ed. (Last J.M., ed). Appleton-Century-Crofts, 1980.

Tagnon, I. et al. "Mesothelioma associated with the shipbuilding industry in coastal Virginia," *Cancer Research,* vol. 40, November 1980, pp. 3875-3879.

Walke, A.M. et al. "Projections of asbestos-related disease 1980-2009," *Journal of Occupational Medicine,* vol. 25(5), 1983, pp. 409-425.

What Are Clinical Trials All About?, * prepared by the Office of Cancer Communications, National Cancer Institute. NIH Publication No. 86-2706.

* The mentioned text is reprinted within this book. See CONTENTS for location.

Chapter 19

Oral Cancers

Description and Function of the Oral Cavity

Cancer may arise in various parts of the oral cavity, most often the lips, buccal mucosa (the tissue lining the inside of the mouth), gingivae (the fleshy tissue covering the border of the teeth), floor of the mouth, tongue, and tonsils. Cancers of the hard palate, soft palate, and adenoids occur less frequently.

The lips, formed by the orbicular muscle, are covered on the outside by skin and on the inside by mucous membrane, the buccal mucosa. Lips get their color from blood vessels that show through the thin layer of cells covering the vermilion, located between the surface of the lip and the soft tissues of the buccal mucosa. The inside of each lip attaches to the gingivae, or gums, which end in the retromolar trigone, a triangular space behind the third molars. The hard palate, made up of the maxilla and palatine bones, separates the mouth from the nose.

The tongue extends across the U-shaped floor of the mouth and attaches by muscles to the lower jaw. Taste buds, located on the upper surface and sides of the tongue, transmit stimuli to the brain that are interpreted as bitter, sour, salty, or sweet.

Throughout the oral cavity, except in the gingivae and the front portion of the hard palate, are many nests of minor salivary glands.

These glands secrete saliva, which moistens the mouth, lubricates food for easier swallowing, and contains an enzyme necessary to begin digestion.

At the back of the mouth is the oropharynx, a passageway for both air and food. The soft palate, an arch-shaped muscular structure in the roof of the mouth, and its fleshy, V-shaped extension, called the uvula, separate the oropharynx from the mouth. In swallowing, the rear edge of the soft palate swings up against the wall of the oropharynx and blocks the passages to the nose. The uvula ("little grape" in Latin), hangs above the base of the tongue and modifies certain speech sounds. On each side of the entrance to the oropharynx are the tonsils and adenoids, which filter bacteria and other foreign material from circulating lymphatic fluid.

Types of Oral Cancers

All of the structures of the oral cavity, like other organs of the body, are composed of individual cells. Normally, these cells divide and reproduce in an orderly way to repair worn-out or injured tissues and to allow for growth. If cell division becomes disordered, abnormal growth takes place, forming masses of tissue known as tumors. These tumors may be benign (noncancerous) or malignant (cancerous). Because they can crowd nearby structures, benign tumors may interfere with normal functions, but they do not spread to other parts of the body and generally do not threaten life. Usually, benign tumors can be removed by surgery and are not likely to recur.

Cancers, by contrast, can invade and destroy normal tissues, and they can extend into surrounding structures. Cancerous cells also can break away from the primary tumor in the mouth and metastasize, or spread, to other parts of the body through the bloodstream or the lymphatic system. When oral cancers spread, they tend to produce secondary (metastatic) tumors in the head and neck region; the lymph nodes in the neck are the most common location of metastasis. Approximately 7.5 percent of oral cancers spread to distant sites of the body, most often to the lungs, liver, and bones. Cancer cells in the secondary tumors usually are identical to those of the primary cancer, and although another part of the body is affected, the disease is still oral cancer.

Almost all oral cancers are squamous cell carcinomas (cancers that arise from the tiny, flat cells that are found in the skin and line the oral cavity). Basal cell carcinomas (cancers that develop in the deepest layer of the skin) can develop on the lip and invade the vermilion. Although rare, melanoma (cancer that affects cells that produce skin pigment) can develop on the gums, as well as on the hard palate, buccal mucosa, and lip.

Incidence

Each year in the United States an estimated 30,000 new cases of oral cancer are diagnosed, representing approximately 3 percent of all cancers in this country. This disease causes about 9,000 deaths every year. Oral cancer accounts for about 4 percent of cancers in men and 2 percent in women. It occurs more frequently in blacks than in whites. More than 90 percent of all oral cancers develop in people over the age of 45. Incidence increases steadily until about age 65, when the rate levels off at about 45 to 50 cases per 100,000 population.

Incidence rates vary widely thoughout the world. In Western countries, oral cancers account for no more than 5 percent of all cancers. In England and Wales, for example, only 2 percent of all cancers develop in the mouth. By contrast, the figure is nearly 50 percent in some parts of India, where people chew a mixture of smokeless tobacco and other substances such as areca nut, catechu, betel leaf, lime, and flavoring agents. Immigrants to the United States have oral cancer rates similar to the rates in their native countries. However, succeeding generations develop oral cancers at the same rate as other Americans.

Causes and Prevention

The primary causes of oral cancers in Americans are tobacco and alcohol use. Certain abnormalities of the mouth, nutritional deficiencies, poor oral hygiene, and exposure to sunlight also are associated with the development of this type of cancer.

Tobacco use—smoking, chewing, and dipping—is the most common risk factor. Tobacco users are 4 to 15 times more likely than nonusers to develop oral cancers, depending on the type and amount of tobacco used. For example, the cancer risk for heavy smokers (those who smoke more than a pack of cigarettes a day) is 6 times greater than for nonsmokers and 1.5 times higher than for light smokers. A number of studies show that cigar and pipe smokers have the same risk of developing oral cancers as cigarette smokers.

The use of smokeless tobacco—chewing tobacco and snuff—is clearly linked to an increased risk of oral cancers. In snuff dipping, the user keeps powdered or finely ground tobacco tucked between the lip and gum, between the cheek and gum, or beneath the tongue. Studies conducted in the southeastern United States indicate that snuff users are 4 times more likely than nonusers to develop oral cancers; among long-term snuff users, the risk of developing cancer of the cheek and gums is 50 times greater. This habit, which was formerly uncommon outside of the South, recently has become more popular among many young Americans in all areas of the country. According to recent surveys, 8 to 36 percent of male high school and college students regularly use some form of smokeless tobacco. Federal law now requires health warning labels on packages of smokeless tobacco.

Although researchers are not certain which substances in tobacco are responsible for the increased rates of oral cancer, a prime suspect is N-nitrosonornicotine. This substance is present in cigarette and cigar smoke, but the amounts are greater in smokeless tobacco. Eliminating tobacco use, whether in the form of cigarettes, pipes, cigars, or snuff, would drastically reduce the incidence of oral cancers.

Chronic or excessive alcohol consumption increases the risk of developing oral cancers, but researchers do not fully understand the exact role that alcohol plays in causing the disease. Animal studies indicate that alcohol by itself is not carcinogenic (cancer-causing). Recent epidemiologic research, however, indicates that the risk of oral cancer is elevated among drinkers even if they do not smoke. In combination, smoking and drinking tend to multiply the harmful effects of each other. The risk of oral cancers among heavy smokers and drinkers exceeds that of abstainers from both products by more than 35-fold. Nutritional deficiencies also may account for some of the increased risk among alcohol abusers, who commonly get 25 to 50 percent or more of their daily calories from alcohol.

Certain nutritional deficiencies unrelated to alcohol use also increase the risk of developing oral cancer. The lack of B vitamins, particularly riboflavin, and vitamin A, as well as Plummer-Vinson syndrome, a condition caused by long-standing iron and multivitamin deficiency, have been linked to oral cancer development.

Oral cancer can arise from previously healthy tissues, or the disease may develop in patients with certain precancerous conditions. In one study, it was reported that about 45 percent of oral cancer patients had a previous history of leukoplakia, a common condition in men over 40. Leukoplakia is a whitish patch that replaces the normal pink mucous membrane of the mouth. Its appearance varies—the growth may be flat or elevated, and its edges may be poorly defined or sharply outlined. Tiny cracks may interlace the surface of larger growths. Leukoplakia may be found in several parts of the mouth, or it may be limited to one small area. Any mucous membrane may be affected; the buccal mucosa is the most common site, followed by the tongue, lips, hard palate, floor of the mouth, and gums.

The causes of leukoplakia are not well understood, but this condition is commonly associated with injury to the mucous membrane and excessive use of tobacco, alcohol, and spicy condiments. Leukoplakia may appear in an area repeatedly injured by the sharp, projecting edge of a tooth. A patch also may develop on the gums of individuals with poorly fitting dentures. The condition often occurs in irritated areas such as the lower lip of pipe smokers and the hard palate of both pipe and cigarette smokers.

Early diagnosis of leukoplakia is important because cancer may develop in some of these whitish patches. Scientists do not know exactly what percentage of cases actually progress to cancer; it has been estimated that about 5 percent of oral leukoplakias become cancerous over a 20-year followup period. However, not every whitish patch in the mouth can be considered precancerous. Another condition that produces growths that look very similar to leukoplakia is lichen planus, which is not precancerous. Lichen planus produces multiple bluish-white patches. The exact nature of a suspicious-looking patch can be established only by a biopsy.

Erythroplakia, or erythroplasia, another precancerous condition, appears as a red patch in the mouth. This condition occurs equally in men and women and develops most often in individuals 60 to 70 years of age. The most common site in women is the gingivae; in men, the floor of the mouth and the retromolar trigone area are most often involved.

Another possible cause of oral cancer is poorly fitting dentures and bridges. In addition, some studies have shown that sharp or broken teeth that produce chronic irritation and/or infection may increase the risk of oral cancers. However, these findings are difficult to evaluate because such dental problems are quite common, and smoking and drinking habits and socioeconomic status may influence study results.

Too much sun is blamed for some cases of cancer of the lower lip, found most often among white men over 40 and often called "farmer's lip" or "sailor's lip." Persons with light-colored skin and those with prolonged exposure to sunlight are most prone to develop lip cancer.

A person who has had one oral cancer has an increased risk of developing a new oral cancer, especially if that individual continues to smoke or drink. Those with oral cancer also appear to be prone to other primary cancers in the pharynx, larynx, esophagus, and lung.

Detection and Diagnosis

Detection

Many deaths from oral cancer could be prevented by early diagnosis. Tissue changes in the mouth that might signal the early beginnings of cancer can be seen and felt easily. A dentist should perform a thorough examination of the soft and hard tissues of the mouth at regular intervals. In addition, oral self-examination, performed in front of a mirror, is an important step in detecting oral cancers. In this procedure, the lips, cheeks, and gums should be checked for color changes. The mouth also should be examined for scabs, cracks, ulcers, swelling, bleeding, or thickenings. The top, bottom, tip, and edges of the tongue should be inspected carefully for white patches, velvety-red spots, ulcers, or swelling, as well as for any lumps. The head can be tilted so the front and back of the roof of the mouth can be seen in the mirror and checked for lumps, swelling, or sores. Finding these or any other changes in the mouth does not automatically mean that cancer is present, but all abnormalities should be checked by a physician or dentist.

Cancer of the lip occurs most often on the lower lip. The most common symptom is an enlarging growth that repeatedly forms a dry crust that bleeds when removed. The growth may not be painful unless it ulcerates (becomes an open sore) and becomes infected. It may develop slowly, after a long history of leukoplakia.

Early cancer of the buccal mucosa is sometimes discovered by a dentist or physician during a routine examination. The most common symptom of this type of cancer is a lump in the cheek that can be felt with the tongue. The lump may not cause pain, even when it grows quite large. However, if a nerve is involved, pain may be felt in the tongue and/or ear. The growth may bleed if it is irritated by chewing or ulcerated by growing against the teeth. Muscle spasms of the jaw may make it difficult to open the mouth. A history of leukoplakia, often quite extensive, is common in patients with cancer of the buccal mucosa.

Toothache, loose teeth, or a sore that does not heal may be warning signs of cancer of the gums. Ill-fitting dentures caused by progressive changes in the gums also may indicate the presence of cancer. Bleeding and mild pain may occur if the area is injured. If the tumor invades the lower jaw, it may involve a nerve, causing partial or complete numbness of the lower lip. Leukoplakia is frequently present.

Cancer of the retromolar trigone may affect nerves, causing pain in the tongue and ear. Muscle spasms can make opening the mouth difficult.

The most common symptom of cancer of the hard palate is a persistent sore. The growth may become ulcerated, causing discomfort. If it involves a nerve, the roof of the mouth may be painful or numb.

Early cancers of the floor of the mouth are not painful. They appear as red, slightly raised areas with ill-defined borders. Leukoplakia also may be present. A lump that can be felt with the tip of the tongue is another warning sign of cancer of the floor of the mouth. Eating or drinking may cause mild soreness. Advanced tumors produce increased pain, bleeding, bad breath, loose teeth, and a change in speech if the tumor grows at the base of the tongue.

Mild irritation is the most common symptom of cancer of the tongue. Pain may occur only during eating or drinking. As ulceration develops, the pain becomes progressively worse and may be felt in the ear. Extensive involvement of the muscles of the tongue affects speech and swallowing. Advanced tumors may produce a foul odor.

The earliest symptom of soft palate cancers is often a sore throat that is made worse by eating or drinking. Discomfort may subside temporarily if antibiotics are given.

As the tumor grows, it interferes with swallowing and causes a voice change. Food and liquid may be misdirected into the nasopharynx and nose if the palate is perforated or destroyed. Earache and headache occur in some patients.

In the early stages of disease, cancer arising in the tonsils often does not produce symptoms. When symptoms do occur, they generally include a sore throat, aggravated by food or drink, and earache. If the tumor involves the hard palate or upper gum, dentures sometimes fit improperly, causing further irritation.

biopsy, a piece of the suspicious area is surgically removed; often an area of nearby healthy tissue also is taken for comparison. In an excisional biopsy, the entire suspicious area is removed along with a margin of surrounding healthy tissue. If the physician or dentist is highly suspicious of cancer but the first surgical biopsy report is negative, the biopsy should be repeated. Needle biopsies may be used for masses in the neck. However, because a needle biopsy may give false-negative results, a negative needle biopsy should be confirmed by a surgical biopsy.

Diagnosis

To diagnose oral cancer, a physician or dentist first carefully examines the mouth. A dental mirror is used to inspect areas that cannot be seen directly. Irregularities in the shape of the neck can be seen readily by comparing both sides of the neck in a good light.

Next, the doctor or dentist carefully feels the inside of the mouth and the neck, paying special attention to any area that appears abnormal on visual inspection. Lymph nodes in the front and back of the neck are checked for swelling or change in consistency.

Biopsy (removal and microscopic examination of tissue) of all suspicious areas is necessary to make a definite diagnosis. In an incisional

Staging

Once oral cancer has been diagnosed, additional tests are needed to determine the extent (stage) of disease. The pretreatment evaluation includes a thorough medical history and physical examination. X-ray studies are an essential part of the staging of patients with oral cancers. In addition to dental x-rays, studies of the skull and chest x-rays may be done. Endoscopy is used to examine other parts of the head and neck area. An endoscope is a special instrument that contains bundles of flexible glass fibers carrying light for visual examination and a tweezer-like instrument for biopsy. If distant metastases are suspected, liver and bone scans also are done.

The staging system used to determine appropriate treatment is the same for all oral cancers. The stage depends on the size of the primary tumor (T), the presence or absence of cancer cells in lymph nodes (N), and whether the cancer has metastasized to distant sites in the body (M).

Oral cancers are classified TX, when the size of the tumor cannot be determined; T0, when there is no evidence of a primary tumor; Tis (tumor in situ), when the tumor is very small and confined to its original location; or T and a number from 1 to 4, reflecting the size of the tumor. Lymph nodes are classified NX, if they cannot be assessed; N0, if the nodes do not contain cancer, or N and a number from 1 to 3, indicating the number and location of the nodes containing cancer. Distant metastases are classified as MX, when the metastases cannot be determined; M0, when there are no known metastases; or M1, when distant disease is found.

Using this system, oral cancer can be classified into four different stages.

Stage I: The tumor is 2 centimeters (about ¾ of an inch) or less and has not spread to lymph nodes or other parts of the body.

Stage II: The tumor is greater than 2 centimeters, but not more than 4 centimeters (about 1½ inches), and has not spread to lymph nodes or other parts of the body.

Stage III: The tumor is greater than 4 centimeters and has not spread to lymph nodes, or the tumor is of any size (except massive) and involves a single lymph node less than 3 centimeters (about 1¼ inches) located on the same side of the neck as the primary tumor.

Stage IV: The tumor measures more than 4 centimeters and deeply invades surrounding tissue; or the tumor involves one lymph node larger than 3 centimeters, one lymph node on the opposite side of the neck from the primary tumor, or multiple nodes; or the tumor has spread to distant parts of the body.

Treatment

Significant advances have been made in recent years in the treatment of oral cancers because of improvements in surgical techniques, radiation therapy procedures, and combination treatment programs. Survival rates are improving, and this trend is expected to continue.

Depending on the location and the extent of the primary tumor and whether cancer has spread to the lymph nodes, cancers in the oral cavity may be treated by surgery alone, radiation alone, or with a combination of these therapies. Small tumors (stages I and II) often may be treated successfully by either surgery or radiation therapy alone. Advanced tumors (stages III and IV) usually require the combination of both treatment methods. Chemotherapy has proved useful in relieving symptoms for patients with recurrent or metastatic disease. In addition, research is under way to evaluate its role when combined with surgery and/or radiation therapy for patients with locally advanced cancers.

The choice of treatment for a patient with oral cancer depends on many factors, including the primary site of the tumor, the extent of disease at the time of diagnosis, the presence or absence of cancer in the lymph nodes in the neck, the age and general health of the patient, and other variables. Because patients with early stage disease usually have a favorable prognosis when treated by either surgery or radiation therapy, treatment decisions may be influenced by the expected functional and cosmetic results of treatment, as well as by the occupation, lifestyle, and preferences of the patient.

Surgery

Surgery is the usual treatment for most oral cancers. Extensive surgery, once the standard method of removing the primary tumor and the lymph nodes in the neck, has recently been replaced by less radical surgery.

In a radical neck dissection, the surgeon removes a block of tissue from the collarbone to the jaw and from the front to the back of the neck. The large muscle on the side of the neck used in rotating, flexing, and extending the neck also is removed, along with the jugular vein. The supraomohyoid neck dissection is a more conservative procedure: only the lymph nodes, fibrous tissue surrounding the nodes, and a muscle at the front of the neck are removed. During surgery this procedure may be changed to a radical neck dissection if extensive disease is found. Another technique, the functional neck dissection, preserves the muscles of the neck, removing only the lymph nodes and the fibrous tissue surrounding them.

Head and neck surgery can result in changes in appearance and can cause problems with chewing, swallowing, and speaking, as well as neck stiffness and difficulty moving the shoulder and arm on the affected side. Rehabilitation is a very important part of the overall treatment plan for patients with oral cancers. In some cases, a plastic surgeon may need to repair the cosmetic and functional disabilities caused by extensive surgery. Surgery to reconstruct the body's natural contours uses the patient's own tissues, including grafts of skin, cartilage, and/or bone. Frequently, however, a prosthesis, or artificial substitute, is used to restore appearance and function in patients with oral and facial defects. Intraoral prostheses can be used to restore the teeth, palate, mandible (jawbone), and other structures inside the mouth. A maxillofacial prosthodontist, a dentist who has had specialized training, constructs the device to be used. It can be made of many different materials; plastic and silicone rubber are the most commonly used.

Radiation Therapy

With the development of megavoltage radiation in the 1950's, radiation therapy became a major treatment for oral cancers, with cure rates of 80 to 90 percent for cancers that are detected at an early stage. Radiation can be given by external beam, using machines located outside the body that deliver x-rays, gamma rays, or electrons to the site of the cancer. Implants of various radioactive isotopes (a form of internal radiation therapy also known as interstitial radiation therapy, endocurie therapy, or brachytherapy) can deliver a higher total dose of radiation to the tumor site than is possible with external radiation therapy. Radium 226, cesium 137, or iridium 192 are radioactive isotopes that may be used.

Radioactive implants place cancer-killing rays as close as possible to the tumor while sparing most of the surrounding healthy tissues. Special instruments or molds also may be used to place radioactive implants next to superficial tumors. This type of radiation therapy is especially useful in treating tumors of the lip and hard palate.

The dose for external radiation is based on the size and location of the tumor. Many patients first receive external beam therapy to a wide area that includes the primary tumor, surrounding areas, and the lymph nodes in the upper part of the neck. After the initial treatments, a smaller area is treated to minimize the side effects caused by radiating a large region. The final treatment area is often quite small; radiation here is referred to as

a "boost" or "booster treatment."
The boost of radiation can be
administered with either external
beam radiation or radiation implants.

A number of new approaches to
radiation therapy are currently
under study in clinical trials, which
are research studies conducted with
patients. (More information about
clinical trials is provided on page
16.) For example, scientists are
comparing the effectiveness of conventional external beam therapy
with particle beam radiation therapy,
which uses fast-moving subatomic
particles (such as neutrons) for
patients with locally advanced
tumors. Investigators also are
studying radiosensitizers (substances
that make cancer cells more susceptible to radiation therapy) such
as SR–2508 and radioprotectors
(drugs that protect normal cells
from radiation damage) such as
WR–2721. Another investigational
approach is the use of hyperthermia
(heat as a cancer treatment) combined with radiation therapy.
Photodynamic therapy is an investigational treatment that uses an
interaction between laser light and
a substance that makes cells more
sensitive to light to destroy tumor
tissue. Researchers are trying to
determine if this treatment may be
of value for patients with oral
cancers that have recurred after
previous treatment or as an addition to the initial treatment for oral
cancers.

In addition to killing cancer
cells, radiation therapy can injure
healthy areas of the mouth, including the teeth, gums, soft tissues,
and jaw. All patients should be
evaluated by a dentist before treatment. A number of measures can
be taken prior to radiation therapy
to prevent complications. If
required, extractions and other
dental work usually are performed
prior to treatment. Patients must
wait approximately 7 to 10 days to
allow the mouth to heal before
radiation therapy can begin. There
is no evidence that this delay
influences the outcome of treatment.

Patients treated with radiation
therapy to the head and neck are at
increased risk of developing
cavities, mainly because the treatment causes saliva to become acidic
and quite thick. Also, patients
sometimes neglect routine dental
care because the tissues are tender,
making it uncomfortable to brush,
floss, and maintain good oral
hygiene. The result is an increased
amount of organic material sticking
to the teeth. Plaque forms, which
rapidly leads to cavities. Dentists
encourage patients to clean their
teeth and gums thoroughly and to
floss between teeth daily. They
may recommend a fluoride gel to
help prevent cavities. In addition to

the gel, patients may use a salt and baking soda mouthwash to refresh the mouth. It is important for patients to see a dentist regularly for cleaning, fluoride applications, early repair of cavities, and other procedures that will preserve their teeth.

Some patients are able to wear their dentures during radiation therapy. However, the gums tend to shrink during treatment and for several months afterward, so dentures may not fit snugly. Following treatment, dentures may need to be relined, or in some cases, replaced.

Some patients complain that their tongue is sensitive following radiotherapy. This side effect usually disappears with time. Taste also may be altered during treatment. Some patients report a bitter taste during the early part of radiation therapy. Loss of taste occurs in many patients, but for most the sense of taste returns within a week to several months after treatment. For some, however, taste is not as keen as before, although usually it is quite adequate. A dry mouth (caused by radiation of the salivary glands) may contribute to the poorer sense of taste. Return of saliva depends on the area treated and the radiation dose to the salivary glands.

Radiation therapy can destroy tissue, a side effect called radiation necrosis. Necrosis usually begins with the breakdown of mucous membranes, leaving a small open sore or ulcer. Ulceration that

occurs on soft tissues that have no underlying bone is referred to as soft tissue necrosis. Treatment may include antibiotics and/or a local anesthetic. Sometimes areas of gingiva shrink, exposing underlying bone. If the gum does not regrow over the exposed area and if a large area is involved, a tissue graft may be necessary to cover the exposed bone. Large doses of radiation can cause osteoradionecrosis, injury to the bone of the jaw. The jaw will tolerate rather large amounts of radiation without serious problems as long as the tissues over the bone remain intact and the bone is not injured. This complication may be prevented with good oral hygiene following treatment. Some patients may require antibiotics and a local anesthetic for pain. In addition, they should not smoke, drink alcohol, or wear dentures. In severe cases, surgery may be needed to remove the injured portion of the bone.

Chemotherapy

The role of chemotherapy in the treatment of oral cancers is under intensive exploration and evaluation. Scientists are studying new drugs, more effective drug combinations, and new dosage schedules. They also are seeking ways to include chemotherapy in treatment programs using surgery and radiation therapy.

Of the many anticancer agents currently available, only a few are effective against oral cancers. Three drugs have shown consistent antitumor activity: methotrexate (MTX), bleomycin (Blenoxane), and cisplatin (Platinol). Methotrexate has been the most carefully studied. It was the first drug found to be truly useful in the treatment of head and neck tumors, and it is still regarded as the standard therapy for recurrent head and neck cancers. In an effort to improve on the effectiveness of methotrexate, researchers are examining the use of high doses of this drug followed by leucovorin, a vitamin-like substance that rescues normal cells from the damaging effects of methotrexate. Scientists believe that cisplatin is as effective as methotrexate, but they are looking for related compounds that produce fewer side effects. Vincristine (Oncovin), vinblastine (Velban), hydroxyurea (Hydrea), cyclophosphamide (Cytoxan), doxorubicin (Adriamycin), and 5-fluorouracil (5FU), alone or in various combinations, also are used to treat oral cancers. In addition, researchers are continuing their search for more effective and less toxic drugs. Some agents currently under study include carboplatin (a drug similar to cisplatin), mitoguazone (methyl-GAG), trimetrexate (a drug similar to methotrexate), and 13-cis retinoic acid (a form of vitamin A that may prevent the development of further cancerous changes in early or precancerous lesions).

Researchers also are studying intra-arterial chemotherapy for advanced oral cancers. This is a technique in which a pump delivers chemotherapy directly into an artery that supplies blood to the tumor. This procedure minimizes exposure of healthy tissues to the drugs and increases the concentration of drugs to the cancer. Induction chemotherapy, or neoadjuvant chemotherapy (chemotherapy administered prior to surgery and/or radiation therapy), is another promising approach for stage III and IV oral cancers. Several studies have confirmed that it is possible to proceed with further treatment without any increase in complications.

Anticancer drugs circulating in the bloodstream can reach and damage normal cells as well as cancer cells. Therefore, chemotherapy can produce a variety of side effects. There may be increased risk of infection due to reduced numbers of blood cells, nausea and vomiting, hair loss, and certain other problems associated with specific drugs. Most of these side effects are temporary and stop following completion of treatment.

Combination Therapy

Combination therapy is used to treat tumors that cannot be controlled by either surgery or radiation therapy alone. Radiation therapy may be administered before or after surgery. In some cases, preoperative radiotherapy makes surgery possible by shrinking a large cancer. Postoperative radiation therapy is used to treat tumors that cannot be completely removed surgically. Physicians also administer radiation to treat rapidly growing tumors and those that have invaded cartilage or bone. In some cases, radiation may decrease the chances of disease recurrence.

In addition, research is under way to evaluate the usefulness of chemotherapy given before surgery or radiation therapy (neoadjuvant therapy) or following these initial treatments (adjuvant therapy).

Immunotherapy

Immunotherapy, sometimes called biotherapy or biologic therapy, is a form of treatment in which the body's immune or defense system is used to help treat cancer. Modern laboratory technology permits researchers to identify and manufacture large amounts of some of the natural substances that the body produces to fight diseases. Some of these substances, known as biological response modifiers (BRMs), are being studied in patients with advanced or recurrent cancers of the mouth. This form of treatment is investigational, and more research is needed before it can be widely used for patients with oral cancers.

Currently, scientists are studying interferon, one of the best-known biological response modifiers, in patients with advanced or recurrent cancer of the mouth. Another BRM, interleukin-2 (IL-2), is also under study in patients with advanced oral cancer. Researchers are evaluating IL-2 used alone and combined with lymphokine-activated killer (LAK) cells. LAK cells are a special type of white blood cell that can be made in the laboratory. To produce LAK cells, IL-2 is given to a patient, whose white blood cells are then removed using a special machine. These cells are treated with IL-2 again to create LAK cells. The LAK cells, along with additional IL-2, are then returned to the patient's body. The IL-2 stimulates the LAK cells to multiply for a short time in the body, thus enhancing their ability to destroy cancer cells. Patients have not been followed long enough to evaluate the long-term effectiveness and safety of these therapies.

Clinical Trials and PDQ

To improve the outcome of treatment for patients with oral cancers, the NCI supports clinical trials at many hospitals throughout the United States. Patients who take part in this research make an important contribution to medical science and may have the first chance to benefit from improved treatment methods. Physicians are encouraged to inform their patients about the option of participating in such trials. To help physicians learn about current trials, the NCI has developed PDQ (Physician Data Query), a database designed to give doctors quick and easy access to:

• Descriptions of ongoing clinical trials, including information about the objectives of the study, medical eligibility requirements, details of the treatment program, and the names and addresses of physicians and facilities conducting the study;

• Up-to-date information about the standard treatment for most types of cancer; and

• Names of organizations and physicians involved in cancer care.

To access PDQ, doctors may use an office computer with a telephone hookup and a PDQ access code or the services of a medical library with online searching capability. Most Cancer Information Service offices (1–800–4–CANCER) provide PDQ searches to callers and can tell doctors how to obtain regular access to the database. Patients may ask their doctor to use PDQ or may call 1–800–4–CANCER themselves. Information specialists at this toll-free number use a variety of sources, including PDQ, to answer questions about cancer prevention, diagnosis, treatment, and research.

Selected References

The materials marked with an * are distributed free of charge by the NCI. Ordering information is provided at the end of this publication. The other items are not available from the NCI. They can be found in medical libraries, many college and university libraries, and some public libraries.

Ariyan, S., ed. *Cancer of the Head and Neck.* St. Louis: C.V. Mosby Company, 1987.

Brady, L., ed. "Head and Neck Cancer," *Seminars in Oncology,* Vol. 15(1), February 1988.

Calabresi, P. et al., eds. *Medical Oncology: Basic Principles and Clinical Management of Cancer.* New York: Macmillan Publishing Company, 1985.

Chemotherapy and You: A Guide to Self-Help During Treatment. Office of Cancer Communications, National Cancer Institute. NIH Publication No. 86-1136.

Connolly, G.N. et al. "The Re-emergence of Smokeless Tobacco," *The New England Journal of Medicine,* Vol. 314(16), April 17, 1987, pp. 1020-1027.

DeVita, V.T. et al., eds. *Cancer: Principles and Practice of Oncology,* Second Edition. Philadelphia: J.B. Lippincott Co., 1985.

Donald, P.J., ed. *Head and Neck Cancer: Management of the Difficult Case.* Philadelphia: W.B. Saunders Co., 1984.

Hamner, J.E. III, ed. *Management of Head and Neck Cancer.* Berlin: Springer-Verlag, 1984.

Haskell, C.M., ed. *Cancer Treatment.* Second Edition. Philadelphia: W.B. Saunders Co., 1985.

The Health Consequences of Using Smokeless Tobacco: A Report of the Advisory Committee to the Surgeon General. U.S. Department of Health and Human Services, NIH Publication No. 86-2874, 1986.

Health Implications of Smokeless Tobacco. National Institutes of Health Consensus Development Conference, January 1986. Office of Medical Applications of Research, National Institutes of Health.

Holland, J. and Frei, E. III, eds. *Cancer Medicine.* Second Edition. Philadelphia: Lea and Febiger, 1982.

Marcial, V. and Pajak, T. "Radiation Therapy Alone or in Combination with Surgery in Head and Neck Cancer," *Cancer,* Vol. 55, May 1985, pp. 2259-2265.

McQuarrie, D.G. et al. *Head and Neck Cancer: Clinical Decisions and Management Principles.* Chicago: Year Book Publishers, Inc., 1986.

Million, R., ed. *Management of Head and Neck Cancer: A Multidisciplinary Approach.* Philadelphia: J.B. Lippincott Co., 1984.

Radiation, Chemotherapy, and Dental Health. National Institute of Dental Research. NIH Publication No. 81-2090.

Radiation Therapy and You: A Guide to Self-Help During Treatment. Office of Cancer Communications, National Cancer Institute. NIH Publication No. 86-2227.

Schottenfeld, D. and Fraumeni, J., eds. *Cancer Epidemiology and Prevention.* Philadelphia: W.B. Saunders Co., 1982.

Winn, D.M. et al. "Snuff Dipping and Oral Cancer Among Women in the Southern United States," *The New England Journal of Medicine,* Vol. 304(13), March 26, 1981, pp. 745-749.

Wolf, G., ed. *Head and Neck Oncology.* Boston: Martinus-Nijhoff Publications, 1984.

* *The mentioned text is reprinted within this book. See CONTENTS for location.*

Chapter 20

Cancer of
the Pancreas

Introduction

This text describes current research on the causes and prevention, symptoms, diagnosis, and treatment of pancreatic cancer. The information presented here came from medical textbooks and recent articles in the medical literature, discussions with National Cancer Institute scientists and other researchers, and various scientific meetings.

Description and Function of the Pancreas

The pancreas is known as a "silent" organ because it is slow to signal disease. Located deep in the abdomen, it is surrounded by the stomach, colon, liver, gallbladder, kidneys, and part of the small intestine called the duodenum.

The pancreas is a spongy, tubular organ about 6 inches long and 2 inches wide. The rounded head, or ampulla, empties into the duodenum on the right side of the body; the narrow tail ends at the spleen on the left.

The pancreas performs two vital functions: it supplies the intestines with enzyme-rich juices that help digest food, and it secretes insulin and glucagon, hormones that control the amount of sugar in the blood. These two functions have led physicians to give the gland two names—the "exocrine pancreas" for the digestive tasks and the "endocrine pancreas" for the hormonal processes.

Both functions are handled by a tightly packed network of cells and ducts. The cells of the exocrine pancreas produce pancreatic juices consisting of salts, enzymes, and water, which flow from small ducts into the main pancreatic duct extending the full length of the gland. This tube joins the common bile duct at the head of the pancreas, and together they carry pancreatic juice and bile into the duodenum to aid in digestion.

In the endocrine pancreas, islet cells secrete insulin and glucagon, hormones that regulate the metabolism of sugar and starches. Insulin causes sugar to enter the body's cells and be converted into energy; it also stimulates the conversion of sugar to glycogen, a starch stored in the liver.

Glucagon triggers the reverse process. When blood sugar levels are below normal, glucagon converts glycogen in the liver back into sugar, or glucose, to increase the sugar content of the blood. The exocrine cells, called acini or acinar cells, outnumber endocrine islet cells about 99 to 1.

Types of Pancreatic Cancer

Normal pancreatic cells divide and reproduce in an orderly manner, replacing worn out and injured tissue. When cell division becomes disordered, abnormal growth takes place, forming masses of tissue known as tumors. These tumors may be cancerous (malignant) or, on rare occasion, benign.

Benign tumors may interfere with the normal functioning of the pancreas and crowd nearby organs, but they do not spread to other parts of the body and generally are not life threatening. Cancerous tumors, however, compress, invade, and destroy normal tissues. Also, cancer cells can break away from a tumor and spread, or metastasize, to other parts of the body where they may form secondary tumors. These secondary tumors, although in another organ, are still called pancreatic cancer and are

treated with therapies that target cancer of the pancreas.

By the time of diagnosis, cancer has often spread beyond the pancreas, first to regional lymph nodes and then to the liver. Pancreatic cancer also may spread to the lungs, abdominal organs, adrenal glands, kidneys, bone, brain, and skin.

Exocrine Cancer

Cancer of the exocrine pancreas accounts for 95 percent of all pancreatic tumors. Most often, these cancers, called ductal adenocarcinomas, arise in the pancreatic duct cell membrane and form hard, irregular tumors.

Rare cancers found in the exocrine pancreas include giant cell carcinoma, with large cells of bizarre shapes and patterns, and acinar cell carcinoma.

Almost three-fourths of exocrine cancers originate in the head of the organ; the rest begin either in the body or tail, although some are diffused throughout the pancreas.

Endocrine Cancer

Cancer of the endocrine pancreas is very rare, accounting for probably several hundred cases a year. Also called "islet cell cancer," these tumors tend to be soft and fleshy. They are slow growing, and the outcome is usually more favorable than for exocrine pancreatic cancer.

Incidence

The incidence (number of new cases in a year) of pancreatic cancer in the United States is about 9 cases per 100,000 people. In 1987 it will account for 3 percent, or 26,000, new cancer cases, putting its incidence well below the rates for cancers of the lung, breast, colon, and prostate.

The incidence rate for pancreatic cancer increases steadily with age; approximately 80 percent of cases occur after the age of 60. Among 80- to 84-year-olds, the annual incidence rate is 100 per 100,000 population, a 50-fold increase over the rate for people 40 to 44 years of age. The disease is 30 percent more common in men, and about 50 percent more common in black versus white Americans. It occurs more frequently in Jews than in Catholics or Protestants, and least among Mormons and Seventh Day Adventists.

Pancreatic cancer is seen more often in developed, industrial countries. The United States and northern European countries, including Great Britain, have high rates; low rates are found in the African nations, South America, the Near East and India, with rates for Europe, Asia, and the Far East in between. Worldwide mortality figures parallel incidence.

Causes and Prevention

The most important known risk factor for pancreatic cancer is cigarette smoking, according to various research studies. One study of American veterans shows that smoking more than two packs of cigarettes a day seems to double the risk of pancreatic cancer. A recent major study of 490 pancreatic cancer patients in Los Angeles County found that smoking a pack or more a day was associated with a fivefold to sixfold increased risk of developing pancreatic cancer. Ten years after stopping smoking, however, the risk dropped to the level of people who never smoked.

Family histories of patients with pancreatic cancer have been examined to identify possible genetic factors for the disease, and some evidence of familial predisposition has been found in some cases. Also, pancreatic cancer has been seen in persons with hereditary pancreatitis (inflammation of the pancreas), Gardner's syndrome (colon polyps, various growths outside the colon, and cysts), and neurofibromatosis, sometimes called "Elephant Man" disease, which is thought to be hereditary. In general, though, the argument that pancreatic cancer may be inherited seems weak, based on available data. Diabetes mellitus has been mentioned as a risk factor, but some researchers believe it follows rather than precedes the cancer.

Numerous studies have been conducted to determine if food and drink can cause pancreatic cancer. Scientists have reported that diets high in meat and total fat intake may be related to the disease. One large study suggested that fruits and vegetables may be protective. Alcohol has been mentioned as a possible cause, but its role has not been established. Another study reported an increased rate of pancreatic cancer among coffee drinkers, but this finding has not been confirmed by later research.

Various occupations in which workers are exposed to known carcinogens have been implicated in isolated studies, but none of these observations has been confirmed. One study reported 56 deaths among members of the American Chemical Society, compared to 35 projected from the national rate. However, in another study, no excess of pancreatic cancer deaths was found among chemists employed by the Du Pont Company. Still, the percentage of pancreatic cancer patients who have worked in occupations where they were exposed to solvents and petroleum compounds is greater than the percentage of patients with other types of cancer who have had similar exposure.

Because radiation is known to cause some types of cancer, researchers have studied pancreatic cancer rates among radiologists and among Japanese atomic bomb survivors. Slightly higher rates among these groups have been reported, but the differences are considered too slight to be significant.

Smoking cessation is probably the single most important step people can take to protect themselves against pancreatic cancer. Although more research is needed to identify risk factors, the NCI suggests these additional guidelines: follow the dietary suggestions given to reduce the risk of other cancers—eat less meat and less fat; eat more chicken and fish, and more fruits, vegetables, and fiber. If you drink alcohol, do so in moderation. Be alert to hazards in the workplace and the environment, and try to avoid them.

Symptoms

Prompt detection of pancreatic cancer is extremely difficult because its early symptoms often resemble those of other digestive disorders, like chronic pancreatitis, hepatitis, hiatal hernia, gallstones, and diabetes mellitus. In the beginning, the patient may complain of vague, ill-defined aches and pains. In fact, a large review of pancreatic cancer cases showed that frequently patients ignore early signs of illness, often for several months.

Pain is the primary symptom of pancreatic cancer. It characteristically comes and goes and gradually grows worse. Sometimes it occurs after meals, once the stomach empties out, resembling ulcer pain. In one-fourth of patients, the pain radiates to the back or is limited to the back, a condition that may prompt extensive and fruitless neurological and orthopedic examinations. Pain is often more severe at night.

Weight loss occurs in nearly all patients before diagnosis. The loss may be rapid, even though the patient has a good appetite and is eating normally. Bowel habits also may be altered: some patients have diarrhea or greasy stools, others have severe constipation.

Jaundice is a frequent symptom, present in 50 percent of pancreatic cancer patients at the time of diagnosis. It is found even more often in patients with cancer at the head of the pancreas. Diabetes that appears suddenly in older patients without a family history of the disease is seen in 10 to 20 percent of patients with pancreatic cancer.

Cancer of the endocrine pancreas has its own set of symptoms. Because the tumor interferes with insulin secretion and sugar regulation, patients may have attacks of hypoglycemia (low blood sugar) with restlessness, irritability, sweating, and flushing. If the hypoglycemia is not treated, the lack of glucose uptake by the central nervous system may result in seemingly irrational behavior.

Diagnosis

As the disease progresses, the symptoms become more pronounced. Even so, physical examination, blood tests, and

333

routine radiologic studies of the gastrointestinal tract may not reveal cancer. Because of its location behind other organs, the pancreas cannot be examined physically without surgery.

As a rule, once pancreatic cancer is suspected, the physician prescribes a "barium swallow," in which the patient swallows a dose of barium sulfate to make the upper digestive tract visible during x-ray examination. But this test rarely identifies early tumors. Several newer tests, including ultrasound, x-ray imaging techniques, and fine-needle biopsy, are usually ordered.

Ultrasonography provides pictures from the echo patterns of soundwaves bounced back from the patient's organs. It has a high rate of accuracy in detecting even small tumors at the head of the pancreas but is less successful in identifying those in the body and tail. Ultrasound patterns help distinguish cancer from pancreatitis; however, both false-positive and false-negative results are fairly common, so this test must be combined with other diagnostic methods.

Computed tomography (CT), or CAT scans, give cross-sectional x-ray images of an organ. It is more accurate than ultrasonography, but it may miss small or early tumors. This technique is good for locating cancers that have deformed the gland and those that have spread beyond its immediate borders.

Endoscopic retrograde cholangiopancreatography (ERCP) is performed by passing a flexible fiberoptic tube down the throat, through the stomach, and into the pancreas. The physician can look through the tube and guide its movement. Dye is injected through the tube into the target area, and an x-ray picture is taken that reveals abnormalities in the organ's shape. This procedure is highly accurate, but it can lead to complications such as infections. ERCP also is used in combination with fine-needle biopsy to withdraw a sample of pancreatic cells for microscopic examination.

Percutaneous transhepatic cholangiography (PTC) is another accurate diagnostic method. A fine-gauge needle punctures the patient's right side to enter the liver and inject a dye. This material spreads through the gallbladder and bile duct systems to reveal blockages caused by a tumor at the head of the pancreas. Complications such as hemorrhage or infection have been reported in some cases.

Finally, *laparotomy,* an operation that permits direct examination of the pancreas, may be needed to give a conclusive diagnosis, to remove the tumor if it appears limited to the organ, or to open blockages caused by the cancer. This operation alone enables the doctor to confirm the site and size of the tumor.

Tumor Markers

The need for better diagnostic tools has stimulated research on tumor markers for pancreatic cancer. Markers are chemical substances in the blood that suggest the presence of disease. They may be used to screen people with no symptoms of the disease, to diagnose cancer in someone suspected of having it, or to monitor the course of the illness.

Several substances found in the blood of patients with pancreatic cancer are being investigated. For example, high levels of carcinoembryonic antigen (CEA), a substance normally present in the human embryo and found only in minute amounts in a healthy adult, may signal disease. Elevated levels of CEA have been reported in more than 80 percent of patients with advanced pancreatic cancer, and it is sometimes used to help confirm radiological and ultrasound tests. However, the level of this blood protein is also high in people with inflammatory conditions of the gastrointestinal tract, other types of cancer, and pancreatitis.

Gastrointestinal cancer antigen (GICA), also under study as a possible marker for this disease, has been detected in patients with cancers of the colon, stomach, and pancreas.

Pancreatic oncofetal antigen (POA), a substance found in the normal fetal pancreas, may be a useful marker for human pancreatic cancer. One group of researchers found high levels of POA in 77 percent of patients known to have this disease.

Several other markers have been successful in identifying small tumors, but with most of the marker techniques, the methods are complex and need further development.

Staging

Staging, or determining the extent of disease, helps the physician choose the best treatment. A full range of tests, including laparotomy to examine the pancreas first hand, may be needed to determine how far the disease has spread.

Stage I: The tumor appears to be confined to the pancreas.

Stage II: The tumor has extended into nearby tissue, but there is no lymph node involvement.

Stage III: The cancer has invaded the regional nodes; the liver and other organs are free of disease.

Stage IV: The disease has spread to the liver or other organs (distant metastases).

Treatment

While cancer of the exocrine pancreas is rarely curable, it can be treated, symptoms can be relieved, and lifespan can be extended. Clinical research studies supported by the National Cancer Institute are taking place at many hospitals throughout the United States in an effort to improve the prognosis for patients with this disease.

Pancreatic cancer may be cured by surgery if the tumor is limited to the pancreas and is

diagnosed early. Discomfort is often relieved by surgically inserting a catheter to drain off the bile that accumulates when the bile duct is blocked by cancer. When cancer blocks the duodenum, the surgeon may bypass it by connecting the common bile duct to another part of the small intestine called the jejunum. Bypass procedures can double the remaining lifespan in many patients.

Radiotherapy is often used for patients with stage II or stage III pancreatic cancer to control the disease, to provide relief of symptoms, and to prolong survival. Until recently, chemotherapy had been reserved for advanced disease. Now, combinations of surgery, radiotherapy, and chemotherapy are being tried for all stages in an effort to extend life.

Surgery

Surgery is the standard treatment for pancreatic cancer. It is, however, a major procedure with potential complications. Some, like hemorrhaging and infection, can be life threatening.

The oldest and least extensive operation for cancer of the pancreas is called the Whipple procedure, by which the head and neck of the pancreas, the duodenum, and adjacent structures are removed. The procedure leaves enough of the pancreas for the organ to continue producing insulin and digestive enzymes. The Whipple procedure leaves behind the regional nodes and major blood vessels, and some clinicians believe that they may harbor additional cancer cells.

Total pancreatectomy, or removal of the entire pancreas, is a more radical technique. It was developed to improve the survival rate of the Whipple procedure and to better assure the removal of all cancer cells. Proponents of total pancreatectomy argue that preserving the organ's function does not justify the risk of leaving stray cancer cells. When the entire pancreas has been removed, patients are given insulin and replacement enzymes. As part of this surgery, the duodenum, bile duct, gallbladder, spleen, and most of the adjacent lymph nodes are removed along with the pancreas.

Regional pancreatectomy, an even more extensive operation, removes the organ, more lymph nodes, and part of the arterial and venous systems. Physicians who favor this procedure believe it offers a better chance of cure.

So far, however, there is little evidence that it achieves longer survival.

Some authorities argue that the high rate of complications and death with only a small chance of cure should rule out surgery altogether. Others note that surgery does provide some relief of pain and prolongation of life. So far, there is little evidence that one type of surgery is better than another.

Radiation Therapy

Radiation therapy helps to ease symptoms in patients whose cancer is localized but for whom surgery is not an option. However, this form of therapy has not yielded any major increase in long-term survival.

With external beam radiotherapy, 4,500 to 5,000 rads are administered at a rate of about 180 to 200 rads a day. At these doses, more than one-third of patients can expect to get pain relief from radiotherapy. When doses in clinical studies were raised to 6,000 and 7,000 rads, more than half of the patients had pain relief, although the higher doses tended to induce nausea, loss of appetite, and diarrhea.

Interstitial therapy involves implanting radioactive materials such as iodine I-125 directly into the tumor. In one study, patients received implants with a dosage of 16,000 to 20,000 rads over a year's time. Most patients had relief from pain, but survival was not improved over the median of 6 months. However, when implants were combined with high-dose external radiation, survival time increased to 11 months.

A third technique, intraoperative radiotherapy (IORT), consists of treating the tumor and possible areas of regional spread with a single large dose of radiation during surgery. Currently, researchers are using surgery and IORT followed by conventional external beam radiation to provide symptom relief and to increase survival.

Another type of radiotherapy is high linear energy transfer of radiation (high LET), which focuses strong doses of neutrons on the tumor. So far, this type of radiotherapy, still experimental, has not significantly improved survival.

Chemotherapy

Anticancer drugs have been used mainly in patients with advanced disease. Because of evidence that drugs can cure pancreatic cancer in animals, some single agents have been tested, with several showing promise. The first to be tried, 5-fluorouracil (5-FU), showed a response, or reduction in tumor size, in 28 percent of patients. Results with the antibiotic mitomycin C were similar. Anticancer drugs have also been tried in various combinations in an attempt to improve survival for exocrine pancreatic cancer, but so far no drug regimen has provided consistently good results.

In a recent NCI trial, 5-FU plus intraoperative and standard radiation therapy led to a median survival of 15 months—a modest but encouraging gain in survival time.

Streptozotocin, which was found to kill islet cell cancer in animals, reduced tumor size in up to 50 percent of islet cell cancer patients and increased survival by a few months. Streptozotocin plus 5-FU are now considered standard treatment for advanced islet cell cancer.

In laboratory research, some investigators are trying to establish the basic order of biochemical events in pancreatic function. Others are exploring ways to harness the body's natural immune defenses against cancer cells, and still others are exploring the resistance of pancreatic cancer cells to drugs. New lines of monoclonal antibodies (pure antibodies produced in large amounts by specially made hybrid cells) are being mass-produced in the laboratory. Designed to attack pancreatic cancer, they are injected into the patient to seek out and destroy cancer cells.

In one small trial at the Fox Chase Cancer Center in Philadelphia, a complete response was reported in several patients receiving a monoclonal antibody. NCI began a study to duplicate these results in inoperable pancreatic cancer. Patients in the study were given one dose of a monoclonal antibody called 17-1-A and are now being followed on a regular schedule. Evaluation of the patients is under way.

Suggestions for Additional Reading

Except as noted, the following materials are not available from the National Cancer Institute (NCI). They can be found in medical libraries, many college and university libraries, and some public libraries.

Cubilla, A.L. and Fitzgerald, P.J., eds. "Cancer of the Exocrine Pancreas: The Pathologic Aspects," *Ca-A Cancer Journal for Clinicians,* Vol. 36 (1), Jan./Feb. 1985, pp. 2-18.

DeVita V.T., Jr. et al., eds. *Cancer: Principles and Practice of Oncology,* 2nd ed. Philadelphia: Lippincott, 1985.

Dobelbower R., Jr. and Milligan, A.J., eds. "Treatment of Pancreatic Cancer by Radiation Therapy," *World Journal of Surgery,* Vol. 8 (6), Dec. 1984, pp. 919-928.

Harvey, J.H. and Schein, P.A., eds. "Chemotherapy of Pancreatic Carcinoma," *World Journal of Surgery,* Vol. 8 (6), Dec. 1984, pp. 935-939.

Holland, J.F. and Frei, E. III, eds. *Cancer Medicine,* 2nd ed. Philadelphia: Lea & Febiger, 1982.

Kent, R.B. et al. "Nonfunctioning Islet Cell Tumors," *Annals of Surgery,* Vol. 193 (2), 1981, pp. 185-190.

Mack, T.M. et al. "Pancreas Cancer and Smoking, Beverage Consumption, and Past Medical History," *Journal of the National Cancer Institute,* Vol. 76 (1), Jan. 1986, pp. 49-60.

Moossa, A. R., ed. "Pancreatic Cancer—Approach to Diagnosis, Selection for Surgery and Choice of Operation," *Cancer,* Vol. 50, Dec. 1982, pp. 2689-2698.

O'Connell, M.J. "Current Status of Chemotherapy for Advanced Pancreatic and Gastric Cancer," *Journal of Clinical Oncology,* Vol. 3 (7), July 1985, pp. 1032-1039.

Chapter 21

Cancer of
the Prostate

Introduction

This Report describes current knowledge of the incidence, possible causes, detection and diagnosis, and treatment of prostate cancer. The information presented here was gathered from medical textbooks, recent articles in the scientific literature, National Cancer Institute (NCI) researchers and other scientists, and the NCI's PDQ (Physician's Data Query) database.

Knowledge about cancer of the prostate is increasing steadily. Up-to-date information on this and other cancer-related subjects is available from the toll-free Cancer Information Service at 1-800-4-CANCER.

Description and Function of the Prostate

The prostate gland and the testes are part of the male reproductive system. The prostate is located inside the body at the base of the penis, just below the bladder and in front of the rectum. It is composed of glandular and fibrous tissue enclosed in a capsule of connective tissue. The prostate surrounds the first inch or so of the urethra, the canal that carries urine from the bladder. Normally, it is about 1½ inches in diameter and about ¾ of an inch thick.

Normal activities of the prostate depend on the presence of the male hormone testosterone, which is manufactured by the testes. The prostate produces semen, the thick, whitish fluid that carries sperm. Other functions of the prostate are not well understood.

Benign Conditions

Like all other tissues and organs of the body, the prostate gland is composed of individual cells. Normally, cells divide and reproduce in an orderly, well-controlled manner to replace worn-out and injured tissue. Sometimes, however, cell division becomes excessive, leading to an overgrowth of tissue. When the overgrowth causes enlargement of the prostate gland, the condition is known as benign hyperplasia (BPH). Enlargement of the prostate is common in older men; it is estimated that more

343

than half of men in the United States above the age of 40 have an enlarged prostate gland.

Sometimes excessive cell division results in the formation of tumors. These tumors maybe benign (non-cancerous) or malignant (cancerous). Both BPH and benign tumors can crowd and press on adjacent organs and may interfere with normal urinary function. However, neither invades neighboring tissue, and neither spreads to other parts of the body. It is rare that either is life-threatening.

Prostate Cancer

By contrast, cancerous growths not only compress but also invade and destroy normal tissue. In addition, cancer cells can break away from the primary tumor in the prostate and spread, or metastasize, through the blood and lymph systems to other parts of the body, where they form secondary (metastatic) tumors. When prostate cancer spreads, it most commonly affects the lymph nodes, bladder, rectum, lungs, liver, and especially the bones—most often the pelvic bone and lower spine. Micro-scopically, the cancer cells of these secondary tumors are identical to those of the primary cancer. As such, they retain many of the characteristics of the original prostate cancer despite being located in the bone, lung, liver, or elsewhere. These secondary tumors are referred to as "metastatic prostate cancer" (rather than bone, lung, or liver cancer) to indicate that they are all part of a single disease and are not new cancers originating in these organs. Treatment for cancer that has spread must take into account the site and type of the primary tumor as well as the location and extent of the metastatic tumors and other factors.

Prostate cancer most often arises from tissue deep within the prostate gland and not in the benign prostatic hyperplastic cells so common in older men. Over 95 percent of prostate cancers are adeno-carcinomas, cancers whose cells, when viewed under a microscope, grow in patterns that resemble disordered glands that invade surrounding normal tissue. The remaining prostate cancers are atypical adeno-carcinomas, sarcomas, peripheral ductal carcinomas, adenoid cystic carcinomas, endometrioid tumors, carcinosarcomas, and malignant lymphomas. These unusual cancers are not discussed in this Research Report.

Incidence and Mortality

The true prevalence of prostate cancer (the total number of cases at a particular time) may be higher than statistics indicate, especially in men over the age of 70. Autopsy examinations of elderly men who die from other causes often reveal previously undiagnosed cancer of the prostate. In addition, unsuspected prostate cancer is often diagnosed during microscopic examination of prostate tissue removed during surgery for other diseases of the prostate. It is not clear what the natural rate of progression would be for these early cancers, but epidemiologic studies have shown that men who have prostate cancer incidently discovered during examination for other reasons have survival patterns similar to those of age-matched members of the general population.

Although the incidence of new cases of prostate cancer has increased steadily over the past 35 years, the mortality rate has increased only slightly. Prostate cancer was responsible for about 28,000 deaths during 1988. The 5-year survival rate for all stages of prostate cancer has improved from 43 percent in 1950 to 73 percent in 1980, due to better understanding of the epidemiology of this disease, more effective screening and detection techniques, and improved treatment.

Black men in the United States have the highest incidence rate of prostate cancer in the world. Although reliable data on black Africans are not readily available, their prostate cancer rates appear to be much lower than those for American blacks. The reasons for this apparent difference are not known. However, it appears that socioeconomic and lifestyle factors, rather than an inherent racial predisposition, explain the difference. Limited access to health care and detection of prostate cancer only after it has produced symptoms and is in an advanced stage contribute to the poor survival from prostate cancer among American black men.

The incidence of prostate cancer varies among population groups and by geographic area.

This cancer is common in Western Europe and North America, but rare in the Near East, in some parts of Africa, and in Central and South America.

Possible Causes

Little is known about the causes of prostate cancer, and it is seldom possible to explain why a man develops this disease. Scientists believe that cancer of the prostate develops over a period of many years as a result of gradual changes in the cells. No single theory explains the development of this disease, but a number of possible causes have been suggested. Investigations have focused on four general areas: genetic predisposition (heredity), hormonal influences, environmental and lifestyle factors, and sexually transmitted agents.

The data from population studies have produced conflicting results. Some studies suggest a genetic predisposition to prostate cancer and an increased risk for blood relatives of men with the disease. However, other studies have not confirmed a genetic link, and data from studies of people migrating

from one geographic area to another point to the importance of environmental factors, including diet, in the development of prostate cancer. Epidemiologic studies suggest that a diet rich in fat may increase the risk of prostate cancer. For example, Japanese in Hawaii have more fat in their diet and a higher incidence of prostate cancer than do their counterparts in Japan. In addition, prostate cancer has been linked with the consumption of animal fat and protein among several other ethnic groups in Hawaii.

Scientists have long suspected that hormones contribute to the development of prostate cancer. When the testicles are removed before puberty, there is little risk that a man will develop this disease, apparently because the primary source of male hormones has been removed. Moreover, researchers can induce prostate cancer in rats by prolonged administration of hormones. However, the precise role of hormones in the development of prostate cancer in humans has been difficult to determine. Currently, scientists are comparing the testosterone production and metabolism in prostate cancer patients and their brothers as well as in men from families who do not have prostate cancer.

Prolonged workplace exposure to cadmium, a metalic element used during welding, electroplating, and the production of alkaline batteries, may increase the risk of prostate cancer. But dietary exposure to cadmium (from oysters, for example) does not have the same effect. Workers in the rubber industry may also be at increased risk. However, the results of these studies are not conclusive.

The possible role of sexually transmitted viral diseases in the development of prostate cancer has been examined by a number of researchers. The work is continuing, but currently there is no firm evidence to link sexually transmitted diseases and prostate cancer. New technology is enabling scientists to further explore the possible of a viral etiology.

Some investigators have suggested a relationship between BPH and prostate cancer, but studies have produced conflicting results. While one large study indicated that men with BPH are at higher risk for prostate cancer, another found no increased risk associated with this condition.

Detection

Since the causes of prostate cancer remain unknown, prevention of the disease is not yet possible. However, when the disease is detected early, more men can be treated successfully. Based on scientific information currently available, the National Cancer Institute has suggested guidelines for the early detection of prostate cancer. They should be considered along with a person's medical history.

Early Detection

The NCI guidelines for early detection of cancer encourage an annual digital rectal examination of the prostate for all men beginning at age 40. At present, this is the most effective way to detect the disease at an early, more curable stage. The location of the prostate in front of the rectum allows the physician to feel irregularities or unusually firm areas. The rectal exam can reveal a cancerous growth before symptoms develop. This examination is also important for early detection of rectal cancer. Some doctors have suggested the use of transrectal ultrasound (see page 350) to screen (detect the disease in men without symptoms) for prostate cancer. Thus far, the value of transrectal ultrasound for this purpose has not been proven.

Symptoms

Most often, there are no symptoms in the early stages of prostate cancer. When symptoms do occur, they depend on the size and location of the growth.

Symptoms that should cause a man to consult a doctor include weak or interrupted urine flow, frequent urination, blood in the urine, or painful or burning urination. Persistent pain in the back, hips, and pelvis may suggest prostate cancer even when other symptoms are absent.

These problems can be caused by a variety of other conditions and diseases, including infections, BPH, and prostate cancer. It is not possible to diagnose cancer from the symptoms alone, so any persistent urinary problems or pain should be evaluated promptly by a physician. A man who is experiencing urinary tract problems may wish to be evaluated by his family doctor or be referred to a urologist, a doctor who specializes in diseases of the urinary and male reproductive systems.

Diagnosis

To determine the cause of any of these symptoms, the doctor begins by taking a careful medical history, performing a thorough physical exam (including a digital rectal examination), and ordering laboratory tests.

Enlargement of the gland and/or the presence of firm or irregular areas in the prostate gland indicate a need for additional tests. These tests usually include urinalysis, blood studies, and x-rays, such as an intravenous pyelogram (IVP). The IVP is a series of x-rays taken after a substance is injected that outlines the kidneys, ureters, and bladder. It can reveal obstructions or abnormalities in these organs and help the doctor determine whether the symptoms are caused by a problem in the prostate or in the urinary tract.

If the doctor suspects prostate cancer, the patient is usually referred to a specialist (such as a urologist or surgeon) for a biopsy, which is the only way to make a definite diagnosis. A small tissue sample is removed for microscopic examination by a pathologist (a doctor who specializes in the diagnosis of disease by studying cells and tissues removed from the body).

In the United States, core needle biopsy and fine needle aspiration biopsy are the two most common biopsy methods. The method chosen for a particular patient depend on his physical condition, the apparent extent of the tumor, and other factors. In core needle biopsy, a tissue sample is removed with a special needle inserted by a trans-perineal (through the area between the scrotum and the anus) or transrectal (through the rectum) route. It can be performed as an outpatient procedure, but may require a local or general anesthetic. In fine needle aspiration, a special needle is inserted into the pro-state through the rectum, and a cell sample is withdrawn. This procudure is performed on an outpatient basis, generally without anesthesia. It is becoming an increasingly common biopsy procedure as more physicians are trained and become experienced in carrying it out and as pathologists develop expertise in its interpretation.

Staging

If the biopsy confirms prostate cancer, the patient may benefit from a review of his case by a medical team composed of a variety of health professionals. A team might include an on-cologist (a cancer specialist) and/or a urologist, radiation therapist, nursing professionals, and rehabilitation specialists. The composition of the team will depend on the patient's needs and the staff of the hospital or treatment center.

The physician conducts addi-tional tests to establish the extent of the disease. This important step, called staging, helps in planning the most appropriate treatment for each patient. Staging procedures include a repeat of the rectal exam. The physician attempts to determine whether the tumor is contained within the gland or has spread beyond the prostate. The physician also feels the nearby lymph nodes for signs of enlargement, which may indicate the presence of cancer cells.

The spread of cancer cells to the lymph nodes is sometimes detectable with lymphography (x-rays taken after a substance is injected that outlines the lymphatic system). However, the most precise way to determine whether cancer is present in lymph nodes is by surgical removal and microscopic examination of the nodes. This is a major surgical procedure with some risk, and doctors are not in agreement about its usefulness for all prostate cancer patients.

Staging Techniques

To stage prostate cancer accurately, other techniques to produce images of the internal organs are used. These may include transrectal ultrasound, computed axial tomography (CT scan), and magnetic resonance imaging (MRI). While each of these tests may contribute valuable information, there is no single best procedure, and none is completely accurate.

Transrectal ultrasound uses sound waves produced by a probe inserted in the rectum. These sound waves bounce off the prostate and produce a pattern of echoes that a computer converts into a picture. This procedure may improve staging by estimating the size of the primary tumor and identifying local spread, but it cannot assess the size of the lymph nodes. This relatively new technique is not available at all treatment centers.

CT scans are a series of x-rays taken as an instrument called a scanner revolves around the patient. A computer receives the x-ray images and creates a cross-sectional picture of the area of the body being examined. While CT scans can detect enlarged nodes, the images they provide of the prostate area are poor.

An MRI scanner contains a powerful electromagnet that excites the hydrogen molecules in water, the main component of all soft tissue. The hydrogen molecules, in turn, give off tiny electrical charges that are picked up by the scanner and transformed into an image of the tissue being examined. It is comparable to the CT scan in detecting enlarged lymph nodes. Currently, however, the cost of MRI and its lack of widespread availability limit its application.

A bone scan can help the doctor determine whether the cancer has spread to the bone. The patient is given an intravenous injection of a mildly radioactive substance that collects in areas of active bone growth and gives off radiation. These radioactive areas are then pinpointed by a scanner and recorded on x-ray film. A bone scan detects bone abnormalities, but it does not always distinguish cancer from other problems such as arthritis, infections, or fractures.

Flow cytometry is a new laboratory procedure that is used to determine how fast a tumor is growing and to measure DNA, the genetic material in cells. This test identifies the cell characteristics that appear to correlate with the aggressiveness (growth rate and potential to metastasize) of the cancer. Research is under way to evaluate how useful flow cytometry will be in planning treatment for prostate cancer patients.

Staging Systems

Several staging systems have been used for prostate cancer.

The widely used American Urologic System divides cancer into stages A, B, C, and D.

□ Stage A: Microscopic clusters of cancer cells are found in tissue samples removed during surgical treatment for benign disease; stage A disease cannot be detected by the physician during rectal examination.

A1: The tumor cells are well differentiated and are found only in one area of the gland.

A2: The tumor cells are poorly differentiated or occur in many areas of the gland.

□ Stage B: Cancer is confined within the capsule of the prostate; it can be felt by the physician during rectal examination.

B1: A single tumor is found in one lobe of the prostate.

B2: The cancer is more extensive, involving one or both lobes.

□ Stage C: The cancer extends outside the prostatic capsule to nearby tissues or organs.

□ Stage D: The cancer has spread to regional lymph nodes or beyond the pelvis to the bone or other organs.

D1: Only regional lymph nodes are involved.

D2: The cancer has spread to the bone, distant lymph nodes, or other distant organs.

Another important part of pretreatment is determining the grade, or degree of differentiation, of the cancer cells. Grading is an effort to predict the aggressiveness of a tumor based on the microscopic appearance of the cancer cells. Well-differentiated cancer cells resemble their normal counterparts, while poorly differentiated cancer cells are disorganized and abnormal looking. Since poorly differentiated cells tend to spread more rapidly than well-differentiated ones, this characteristic helps the physician make recommendations about treatment.

The widely known Gleason grading system is one of a number of different strategies that classify cancer cells based on their microscopic appearance. Lower Gleason scores (1 through 4) indicate well-differentiated cells. Intermediate scores (5 through 7) denote tumors with moderately differentiated cells. Higher scores (8 through 10) describe poorly differentiated cells.

Tumor Markers

Additional laboratory tests, including identification of substances known as tumor markers, can help define the extent of the cancer. Tumor markers are substances detectable in the blood or urine that suggest the presence of cancer. One of these is prostatic acid phosphate (PAP), an enzyme found in the blood. A certain amount of this enzyme is normally secreted by the prostate after puberty. In many men with prostate cancer, the enzyme level rises above normal when tumor tissue extends beyond the capsule of the prostate. Thus PAP determinations may help to identify patients with metastatic disease. However, this test is not entirely reliable because elevated PAP levels may be observed in men with non-cancerous diseases and do not always occur in those with prostate cancer.

The serum prostate-specific antigen (PSA) is another tumor marker. This protein is produced by cells in normal, benign hyperplastic and malignant prostate tissues. The level of PSA in the blood goes up in men with prostate cancer and other diseases of the prostate. According to recent research, this marker may be more reliable than prostatic acid phosphatase. Thus far, no large-scale studies have evaluated PSA, but it seems likely that PSA and PAP will be used together to help stage prostate cancer as well as to assess the patient's response to treatment.

Treatment

The outlook for patients with prostate cancer has improved steadily since 1950. While the incidence of the disease has been increasing, mortality rates have remained relatively constant. This pattern can probably be explained by a combination of factors: more frequent diagnosis of very early cancers, diagnosis at earlier stages of disease, and improvements in treatment.

Although the growth rate of prostate cancer varies somewhat unpredictably from case to case, doctors generally recommend therapy based on the stage of the disease and certain characteristics of the cells. They also take into account the patient's age and medical history, as well as the probable risks and benefits of the treatment.

Prostate Cancer Therapies

Surgery is used to treat both benign prostate enlargement and prostate cancer. Transurethral resection of the prostate (TUR or TURP) is the most common procedure used to relieve urinary obstruction when the gland is slightly or moderately enlarged. This technique may also be used to remove small cancers. During TURP, an instrument inserted through the penis trims away excess prostate tissue. Tissue removed during surgery is examined by a pathologist.

Radical prostatectomy is a more extensive procedure. It involves the removal of the entire prostate gland and surrounding tissues. Surgeons use several different techniques to remove the prostate gland. In retropubic prostatectomy, an incision is made from the navel to the pubic bone to permit removal of the prostate and pelvic lymph nodes. In perineal surgery, the incision is made between the scrotum and the anus. The perineal approach requires less operating time, but it does not give the surgeon access to the pelvic lymph nodes. In patients with medical conditions such as heart or lung disorders, the perineal technique may be safer. If necessary, lymph nodes can be removed during another procedure.

In the past, impotence was a side effect for nearly all patients undergoing radical prostatectomy. However, improved surgical techniques can often spare potency by bypassing the nerves necessary for erection. This procedure is being widely adopted, but doctors agree that attempts to preserve potency are secondary and that complete removal of the tumor is most important. Urinary incontinence and stricture (narrowing of the urethra) are two other possible side effects of radical prostatectomy, but they are not common.

Radiation therapy, the application of high-energy rays to destroy cancerous tissue, has been used to treat prostate cancer since the early 1900s. While early efforts were limited by radiation damage to normal tissues, advances in technology have given radiation therapy an important role in the treatment of this disease. The radiation may be delivered by machine (external beam radiation) or may come from radioactive material implanted in the body (interstitial radiation therapy).

External beam radiation can be sharply focused on localized tumors, sparing normal tissues in the area. Usually, treatment is administered over 6 to 7 weeks. when used to treat a wider area to which cancer cells may have spread, such as the pelvic lymph nodes, the treatment is called "extended field radiation."

Radiation therapy commonly produces certain side effects, including inflammation of the bladder and bowel. These problems are managed with medication and are usually temporary. Some patients experience a gradual loss of sexual potency following treatment. Side effects of radiation therapy can be minimized with careful treatment planning and the use of sophisticated radiation techniques, including linear accelerators, which produce high-energy x-ray beams.

Interstitial irradiation, also called brachytherapy, may be used alone or along with external beam radiation. The treatment involves temporary implantation of radioactive isotopes of gold (Au198), iodine (I125), or iridium (Ir192) directly into the tumor. Used alone, interstitial irradiation affects only the prostate gland and the immediate area around it. The side effects of radiation implants vary with the isotope chosen. Not every patient experiences side effects. Some men have temporary urinary tract symptoms, and a small number become incontinent. While sexual potency may be decreased somewhat, most men are able to have sexual intercourse.

Hormone therapy is the standard treatment when prostate cancer has spread to distant parts of the body, when the disease recurs, or, in some cases, when the tumor is locally advanced. For years, scientists have known that prostate cancer cells depend on male sex hormones known as androgens for their growth. The purpose of hormone therapy is to deprive the tumor of the predominant circulating male hormone, called testosterone. While hormone therapy is not a cure, it usually arrests the disease for prolonged periods and often relieves pain and other symptoms caused by the cancer.

Doctors use a number of different hormone therapies to prevent the action of male hormones on the prostate gland. Surgical removal of the testes, an operation called orchiectomy, is the oldest and most widely used form of hormone therapy. This procedure, which is a low-risk operation, eliminates the major source of testosterone. However, some patients and doctors find this procedure psychologically unacceptable, as it causes a loss of libido (sex drive) and impotence. In addition, a small number of patients have hot flashes.

Another hormone approach is the administration of estrogen, a female hormone that reduces or eliminates the body's production of testosterone. Diethylstilbestrol (DES) is a synthetic estrogen frequently prescribed to treat advanced or recurrent prostate cancer.

As with most types of hormone therapy, estrogen administration has some undesirable side effects. Long-term effects may include loss of libido, impotence, and breast enlargement or tenderness. Radiation to the breasts prior to estrogen treatment can prevent this problem, but it appears that radiation therapy is ineffective once breast enlargement has occurred. Administration of high doses of estrogen is also known to increase the risk of heart and circulatory disorders in men. However, studies indicate that reducing the diethylstilbestrol dose to 1 milligram (mg) per day lowers the risk of cardiovascular effects while maintaining the effectiveness of the treatment.

Most studies report no added benefit from combining orchiectomy with estrogen therapy. Use of one or the other, though, helps about 70 percent of patients, with benefits sometimes lasting several years.

Another approach to reducing testosterone levels is the use of LHRH agonists. LHRH (luteinizing hormone-releasing hormone) is a hormone that controls the production of sex hormones in men and women. (Scientists also refer to it as gonadotropin-releasing hormone.) Agonists of LHRH—compounds that are structurally similar to LHRH—are given in large doses on a long-term basis to suppress the production of testosterone. LHRH agonists are apparently as effective as estrogen therapy or orchiectomy in blocking the testicular production of male hormones.

Leuprolide (Lupron), an LHRH agonist, was approved in 1985 by the U.S. Food and Drug Administration (FDA) as a form of hormone treatment for advanced prostate cancer. Currently, this treatment is given by daily injection. As with other treatments that suppress testosterone, impotence is common, and patients often experience hot flashes. Also, leuprolide may temporarily stimulate tumor growth and symptoms, a phenomenon known as "tumor flare," which may limit its usefulness in some patients.

Other LHRH agonists being

tested include Buserelin, Zoladex, Nafareline, and D-Trp-6-LHRH. These drugs are administered by nasal spray or by injection; the injection method is preferred because the drug is better absorbed. Recently, researchers have been experimenting with a new method of administration for these drugs and for leuprolide. A pellet of the drug, called a depot, is injected beneath the skin of the abdomen, and the drug is slowly released over a period of 1 to 3 months. The FDA has not yet approved this method for general use.

Antiandrogen compounds are another type of hormone treatment. They function by inhibiting the action of testosterone on the prostate. Antiandrogens can be divided into two types: steroidal agents and nonsteroidal agents. Megestrol acetate (Megace), cyproterone acetate, and medroxyprogesterone acetate (Depo-Provera and several other brands) are examples of progestational agents (steroids) that function as antiandrogens. The activity of these steroidal agents varies, and their usefulness can be limited by their tendency to lose effectiveness with long-term administration. Few significant side effects have been noted with this treatment. Nonsteroidal agents include Anadron (RU 23908) and flutamide.

Research has shown that a combination of LHRH agonists and flutamide can block the small amount of androgens produced by the adrenal glands and improve response to hormone therapy. In 1989, the FDA approved the use of flutamide (Eulexin) in combination with leuprolide for the treatment of advanced prostate cancer. The FDA's approval was based on the results of recent clinical trials. In an NCI-sponsored trial carried out at five medical centers, patients treated with the combination of leuprolide and flutamide have survived for an average of about 7 months longer than those who received leuprolide alone. Moreover, the combined therapy has been well-tolerated by patients participating in this study. Their records will be reviewed regularly to evaluate the effectiveness of the combined therapy.

Chemotherapy (treatment with anticancer drugs) may benefit patients who have relapsed after hormone therapy. In such cases, efforts to control the disease with additional hormonal approaches are usually not successful, probably because of the presence of cancer cells that do not depend on hormones to grow. Doctors are studying the value of various anticancer drugs used individually and in combination. They are also investigating the timing of therapy for the best effect and the possibility of combining chemotherapy with hormone therapy.

Biological therapy, also known as biotherapy or immunotherapy, is the use of biological agents to fight cancer. It is a new form of cancer treatment based on knowledge and tools of modern molecular biology, immunology, and genetics. Biological therapy works either directly against the cancer or indirectly to modify the relationship between the tumor and the patient. It may enhance a cancer patient's immune system so that the system will fight the growth of cancer cells, eliminate or suppress body responses that permit cancer growth, or make a cancer cell more sensitive to destruction by the patient's immune system. Interferons, interleukin-2 (IL-2), tumor necrosis factor, interferon inducers, monoclonal antibodies, differentiation agents, and adoptive cellular therapy with lymphokine-activated killer (LAK) cells and interferon-activated macrophages are among the many approaches being tested in patients with cancer.

Treatment Planning

The choice of treatment depends on many factors. These will include the stage of the disease, the patient's age and other medical conditions, the anticipated side effects, the patient's ability to comply with treatment, and the preference of the patient and his doctor.

In addition to the therapies currently in general use, doctors are seeking new and better ways to treat prostate cancer. Treatments that have shown promise in the laboratory and in animal studies are evaluated in clinical trials with cancer patients. Clinical trials (investigational protocols) are designed to answer specific scientific questions and to determine whether a new treatment is safe and effective for patients. Many of the current standard treatments for cancer patients were developed in such clinical studies. Clinical trials are available for patients with all stages of prostate cancer. The NCI encourages patients and their doctors to consider this possibility when selecting treatment for prostate cancer. Information about how patients and their doctors can learn about current clinical trials is found on page 511.

The following is a general description of treatment options by stage of disease.

Stage A

Older patients diagnosed with stage A1 prostate cancer that was found during TURP for treatment of a non-cancerous prostate condition usually require no further treatment. Generally, the patient is advised to return for regular examinations. Active treatment may be considered for stage A1 prostate cancer in younger men (ages 50-60).

Because patients diagnosed with stage A2 prostate cancer are somewhat higher risk of having their disease spread, radiation therapy or surgical removal of the prostate may be recommended. The outlook for stage A1 patients is excellent;

their survival usually equals that of the general population of the same age.

In investigational protocols for patients with stage A disease, researchers are trying to learn whether hormone therapy is useful in preventing the cancer from recurring.

Stage B

When prostate cancer has not spread beyond the capsule, the disease can be treated effectively with either radiation therapy or surgery (removal of the prostate and pelvic lymph nodes). Ten-year follow up studies indicate that survival rates are about the same for patients treated by either external beam radiation or surgery. Because primary radiation therapy has not been in general use as long as prostatectomy, patients treated with radiation are still being followed to determine whether the similarity in survival persists after 15 years.

Clinical trials for patients with stage B disease include studies of new types of radiation therapy and drugs that may make prostate cancer cells more vulnerable to radiation treatment.

Stage C

Stage C prostate cancer is usually treated with external beam radiation therapy, but surgery or interstitial radiation may be recommended for some patients. Primary radiation treatment is delayed 4 to 6 weeks after TURP to reduce the risk that the urethra will close.

For patients who undergo radical prostatectomy, post operative radiotheraphy may be suggested if the tumor extends beyong the capsule of the prostate or if the seminal vesicles are involved. Radiotherapy may also be suggested for patients who have a detectable level of PSA more than 3 weeks after surgery. Further study is needed to clarify the value of postoperative radiotherapy.

Because hormone treatment has side effects, doctors usually do not recommend it for patients with stage C prostate cancer, and currently there is no evidence that survival time is improved by beginning treatment before the patient experiences symptoms. However, some stage C patients do have urinary problems or other discomfort because of their disease. In these situations the doctor may suggest radiation, TURP or other surgery, or hormone treatment to relieve symptoms.

For stage C patients, researchers are investigating new methods of radiation therapy combined with the use of hormones to control the growth of the cancer.

Stage D

Hormone therapy is the mainstay of treatment for patients with stage D prostate cancer. Although cure is seldom, if ever, possible, most patients respond favorably initially. When hormone therapy begins, most patients experience pain relief and prompt improvement of their other symptoms. Laboratory test results often return to normal, the primary tumor may shrink, and secondary tumors may decrease in size and number. Some physicians delay hormone therapy until symtoms (such as bone pain or bladder obstruction) occur, while others administer hormone therapy when the diagnosis of stage D, especially stage D2, cancer is made. TURP is sometimes done to relieve localized problems.

Investigational protocols for stage D patients include experimental forms of radiation therapy, combining chemotherapy with hormone therapy, single- and mutiple-agent chemotherapy regimens, and biological therapies.

Recurrent Prostate Cancer

When patients receiving hormone therapy relapse, additional hormone therapy is usually prescribed. However, one study has reported that chemotherapy is superior to further hormonal approaches in such situations. Clinical trials investigating new hormonal and chemotherapeutic agents or biological treatments are often considered for patients with recurrent prostate cancer.

Clinical Trials* and PDQ

To improve the outcome of treatment for patients with prostate cancer, the National Cancer Institute supports clinical trials at many hospitals throughout the United States. Patients who take part in this research make an important contribution to medical science and may have the first chance to benefit from improved treatment methods. Physicians are encouraged to inform their patients about the option of participating in such trials. To help patients and doctors learn about current trials, the NCI has developed PDQ (Physician Data Query), a database designed to give doctors quick and easy access to:

- descriptions of current clinical trials that are accepting patients, including information about the objectives of the study, medical eligibility requirements, details of the treatment program, and the names and addresses of physicians and facilities conducting the study;

- the latest treatment information for most types of cancer; and

- the names and addresses of physicians and organizations involved in cancer care.

To access PDQ, doctors may use any office computer with a telephone hookup and a PDQ access code, or the services of a medical library with online searching capability. Most Cancer Information Services offices (1-800-4-CANCER)

---

*For in-depth discussion of clinical trials see chapter entitled, Clinical Trials: What Are They All About? See CONTENTS for location.

provide physicians with free PDQ searches and can explain how to obtain regular access to the database. Patients may ask their doctors how to use PDQ or may call 1-800-4-CANCER themselves. Information specialists at this toll-free number use a variety of sources, including PDQ, to answer questions about cancer prevention, diagnosis, treatment, and research.

Selected References

Bruce, A.W. and Trachtenberg, J., eds. *Adenocarcinoma of the Prostate.* London: Springer-Verlag, 1987.

Chemotherapy and You: A Guide to Self-Help During Treatment. Office of Cancer Communications, National Cancer Institute, NIH Publication No. 86-1136.

deKernion, J.B. and Paulson, D.F., eds. *Genitourinary Cancer Management.* Philadelphia: Lea and Febiger, 1987.

deVere White, R.W. and Palmer, J.M., eds. *New Techniques in Urology.* Mt. Kisco, New York: Futura Publishing Co., 1987.

DeVita, V.T. et al., eds. *Cancer: Principles and Practices of Oncology.* 2nd ed. Philadelphia: J.B. Lipincott., 1985.

Gillenwater, J.Y. et al., eds. *Adult and Pediatric Urology.* Chicago: Year Book Medical Publishers, 1987.

Grayhack, J.T. et al. "Carcinoma of the Prostate: Hormonal Therapy," *Cancer,* Vol. 60(3), Supplement, August 1987, pp. 589-601.

Heinrich-Ryhnning, T. "Prostatic Cancer Treatments and their Effects on Sexual Functioning," *Oncology Nursing Forum,* Vol. 14(6), November/December 1987, pp. 37-41.

Labrie, F. et al. "Flutamide Eliminates the Risk of Disease Flare in Prostatic Cancer Patients Treated with Luteinizing Hormone-Releasing Hormone Agonist," *7The Journal of Urology,* Vol. 138(4), October 1987, pp. 804-806.

Lange, P.H. and Winfield, H.N. "Biological Markers in Urologic Cancer," *Cancer,* Vol. 60(3), Supplement, August 1987, pp. 464-472.

Management of Clinically Localized Prostate Cancer. National Institutes of Health Consensus Development Conference, June 1987. Office of Medical Applications Research, National Institutes of Health.

Radiation Therapy and You: A Guide to Self-Help During Treatment. Office of Cancer Communications, National Cancer Institute, NIH Publication No. 86-2227.

Schover, L.R. "Sexuality and Fertility in Urologic Cancer Patients," *Cancer,* Vol. 60(3), Supplement, August 1987, pp. 553-558.

Schover, L.R. and Randers-Pehrson, M.B. - *Sexuality and Cancer: For the Man Who Has Cancer and His Partner.* American Cancer Society. 1988.

Stamey, T.A. et al. "Prostate-Specific Antigen as a Serum Marker for Adenocarcinoma of the Prostate," *The New England Journal of Medicine,* Vol. 317(17), October 1987, pp. 909-916

What are Clinical Trials All About? Office of Cancer Communications, National Cancer Institute. NIH Publication No. 86-2706.

Walsh, P.C. et al., eds. *Campbell's Urology.* 5th ed. Philadelphia: W.B. Saunders, 1986.

Williams, R.D., ed. *Advances in Urologic Oncology.* New York: Macmillan Publishing Co., 1987.

---

* The mentioned text is reprinted within this book. See CONTENTS for location.

Chapter 22

Nonmelanoma Skin Cancers

Basal and Squamous Cell Carcinomas

Introduction

This text describes current knowledge on the causes, prevention, detection and diagnosis, and treatment of basal and squamous cell carcinomas, the two most common types of skin cancer. The information presented here came from medical textbooks, recent articles in the scientific literature, discussions with National Cancer Institute (NCI) scientists, and various scientific meetings.

Description and Function of the Skin

The skin is the body's outer covering. It protects the body from heat and light, injury, infection, and many chemicals. The largest organ of the body, it also regulates body temperature, stores water and fat, and helps to make vitamin D. By sending information to the brain about temperature, pressure and vibration, pain, and touch, the skin also acts as a sensor to the environment.

The skin has two main layers—the inner dermis and outer epidermis. The dermis is divided into an upper part called the papillary dermis and a lower portion named the reticular dermis. The dermis contains blood and lymph vessels, sweat and sebaceous glands, and the follicles, or hair shafts, in which hair grows. Blood vessels in the dermis reach up into the epidermis to supply it with nutrients. Sweat produced by glands evaporates, thereby cooling the skin and regulating body temperature. The sebaceous glands produce sebum, an oily substance that keeps the skin from drying out. Sweat and sebum reach the skin's surface through tiny openings, or pores.

The epidermis, the outermost layer of the body, is mostly made up of flat, scale-like cells called squamous cells. Less common are the spherical-shaped basal cells, which are found mainly in the lowest part of the epidermis. The deepest part of the epidermis also contains melanocytes, the cells that produce the pigment called melanin. The amount of melanin in the skin accounts for variations in skin color in different people and different races.

Skin cell growth begins deep in the epidermis. New cells push mature cells upward to the skin's surface, where they die and flake off. In this way, the skin is constantly repairing itself, with new cells growing and multiplying in an orderly manner to replace dying ones.

Sometimes, though, cell growth becomes disordered, and a mass of tissue known as a tumor develops. Tumors can be either benign or malignant. Benign tumors are not cancers. They do not spread and are seldom a threat to life. Usually, benign tumors can be removed and are not likely to return. Malignant tumors are cancer. They can invade and destroy healthy tissue and extend into nearby tissues and organs. Cancer cells also can break away from the original (primary) tumor and spread, or metastasize, through the bloodstream or lymphatic system to form secondary (metastatic) tumors in distant organs. Cancer cells that make up these secondary tumors are usually identical to those of the primary cancer and, although another organ of the body is affected, the disease is still skin cancer.

Types of Skin Cancer

The most common type of skin cancer is basal cell carcinoma,

which arises from basal cells. Squamous cell carcinomas are the other principal skin cancer type. These cancers begin in the squamous cells. ("Carcinoma" is cancer that starts in the lining or covering of an organ.) Basal cell and squamous cell carcinomas are often diagnosed and treated in the same way and usually can be cured. They are also called nonmelanoma skin cancers to distinguish them from melanoma of the skin.

Melanoma is another, more serious type of cancer that develops in the melanocytes. Although melanoma most often affects the skin, it also can occur in other organs. Other, less common types of cancer that can affect the skin include Kaposi's sarcoma and cutaneous T-cell lymphoma (also called mycosis fungoides); melanoma and these other cancers are not discussed in this Research Report.

Incidence

More than 500,000 new cases of nonmelanoma skin cancer are estimated to occur in the United States each year, and the number is rising. Forty to fifty percent of people who live to age

65 will have at least one skin cancer. Basal cell carcinoma is the most common form, account ing for 75 percent of all skin cancers in the southern United States and 90 percent in the northern States. It occurs almost twice as often in men as in women. Squamous cell carcinoma is 2-to-3 times more common in men than in women. Both types usually develop on areas of the skin exposed to sunlight, including the face, head, neck, arms, hands, and back. However, they can appear anywhere on the body.

Nonmelanoma skin cancer is the most common cancer among whites in the United States. The disease occurs less often in Asians and least often among blacks. A 1977-1978 NCI survey showed that, among whites, 232.6 of 100,000 developed skin cancer per year, while only 3.4 of 100,000 black people developed the disease. Worldwide, the highest rates of skin cancer have been recorded among whites in South Africa and Australia.

Basal cell carcinoma is seldom fatal, causing only approximately 1,900 deaths per year. The highest mortality rates occur in whites, specifically white males, because they have the highest in-cidence of the disease. Squamous cell carcinoma also leads to a small number of deaths and, unlike basal cell, it is a fast-spreading disease and is quite serious unless treated early.

Causes and Risk Factors

Ultraviolet (UV) radiation from the sun is the main cause of skin cancer. The amount of solar radiation reaching the earth in-creases at higher altitudes and decreases with distance from the equator. When skin cancer in-cidence is compared for major United States cities, those cities receiving higher levels of UV radiation have more skin cancer cases.

The earth's ozone layer helps protect us from the sun's UV radiation. During the last 10 years, there has been increasing concern that the ozone layer is being depleted by certain man-made products known as chloro-fluorocarbons, such as Freon. These products are used as pro-pellants in aerosol spray cans and as cooling agents in refriger-ators and air conditioners. As the ozone layer shrinks, more UV radiation reaches the earth, raising the risk of developing skin cancers. Studies are now investigating the relationship between ozone depletion and increased incidence and mortality rates from skin cancer.

The risk of getting skin cancer is related to the amount of sun exposure and the degree of skin pigmentation. Individuals at highest risk live in sunny climates and are fair skinned. This link with sunlight also is supported by the appearance of cancers mainly on sun-exposed parts of the body, like the face, head, or neck. Women have higher rates of nonmelanoma skin cancers on the legs than men, and men develop more cancers on the trunk.

Anyone can get skin cancer, but people at greatest risk have red or blond hair, blue or light-colored eyes, and fair skin that tends to freckle or burn rather than tan. Blacks have a much lower incidence of skin cancer than whites because they have a higher concentration of melanin, which protects the skin from the effects of UV radiation.

Also at increased risk for skin cancer are people with actinic, or solar, keratosis. This precancerous condition, which causes scaling on sun-exposed skin, sometimes develops into squamous cell carcinoma.

Three rare hereditary disorders—multiple basal cell carcinoma syndrome, xeroderma pigmentosum, and albinism—increase the risk of developing skin cancer. These conditions cause the skin to be very sensitive to the effects of UV radiation. People with multiple basal cell carcinoma syndrome have a genetic tendency to develop tumors that is increased by sun exposure; they develop these skin cancers on many areas of the body, including those not usually affected, such as the palms of the hands and the soles of the feet. Xeroderma pigmentosum causes thinning of skin areas that are exposed to the sun. People with this disease have many pigmented spots that look like freckles, and they often develop many skin cancers at an early age. People with albinism have very small amounts of melanin, making them more sensitive to the UV radiation from the sun and placing them at a high risk of getting skin cancer.

Other risk factors for nonmelanoma skin cancers include exposure to ionizing radiation (from x-rays or uranium) and to a variety of chemicals. Coal tars, pitch, asphalt, soot, creosotes, paraffin waxes, and lubricating and cutting oils contain polycyclic aromatic hydrocarbons (PAH), which have been shown to cause skin cancer in animals. Several studies have found an increased risk of squamous cell carcinoma among workers exposed to PAH—including shale oil workers, jute processors, tool setters who operate automatic lathes, and wax pressmen. Chronic exposure to arsenic also is known to cause skin cancer.

Prevention of Skin Cancers

The easiest and most effective protection against all skin cancers is to reduce exposure to the sun and other known causes. The harmful effects of sun exposure begin in childhood and may be severe by age 20. Unfortunately, many people do not take measures to prevent skin cancer until they develop the disease, which is usually after age 50.

Ultraviolet radiation exposure can be reduced 50 percent by avoiding the sun between the hours of 11 a.m. and 1 p.m. (12 p.m. and 2 p.m., daylight saving time). Wearing protective clothing (such as hats and long sleeves) and using an effective sunscreen are also important. Sunscreens that block harmful UV radiation contain para-aminobenzoic acid (PABA) or related compounds; they are rated in strength from 2 to 15 or higher. This rating, or solar protection factor (SPF), must be printed on the container. The higher the rating, the greater the amount of UV radiation that will be blocked.

"Extra" UV radiation exposure from artificial sources, such as sunlamps or tanning booths, also can cause skin cancer. The UV radiation used in tanning beds is different from and doesn't burn the skin like the UV radiation used in tanning booths and sunlamps. However, this type of radiation penetrates the skin more deeply, damages the skin, and may cause skin cancer. Its long-term effects are unknown.

People should also avoid unnecessary x-rays in order to reduce exposure to ionizing radiation. In addition, people who work with substances known to cause skin cancer should take appropriate precautions, such as wearing proper clothing and protective equipment, to reduce their exposure.

The NCI is supporting research in the area of chemoprevention of skin cancer. Chemoprevention is the use of natural and man-made substances to prevent cancer. Studies are currently evaluating the effectiveness of natural and man-made forms of vitamin A and its precursor beta-carotene. Vitamins C and E are also being evaluated to determine if they can reduce the incidence of skin cancer in persons who have a higher-than-average risk of developing the disease, including people with albinism, patients with actinic keratosis, and those already treated for skin cancer. The results of these studies are not yet available, and because some of these substances can be extremely toxic in high doses, they should be taken only under the direction of a physician.

It is important to detect skin cancers at an early stage when they are curable. Doctors should examine any new growth, particularly an existing sore that does not heal or a mole that changes in appearance. A dermatologist, a doctor who specializes in skin diseases, is most familiar with abnormal growths on the skin. Family practitioners, general surgeons, internists, and plastic surgeons with a special interest in skin problems also diagnose and treat skin disorders.

Detection and Diagnosis

Detection

Since most changes on the skin are easily seen, nonmelanoma skin cancers usually are detected and treated early in their development, greatly improving the chances for cure. Basal and squamous cell cancers have many different appearances. Either may start as a small, smooth, shiny, pale or waxy lump, which sometimes bleeds or develops a crust; as a flat, red spot, either scaly and crusty or smooth and shiny; or as a firm, red lump.

Changes on the skin also can be caused by actinic keratosis. These rough, red or brown, scaly patches appear on sun-exposed skin. Because actinic keratosis sometimes precedes squamous cell carcinoma, people with this condition should be examined regularly.

Diagnosis

Diagnosis of skin cancer starts with a physician's careful examination of any areas on the skin that look abnormal. If cancer is suspected, the patient has a biopsy, which is the only way to make a definite diagnosis. The biopsy can usually be performed under local anesthesia in a doctor's office. For this test, part or all of the growth is removed and examined under a microscope by a pathologist or dermatologist.

Staging

When cancer is diagnosed, the physician needs to know the stage or extent of the disease. Doctors generally classify nonmelanoma skin cancer as localized (affecting only the skin) or metastatic (spreading beyond the original area of growth). Basal cell carcinoma rarely metastasizes; therefore, other than a biopsy, no special staging tests are done unless the growth is very large or has been present for a long time. Squamous cell carcinoma also rarely spreads, although it does so more often than basal cell carcinoma. In advanced stages, squamous cell carcinoma may involve other organs, such as the lungs or liver. If metastasis is suspected, staging tests for squamous cell carcinoma may include various x-rays, such as a chest x-ray and/or a liver scan.

Treatment

More than 95 percent of patients with nonmelanoma skin cancer are completely cured. The cure rate could be even higher— perhaps 100 percent—if all skin cancers were brought to the attention of a physician before they had a chance to spread.

Several types of treatment are effective against these cancers. The choice of treatment is based on several factors, including size, location, and type of cancer, as well as its potential for spread. The objective is to select a method that will completely destroy the cancer while causing as little scarring as possible.

Surgery

Surgery, usually performed with local anesthesia, is used to remove many skin cancers. Often the cancer is completely removed at the time of biopsy, and no further therapy is necessary. An advantage of surgery is that it allows microscopic examination of the growth's edges to determine the exact size of the cancer and whether it was entirely removed.

All cancer cells must be removed to prevent a recurrence. In some cases, cancers are larger than they appear on the skin's surface and, therefore, more tissue must be cut out than might seem necessary. When the incision is large or cannot be closed without damaging the surrounding tissue, a skin graft or flap may be needed. For a graft, healthy skin is taken from one area of the body and moved to another. For the best cosmetic result, grafted skin should be as similar as possible to the skin being replaced. Grafts for the face, for example, are often taken from behind the ear. Flaps of skin can sometimes be shifted without being completely detached. A flap has its own blood supply and, thus, is able to survive in areas where grafts might fail, such as over tissue that is severely damaged from a burn.

Curettage

Curettage is the procedure most often used to treat basal cell carcinomas. Anesthetic is injected to numb the area, and the cancer is scooped out with a curette, an instrument with a sharp spoon-shaped end. The area may then be treated by electrodesiccation (application of electric current from a special instrument to control bleeding and kill any

remaining cancer cells). The combination of curettage and electrodesiccation, known as electrosurgery, often causes a white scar, which is less noticeable on people with fair skin.

Cryosurgery

Both precancerous skin conditions (such as actinic keratosis) and nonmelanoma skin cancers can be treated by cryosurgery. Liquid nitrogen is sprayed on the growth to freeze and kill the tissue. The dead tissue then thaws and flakes away. More than one freezing may be needed to completely remove the cancer. Healing takes at least 3 to 4 weeks, depending on the part of the body treated. As with curettage, a white scar commonly forms in the treated area.

Mohs' Technique

Mohs' technique is a highly specialized type of surgery used to treat patients with large or recurrent cancers or when the exact extent of cancer is not clear. This treatment is sometimes referred to as chemosurgery because when it was first used, the growth was treated with a chemical (often zinc chloride paste) before surgery. As currently practiced, Mohs' technique is a precise method of surgically removing a cancer one thin layer a time, until only healthy tissue remains. This method ensures that the entire cancer is removed while taking as little healthy tissue as possible. Mohs' technique should only be performed by doctors who are specially trained in this procedure.

Radiation Therapy

Nonmelanoma skin cancers, especially those that occur on the head and neck area, respond well to radiation therapy. This treatment method is often used to treat cancer that occurs in areas that would be noticeably scarred after treatment with other techniques. For example, radiation therapy might be used to treat skin cancers of the eyelid, tip of the nose, and ear. Radiation therapy is also effective for cancers that have grown deep into tissue, are too large to be removed completely by other means, or have recurred. Several treatments may be needed to kill all of the cancer cells. During treatment, patients may notice skin reactions, such as rashes or red areas, in the site being treated. Changes in skin color and texture may occur and become more noticeable many years after treatment, factors

that are especially important to consider in younger patients.

Topical Chemotherapy

Actinic keratosis can be treated effectively with the anticancer drug 5-fluorouracil (5-FU). The 5-FU cream or solution is applied daily for several weeks to the areas of abnormal growth. In rare cases, basal cell carcinoma also has been treated with topical 5-FU. Although inflammation is common during treatment, scars usually do not occur.

Investigational Therapies

Even though the cure rate for nonmelanoma skin cancer approaches 100 percent with current treatment methods, new approaches are being investigated for patients with hard-to-treat or widespread disease. For example, studies are under way to evaluate photodynamic therapy in patients who have large or multiple basal cell and/or squamous cell skin cancers that have recurred after previous therapy. In photodynamic therapy, hematoporphyrin derivative (HPD), a nontoxic dye that fluoresces under light and is attracted to cancer cells, is injected into the patient. Light from a laser, a device that produces a powerful, narrow beam of light at one wavelength, is then directed at the area to be treated. The HPD absorbs the light and causes a reaction that kills cancer cells.

Followup Care

Because people who have had skin cancer are at risk of recurrence of the original cancer and development of new cancers, they should be examined by a physician regularly. In addition, patients should also routinely examine their own skin for new growths or other changes. Any suspicious-looking areas should be brought promptly to the attention of a physician, since early detection is the key to successful treatment of skin cancer.

Selected References

The materials marked with an * are distributed free of charge by the NCI. The other items are not available from the NCI; they can be found in medical libraries, many college and university libraries, and some public libraries.

*"Cancer Prevention Research: Chemoprevention and Diet." Prepared by the Office of Cancer Communications, National Cancer Institute. February 1987.

*Cancer Rates and Risks.*Prepared by the Office of Cancer Communications, National Cancer Institute. NIH Publication No. 85-691.

*"Center Briefs Media on Harmful Effects of Newer Suntanning Equipment," Radiological Health Bulletin, Vol. 20(3), Apr./May 1986, p. 1.

*Chissler, P. and Thompson, R. "Tanning Beds Are Not Without Drawbacks." Prepared by the U.S. Food and Drug Administration. HHS Publication No. (FDA) 84-8228.

DeVita, V.T., Jr. et al., eds. Cancer: Principles and Practice of Oncology. 2nd ed. Philadelphia: J.B. Lippincott Co., 1985.

Haskell, C.M., ed. Cancer Treatment. 2nd ed. Philadelphia: W.B. Saunders, 1985.

Holland, J.F. and Frei, E., eds. Cancer Medicine. 2nd ed. Philadelphia: Lea and Febiger, 1982.

Incidence of Nonmelanoma Skin Cancer in the United States. Prepared by the Biometry and Environmental Epidemiology Branches, National Cancer Institute. NIH Publication No. 83-2433.

*Radiation Therapy and You: A Guide to Self-Help During Treatment. Prepared by the Office of Cancer Communications, National Cancer Institute. NIH Publication No. 86-2227.

Schottenfeld, D. and Fraumeni, J.F., Jr. eds. Cancer Epidemiology and Prevention. Philadelphia: W.B. Saunders, 1982.

*The mentioned text is reprinted within this book. See CONTENTS for location.

Chapter 23

Cancer of the Stomach

Introduction

This *Report* describes current research on the incidence, possible causes, detection and diagnosis, and treatment of stomach (gastric) cancer. The information presented here was gathered from medical textbooks, recent articles in the medical literature, researchers at the National Cancer Institute (NCI), and various scientific meetings.

Description and Function of the Stomach

The stomach, a J-shaped muscular sac located between the esophagus and the small intestine, prepares food mechanically and chemically so that it can move into the small intestine for further digestion and absorption by the body. The stomach slants from the upper left portion of the abdomen downward across the body to the right side just below the liver. The size of the stomach continually changes. When it is empty, the stomach is about the size of a large sausage; however, it can stretch to hold large amounts of food.

Muscular rings, or sphincters, control the openings at each end of the stomach. After food is swallowed, the esophageal sphincter contracts and relaxes to allow the food to move from the esophagus into the stomach. The pyloric sphincter permits food to pass from the stomach into the duodenum, the first division of the small intestine.

The stomach is divided into four regions: the cardia, which surrounds the esophageal sphincter; the fundus, or rounded portion above and to the left of the cardia; the body, the large central area of the stomach; and the pylorus, or pyloric antrum, which opens into the pyloric sphincter. The shorter bend of the stomach is called the inner or lesser curvature; the longer, outer bend is the greater curvature.

Layers of mucosa, submucosa, tunica muscularis (smooth muscle tissue), and serosa form the stomach wall. Glands found in the mucosa, or lining of the stomach, secrete gastric juice made of a mixture of enzymes (substances that start and accelerate chemical reactions) and hydrochloric acid, which is needed to digest food. Mucus, also secreted by the mucosa, protects the stomach from the damaging effect of these chemicals. The

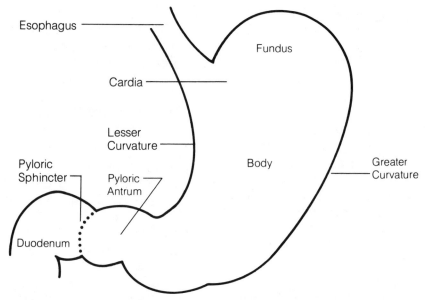

submucosa, loose connective tissue containing blood vessels, lymphatic channels, and nerves, lies between the mucosa and the tunica muscularis. Smooth muscle tissue arranged in an inner diagonal layer, a middle circular layer, and an outer lengthwise layer make up the tunica muscularis. This arrangement of muscles enables the stomach to contract in a variety of ways to churn food, break it into small pieces, and mix it with gastric juice. The serosa, which covers the outside of the stomach, is part of the peritoneum, or membrane lining the abdominal cavity.

Several minutes after food enters the stomach, gentle, rippling movements begin. These waves create an agitation similar to that in a washing machine, mixing food and gastric juice together. Wavelike contractions, known as peristalsis, reduce food to a thick liquid. As digestion continues, more vigorous mixing waves start at the body of the stomach and intensify as they approach the pylorus. When food reaches the pylorus, each wave forces a small amount through the pyloric sphincter into the duodenum. The stomach empties its contents within 2 to 4 hours after eating. Muscular contractions that continue when the stomach is empty are responsible for "hunger pangs."

The principal chemical activity of the stomach is to begin protein digestion, which is accomplished through the action of gastric juice. The chemical component of gastric juice primarily responsible for digestion is the enzyme pepsin. To prevent it from digesting protein in the cells lining the stomach, gastric glands make an inactive form of pepsin called pepsinogen. When pepsinogen is released into the stomach and comes in contact with hydrochloric acid, it is converted into active pepsin. The stomach also secretes intrinsic factor, a sugar-protein compound that influences the absorption of vitamin B_{12} from the small intestine.

Types of Stomach Cancer

Like other tissues and organs of the body, the stomach is made up of individual cells. Normally, cells divide and reproduce in an orderly way to repair worn-out or injured tissues and to allow for growth. When cell division becomes disordered, abnormal growth takes place and masses of tissue known as tumors form. Tumors may be benign (noncancerous) or malignant (cancerous). Benign tumors may interfere with normal function by crowding nearby structures, but they do not spread to other parts of the body and generally are not life threatening.

Cancers can invade and destroy the normal tissues in which they arise and can extend into surrounding structures. Cancerous cells also can break away from the original (primary) tumor and metastasize, or spread, through the lymphatic system and the bloodstream. Cells that migrate to other parts of the body can continue to divide abnormally and form metastatic (secondary) tumors. Although another organ is affected, the disease is still called stomach cancer.

Stomach cancer may grow along the stomach wall into the esophagus or small intestine, or, more often, it may extend through the wall of the stomach into nearby organs and tissues such as the liver, pancreas, colon, and peritoneum. In women, stomach cancer can also spread to the ovaries and to the pouch of Douglas, the fold of peritoneum between the uterus and rectum. Cancerous cells often enter the lymphatic system and become lodged in nearby or distant lymph nodes. They also may travel through the bloodstream to the liver, lungs, bone, and brain. In the late stages of the disease, stomach cancer may spread to any organ in the body.

The term stomach cancer generally refers to adenocarcinoma (cancer that arises in glandular tissue). These tumors account for 97 percent of all cancers that develop in the stomach. The adenocarcinomas are often classified as intestinal type or diffuse, depending on their appearance when examined under a microscope and their pattern of growth in the stomach.

- Intestinal stomach cancer cells are large cells that attach to each other to form well-defined, tubular structures. This form of stomach cancer is called "intestinal" because it is similar to cancers that develop in intestinal organs. This disease is found more often in men than in women and usually occurs in older persons.

- Clusters of small cells that infiltrate the lining of the stomach without a well-defined border are called diffuse, or infiltrating, stomach cancers. This type of stomach cancer is found equally in men and women and tends to develop most often in younger people.

Some stomach tumors are classified as "adenoacanthomas,"

squamous cell carcinomas, lymphomas, small cell carcinomas, and carcinoid tumors; however, each of these diseases accounts for less than 1 percent of all stomach cancers. Leiomyosarcomas, cancers that develop in the muscular tissue of the stomach, comprise 2 percent of stomach cancers. These rare types of stomach cancer are not discussed in this *Report*.

Incidence

While the incidence of other cancers has increased or remained the same, the number of new stomach cancer cases in the United States has declined remarkably from 33 per 100,000 individuals in 1930 to its present level of 8 per 100,000. Roughly 24,000 new cases of stomach cancer are diagnosed each year.

Residents of Japan, Singapore, Colombia, Chile, Costa Rica, and Iceland have the highest rates of stomach cancer in the world, while people who live in Nigeria, India, and the United States have the lowest. During the last several decades, cancer of the stomach has become more prevalent in Japan, Chile, and Scandinavia, but its incidence has generally decreased elsewhere in the world.

Stomach cancer is generally a disease of middle and later life, with a peak incidence in the 50- to 60-year age group. Nonwhites develop the disease twice as often as whites.

Cancer does not arise with the same frequency in all parts of the stomach. Most cancers develop in the pylorus, or lower portion of the stomach. The disease is less common in the body of the stomach and least common in the top portion, or cardia. In recent years, however, the number of cancers occurring in the upper part of the stomach appears to be increasing.

In 1930, stomach cancer was the leading cause of cancer death among men in the United States. Among women, it was third, surpassed only by breast and uterine cancers. Although it remains the sixth most common cause of cancer deaths in the United States, the mortality rate from this disease is declining. The decrease has been steepest in older persons, women, and whites. This drop in the death rate is primarily due to a decline in the incidence of stomach cancer rather than to improvements in treatment. Each year about 14,000 people die of stomach cancer.

Causes

In spite of extensive research, the exact cause of stomach cancer remains unknown. Studies suggest that a number of factors may play a role in the development of the disease, including environmental influences, socioeconomic status, heredity, certain noncancerous stomach conditions, history of previous stomach surgery, and others.

Several types of studies suggest that environmental factors may influence stomach cancer development. For example, research shows that immigrants to the United States have stomach cancer rates more like the rates in their country of origin than in the general population of the United States. However, their descendants born in the United States have stomach cancer rates similar to those of other Americans. These studies suggest that environmental exposures early in life may be related to the development of stomach cancer.

Population studies have shown that all races are susceptible to developing stomach cancer. The varying incidence rates in different parts of the world may be related to differences in diet. Populations with a high frequency of stomach cancer, such as the Japanese, Scandinavians, and Latin Americans, have vastly different diets. No single food is common to these groups; however, they share a pattern of food consumption. These groups eat small amounts of fresh fruits and vegetables, animal fat, and protein, and large amounts of complex carbohydrates, salt, and nitrates.

Investigators have observed that populations at high risk of stomach cancer often use chemicals to preserve their food. A number of studies suggest an association between nitrogen-containing compounds and the development of stomach cancer. Nitrate is a preservative that is added to cured meats and some cheeses to prevent bacterial contamination. Nitrate is converted into nitrite spontaneously at room temperature and when it is combined with normal bacteria in the mouth. Nitrites then can combine with other nitrogen-containing compounds to form nitrosamines, potent carcinogens (cancer-causing agents). Researchers have found that ascorbic acid (vitamin C) prevents the formation of nitrosamines. The protective effect of fruits and vegetables is attributed to their vitamin C content. In this country, the levels of nitrate in prepared meats are controlled by the Food and Drug Administration and have been reduced to the minimum needed to prevent

food contamination; vitamin C and other substances are also added to prevent the formation of nitrosamines.

Because spontaneous conversion of nitrate to nitrite is almost completely inhibited at very low temperatures, it has been suggested that the widespread use of refrigeration might be partly responsible for the decrease in stomach cancer incidence in developed countries. The availability of refrigeration also lessens the need for chemical preservatives and provides year-round access to fresh fruits and vegetables.

A few reports in the medical literature have described familial clustering of stomach cancer. In these studies, risk appeared to be highest in first-degree relatives of patients who developed stomach cancer at an early age. This research suggests that genetic susceptibility may play a role in the development of stomach cancer in a relatively small group of individuals. At present, the reason for increased familial risk cannot be explained. Because families share the same environment, it is difficult to distinguish between environmental and genetic influences.

Individuals with certain non-cancerous conditions that affect the lining of the stomach may have an increased risk of developing stomach cancer. One such condition is pernicious anemia, which is caused by the lack of intrinsic factor, a substance that is essential to the absorption of vitamin B_{12} and the maturation of red blood cells and other cells. The incidence of stomach cancer in patients with pernicious anemia is estimated to be about 10 percent. Some researchers believe that because the concentration of nitrite is increased in the gastric juice of patients with pernicious anemia, excess nitrosamine production may be responsible for the development of stomach cancer in these individuals.

Chronic atrophic gastritis, a condition that destroys stomach glands, changes gastric juice secretions, and causes the stomach lining to become inflamed, has been linked to stomach cancer. Chronic gastritis may not produce any symptoms, or it may cause vague stomach discomfort, nausea, and vomiting, also known as dyspepsia. This condition is always found in individuals with pernicious anemia. The incidence of both gastritis and stomach cancer increases with age. Although a causal relationship between gastritis and stomach cancer has not been established, gastritis is known to occur before stomach cancer develops.

The exact role of intestinal metaplasia in the development of stomach cancer also has not been determined. In this condition, the lining of the stomach is replaced by intestinal-like tissue. Intestinal metaplasia is seen most frequently in countries with a high incidence of stomach cancer and chronic gastritis. In animal studies, researchers have used known carcinogens to induce intestinal metaplasia, which later developed into stomach cancer. However, more recent animal studies have shown that metaplasia is not necessarily an intermediate stage in the development of stomach cancer.

The relationship between gastric polyps and the development of stomach cancer has been debated for many years. The term polyp refers to any growth that protrudes from a mucous membrane. Hyperplastic polyps are the most common polyps found in the stomach, accounting for about 75 to 80 percent of stomach polyps, and it appears that these growths do not become malignant. Approximately 5 percent of stomach polyps are adenomas, which may become cancerous.

Followup of patients treated with partial gastrectomy (surgical removal of a portion of the stomach) for noncancerous stomach conditions has revealed that these patients may be at increased risk of developing cancer. The reason for this association remains unknown. Some gastrectomy techniques cause bile to flow backward from the small intestine into the stomach, where it might react with nitrite to produce carcinogens. The risk of stomach cancer increases with time after surgery; the length of time between surgery and the development of cancer generally ranges from 15 to 40 years.

Controversy exists concerning the association between stomach ulcers and cancer. Ulcers produce sporadic pain, which varies in location and intensity. This pain usually is described as gnawing, aching, or burning and typically occurs after eating. Studies done in the United States support the theory that ulcers rarely, if ever, become cancerous. Recent Japanese studies have confirmed this research and

suggest that the risk of stomach cancer in individuals with ulcers is small.

Detection and Diagnosis

Detection

Early detection of stomach cancer is difficult because tumors can grow very large and can be present in the stomach for long periods of time before they cause significant symptoms. Individuals often ignore the warning signs of the disease until they become persistent and severe.

The first description of the symptoms of stomach cancer was recorded in the 11th century and remains accurate today. Indigestion and abdominal discomfort are the most common, and usually the earliest, symptoms of stomach cancer. Often, the person tries to relieve discomfort by belching, using antacids, or changing his or her diet. Early in the development of stomach cancer, these attempts may be successful, but as the disease progresses, the discomfort usually becomes more intense.

Loss of appetite, a bloated feeling after eating, mild stomach pain, heartburn, weight loss, and fatigue are the next most frequent stomach cancer symptoms reported to physicians. Often these symptoms are more apparent to an observant family than to the patient. Symptoms may progress to include mild nausea and periodic bouts of vomiting, particularly after a heavy meal. Abdominal pain, changes in bowel habits (such as constipation or diarrhea), or blood in the stool may occur. Difficulty swallowing is noticed by some patients.

Diagnosis

Early diagnosis can increase the survival rate for patients with stomach cancer. Procedures used to diagnose cancer in the stomach include careful physical examination, upper gastrointestinal x-rays, and gastroscopy with biopsy. These techniques used together can increase the accuracy of preoperative stomach cancer diagnosis to almost 100 percent.

Upper gastrointestinal x-rays, also called an upper GI series or barium swallow, is one of the first procedures used to diagnose stomach cancer. The patient swallows a barium sulfate solution that coats the stomach lining, which makes it more visible on x-ray. X-rays are taken as the barium passes through the esophagus, stomach, and small intestine. The accuracy of this procedure can be improved by using a double-contrast technique, in which air is pumped into the stomach to produce a sharper outline on the x-ray. The double-contrast study also allows a careful evaluation of the cardia, where cancers can be missed by conventional barium studies. Multiple x-rays are taken so that the entire stomach can be evaluated.

Gastroscopy, the use of an instrument to view the inside of the stomach, also can be useful in diagnosing stomach cancer. After the throat is numbed with an anesthetic, the patient swallows a thin, lighted tube. The physician can look through the gastroscope at the inside of the stomach and can collect tissue samples for microscopic examination (biopsy). A small brush and a suction tube in the gastroscope can be used to remove cells shed by the lining of the stomach. Gastroscopy is more than 90 percent accurate, and improvements in gastroscopes—including the development of a thinner, more flexible instrument and ways to change the direction of the viewing lens—have greatly improved the usefulness and accuracy of this procedure.

Additional tests may be needed to evaluate patients with suspected stomach cancer. They include computed tomography (CT) scanning, which combines x-rays and computerized processing of the x-ray pictures, and ultrasonography, in which high-frequency soundwaves are projected into the body and the echoes produced are converted by a computer into a picture. A CT scan can provide more information about the extent of disease than any other technique short of surgery. For example, CT scanning can detect tumor extension into nearby organs, regional lymph node enlargement, and liver metastases.

Investigators continue to search for substances that may signal the presence of stomach cancer. These substances, known as tumor markers, circulate in the blood and might prove useful in diagnosing stomach cancer or detecting a recurrence of the disease. One tumor marker under study measures the levels of carcinoembryonic antigen (CEA), a protein normally found in small amounts throughout the digestive tract. Elevated levels of CEA can be detected in the gastric juice and blood of some stomach cancer patients.

However, this test cannot be used to diagnose stomach cancer because elevated levels of CEA also can be found in cigarette smokers and in patients with noncancerous tumors, inflammatory disorders, liver disease, and lung infections. When the CEA level is elevated preoperatively and falls to normal levels after surgery, it may be useful in following patients to detect a recurrence of cancer.

Researchers also have attempted to use changes in gastric secretions as a marker for stomach cancer; however, variations in gastric acid production occur normally as people age, and varying degrees of decreased stomach acidity accompany gastritis as well as stomach cancer. A mucus component, fetal sulfoglycoprotein antigen (FSA), has been found in mucus-producing gastric cancer cells. Unfortunately, this is not a specific marker for stomach cancer because patients with ulcers, gastritis, and a variety of other noncancerous stomach conditions also may produce FSA. Alpha-fetoprotein, another protein that is found in the blood, is elevated in 15 to 20 percent of patients with stomach cancer, but it also may be elevated in patients with primary liver cancer and in people with noncancerous diseases, including cirrhosis and hepatitis. At this time, tumor markers are of limited value in diagnosing stomach cancer.

Staging

The extent (stage) of disease at the time of diagnosis is a major factor for selecting treatment and estimating the prognosis of patients with stomach cancer. Physical examination, x-rays, gastroscopy, surgical exploration of the abdomen, and scans of the liver, spleen, and bones are used to determine the stage of disease.

In order to document progress in the treatment of stomach cancer and to ensure that research results are comparable, the American Joint Committee on Cancer (sponsored by the National Cancer Institute, the American Cancer Society, and the American Colleges of Pathologists, Physicians, Radiology, and Surgeons) has established a staging system for stomach cancer. This system is based on the extent of tumor penetration through the stomach wall, the extent of lymph node involvement, and the presence or absence of distant metastases.

The amount of stomach wall invasion determines the stage of the primary tumor (T). Stomach cancer is classified TX, when this factor cannot be assessed; T0, when there is no evidence of primary tumor; Tis, or carcinoma in situ, when the disease is limited to the mucosa; or T and a number from 1 to 4b, depending on the extent of penetration. Lymph nodes (N) are classified NX, if they cannot be assessed; N0, if no cancer cells are found; or N and a number from 1 to 3, depending on the location of the nodes involved. Distant metastases (M) are classified as MX, when the metastases cannot be assessed; M0, when no distant disease is found; or M1, when distant metastases are present.

Using this system, stomach cancer can be classified into five different stages:

Stage 0:   This is very early stomach cancer that has not spread beyond the mucosa (Tis, N0, M0).

Stage I: Cancer is confined to the inner layers of the stomach wall (T1, N0, M0).

Stage II: Cancer is confined to the stomach wall but does not involve adjacent tissues (T2-3, N0, M0).

Stage III: Cancer involves tissues adjacent to the stomach and/or regional lymph nodes (T1-3, N1-2, M0; or T4a, N0-2, M0).

Stage IV: Cancer has spread locally or distantly. Most commonly the cancer has spread to the liver or other organs or has penetrated through the entire stomach wall (T1-3, N3, M0; or T4b, any N, M0; or any T, any N, M1).

Treatment

Surgery, radiation therapy, and chemotherapy, alone or in various combinations, are used to treat stomach cancer. The choice of therapy for an individual patient depends on a number of factors, including the stage of disease at the time of diagnosis, the age and general health of the patient, and other variables. For patients with early, localized stomach cancer, surgery is the usual treatment. These patients also may receive radiation therapy or chemotherapy. Patients with advanced stomach cancer may be treated with chemotherapy, with or without radiation therapy, or may have surgery to relieve symptoms of the disease.

Surgery

At this time, surgery is the only potentially curative treatment for patients with stomach cancer. The first successful surgery to remove part of the stomach (partial gastrectomy) was performed by Dr. Theodore Billroth in 1880, and modifications of his surgical procedure are still used today.

The type of surgery chosen depends on the extent of the tumor and its location in the stomach. Because it is not a vital organ, part or all of the stomach can be removed. The connecting portion of the esophagus or small intestine, spleen, and areas of the liver and colon also may be removed without jeopardizing the patient's long-term survival.

For most patients with stomach cancer, the preferred procedure is some form of subtotal gastrectomy. In this operation, 80 to 85 percent of the stomach is removed, along with a portion of the peritoneum, a portion of the esophagus or the first part of the small intestine called the duodenum (depending on the site of the tumor), and nearby lymph nodes. The spleen is removed if it contains evidence of cancer or if cancer is found in the part of the stomach that lies next to the spleen. Tumor that extends directly into adjacent organs, such as the liver or colon, also is removed. A replacement stomach may be made by gastroduoden-ostomy (connecting the stomach remnant to the duodenum), or by gastrojejunostomy (connecting the stomach remnant to the je-junum, or second segment of the small intestine).

If cancer is widespread throughout the stomach, total gastrectomy is necessary. In this procedure, the entire stomach, portions of the esophagus or small intestine, the obvious sites of metastases, and part of the peritoneum are removed. The spleen also may be removed in some cases. A substitute stomach may be made by esophagoduo-denostomy (connecting the esophagus to the duodenum) or by esophagojejunostomy (con-necting the esophagus to the jejunum). The new stomach may be formed during the initial operation, or it may be made after the patient has had time to recover from the original surgery.

Surgery also may be done to relieve symptoms, reduce the risk of bleeding, or remove an ob-structing tumor. Usually, some form of subtotal gastrectomy is performed.

One of the most common complications following extensive stomach surgery is known as the "dumping syndrome." Patients with this syndrome may feel full after eating only small amounts, and they may have rumbling noises, cramps, and diarrhea soon after eating. Other com-plaints may include rapid heart-beat, sweating, weakness, and dizziness. These symptoms may be worse after high-carbohydrate meals. The dumping syndrome is caused by the rapid emptying of the stomach contents into the small intestine. Eating frequent, small meals of low-carbohydrate, high-protein foods and limiting the intake of salt and liquids may relieve these symptoms.

All patients who have had gastrectomy eventually become deficient in vitamin B_{12}. Monthly injections of the vitamin can replace normal levels.

Patients with stomach cancer who have significant malnutrition following surgery may require nutritional support. Nourishment may be given through a nasogastric tube (a thin tube inserted through the nose and throat into the stomach), or a tube may be surgically implanted directly into the stomach (gastric tube). In total parenteral nutrition, nutrients are given through a catheter placed in a vein, often in the upper chest.

Radiation Therapy*

Although stomach cancer cells are sensitive to radiation, radiotherapy cannot be used alone to treat this disease because nearby tissues and organs (particularly the small intestine, liver, kidneys, and spinal cord) cannot withstand the large amounts of radiation required to destroy the cancer cells. Its use is further limited because stomach cancer usually has spread to other areas by the time it is diagnosed. However, radiation therapy is useful in treating residual disease following surgery. In addition, radiotherapy, usually in conjunction with chemotherapy, plays a major role in treating patients with advanced or recurrent stomach cancer.

Surgery and radiation therapy can be combined in a number of ways to treat patients with stomach cancer. Radiation may be given before surgery to shrink a tumor and make it easier to remove. Postoperative radiotherapy may be used to treat tumor cells that cannot be removed. During surgery, the cancerous tissue that cannot be removed is outlined with metal clips. Postoperative radiation therapy is planned so that the marked tissue, which can be seen on an x-ray, is included in the radiation field (the area treated by radiotherapy).

Another promising technique under study is intraoperative radiotherapy (IORT), in which radiation is given during surgery. One possible advantage of this procedure is that healthy tissues can be spared by moving them out of the radiation field. In a large multi-institution study conducted in Japan, approximately 200 stomach cancer patients were treated with surgery and IORT. An increase in survival rates was seen in some groups of patients, and no serious complications were reported. This study suggests that IORT might be useful, but it is not clear whether these results are better than those that might be obtained with conventional postoperative radiotherapy. The National Cancer Institute currently is studying IORT to

---

* See chapter entitled, **Radiation Therapy and You.** Consult CONTENTS for page location.

learn more about the side effects of this procedure and its ability to control stomach cancer.

The side effects of radiotherapy vary from patient to patient. The most common complications include skin problems in the treated area, fatigue, and loss of appetite. Nausea, vomiting, and diarrhea may begin in about 1 week and persist to a diminishing degree for a month or more following treatment.

Chemotherapy*

Chemotherapy is used to relieve the symptoms of patients with advanced or recurrent stomach cancer. In addition, researchers are studying the possible benefits of adjuvant chemotherapy, the use of drugs soon after surgery or radiation therapy in an effort to kill undetectable cancer cells that may remain after initial treatment. They also continue to look for new single agents and combinations of drugs that might be effective against metastatic and recurrent stomach cancer.

The most extensively studied and probably the most useful single agent is 5-fluorouracil (5-FU). Other drugs that have been studied include doxorubicin (Adriamycin), mitomycin C,

BCNU (Carmustine), and methyl CCNU (Semustine). Hydroxyurea, mechlorethamine, DTIC, and chlorambucil (Leukeran) also have shown some activity against stomach cancer.

In numerous attempts to develop more effective chemotherapy, researchers have studied combinations of drugs. Two promising regimens that have been tested extensively in the United States combine 5-FU with either BCNU or methyl CCNU. Another combination under investigation is FAM, which combines 5-FU, Adriamycin, and mitomycin C.

Postoperative adjuvant chemotherapy is an area of active research. Early results have been promising, but it is too soon to tell whether the addition of chemotherapy to primary therapy will improve disease-free or overall survival rates in patients with stomach cancer. Researchers have studied adjuvant chemotherapy using 5-FU and methyl CCNU. Results of these studies differed, with one trial showing a statistical benefit for patients treated with these drugs, while another did not.

Adjuvant combination chemotherapy also is being evaluated as

---

* See chapter entitled, **Chemotherapy and You.** Consult CONTENTS for page location.

treatment for patients who have had initial treatment with surgery or radiation therapy. Combinations currently under study include FAM and 5-FU plus Adriamycin. Additional research is needed to determine the exact role of adjuvant chemotherapy in the treatment of patients with stomach cancer.

Clinical trials also are under way to evaluate the benefit of chemotherapy for patients with metastatic stomach cancer. Studies are being conducted with FAM, FAME (5-FU, Adriamycin, and methyl CCNU), 5-FU alone, and BCNU alone. (Additional information about clinical trials appears below).

The drugs used to treat cancer interfere with the growth of rapidly dividing cancer cells. Because some normal cells also grow quickly, they also can be affected by chemotherapy. The type and intensity of the side effects of this type of treatment depend on the drug or drugs used and the response of the individual patient. Common side effects include nausea and vomiting, increased susceptibility to infection, mouth and throat problems, and hair loss. Anticancer drugs also may cause muscle weakness, nerve effects, and heart complications.

While it may be another decade before the results of current stomach cancer research are available, a number of advances already have been made in treating this disease. A better understanding of the routes of tumor spread has led to a number of improvements in the surgical procedures used to remove stomach cancer. Studies conducted with cancer patients have suggested that the combination of surgery and radiation therapy may be effective in controlling microscopic residual disease. In addition, careful followup evaluation and attention to nutrition may improve the quality of the patient's life.

Clinical Trials*and PDQ

To improve the outcome of treatment for stomach cancer, the NCI supports clinical studies at many hospitals throughout the United States. Patients who take part in this research make an important contribution to medical science and may have the first chance to benefit from improved treatment methods. Physicians are encouraged to inform their patients about the option of participating in such studies.

---

*For in-depth discussion of clinical trials see chapter entitled, Clinical Trials: What Are They All About? See CONTENTS for location.

To help patients and doctors learn about current trials, the NCI has developed PDQ (Physician Data Query), a computerized database designed to give doctors quick and easy access to:

- the latest treatment information for most types of cancer;

- descriptions of current clinical trials that are accepting patients; and

- names of physicians and organizations involved in cancer care.

To access PDQ, doctors may use an office computer with a telephone hookup and a PDQ access code or the services of a medical library with online searching capability. Most Cancer Information Service offices (1-800-4-CANCER) provide PDQ searches and can tell doctors how to obtain regular access to the database. Patients may ask their doctor to use PDQ, or they may call 1-800-4-CANCER themselves to request a search. Information specialists at this toll-free telephone number use a variety of sources, including PDQ, to answer questions about cancer prevention, diagnosis, treatment, and research.

Selected References

The materials marked with an * are distributed free of charge by the NCI. The other items are not available from the NCI; they can be found in medical libraries, many college and university libraries, and some public libraries.

Cancer Rates and Risks. Prepared by the Office of Cancer Communications, National Cancer Insitute. NIH Publication No. 85-691.

Caygill, C.P. et al. "Mortality From Gastric Cancer Following Gastric Surgery for Peptic Ulcer," *The Lancet,* Vol. 1, April 26, 1986, pp. 929-931.

Chemotherapy and You: A Guide to Self-Help During Treatment. Prepared by the Office of Cancer Communications, National Cancer Institute. NIH Publication No. 86-1136.

Correa, P. "Precursors of Gastric and Esophageal Cancer," *Cancer,* Vol. 50(11), December 1982, pp. 2554-2565.

Correa, P. et al. "Epidemiology of Gastric Carcinoma: Review and Future Prospects," *National Cancer Institute Monograph,* No. 62, December 1982, pp. 129-134.

DeVita, V.T., Jr. et al., eds. *Cancer: Principles and Practice of Oncology.* 2nd Edition. Philadelphia: J.B. Lippincott Co., 1985.

Diet, Nutrition and Cancer Prevention: The Good News. Prepared by the Office of Cancer Communications, National Cancer Institute. NIH Publication No. 87-2878.

---

* The mentioned text is reprinted within this book. See CONTENTS for location.

DuPont, B.J., Jr. and Cohn, I., Jr. "Gastric Adenocarcinoma," *Current Problems in Cancer,* Vol. 4(8), February 1980, pp. 1-46.

Haskell, C.M., ed. *Cancer Treatment.* 2nd Edition. Philadelphia: W.B. Saunders Co., 1985.

Hattori, T. "Development of Adenocarcinomas in the Stomach," *Cancer,* Vol. 57 (8), April 1986, pp. 1528-1534.

Holland, J. and Frei, E., III, eds. *Cancer Medicine.* 2nd Edition. Philadelphia: Lea and Febiger, 1982.

Howson, C.P. et al. "The Decline in Gastric Cancer: Epidemiology of an Unplanned Triumph," *Epidemiologic Reviews,* Vol. 8, 1986, pp. 1-24.

Radiation Therapy and You: A Guide to Self-Help During Treatment. Prepared by the Office of Cancer Communications, National Cancer Institute. NIH Publication No. 86-2227.

Schein, P.S. et al. "Gastric Cancer," *Seminars in Oncology,* Vol. 12(1), March 1985, pp. 1-53.

Schottenfeld, D. and Fraumeni, J., eds. *Cancer Epidemiology and Prevention.* Philadelphia: W.B. Saunders Co., 1982.

What Are Clinical Trials All About? Prepared by the Office of Cancer Communications, National Cancer Institute. NIH Publication No. 86-2706.

* The mentioned text is reprinted within this book. See CONTENTS for location.

Chapter 24

Testicular Cancer

Introduction

This *Research Report* describes current research on the causes, symptoms, diagnosis, and treatment of cancer of the testis. The information presented here came from medical textbooks, recent articles in the scientific literature, discussions with National Cancer Institute (NCI) scientists and other researchers, and various scientific meetings.

Description and Function of the Testes

The testicles, or testes, are the male gonads. Formed in the abdominal cavity early in the development of a male fetus, they normally descend into the scrotum before or soon after birth. In addition to producing spermatozoa, the testes are the principal source of male hormones called androgens. These hormones control the development of the reproductive organs and secondary sex characteristics. Androgens also are responsible for the sex drive.

Inside each testicle is a mass of narrow, tightly coiled tubes, called seminiferous tubules, which manufacture sperm. As sperm are produced, they move to the epididymis, a larger tube at the back of the testicles, where they are temporarily stored. Upon ejaculation, sperm leave the epididymis through a duct known as the vas deferens and are mixed with fluids produced by the seminal vesicles, the prostate gland, and Cowper's gland. The seminal fluid is then forcibly propelled out through the urethra, the same duct that carries urine from the bladder.

Like all other tissues and organs, the testes are composed of individual cells. Normally, cells divide and reproduce in an orderly way as they are needed to carry out their proper functions in the body. Cancers in the testes, as in other organs, result from the uncontrolled multiplication and accumulation of defective cells. The growing mass of abnormal tissue eventually crowds out and destroys nearby healthy tissue. In addition, cancer cells can break away from the tumor and metastasize, or spread, through the lymphatic system and the bloodstream, to other parts of the body. Testicular cancer cells tend to migrate to the lungs, bone, liver, and brain, where they can continue to reproduce excessively and form secondary tumors. Cancer cells found in these secondary tumors are usually identical to those of the primary cancer, and although another organ of the body is affected, the disease is still called testicular cancer. The secondary tumors are treated by methods appropriate for metastatic testicular cancer, rather than for cancer that originates at the site of the metastasis.

Incidence

Cancer of the testis accounts for only about 1 percent of all male cancers, but unlike most other cancers, this disease is generally found in relatively young men. It is the most common cancer in white men between 20 and 34 years of age, the second most common from 35 to 39, and the third most common from 15 to 19. This type of cancer is 4.5 times more common among white men than black, with intermediate incidence rates for Hispanics, American Indians, and Asians. Overall, about 3 American men in 1,000 develop testicular cancer at some time in their lives. It is estimated that about 5,100 new cases of testicular cancer will be diagnosed in the United States in the current year.

Cause and Prevention

The causes of cancer of the testis are not well understood, and scientists cannot yet explain why some men develop the disease while others do not. Congenital abnormalities, hormonal drugs, certain diseases, and trauma have been suggested as factors that could increase a man's risk of developing testicular cancer.

One known risk factor for this type of cancer is a congenital condition known as cryptorchidism (failure of one or both testes to descend into the scrotal sac). Approximately 1 testicular cancer patient in 10 has a history of this developmental abnormality. Recent studies indicate that men born with undescended testes have 3 to 17 times the average risk of developing testicular cancer later on, particularly if the condition is not surgically corrected in early childhood. The results of one study suggest that there may be no appreciably increased risk if the surgical repair is performed before the age of 6.

In laboratory experiments, pregnant mice injected with estrogen (a female hormone) or with DES (the synthetic estrogen diethylstilbestrol) gave birth to male offspring with testicular abnormalities. In humans, prenatal exposure to DES, taken in the past to prevent miscarriage, is known to increase the risk of structural abnormalities of the reproductive tract and vaginal cancer in daughters. Such exposure also has been associated with certain testicular abnormalities in sons, but whether prenatal exposure to DES or other forms of estrogen increases the risk of testicular cancer in sons is not known.

Studies have demonstrated a link between testicular cancer and certain rare congenital conditions. These include chromosomal abnormalities, such as Klinefelter's syndrome, as well as abnormalities in fetal development of the reproductive tract, such as gonadal aplasia (failure of the testes to develop) or various forms of hermaphroditism (development of both male and female sex characteristics in the same individual).

Because some testicular cancer patients report a history of infectious diseases affecting the testes, some scientists speculate that damage to testicular tissue from viral infections such as mumps may increase the risk of testicular cancer years later, but this possibility has not been confirmed. Similarly, a history of scrotal injury is encountered in some men with cancer of the testis, but it is not clear whether these problems actually cause the disease or simply call attention to a tumor that already exists.

Detection and Diagnosis

In recent years, because of remarkable advances in the management of testicular cancer, this has become one of the most curable of all cancers, especially if it is found at an early stage. It is extremely important, therefore, that the condition be detected early and treated promptly.

Detection

Most testicular cancers are discovered by patients themselves, by accident or by practicing a simple technique known as testicular self-examination. This procedure is best performed once a month, during or soon after a warm shower or bath, when the scrotal wall is relaxed and abnormalities are easy to feel. While standing, the man gently rolls one testicle between his thumb and fingers, checking for lumps, swelling, or other changes. The process is repeated with the other testicle. The normal testicle feels smooth, egg-shaped, and rather firm.

The most common sign of cancer of the testis is a small hard lump, about the size of a pea, but any abnormality (particularly scrotal enlargement, unusual tenderness, pain, or a feeling of heaviness) should be reported to a physician without delay. Such symptoms can be caused by various conditions other than cancer, and only a doctor can make a diagnosis.

Diagnosis

If infection and other diseases are ruled out by physical examination and medical tests, symptoms such as those described above can generally be attributed to the presence of a tumor. Because most tumors in the testes are malignant (cancerous) rather than benign (noncancerous), the standard procedure for a suspicious lump in the scrotum is surgical removal of the entire affected testis. This is accomplished through an incision in the groin, a procedure known as inguinal orchiectomy. Removing the testicle provides a diagnosis, prevents further growth of the primary tumor, and when performed at an early stage, may stop the spread of the cancer to other parts of the body. (A biopsy is *not* performed through the scrotal sac because this procedure would entail cutting through the tunica albuginea, the tough, fibrous outer capsule of the testis, and could contribute to the spread of cancer cells.)

Microscopic examination of the tissue enables a pathologist to make a diagnosis and, if the disease is cancer, to identify the particular type of cells that make up the tumor. Nearly all testicular cancers arise from germinal cells, the special sperm-forming cells in the testes. (Nongerm cell cancers of the testes are quite rare and are not dealt with in this Research Report.)

Germ cell cancers are classified as *seminomas* and *nonseminomas*. Seminomas, which account for about 40 percent of all testicular germ cell cancers, are composed of undifferentiated cells; that is, cells in a very early stage of development. Nonseminomas, made up of more specialized cells, include embryonal carcinoma, teratoma, yolk sac carcinoma, choriocarcinoma, and tumors that contain more than one type of cancer cell.

Staging

The stage of the disease indicates whether the cancer has spread beyond the testis, where, and to what extent. Stage I refers to testicular cancer that appears to be confined to the testis; stage II means the disease has spread to the abdominal lymph nodes; and stage III indicates the cancer has metastasized beyond these nodes. Physicians use imaging techniques, serum markers, and surgical procedures to make staging more accurate and subsequent choice of treatment more precise.

Imaging techniques include conventional X-rays and several recently developed procedures such as computerized tomography (CT) scans (detailed X-ray pictures of cross-sections of the body), lymphangiography (X-rays of the lymph system taken after a dye is injected into a lymph vessel), and intravenous pyelography (X-ray studies of the kidneys and urinary system following an injection of dye into a vein). Ultrasound studies, which produce a visual image of sound waves and their echoes passing through tissue, may also be used to help determine whether the cancer has spread.

Serum markers are proteins that frequently are present in abnormal amounts in the blood of cancer patients. Alpha-fetoprotein (AFP) and the beta subunit of human chorionic gonadotropin (HCG) are the most dependable markers for nonseminomatous testicular cancers. Studies have shown that most patients with nonseminomas of the testis have elevated levels of AFP and/or HCG. The levels of these blood proteins are measured before and after surgery; comparing the pre- and postoperative test results helps determine whether any cancer cells remain. AFP and HCG levels return to normal when the cancer has been entirely removed or has completely regressed. If the disease recurs, marker levels often become elevated again months before X-rays or physical examination can detect the problem. Thus, measuring these serum markers helps to establish the stage of the cancer, as well as to monitor the patient's response to treatment and to detect a relapse if it occurs.

By contrast, among patients with seminomas, only about 10 to 20 percent have abnormal HCG levels, and all have normal AFP levels. If AFP levels are elevated in seminoma patients, it is assumed that the tumor type is actually mixed, containing some nonseminomatous cells. These patients are then treated as having nonseminomas.

Less specific markers, such as lactic dehydrogenase (LDH), carcinoembryonic antigen (CEA), placental alkaline phosphatase, ferritin, and others, may also be indicators of testicular cancer, but their value in the clinical management of patients remains to be defined.

Surgery to remove the abdominal lymph nodes and microscopic examination of this tissue is necessary in some patients for accurate appraisal of the stage of the disease. In addition, since testicular cancer spreads first to the retroperitoneal lymph nodes (the nodes deep in the abdomen below the diaphragm), this surgical staging procedure is believed to help control the disease by removing any involved nodes.

At this time, removal of the abdominal lymph nodes is generally recommended for patients with nonseminomas to determine whether the disease is in stage I or stage II. However, because of improvements in staging and diagnostic techniques and advances in the treatment of recurrent testicular cancer, clinical studies now in progress are attempting to determine whether lymph node removal is routinely necessary. These studies may show that the procedure can be omitted in nonseminoma patients who have negative CT scans and lymphangiograms, as well as certain other favorable prognostic factors, and who agree to a program of thorough monthly checkups. In the event that physical examination and imaging procedures indicate that stage II patients have extensive cancer in their lymph nodes, chemotherapy may be initiated without removing the nodes.

The lymph nodes of early-stage seminoma patients are not removed. Orchiectomy followed by radiation therapy to destroy cancer cells in the lymph nodes is highly curative in stage I and most stage II patients with this type of testicular cancer, so it is not necessary for the physician to determine whether the lymph nodes are affected.

Lymph node removal is not performed in advanced testicular cancer (stage III) of either cell type. This procedure is unnecessary when other staging procedures indicate that the cancer has spread to lymph nodes above the diaphragm, to the lungs, or to other organs.

Treatment

Achievements in the treatment of testicular cancer have been impressive. More effective chemotherapy—notably cisplatin in combination with other anticancer drugs—improved diagnostic tools such as serum markers and better imaging techniques, and a better understanding of the disease have contributed to significant improvement in patient survival.

Only a decade or two ago, the outlook for patients with advanced nonseminomatous testicular cancers was particularly poor, with fewer than 10 percent of patients living 5 years after their diagnosis. Now, 70 percent or more can expect to remain free of disease for at least 5 years. The 5-year survival rate for patients with early-stage nonseminomas has also improved since 1970, from as low as 50 percent at that time to over 95 percent expected in patients diagnosed in 1981.

Information about testicular cancer patients diagnosed between 1976 and 1981 has been collected and analyzed by the Surveillance, Epidemiology and End Results (SEER) Program of the National Cancer Institute. Combining all stages of both seminoma and nonseminoma, the overall 5-year survival rate is now 86 percent, and this rate is continuing to improve.

Seminomas and nonseminomas differ in cellular composition and in their tendency to metastasize, pattern of metastasis, and response to radiation therapy. Physicians make treatment decisions after the cell type has been identified and staging procedures have determined the extent of the disease.

Seminoma

These cancers tend to remain localized; the vast majority of seminomas are diagnosed in stage I or stage II. For patients with early-stage seminomas, surgery is usually limited to the orchiectomy. As mentioned above, the removal of abdominal lymph nodes to control metastasis is not warranted because seminomas are highly sensitive to radiation. Radiotherapy is routinely directed to the retroperitoneal lymph nodes to eliminate any clusters of cells that may be present but too small to be detected (stage I); radiation is also used to destroy cancer discovered in these nodes in the staging process (stage II). As a preventive measure, lymph nodes above the diaphragm and in the groin are sometimes irradiated as well.

Seminoma patients with large tumors but no evidence of spread beyond the lymph nodes in the abdomen (known as "bulky" stage II tumors) and those with disseminated cancer (stage III) are generally treated with combination chemotherapy (often the same drugs used for nonseminomas, described below), sometimes in combination with radiotherapy.

Nonseminoma

In contrast to seminomas, most nonseminomas are not diagnosed in an early stage. About 65 percent of men with nonseminomatous testicular cancer have some degree of metastasis when first seen by a physician.

When removal of the retroperitoneal lymph nodes confirms that a nonseminomatous tumor is confined to the testis (stage I), the patient receives no further treatment. The small number (about 10 percent) of stage I patients who have recurrences later on are treated with chemotherapy.

Similarly, stage II patients whose tumor marker levels return to normal after orchiectomy and lymph node removal may require no additional treatment. Another option in the treatment of stage II patients with no evidence of cancer after surgery is to administer a short course of adjuvant chemotherapy (anticancer drugs given soon after surgery) to reduce the risk of recurrence. Clinical studies are in progress to compare the effects of these two treatment approaches on long-term survival; preliminary data indicate excellent results for both options.

For stage II patients whose tumor markers remain elevated after removal of the cancerous testicle and retroperitoneal lymph nodes, and for those with stage III nonseminomas, anticancer drugs are administered. Dramatic progress has been made in the treatment of these patients. Combination chemotherapy for nonseminomatous testicular cancer was used as early as 1960 but produced complete remissions in only about 12 percent of patients with metastatic cancer. At that time, only half of those achieving complete remission lived longer than 2 years. In 1970, research physicians began using a combination of vinblastine and bleomycin, which improved complete remission rates to about 40 percent. Given together, these two drugs had a synergistic effect that enhanced their potency as anticancer agents. Today, drug combinations that include cisplatin are producing even better results.

The ability of the metal compound cisplatin to block cell division was first observed in 1961. Since this drug (also called DDP, Platinol, or cis-platinum) became available for clinical study in 1974, the combination of cisplatin, vinblastine, and bleomycin (called PVB) has led to greatly improved results in nonseminoma patients, with complete remission rates of 60 to 80 percent in men who have had no previous treatment. Cisplatin given with cyclophosphamide, vinblastine, actinomycin-D, and bleomycin (a variation of a combination known as VAB) has also produced good results. In 1978, after its efficacy was demonstrated in clinical trials, cisplatin was approved by the U.S. Food and Drug Administration (FDA) for the treatment of testicular cancer.

Despite the success of cisplatin combinations in nonseminomatous testicular cancer, however, about 20 percent of patients with metastatic disease achieve only a partial response and do not have a long-term survival. Moreover, some patients (about 5 to 10 percent) relapse after achieving complete remission. A new drug called etoposide (also known as VP-16 and VePesid) appears to improve the prognosis for these patients.

Since 1977, etoposide has been used alone and in combination with other drugs, particularly cisplatin and bleomycin, in the successful treatment of patients who were not cured by PVB. The National Cancer Institute has studied etoposide in combination with cisplatin, vinblastine, and bleomycin. Results suggest that this four-drug regimen may benefit patients with large tumors or advanced disease, who would have a poor prognosis with standard PVB therapy. In 1983, etoposide received FDA approval for the treatment of testicular cancer that has not responded well to previous treatment with surgery, chemotherapy, and radiation.

In patients with metastatic nonseminomas, sometimes a mass of tissue is still present after treatment with combination chemotherapy. This mass is not always cancerous; it may be comprised of dead tissue or abnormal, noncancerous tissue. Elevated tumor marker levels after four cycles of chemotherapy indicate that cancer is still present, and additional chemotherapy is required. On the other hand, if marker levels are not elevated, surgery is usually performed to determine whether cells in the remaining mass are or have the potential to become cancerous, so that the best treatment strategy can be selected. If surgery reveals that cancer cells are present, further chemotherapy is required. Removing potentially cancerous tissue may contribute to disease control in some patients. When tumor markers are normal and no cancer cells are apparent at surgery, further chemotherapy is not necessary.

Side Effects of Treatment

Every form of cancer treatment can be accompanied by various undesirable side effects, but all patients do not have the same problems, nor do they experience difficulties to the same degree. In general, men with testicular cancer—who are usually in their 20's, 30's, and 40's—may be better able to tolerate side effects than older patients. Young men are likely to be particularly concerned, however, about the effects that treatment may have on their sexual and reproductive abilities.

Surgery

Orchiectomy (the removal of one testicle) does not impair either fertility or sexual function. The remaining testicle can produce adequate amounts of both sperm and hormones. Patients concerned about their appearance may consider having an artificial testicle implanted in the scrotum. A gel-filled implant, which has the weight, shape, and texture of a normal testicle, may be inserted at the time of the orchiectomy or at a later time.

Lymph node removal seldom affects a man's ability to have erections and orgasms. However, the surgical technique generally performed to remove abdominal lymph nodes often results in infertility because of impaired ejaculation.

As mentioned above, lymph node surgery has been part of the standard treatment of patients with nonseminomas, but research physicians currently are trying to learn whether improvements in staging techniques and better chemotherapeutic drugs can make lymph node surgery unnecessary for some patients. Scientists are also exploring new surgical techniques that may be just as effective against the cancer without impairing normal ejaculation.

Radiotherapy

Because radiation affects normal as well as cancerous cells, radiotherapy can cause a number of side effects. Many patients experience fatigue and lowered blood counts. Some also have diarrhea, nausea, and vomiting, but these problems are generally neither severe nor long lasting. They can usually be alleviated with medication.

Irradiation of the lymph nodes does not affect sexual function but does interfere with sperm production. With proper shielding of the normal testicle and other parts of the reproductive tract, infertility is temporary. Most patients regain fertility within a matter of months.

Chemotherapy

Anticancer drugs circulating in the bloodstream can reach and damage normal cells as well as cancer cells. Therefore, chemotherapy can produce a variety of side effects. There may be increased risk of infection due to reduced blood cell counts, nausea and vomiting, hair loss, and certain other problems associated with specific drugs.

Most men receiving chemotherapy remain capable of having sexual relations. For some, however, the general side effects of chemotherapy, such as fatigue and a decreased sense of well-being, may temporarily interfere with ability or desire.

Some anticancer drugs can cause infertility. Unfortunately, most patients with testicular cancer are ineligible for sperm banking before chemotherapy because they already have impaired sperm production as a result of the disease itself. Recent studies have shown, however, that many men recover their fertility 2 to 3 years after completing chemotherapy.

407

Severe nausea and vomiting are common for testicular cancer patients receiving cisplatin, but physicians can ease these problems with appropriate medications, such as metoclopramide. During cisplatin treatment, some patients experience hearing problems, which may diminish once the drug is stopped. Lowered blood counts are another significant side effect of this drug.

The major drawback of cisplatin has been its toxic effect on the kidneys. Investigators have learned to combat this problem in two ways: They maintain the patient's fluid flow through the kidneys before and during treatment with large volumes of intravenous saline (salt) solution and diuretics, and they administer the drug in concentrated saline. Clinical studies have shown that cisplatin mixed with a 3-percent saline solution can be given at twice the usual dose without increasing the risk of kidney damage. Doubling the dosage appears to improve the effectiveness of the drug.

In an effort to develop effective drugs with fewer undesirable side effects, scientists are investigating several substances that are chemically related to cisplatin. One promising analog of cisplatin is diaminocyclobutyldicarboxylateplatinum(II), also known as CBDCA. This investigational drug has been found to be far less toxic to kidney tissue in animals; it is now being tested in cancer patients.

Followup Care

Once a testicular cancer patient has completed his course of therapy, continuing medical care is vital. To identify relapses and initiate treatment as soon as possible, followup should include monthly measurement of serum marker levels, and regular X-rays and scans during the first 2 years, when the risk of recurrence is highest. After that, checkups are scheduled just once or twice a year. Nearly all patients who remain free of disease for 3 years can be considered cured.

In the past, monthly maintenance doses of anticancer drugs were given to patients in complete remission to prevent recurrence of testicular cancer. Recent clinical research indicates, however, that continuation of chemotherapy for patients in remission after treatment for disseminated disease is not necessary. An important study compared patients in complete remission who received maintenance doses of vinblastine with those who did not; there was no difference in the relapse rates of the two groups. Thus, the study demonstrated that testicular cancer patients who achieve a complete remission with their initial chemotherapy do not need maintenance therapy. Additional treatment is necessary only if the cancer recurs later.

Patients who have been treated for testicular cancer have roughly a 1 percent risk of developing cancer in the remaining testicle. If cancer appears in the second testicle years later, it is, in all likelihood, a new disease and not metastasis from the previous tumor. As with the first cancer, early detection significantly enhances the probability of cure. For that reason, these men should be conscientious about performing testicular self-examination and should also continue to be examined periodically by a physician.

PDQ

The National Cancer Institute has developed PDQ (Physician Data Query), a computerized database designed to give doctors quick and easy access to:
• The latest treatment information for most types of cancer;

• Descriptions of clinical trials that are open for patient entry; and
• Names of organizations and physicians involved in cancer care.

To get access to PDQ, a doctor may use an office computer with a telephone hookup and a PDQ access code or the services of a medical library with online searching capability. Most Cancer Information Service offices (1-800-4-CANCER) provide a physician with one free PDQ search, and can tell doctors how to get regular access to the database. Patients may ask their doctor to use PDQ or may call 1-800-4-CANCER themselves. Information specialists at this toll-free number use a variety of sources, including PDQ, to answer questions about cancer prevention, diagnosis, and treatment.

Suggestions for Additional Reading

Except as noted, the following materials are not available from the National Cancer Institute (NCI). They can be found in medical libraries, many college and university libraries, and some public libraries.

"Anticancer Drug VP-16," prepared by the Office of Cancer Communications, National Cancer Institute, May 1984.

Cancer Rates and Risks, prepared by the Office of Cancer Communications, National Cancer Institute. NIH Publication No. 85-691.

Carter, S.K. "The Management of Testicular Cancer," *Recent Results in Cancer Research,* vol. 85, 1983, pp. 70-122.

Chemotherapy and You: A Guide to Self-Help During Treatment, prepared by the Office of Cancer Communications, National Cancer Institute. NIH Publication No. 85-1136.

DeWys, W.D. et al. "Adjuvant Chemotherapy of Testicular Cancer," *Adjuvant Therapy of Cancer IV,* Jones, S.E. and Salmon, S.E., eds. New York: Grune and Stratton, 1984, pp. 529-537.

DeVita, V.T., Jr. et al., eds. *Cancer: Principles and Practice of Oncology,* second edition. Philadelphia: Lippincott Co., 1982.

Drasga, R.E. et al. "The Chemotherapy of Testicular Cancer," *Ca--A Cancer Journal for Clinicians,* March/April 1982, pp. 66-77.

Drasga, R.E. et al. "Fertility After Chemotherapy for Testicular Cancer," *Journal of Clinical Oncology,* March 1983, pp. 179-183.

Einhorn, L.H., ed. *Testicular Tumors: Management and Treatment.* New York: Masson Publishing USA, Inc., 1980.

Einhorn, L.H. "Testicular Cancer as a Model for a Curable Neoplasm: The Richard and Hinda Rosenthal Award Lecture," *Cancer Research,* Sep. 1981, pp. 3275-3280.

Haskell, Charles M., ed. *Cancer Treatment,* second edition. Philadelphia: W.B. Saunders, 1985.

Holland, J.F. and Frei, E., eds. *Cancer Medicine,* second edition. Philadelphia: Lea and Febiger, 1982.

Hubbard, S.M. and Jenkins, J. "An Overview of Current Concepts in the Management of Patients with Testicular Tumors of Germ Cell Origin. Part I: Pathophysiology, Diagnosis, and Staging," *Cancer Nursing,* February 1983, pp. 125-139.

Hubbard, S.M. and Jenkins, J. "An Overview of Current Concepts in the Management of Patients with Testicular Tumors of Germ Cell Origin. Part II: Treatment Strategies by Histology and Stage," *Cancer Nursing,* April 1983, pp. 125-139.

Huben, R.P. and Pontes, J.E. "Advances in the Treatment of Testicular Tumors," *International Advances in Surgical Oncology,* vol 7, 1984, pp. 355-372.

Javadpour, N., ed. *Principles and Management of Urologic Cancer,* second edition. Baltimore: Williams and Wilkins, 1983.

Johnson, D.H. et al. "Testicular Function Following Combination Chemotherapy with Cis-Platin, Vinblastine, and Bleomycin," *Medical and Pediatric Oncology,* vol. 12, 1984, pp. 233-238.

Li, F.P. et al. "Improved Survival Rates Among Testis Cancer Patients in the United States," *Journal of the American Medical Association,* Feb. 12, 1982, pp. 825-826.

Ostrow, S.S. "The Management of Nonseminomatous Testicular Cancer: Current Therapy and Future Directions," *American Journal of Medical Science,* Jan./Feb. 1983, pp. 24-37.

Ozols, R.F. et al. "Randomized Trial of PVeBV [High Dose (HD) Cisplatin (P), Vinblastine (Ve), Bleomycin (B), VP-16 (V)] Versus PVeB in Poor Prognosis Nonseminomatous Testicular Cancer (NSTC)," *Proceedings of the Annual Meeting of the American Society of Clinical Oncology,* vol. 3, 1984, p. 155.

Paulson, D.F. "Testicular Carcinoma," *Current Problems in Cancer,* May 1982, pp. 1-44.

Radiation Therapy and You: A Guide to Self-Help During Treatment, prepared by the Office of Cancer Communications, National Cancer Institute. NIH Publication No. 85-2227.

Richie, J.P. and Garnick, M.B. "Changing Concepts in the Treatment of Nonseminomatous Germ Cell Tumors of the Testis," *Journal of Urology,* June 1984, pp. 1089-1092.

Schottenfeld, D. and Fraumeni, J.F., Jr. eds. *Cancer Epidemiology and Prevention.* Philadelphia: W.B. Saunders, 1982.

Schover, L.R. and von Eschenbach, A.C. "Sexual and Marital Counseling of Men Treated for Testicular Cancer," *Journal of Sex and Marital Therapy,* Spring 1984, pp. 29-40.

Testicular Self-Examination, prepared by the Office of Cancer Communications, National Cancer Institute. NIH Publication No. 85-2636.

Tollerund, David J. et al. "Familial Testicular Cancer and Urogenital Developmental Anomalies," *Cancer,* vol. 55, April 15, 1985, pp. 1849-1854.

What Are Clinical Trials All About?,* prepared by the Office of Cancer Communications, National Cancer Institute. NIH Publication No. 86-2706.

What You Need to Know About Cancer of the Testis, prepared by the Office of Cancer Communications, National Cancer Institute. NIH Publication No. 86-1565.

Williams, S.D. and Einhorn, L.H. "Clinical Stage I Testis Tumors: The Medical Oncologists's View," *Cancer Treatment Reports,* Jan. 1982, pp. 15-18.

---

* The mentioned text is reprinted within this book. See CONTENTS for location.

Chapter 25

Cancer of
the Uterus

Introduction

This *Research Report* describes current research on the causes and prevention, symptoms, diagnosis, and treatment of cancers of the *uterine cervix* and the *uterine corpus,* or endometrium. The information presented here was obtained from recent articles in the scientific literature, discussions with National Cancer Institute (NCI) scientists and other researchers, and various scientific meetings.

Description and Function of the Uterus

The uterus, or womb, is located in the female pelvis. Under normal circumstances, the uterus is hollow and about the size and shape of an inverted pear. The broad upper part is called the corpus; the lower, narrow end is the cervix. During pregnancy, the uterus expands as the fetus grows within it.

The walls of the uterus are composed of muscular tissue called the myometrium, which is lined with a membrane called the endometrium. Cancer of the uterus most often develops in the cervix or in the endometrium of the corpus.

Endometrial and cervical cells normally grow and are replaced in an orderly, controlled pattern. When cell division is disordered, masses of tissue, called tumors, begin to grow. Such tumors may be benign or cancerous.

Benign uterine tumors, or fibroids, do not spread to nearby tissues or organs. They often cause no symptoms and require no treatment. If fibroids cause pain or bleeding, they may be removed completely by surgery.

In contrast, endometrial and cervical cancers invade and destroy nearby tissues and organs and can spread, or metastasize, to other parts of the body. When they begin to spread outside of the uterus, these cancer cells usually travel through the lymphatic system rather than the bloodstream. Lymph nodes scattered along the vessels of the lymphatic system collect and filter lymph fluid. The nodes filter out abnormal substances, including cancer cells. For this reason, lymph nodes near the tumor site are often removed during surgery so that a pathologist can examine them for evidence of cancer cells.

Cancer of the Cervix

Incidence

Cancer of the cervix accounts for 6 percent of all cancers in women and occurs most often in women between the ages of 40 and 60. In 1986, about 14,000 cases of cervical cancer will be diagnosed in the United States, and the disease will cause approximately 6,800 deaths. From 1950 to 1970, the incidence and mortality rates of invasive cervical cancer fell by more than 50 percent. Both rates have continued to drop since 1970, due mainly to the success of screening programs in bringing about earlier detection and treatment.

Cause and Prevention

Some women are more likely than others to develop abnormal cervical cells. Such women are considered to be "at risk," which means that their chances of developing cervical cancer are higher than average. The incidence of cervical cancer is higher than average among women of low income, women who began having sexual intercourse before age 18, and women who have had many sex partners. The daughters of women who took the drug diethylstilbestrol (DES) during pregnancy are also at risk. In a small number of such daughters, DES and some similar drugs have been linked to abnormal tissue formations in the vagina and cervix, including a rare type of vaginal and cervical cancer. Women on menopausal estrogen therapy and women who have had no children have a lower-than-average risk of developing cervical cancer.

There is also some suspicion that cervical cancer may be associated with venereal disease. This suspicion has been strengthened by the finding that increased levels of antibodies to genital herpes virus have been found in some women with cervical cancer, indicating that they were exposed to the virus.

Recent research indicates that another type of virus, a papillomavirus, may play a role both in the development of cervical dysplasia (abnormal cells) and the transformation of dysplasia into cancer. Papillomavirus infection is associated with flat genital warts, or condylomas, which may be precursors of dysplasia. In addition, papillomavirus proteins have been found in a large percentage of dysplastic tissue samples. Most scientists believe that several agents are necessary to cause dysplasias to progress into cancers, but some now believe that the initiating factor may be the human papillomavirus.

Type of contraception is related to cervical cancer incidence: more cervical cancer is seen among women who use oral contraceptives, less among those who use barrier methods, like the diaphragm. This may be because barrier methods protect against venereal infection, or because women who use oral contraceptives may be more sexually active.

The circumcision status of a sexual partner has not been found to increase cervical cancer risk.

Smoking does increase risk, although scientists are unable to explain how this occurs biologically.

In studies with laboratory animals, scientists have discovered that vitamin A plays a role in arresting or preventing cancerous changes in epithelial cells, the cells that line the interior and exterior surfaces of the body. Synthetic forms of vitamin A (retinoids), which produce fewer side effects than vitamin A when given in large doses, are currently being tested in populations at high risk of developing cancer. In one such study, women with cervical dysplasia, who are at high risk of developing invasive cervical cancer, are receiving a retinoid-containing vaginal salve. Although studies like these may lead to new methods of preventing cervical cancer, presently the most effective means of prevention is the surgical removal of precancerous tissue.

Detection of Cervical Cancer

Often, cervical cancer does not have any symptoms. The most common symptom is abnormal vaginal bleeding (bleeding that starts and stops between regular menstrual periods or bleeding that occurs after intercourse or after a gynecological examination). An increased vaginal discharge is another common symptom. These are not sure signs of cancer, but they do indicate the need for further tests, including a complete pelvic examination and Pap smear.

Regular, complete pelvic examinations and Pap smears are the best way to detect cervical cancer and precancerous conditions early. A pelvic exam involves physical examination of the organs in the pelvic area, including the uterus, vagina, ovaries, fallopian tubes, bladder, and rectum. A speculum is used to hold the vagina open so that the physician can view the upper portion of the vagina and the opening of the cervix. A Pap test consists of the collection of a sample of cells (a smear) from the cervix and examination of these cells under a microscope. The presence of abnormal cells is not proof of cervical cancer or even of a precancerous condition, but it does indicate the need for further tests.

A National Institutes of Health Consensus Development Conference recommended that all women who have had sexual intercourse should begin a regular screening program for cervical cancer. If the first Pap smear does not show any abnormal cells, it should be repeated in 1 year. If the second smear also is negative, the test should be repeated at regular intervals of 1 to 3 years. The decision on how often to retest should be made jointly by a woman and her physician. With the exception of DES daughters, who should be examined at least once a year after the onset of menstruation, virgins need not be screened for cervical cancer.

The Pap test sometimes fails to pick up cancer cells. The possibility of such "false negative" results is one reason why women should have Pap tests and pelvic exams regularly. The Pap test can detect dysplasia and carcinoma *in situ,* two symptom-free conditions that sometimes develop into invasive cervical cancer. Both conditions are almost 100 percent curable if treated promptly. Dysplasia and carcinoma *in situ* are types of cervical intraepithelial neoplasia (CIN). Mild dysplasia is classified as CIN I, moderate dysplasia as CIN II, and severe dysplasia and carcinoma *in situ* as CIN III. A pathologist classifies dysplastic cells on the basis of microscopic cellular characteristics.

Dysplasia, the development of abnormal cells, is not a cancerous condition. Although dysplastic cells have the same general microscopic appearance as cancerous cells, dysplastic cells do not invade underlying tissue. The term "atypical hyperplasia" is sometimes used to indicate the proliferation of dysplastic cells. Dysplasia occurs most often in women between the ages of 25 and 35, but it can appear in younger women.

Mild dysplasia may not require treatment, but it should be checked regularly for an increase in severity. Moderate dysplasia is usually treated by cryotherapy or cauterization. Cryotherapy destroys abnormal tissue by freezing it; cauterization involves the use of heat. Severe dysplasia may require the surgical removal of abnormal tissue in a procedure called conization, the excision of a small cone-shaped piece of tissue from the cervix. These procedures are frequently done in the doctor's office and do not require a hospital visit.

Carcinoma in situ, also called very early cancer, is cancer that has not spread below the lining of the first layer of cervical tissue. Carcinoma *in situ* is the earliest form of cervical cancer that can be detected. It is most common in women between the ages of 30 and 40, although it can develop in women of other ages.

Cryosurgery, cauterization, or surgical conization may be used to treat carcinoma *in situ.* Conization is the usual treatment for young women who wish to have children. In women who no longer wish to bear children, a hysterectomy, the surgical removal of the uterus, may be performed. This surgery eliminates the possibility that uterine cancer will develop later in life.

Recently, lasers have been used to destroy abnormal cervical tissue. (The word "laser" stands for "light amplification by stimulated emission of radiation.") The laser is a device that transforms light waves into a powerful beam that can be used in some surgical procedures instead of a scalpel. Although preliminary results have been very good, the evidence is not yet conclusive that laser surgery is better than current methods of treatment for early cervical cancer.

Diagnosis of Cervical Cancer

If the doctor's inspection or the Pap smear shows any abnormality, a biopsy—the removal of a tiny amount of suspicious tissue—is usually done. Doctors use several methods to identify areas of suspicious tissue for biopsy. With the Schiller's test, iodine is applied to the surface of the cervix. Normal cells are stained by the iodine; areas not stained are then biopsied. Doctors may also use a colposcope, which magnifies the view of the cervix and vagina, to inspect suspicious areas more closely. If a vaginal infection is suspected as the cause of the abnormal smear, the smear may simply be repeated after treatment of the infection.

If the biopsy and Pap smear results are abnormal, or if the

two tests give conflicting results, larger tissue samples may be required for an accurate diagnosis. These are obtained most often by conization or dilatation and curettage (D and C). In a D and C, the cervix is dilated to permit insertion of a curette, a small instrument that gently scrapes material from the uterine lining.

Examination of tissue samples from biopsy, conization, or D and C may reveal dysplasia, carcinoma *in situ,* cervical cancer, or other diseases. If evidence of cancer is found, further tests are done to determine its extent. The most important of these tests is a more thorough pelvic examination, including inspection of the abdomen, vagina, and rectum. A doctor can often feel a tumor or detect tenderness caused by a tumor in these areas. Cancer spreads to distant parts of the body, most often to the lung, in only about 15 percent of cervical cancer patients. Staging is a system used to describe the degree to which the cancer has spread:

Stage 0: Carcinoma *in situ*

Stage I: Carcinoma confined to the cervix

Stage II: Carcinoma extends beyond the cervix but not to the pelvic wall

Stage III: Carcinoma extends to the pelvic wall

Stage IV: Carcinoma extends beyond the pelvis or invades the bladder or rectum

Almost all cervical cancers are squamous cell carcinomas. Squamous cells are a type of epithelial cell; any cancer that originates in epithelial cells is called a carcinoma.

Treatment of Cervical Cancer

The choice of treatment for cervical cancer depends on the patient's general condition and on the stage of the disease. In its early stages, cervical cancer is usually treated with surgery or radiation or a combination of the two. Chemotherapy (treatment with anticancer drugs) is often recommended for later stages of the disease.

Stage I cervical cancer can be effectively treated with either surgery or radiation therapy. Surgery is often selected in younger women because it preserves the hormone-producing function of the ovaries. Surgical treatment consists of a hysterectomy, the removal of the entire uterus, including the cervix. The two types of treatment are equally effective, with cure rates of 85 to 90 percent.

In older women, radiation may be selected because it is more easily tolerated than surgery, particularly if other medical problems are present. Surgery may also be used in combination with radiotherapy if the shape of the tumor in the cervix makes insertion of radioactive implants (described below) difficult.

Most patients in whom the disease has progressed beyond stage I are treated with radiotherapy alone. However, if the cancer has spread minimally to the vagina (early Stage II), surgery may be selected for patients who are young and in good general health. The surgical procedure most often used is the radical hysterectomy, involving removal of the upper part of the vagina and nearby tissues and lymph nodes as well as the uterus.

Radiation treatment usually consists of a combination of external and internal radiation. X-rays from a linear accelerator or gamma rays from a cobalt source may be beamed through the body to the tumor site. Treatments of this kind are usually given (on an outpatient basis) over a period of several weeks.

Radiation may also be applied directly to the cervix by inserting, through the vagina, tiny metal cylinders containing a radioactive element, such as radium or cesium. The cylinders are usually left in place for 2 or 3 days. Patients receiving internal irradiation are hospitalized for several days.

If the cancer has spread extensively or has reappeared after initial treatment with surgery or radiation therapy, chemotherapy may be prescribed. In such cases, anticancer drugs frequently are injected into the bloodstream, often in an outpatient setting. There is currently no standard treatment for stage IV cervical cancer, but many new regimens are being evaluated in clinical trials.

Several current studies are evaluating the effectiveness of various anticancer drugs, alone and in combination with other drugs and/or radiation. Drugs used in combination chemotherapy protocols, or research programs, include cisplatin (Platinol), bleomycin, mitomycin (Mitomycin-C), vincristine, methotrexate, and doxorubicin (Adriamycin), usually in combinations of two or three.

Other investigational treatments of cervical cancer include immunotherapy and the use of radiation sensitizers. Immunotherapy is the use of drugs that stimulate the body's immune system to fight off disease. In treating cervical cancer, the immunotherapeutic agent most often used is the bacterium *C. parvum*. Immunotherapy is usually given in combination with radiation or chemotherapy. Radiation sensitizers are drugs such as misonidazole and hydroxyurea which, when given before the administration of radiation, are believed to make cancerous cells more sensitive to the radiation.

Endometrial Cancer

Incidence

Endometrial cancer occurs most often in women between the ages of 55 and 70 and accounts for 13 percent of all cancers in women. In the United States, an estimated 36,000 new cases of endometrial cancer will be diagnosed in 1986, and the disease will cause around 2,900 deaths. From 1950 to 1970, the death rate from endometrial cancer fell more than 50 percent; since then, it has continued to decline. The incidence, which increased fairly rapidly from 1969 to 1976, has since been falling. This observation has

been explained by a similar rise and fall in the use of menopausal estrogen therapy, which has since been shown to increase the risk of endometrial cancer.

Cause and Prevention

Although no direct cause of endometrial cancer has yet been found, a variety of factors appear to increase a woman's chances of developing endometrial cancer. Among these so-called risk factors are obesity, diabetes, infertility, and late menopause. As mentioned above, there is also a small but significant increase in risk associated with the use of estrogen replacement therapy to relieve the symptoms of menopause.

The use of certain oral contraceptives actually appears to lower the risk of endometrial cancer. The rate of endometrial cancer among women who have used oral contraceptives containing both estrogen and progesterone, two female hormones, is only about half the rate of women who have never used these drugs. The risk appears to decline with increasing duration of contraceptive use, and the reduced risk seems to persist for several years after use. The reduction in overall incidence is small, however, because endometrial cancer is uncommon in women of childbearing age.

As with cervical cancer, the most promising method of preventing invasive endometrial cancer is early detection and treatment of precancerous conditions. The most common precursor of invasive endometrial cancer is endometrial hyperplasia.

Detection of Endometrial Cancer

Abnormal vaginal bleeding after menopause is the most common symptom of endometrial cancer. The bleeding may start as a watery, blood-streaked discharge, but it eventually contains more blood. A bloody discharge does not always mean that cancer is present, but it does indicate the need for further tests to rule out the possibility of cancer.

Endometrial hyperplasia, the proliferation of endometrial tissue, is generally considered a precancerous condition similar to cervical dysplasia. The usual symptom of hyperplasia is irregular and occasionally profuse uterine bleeding. Like dysplasia, hyperplasia may be mild, moderate, or severe. Severe hyperplasia is often called carcinoma *in situ* of the endo-

metrium. Unlike cervical dysplasia, however, there is no reliable method of screening symptom-free women for endometrial hyperplasia, so this condition is usually not detected until symptoms are present. The Pap smear is not an accurate test for hyperplasia or endometrial cancer, because abnormal endometrial cells often lose their characteristic features before they reach the vagina, where cells for the Pap smear are collected. The American Cancer Society recommends that women at high risk of endometrial cancer have an endometrial biopsy at menopause.

Treatment of endometrial hyperplasia depends largely on the stage of the disease and the age of the patient. In young women, endometrial hyperplasia often is associated with irregular menstrual cycles. These patients are usually given female hormones to induce regular cycles, and the endometrial tissue is sampled frequently to monitor the success of the treatment.

Endometrial hyperplasia in women near menopause is treated with progesterone if the condition is not severe. Hysterectomy, surgical removal of the uterus, is the usual treatment for severe cases, and is also recommended for postmenopausal women with hyperplasia. If other medical problems make the patient a poor candidate for surgery, progesterone therapy usually is prescribed.

Diagnosis of Endometrial Cancer

When symptoms suggest endometrial cancer, a biopsy or D and C usually is performed. A biopsy entails the removal of a small amount of suspicious tissue, while dilatation and curettage (D and C) is used to obtain a larger tissue sample. The D and C entails dilating the cervix and removing a small sample of tissue from the lining of the uterus. Examination of tissue samples from a biopsy or D and C may reveal hyperplasia, endometrial cancer, or other diseases. If there is evidence of cancer, other tests are performed to determine the extent of the disease.

Results of a D and C may indicate that the cancer has spread to the cervix; this occurs in 10 to 15 percent of women with endometrial cancer. If the cancer has spread further, the extent of metastasis is determined by a thorough pelvic exam and the use of endoscopic techniques, which allow a doctor to look directly at tissues within the body, and radiographic techniques, such as X-rays. Metastases to distant parts of the body are uncommon in endometrial cancer. Tumors in the lung, the most common site of distant metastasis, appear in only 2 to 3 percent of patients. The following staging system is used to describe the degree to which the cancer has spread:

Stage 0: Carcinoma *in situ*

Stage I: Carcinoma is confined to uterine corpus

Stage II: Carcinoma involves corpus and cervix but has not extended outside the uterus

Stage III: Carcinoma extends beyond the uterus but not outside the pelvis

Stage IV: Carcinoma extends beyond the pelvis or involves the bladder or rectum

Five cell types of endometrial carcinoma have been reported, but one type, adenocarcinoma, accounts for more than 90 percent of all cases.

Treatment of Endometrial Cancer

The choice of treatment for endometrial cancer depends on the patient's general condition and on the stage of the disease. In its early stages, endometrial cancer is usually treated with surgery or radiation or a combination of the two. Hormone therapy is often recommended for later stages of the disease.

Surgery for endometrial cancer entails not only the removal of the uterus (hysterectomy), but often the removal of the ovaries and fallopian tubes as well, a procedure called bilateral salpingo-oophorectomy. Surgery is the usual treatment for stage I endometrial cancer, with radiation therapy given in addition if the tumor is growing rapidly.

If the cancer has spread to the cervix (stage II), some physicians recommend radiation therapy to the entire pelvis followed by a hysterectomy. Others prefer to evaluate the surgical specimen and recommend postoperative irradiation for patients whose tumors appear likely to recur.

As with cervical cancer, radiation for endometrial cancer may be administered either externally or internally. External irradiation usually consists of X-rays or gamma rays, which may be beamed through the body to the tumor site. These treatments are most often given on an outpatient basis over a period of several weeks.

Patients receiving internal irradiation are usually hospitalized during treatment. This form of radiotherapy is delivered by inserting, through the vagina, tiny metal cylinders containing a radioactive element such as radium or cesium. The cylinders are usually left in place for 2 or 3 days.

In stage III, when the tumor extends outside the uterus but is still confined to the pelvis, standard treatment involves radiation. Patients who are not candidates for surgery or radiotherapy often benefit from progesterone.

Administration of progesterone is the traditional treatment for metastatic endometrial cancer; approximately 30 to 40 percent of patients respond, with responses sometimes lasting years. Synthetic forms of progesterone include hydroxyprogesterone (Delalutin), medroxyprogesterone (Provera), and megestrol (Megace).

Treatment with anticancer drugs (chemotherapy) for patients with advanced disease currently is being tested. Doxorubicin (Adriamycin) appears to be the single most effective drug. Studies of several combinations of commonly used drugs, including doxorubicin and cyclophosphamide (Cytoxan), have also produced encouraging results.

Suggestions for Additional Reading

Chemotherapy and You: A Guide to Self-Help During Treatment, prepared by the Office of Cancer Communications, National Cancer Institute. NIH Publication No. 85-1136.

Creasman, W.T. and Weed, J.C., Jr. "Cancer of the Endometrium," *Current Problems in Cancer,* 5(2), 1980, pp. 1-33.

DeVita, V.T., Jr. et al., eds. *Cancer: Principles and Practice of Oncology, Second Edition,* Philadelphia: J.B. Lippincott, 1985..

DiSaia, P.J. and Creasman, W.T. *Clinical Gynecologic Oncology,* C.V. Mosby, 1981.

Holland, J.F. and Frei, E. III, eds. *Cancer Medicine,* Philadelphia: Lea and Febiger, 1982.

Nelson, J.H., Jr. et al. "Detection, Diagnostic Evaluation and Treatment of Dysplasia, Carcinoma in situ and Early Invasive Cervical Carcinoma," *Ca—A Cancer Journal for Clinicians,* 29(3), 1979, pp. 174-192.

Oral Contraceptives and Cancer Risk, a Fact Sheet prepared by the Office of Cancer Communications, National Cancer Institute, 1985.

*Radiation Therapy and You: *A Guide to Self-Help During Treatment,* prepared by the Office of Cancer Communications, National Cancer Institute. NIH Publication No. 85-2227.

Tsukamoto, N. "Treatment of Intraepithelial Neoplasia with the Carbon Dioxide Laser," *Gynecologic Oncology,* 21(3), 1985, pp. 331-336.

What Are Clinical Trials All About?, * prepared by the Office of Cancer Communications, National Cancer Institute. NIH Publication No. 85-2706.

---

* *The mentioned text is reprinted within this book. See CONTENTS for location.*

PART II—
TREATMENTS and THERAPIES

Chapter 26

Radiation Therapy and You

A Guide to Self-Help During Treatment

Radiation Therapy and You

Introduction

This text was written to help people who are having radiation therapy (RT) for cancer. It describes the two most common types—external RT and radiation implants — and how they work. The main purpose of this text, though, is to help you know what to expect during the course of treatment and how to care for yourself so you get the most benefit.

You may not want to read the entire text in one sitting. Flip through it, read the sections that are of interest to you right now, and refer to others as needed. Included is information on RT methods and the general effects of treatment. There are also self-help "pointers" that relate to specific treatment sites.

The information offered here reflects current RT practices of the National Cancer Institute. Treatment practices can vary among physicians and hospitals, though. You should not be concerned if your treatment program or the advice of your doctor (the radiation therapist) differs from what you read here.

Since your treatment will be tailored to your general health and type of cancer you have, some sections of this text will not apply to you. On the other hand, you are likely to have some questions and concerns that are not covered here. Be sure to discuss these with your radiation therapist or nurse, and ask if they have other educational materials that might help you.

It is suggested that you make notes while you read this text, so you can write down questions, as you think of them, to ask at your next treatment or office visit. Also, please note there is a list of words that relate to radiation therapy and other aspects of cancer care (see, "Glossary") to help you understand more about your illness and the many people involved in your care.

Further information for patients, their families, and others is easy to obtain. The National Cancer Institute has booklets such as *Taking Time, Eating Hints, and Chemotherapy and You*, that may be of help to readers of this text. These and other publications, available at no cost, are listed in the section titled "Resources."

The Cancer Information Service has a toll-free number (1-800-4-CANCER) that you can call to learn more about types of cancer, their treatment, and services for cancer patients. Also, there are large volunteer groups nationwide that can provide information or services. Details appear later in this text.

Radiation in Cancer Treatment

How Does Radiation Therapy Work?

Not long after doctors first knew that radiation (X-rays) would let them see inside the body and *find* disease, they learned how to use the same rays to *treat* disease as well. Radiation at high levels—tens of thousands of times the amount used, for instance, to produce a chest X-ray—destroys the ability of cells to grow and divide. Both normal and diseased cells are affected, but most normal cells are able to recover quickly.

By carefully aiming and timing the high-energy rays, doctors use radiation as an effective tool in cancer treatment. RT is sometimes called radiotherapy, X-ray therapy, cobalt treatment, or irradiation. Half of all people with cancer are treated with it at some point. For many of these patients, RT is the only kind of therapy needed to destroy the cancer.

What Are the Benefits of Radiation Therapy?

Doctors are using radiation to treat cancer in almost every part of the body where it can occur. Sometimes RT is used before surgery, to shrink a cancerous tumor. After surgery, it may be used to stop the growth of any cancer cells that remain. In some cases, doctors prefer to use radiation and anticancer drugs, rather than surgery, to destroy a cancerous growth and prevent its reappearance.

The number of cancers that can be cured is rising every day, and RT plays an important part. In 1980, 136,000 cancer patients were reported to be free of the disease for 5 years or more after having radiation treatments alone or combined with other therapies.

In cases of advanced disease, when a cure of the cancer is not likely, radiation therapy can still bring a large measure of relief. Many patients find the quality of their lives improved when RT is used to shrink tumors and reduce pressure, bleeding, pain, or other symptoms.

Are There Risks Involved?

As with any other treatment for disease, there are risks in radiation therapy. RT uses brief, high-level doses of radiation to destroy cells. The risk of destroying some healthy cells (that is, the risk of side effects) is usually outweighed by the benefits of killing cancer cells, however.

X-rays and gamma rays can eventually cause cancer in people who are exposed to them over a very long time. For this reason, people who work around radiation sources every day—such as your radiation treatment team—are protected against long exposure.

432

Your doctor will not advise you to have any treatment unless the benefits you expect—control of disease and relief from symptoms—exceed the known risks. It will be decades before we can know all the possible negative effects, but we know now that RT can reduce cancer and prevent its spread though your body.

How Is the Therapy Given?

You might have radiation therapy in one or both of its forms: external and internal. In external therapy, a machine directs the high-energy rays to the cancer and some of the tissue around it. The various machines that direct radiation to the cancer (the cobalt 60, linear accelerator, betatron, etc.) work in slightly different ways. Some are better for treating cancers near the skin surface; others work best on cancers deeper in the body.

Most people having RT for cancer have the external type, given during outpatient visits to a hospital or treatment center. For most patients having internal therapy, small containers of radioactive material (implants) are placed in body cavity or directly into the cancer. If you have this type of treatment, you will probably need to stay in the hospital for several days.

Who Gives Radiation Treatments?

Your family doctor will refer you to a cancer specialist—a radiation therapist—who can prescribe the type and amount that best suits your needs. The radiation therapist (or radiation oncologist) is the person referred to as "your doctor" throughout this text.

The radiation therapist heads up a highly trained team of cancer care professionals. Your RT team might include:

- The radiation physicist or dosimetrist, who helps to compute the dosage of radiation needed and ensures that the machines deliver each dose properly;

- The RT nurse, who works closely with the doctor to help you throughout treatment;

- The RT technologist, who delivers the prescribed treatment and assists before and after each treatment session.

You may also, at some point, use the services of a dietitian, a physical therapist, a social worker, or other health care personnel.

Is Radiation Therapy Expensive?

Treatment of cancer with radiation can be costly. It involves very complex equipment as well as the services of many health care professionals. The

433

exact cost of RT varies, of course, with the type and number of treatments required.

Most health insurance policies, including Part B of Medicare, cover charges for RT. You will need to discuss your policy and expected costs with the doctor's office staff or the hospital business office.

In some states, the Medicaid program may help you pay for therapy. Contact the office that handles social services in your city or county or find out if you are eligible for Medicaid and whether your RT is a covered expense.

If you need financial aid, contact the hospital social services office, the Cancer Information Services, or the local office of the American Cancer Society. They may be able to direct you to sources of help.

External Radiation Therapy: What to Expect

How Long Does the Treatment Take?

RT is usually given 5 days a week for several weeks. This schedule helps to protect healthy body tissues by spreading out the total dose of radiation and giving weekend rest breaks in which normal cells can rebuild.

The total dose of radiation and the number of treatments you need will depend on a set of highly individual factors. Your doctor must consider the size and location of your cancer, your general health, and any other treatment you're having, for example. On you first RT visit, in fact, you most likely won't have a treatment because you doctor must first decide how RT can best be used for you.

How Does the Doctor Choose the Best Treatment?

After talking to you about your medical history, the radiation therapist may need some X-rays or other tests to pinpoint the location and size of the cancer. In a process called "simulation" (a major step in planning your treatment), you will be asked to lie very still on a table while technologist uses a special machine to X-ray the cancer and locate your "treatment port." This is the exact place on your body where the high-energy rays will be aimed. Simulation may take from a half-hour to about 2 hours.

After locating the treatment port, the technologist will mark you skin with tiny tatoo dots or colored, indelible ink to define the treatment area. The ink marks must **not** be washed off until your full course of treatment is over.

Using the knowledge gained from the simulation and your medical background, your doctor may consult with a radiation physicist or dosimetrist. Together they can decide how much radiation is needed and how many treatments you should have.

After you have started the treatments, your radiation therapist will watch over your progress, checking the cancer's response to treatment and your overall well-being at least once a week. The treatment plan may be revised by your doctor, as needed, and it's very important that you stick to the schedule to get the most benefit.

What Happens During a Treatment Visit?

Before your treatment is given, you will probably need to change into a hospital gown or robe. It's best to wear few items of clothing, mostly things that are quick to take off and put on again.

In the treatment room, the RT technologist will use the ink marks on your skin to help you get in place on a table or in a chair. You will lie or sit very still beneath the treatment machine. For each external RT session, you will be in the treatment room about 15 to 30 minutes, but you will be getting a dose of radiation for only 1 to 5 minutes of that time.

After you're in place, the technologist may put special lead shields between the machine and certain parts of your body to help protect normal tissues and organs. There might also be plastic or plaster forms to help you stay exactly in place. You will need to remain very still during the treatment so that the radiation reaches only the area where it's needed and the same area is treated each time.

The technologist will move to a nearby room before turning on the machine. From there he or she can control the machine and watch you on a TV screen or through a window. You may feel very much alone for the next few minutes. Keep in mind that your treatment is constantly checked, however, and that you can talk with the RT technologist through a speaker between the rooms.

The machines used for radiation treatment are very large, and they may make noises something like a vacuum cleaner as they move around to aim at the cancer from different angles. Their size and motion may be frightening at first. Remember that machines are under the technologist's control and that they are constantly checked to be sure they're working right. If you are confused or frightened by anything that happens in the treatment room, ask the RT technologist to explain.

You will not see or hear the radiation and you most likely won't feel anything. Some patients have said they feel a warmth or tingling in the area being treated, but you should not have any discomfort. If you feel ill or very uncomfortable during the treatment, tell the technologist at once.

What Are the Effects of Treatment?

After you have had several treatment sessions, your doctor will begin checking you regularly to find out how well the treatment is working. Your own reports of how you feel may be the best sign of the therapy's progress. You may not be aware of changes in your cancer, but you will be able to notice any decrease in pain, bleeding, or other discomforts you may have had.

For some cancers, the doctor can use regular X-rays to see whether the tumor is shrinking. Your doctor will probably also recommend some test to be sure that the radiation is causing as little damage to normal cells as possible. For instance, you may have blood tests to check the level of white blood cells and platelets, which may be reduced during treatment.

You may need other tests if serious side effects appear. Your doctor will advise you about what problems, if any, you need to watch for and how you should deal with them. As a rule, all patients should contact the doctor or RT nurse if they have any cough, sweating, fever, or unusual pain over the course of their treatment.

Most side effects that occur during radiation therapy, although unpleasant, are not serious. They usually disappear within a few weeks after treatment ends. Some RT side effects are more lasting. Many patients have no side effects at all.

In another section of this text (see "Managing Side Effects"), you will find advice on various side effects that might occur during and after your therapy.

Do the Side Effects Limit Activity?

Many patients are able to work, keep house, and enjoy leisure activities as usual while they are having RT. Others find that they need more rest and therefore can not do as much. In general, it's best to pursue the normal activities that you want to and can keep up with.

There is no need to avoid being with other people because of external RT. Your body will not contain any radioactive substance, so you are not a hazard to others—even in intimate contact.

Your desire for physical intimacy may be lower because RT can effect hormone levels and often causes some fatigue. Treatment to organs in the pelvic area can limit sexual activity. In most cases, though, you can have sexual relations if you wish. Sexual function is discussed further under "Managing Side Effects."

Your doctor may suggest that you limit any activities, such as sports, that might irritate the area being treated. Generally, any restrictions you will need will result not from the fact that you're having RT but from the ways that your body responds to it.

What Can I Do To Take Care of Myself?

Each patient's body responds to radiation therapy in its own way. That's why the doctor must plan—and sometimes adjust—your treatment to fit your individual situation. In addition, your doctor or RT nurse may give you specific instructions for at-home care to suit your treatment and the side effects that might result.

Nearly all cancer patients having RT need to take a few extra measures to protect their overall health and help the treatment succeed. Some guidelines to remember are given below.

■ Be sure to get plenty of rest. Sleep as often as you feel the need. Your body will use a lot of extra energy over the course of treatment. Unusual fatigue is discussed under "Managing Side Effects."

■ Good nutrition is a must. Try to maintain a balanced diet that will prevent weight loss. For patients who have problems in eating or diet planning, the section titled "Managing Side Effects" offers practical tips.

■ Do not remove the ink marks from your skin until your full course of treatment is completed. If the line marking the treatment area begin to fade, tell the technologist at your next treatment visit. Do *not* try to draw over faded lines at home

unless they would otherwise be completely gone before your next visit. If your have to replace the marks, tell the RT technologist what you have done.

■ Avoid wearing tight clothing, such as girdles or close-fitting collars, over the treatment area. Since some of the ink marks may rub off on your cloths, it's best to wear loose, soft, older garments that will feel good and that you can discard if they get stained.

■ Be *extra* kind to the skin in your treatment area.

— Wear soft cotton clothing.

— Do not rub or scrub treated skin.

— Do not use any soaps, deodorants, medicines, perfumes, cosmetics, or other substances without the doctor's approval.

— Do not apply extreme heat or cold (heating pad, ice pack, etc) to the treatment area. Even hot water can injure your sensitive skin, so use only lukewarm water for bathing.

— Use an electric shaver if you *must* shave the area—but only after checking with your doctor or nurse.

— Protect the area from the sun. If possible, cover treated skin with light clothing before going outdoors; otherwise, use a PABA sunscreen (protection factor 15) or a sun-blocking product.

- Be sure the radiation therapist knows about any medicines you were taking before starting treatment. If you need to start taking any medicines—even aspirin—let your doctor know before you start.

- Above all, feel free to ask your doctor or RT nurse any questions you may have. They are the only ones who can properly advise you about your treatment, side effects, at-home care, and any other concerns you may have.

Implant Therapy: What to Expect

When Are Implants Used?

Radiation therapy with implants (a form of internal RT) is often used for cancers of the head and neck, breast, uterus, and prostate. Your doctor may recommend treatment with an implant alone or combined with external therapy.

An implant of radioactive material puts cancer-killing rays as close as possible to the tumor while sparing most of normal tissue around it. By using an implant, the doctor can give a higher total dose of radiation than is possible with external RT. The substances used in implants include radium, cesium, iridium and others.

How Is the Implant Placed In the Body?

For almost any type of implant, you will need to be in the hospital and have general or local anesthesia while the doctor places the radioactive material in your body. Usually there is no need to have an anesthetic for removal of the implant. Most can be removed in the patient's room.

The type of implant and the method of placing it can vary with the size and location of the cancer. To get extremely close to the cancer, doctors use implants in the form of needles, wires, seeds, capsules, wax molds, and other devices. For example, needle implants, which the doctor can insert directly into a tumor, are often used for treating the mouth and tongue. In other cases, such as uterine cancer, an applicator holds the implant against the surface of the tumor.

How Long Does the Implant Stay in Place?

Generally, implants are left in place from 1 to 6 days. Your treatment schedule will depend on the type of cancer, its location, your general health, and other cancer treatments you have had. While you're having implant therapy, the hospital may require you to remain in a private room. Depending on the implant's location, you may have to stay in bed and lie fairly still to keep it exactly in place.

For treating some cancer sites—for example, the prostate—the implant may be left in place permanently. If you receive a permanent implant, you may need to stay in an isolated room for a few days while the radiation is most active. The implant will lose energy a little each day, so by the time you are ready to go home, the radiation in your body will be much weaker. Your doctor will advise you if there are any special precautions you need to use at home.

Does an Implant Spread Radiation to Others?

The radioactive substance in your implant may transmit rays into the area around your body. For this reason, hospitals have special rules to protect their staff (who deal with radiation every day) from the risk of unnecessary exposure while your implant is in place.

The nurses and other people caring for you will not be able to spend a long time in your room. They will provide all of your required care—and you should call for a nurse when you need one—but expect your nurses to work quickly and to speak to you from the doorway more often than at your bedside.

There also will be limits on visitors while your implant is in place. Most hospitals do not permit children under 18 or pregnant women to visit implant patients. Approved visitors can sit a distance from your bed (at least 5 feet) for a short time each day.

Are There Any Side Effects?

You are not likely to have severe pain or feel ill during implant therapy. If there is an applicator holding your implant, it may be somewhat uncomfortable. The doctor can order medicine to relax you or to relieve pain if you need it. Some patients feel weakened after having anesthesia, but this effect does not last long.

Be sure to tell the nurse if you have any side effects such as burning, sweating, or other unusual symptoms. In the section of this text headed "Managing Side Effects," you will find tips on skin care and what you can do about problems that might occur after implant therapy.

The area that is treated with an implant may be sore or sensitive for some time after therapy. Your doctor might advise that you limit sports and sexual activity for awhile to avoid irritating the treatment area.

What Happens After the Implant Is Removed?

If you need to stay in bed during implant therapy, you could have an extra day or so in the hospital after the implant is removed. General anesthesia followed by a few days in bed can cause you to feel weak when you get up again. The nurse will help you through gradual stages of activity—sitting, standing, walking—until you're ready to be on your own.

Once the implant is removed, there is no longer a danger of your giving off radiation. The nurses and your visitors will not have to observe any special rules.

Your doctor will advise you if there is any need to restrict your activities after you are discharged. Most patients are allowed to do as much as they feel like doing. You may need extra sleep or rest breaks in your first days at home, but you will regain strength quickly.

Managing Side Effects

Are Side Effects the Same for Everyone?

The extent of radiation therapy side effects varies from patient to patient. Some people have few or no side effects through their course of treatment. Other have serious problems.

The side effects that you might have depend mostly on the treatment dose and what part of your body is treated. Your general health can also affect how your body reacts to RT. Some side effects can result from radiation to any treatment site; the most common ones are fatigue, skin problems, and loss of appetite. Other side effects are related to treatment of specific areas, such as hair loss with treatment to the head.

Fortunately, most side effects will go away in time, and there are ways to reduce the discomfort they may cause. If you should have a side effect that is particularly severe, the doctor may prescribe a break in your treatment or change the kind of treatment you're having.

Tell your doctor or RT nurse of any side effects that you notice. They can help you with treatment measures and ways to prevent further occurrences. The information given here can serve as a guide to handling some side effects, but it cannot replace discussion with the doctor or nurse.

What Causes Fatigue?

During radiation therapy, the body uses a lot of energy. Stress related to your illness, daily trips for treatment, the effects of radiation on normal cells—all may contribute to fatigue. Most people feel unusually tired after a few weeks of RT. Feelings of weakness or weariness will gradually go away after your treatment is finished.

You can help yourself during RT by asking less of your body. If you feel tired, limit your activities and use your leisure time in a restful way. Do not feel that you have to do all the things you did before. Try to get more sleep at night and take naps during the day if you can.

If your have been working a full-time job and want to stay with it, by all means try to do so. Although treatment visits are time-consuming, you can ask your doctor's office or RT department to help by trying to schedule treatments with your work day in mind.

Some patients prefer to take a few weeks off from work while they're having RT. Others work a reduced number of hours. You should speak frankly with your employer about your needs and wishes during this time. You may be able to agree on a part-time schedule, or perhaps you can do some of your work at home.

Whether you're working or not, it's a good idea to ask family members or friends to help with shopping, child care, housework, or driving. Neighbors may be able to help by picking up groceries for you when they do their own shopping. You could also ask a friend to drive you to and from your treatment visits to help conserve your energies.

How Are Skin Problems Treated?

You are very likely to notice dry or itchy skin in any area getting radiation treatment. It is crucial that you not rub, scrub, or scratch any sensitive spots. Ask your RT nurse or technologist for advice about lotion you can use.

Don't try any powders, creams, salves, or other home remedies while you're being treated or for several weeks afterward (unless approved by your doctor). Many over-the-counter products for the skin, such as lotions or petroleum jelly, leave a coating that can interfere with RT. Often radiation therapists and nurses suggest using a light baby oil for dry skin or dusting with cornstarch if excess moisture is a problem, but you should check with your doctor before trying these methods.

You may develop a sunburned look—redness or tanning—and you skin may turn a shade darker than normal. You should avoid exposing treated area to the sun both during and after treatment. Always tell your doctor or RT nurse if you expect to be in the sun for any length of time, such as during a vacation.

The majority of skin reactions to RT should go away a few weeks after treatment is finished. In many cases, though, darkened skin areas will remain. Tell your doctor at once if your skin cracks, blisters, or becomes too moist. Your RT team will also watch closely for symptoms that could mean a change in treatment is needed.

What Can Be Done About Hair Loss?

If you have hair in the area being treated, you may lose some or all of it during RT. Most patients will find their hair growing back again after the treatments are finished, but the loss of hair—whether from scalp, face, or body—can be hard to adjust to.

You may want to cover your head with a hat, turban, or scarf while you're in treatment. Some people prefer a wig or toupee. A hairpiece that you need because of cancer treatment is a tax-deductible expense and may be covered by your health insurance. If you plan to buy a wig, it's a good idea to select it early in your therapy so that you have the option of matching the color and style to your own hair.

Is Loss of Appetite a Serious Problem?

You may lose interest in food during course of radiation therapy. Loss of appetite (anorexia) can occur when changes to normal cells result in nausea, stomach pain, changes in taste, difficulty in swallowing, or other problems. Some people just don't feel like eating because of stress related to their illness and treatment.

Patients having external RT cannot afford weeks of poor nutrition. Even when your desire for food lags, it's important that you make every effort to keep your protein and calorie intake high. If you're not well nourished, you may not have all the strength you need for healing and building new tissues.

Try to keep in mind that your diet is one area in which you can control what's happening to your body. You might feel, at times, that your illness and its treatment are out of your hands, but you may improve the course of your therapy by feeding yourself well. Doctors have found that patients who eat well can better withstand both their cancer and the side effects of treatment.

What If I Don't Feel Like Eating?

The list below suggest ways to perk up your appetite when it's poor and to make to most of it when you *do* feel like eating.

■ Take a walk before meals to increase your appetite.

■ Eat when you are hungry, even if it is not mealtime.

■ Eat frequent small meals during the day rather than three large ones.

■ Create a pleasant dining atmosphere; use soft light, quite music, brightly colored table settings, or whatever helps you feel good while eating.

■ Vary your diet and try new recipes.

■ If you enjoy company while eating, try to have meals with family or friends, or turn on the radio or TV.

■ Ask your doctor or nurse if you can have a glass of wine or beer with your meal to increase the appetite.

■ When you feel like thinking about food, make some simple

442

meals in batches and freeze them to use later.

■ Keep healthful snacks close by for nibbling when you get the urge.

■ If you live alone, you might want to arrange for "Meals on Wheels" to bring meals to you. Ask your doctor, nurse, local American Cancer Society, or the Cancer Information Service about "Meals on Wheels." This service is active in most large communities.

If you are not able to eat much food because of poor appetite or discomfort, the food that you *can* eat must be highly nutritious. When you eat only small amounts of food, try to increase the calories per serving:

■ Add butter or margarine if you like the flavor.

■ Mix canned cream soups with milk or half-and-half rather than water.

■ Drink eggnogs, milkshakes, or prepared liquid supplements between meals.

■ Add cream sauce or melted cheese to your favorite vegetables.

Some people find they can handle large amounts of liquids even when they don't feel like eating solid foods. If this is the case for you, try to get the most from each glassful by having drinks enriched with powered milk, yogurt, eggs, honey, or prepared liquid supplements. A National Cancer Institute booklet, *Eating Hints*, provides further tips to help you enjoy eating, and it includes recipes designed to boost food value.

What Problems Can Occur in Treatment for Breast Cancer?

During the third or fourth week of external RT you may develop tender, moist, dry, or itchy skin under the breast or in the armpit. If itching persists, the doctor or nurse can suggest a treatment to relieve it. You should not use any lotions, oils, or other products for skin problems without your doctor's approval.

Other side effects that might appear are soreness and swelling from fluid buildup in the treated area. These side effects, as well as the skin problems described above, will most likely disappear in 4 to 6 weeks. If fluid buildup continues to be a problem, your doctor will tell you what steps to take.

One long-term side effect of radiation treatment to the breast is a change in size. Because women are so varied, it is not possible to predict the degree of change or whether the breast will become smaller or larger. But, like the skin darkening mentioned earlier, the change is usually slight and will not be noticeable when you are clothed.

Your RT plan could include an implant a week or two after external treatment is completed. There may be some tenderness or a feeling of tightness while the implant is in the breast. After it is removed, you are likely to notice some of the same effects that occur with external treatment. If so, follow the advice given above, and let your doctor know about any problems that persist.

What About Stomach and Bowel Problems?

If you are having radiation treatment to the stomach or some portion of the lower abdomen, you may have to deal with an upset stomach or diarrhea. Your doctor can prescribe medicines to relieve these problems. Do not take any home remedies during your treatment unless you first check with your doctor or RT nurse.

Managing Nausea—Some patients report feeling queasy for a few hours right after an external radiation treatment. If you have the same problem, try not eating for several hours before your treatment time. You may find you can handle the treatment better on an empty stomach. If the problem persists, ask your doctor to prescribe a medicine to prevent nausea. If your stomach feels upset right before your treatment, try eating a bland snack such as toast or crackers and apple juice before your appointment. This type of side effect may have to do with your emotions and attitude toward treatment. If you have to spend time in a waiting room before your treatment, you can use that time to unwind a bit. Reading a

book, writing letters, or working a puzzle may help you torelax while waiting.

Here are some brief tips to help an unsettled stomach:

- Stick to any special diets that your doctor or dietitian gives you.

- Try to eat and drink slowly.

- Avoid fried foods and others with a high fat content.

- Limit yourself to foods that have only a mild aroma and those that can be served cool or at room temperature.

- Don't try to eat more at one sitting than you're comfortable with.

- For severe upsets, try a clear liquid diet (broth and juices) or bland foods that are easy to digest (such as dry toast and gelatin).

How to Handle Diarrhea—Diarrhea, when it occurs, most often begins in the third or fourth week of external therapy. Even if your doctor has ordered a medicine to help with the problem, you might do well to try some diet control measures also:

- Try a clear liquid diet as soon as diarrhea starts or when you feel that it's going to start.

- Ask your doctor or nurse to advise you about liquids that won't make your diarrhea worse. Apple juice, peach nectar, weak tea, and clear broth are frequent suggestions.

- Avoid foods that can cause cramps or a gassy feeling (for instance, coffee, beans, cabbage, sweets, and spicy dishes).

- Try eating frequent small meals.

- Avoid milk and milk products if they irritate your bowels.

- When the diarrhea starts to improve, try eating small amounts of low-fiber food such as rice, bananas, applesauce, mashed potatoes, and dry toast.

- Be sure your diet includes foods that are high in potassium (bananas, potatoes, apricots), a vital mineral that you may lose through diarrhea.

Diet planning is a crucial part of treatment of the stomach and abdomen. Although you may have trouble with eating, you will need to keep up your intake of calories and vital nutrients. Keep in mind that these problems will be greatly reduced when treatment is over. In the meantime, try to pack the highest possible food value into even small meals.

What Are the Effects on Reproductive Organs?

If you are having RT to any part of the pelvis, you might have one or more of the digestive tract problems described above. There are also certain side effects that occur only in reproductive organs.

The effect of RT on sexual and reproductive functions depend on which organs are treated. Some of the more common side effects for both men and women do not last long after treatment. Others may be long-term or permanent. Your doctor should advise you, before your treatment begins, about possible side effects and how long they might last.

Effects on Fertility—The ways that radiation treatment might affect fertility are under continuing study. In the meantime, RT technologist use lead shields as often as they can to protect the reproductive organs.

Radiation treatment to an area that includes the testes can reduce both the number of sperm and their ability to fertilize. This does not mean that conception cannot occur, however. If you're having this type of treatment, you'll need to continue (or alter) your birth control practices accordingly. Discuss your needs and concerns frankly with your doctor. If you want to father a child and are concerned about reduced fertility, you can look into the option of banking your sperm for future use.

Women having RT in the pelvic area can expect to stop menstruating and may have other symptoms of menopause. Treatment can also result in vaginal itching, burning, and dryness. You should report any of these symptoms to your doctor or nurse for prompt treatment.

Sexual Relations—During treatment to the pelvis, many women are advised not to have intercourse.

445

Others may find that intercourse is painful. You will most likely be able to resume having sex within a few weeks after your treatment ends.

Some shrinking of vaginal tissues occurs during RT. Your doctor will instruct you about sexual intercourse and using a dilator, if necessary, after your RT is finished.

With most types of RT, neither men nor women are likely to suffer any decrease in their ability to enjoy sex. Both sexes, however, may notice a change in level of desire. This effect will most likely subside when the treatment ends, so it should not become a major concern.

What Side Effects Occur with RT to the Head and Neck Area?

Many people have had radiation treatments for cancer of the head and neck area with excellent results. Because this type of treatment is used so often, doctors have had a good chance to observe the range of possible side effects and learn how to handle them.

Anyone planning to have radiation therapy to the brain, mouth, neck, or upper chest should be prepared for a strict program of oral health care. Side effects from treatment to this area most often involve the teeth, gums, and other tissues of the mouth.

There are a few precautions that will help you prevent or control mouth problems:

Avoid spices and coarse foods such as raw vegetables, dry crackers, and nuts.

■ Stay away from sugary snacks that promote tooth decay.

■ Clean your mouth and teeth often, using the method your dentist recommends.

■ Do not use a commercial mouthwash; the alcohol content has a drying effect on mouth tissues.

Other problems that could occur during treatment to the head and neck are earaches (caused by hardening of the ear wax) and swelling or drooping of skin under the chin. There may also be changes in your skin texture. Report any side effects to your doctor, and ask what you should do about them.

Dental Care—Mouth care designed to prevent problems will be an important part of your treatment. Before starting radiation therapy, see your dentist for a complete dental/oral checkup, including X-rays if needed. You should tell your dentist that you will be having RT and ask that he or she consult with the radiation therapist about any dental work you need before your radiation treatments begin.

Your dentist will probably want to see you often over the course of your RT. Radiation treatments can increase your chance of getting cavities. The preventive measures that your dentist suggests will not only reduce the risk of tooth decay but will also help you deal with possible problems such as mouth sores.

The dentist can give you very detailed instructions about caring for your mouth and teeth. It is very important to your total well-being that you follow the dentist's advice while you're having RT. Most likely, you will be advised to:

- Clean teeth and gums thoroughly with a soft brush after meals and at least once more each day.

- Use a fluoride toothpaste that contains no abrasives.

- Floss between teeth daily.

- Use a disclosing solution or tablet after brushing to reveal plaque that you've missed.

- Rinse your mouth well with a salt and baking soda solution after you brush.

- Apply fluoride regularly.

Your dentist can explain how to use disclosing tablets, how to mix the baking soda mouthwash, and how to use the fluoride treatment method that best suits your needs. Most likely you can get printed instructions at the dentist's office. Brochures on oral care for cancer patients are available through the Cancer Information Service.

Handling Mouth or Throat Problems—Soreness in your mouth or throat could appear in the second or third week of external RT. It is likely to decrease from the fifth week on, and end a month or so after your treatment ends. You may also have trouble with swallowing during this time because of a lump-like feeling in the throat. Your radiation therapist or dentist can prescribe medicine for painful sores and advise you about products to relieve other mouth problems.

Your glands may produce less saliva than usual, making your mouth feel dry. It's helpful to suck on ice chips and sip cool drinks often throughout the day. Sugar-free candy or gum may also help. Avoid tobacco and alcoholic drinks because they will dry your mouth tissues even more. If these measures are not enough, ask your dentist about artificial saliva.

Tips on Eating—Any discomfort in your mouth or throat can make eating difficult. Pain relief will help you maintain good intake of protein and calories. Choosing foods that taste good and are easy to eat will also help.

If your sense of taste changes during RT, try some different methods of food preparation.

- If meats taste bitter to you, try soaking them in teriyaki sauce, fruit juice, or wine before cooking.

- Try eating high-protein foods cold or at room temperature (tuna salad, deviled eggs, and puddings are good choices).

- Select foods with mild aroma and flavor, such as soft cheeses, fresh fruits, chicken, eggs, and the more delicate types of fish.

- Add a little extra salt (unless your diet is salt-restricted) or try using more seasonings such as basil, tarragon, mint, etc.

If chewing and swallowing are painful, try to have more liquid and semisolid meals.

- Cook solid foods until they are tender but not overdone, then toss them into a blender for smoothing.

- Moisten small bites of solid food with gravy, salad dressing, or yogurt.

- Plan menus to include frequent servings of applesauce, cooked cereal, cream soup, custard, soft-cooked eggs, mashed potatoes, and smooth ice cream or sherbet.

- Try to avoid spices; you can add flavor to a bland dish with delicate herbs.

- Try a prepared high-protein liquid blended with ice cream as a drink with meals or as a snack between.

Does RT Affect The Emotions?

All patients having treatment for cancer are likely to feel some degree of emotional upset. While radiation therapy may affect the emotions indirectly, through fatigue or changes in hormone balance, the treatment itself is not a direct cause of mental distress.

Some patients report feeling depressed or nervous during their therapy. Their feelings may have a number of sources: the need to change daily routines, new limits of physical ability, or fear about the disease. Such feelings are not at all rare in the course of adjusting to a diagnosis of cancer.

If you find yourself feeling especially unhappy or nervous while you're in treatment, try to keep in mind that positive outlook could affect the body's functions. Many believe that using up your energies with unproductive emotions can only detract from the resources your body needs for healing itself.

Many patients have helped themselves by talking about their feelings with a close friend, family member, chaplain, or a nurse or social worker with whom they feel at ease. You may want to ask your doctor or nurse about meditation or relaxation exercises that could help you to unwind and feel better.

Nationwide programs such as CanSurmount and I Can Cope, sponsored by the American Cancer

Society, can provide much-needed support. Groups such as the United Ostomy Association, the Lost Chord Club, and Reach to Recovery offer a chance for you to meet with other people who share your problems and concerns. Some medical centers have formed peer support groups so that patients can meet to discuss their feelings and inspire each other. Many people with cancer feel they have benefited by simply reaching out to help another patient.

There are a number of helpful books and other materials in this subject area. The Cancer Information Service can direct you to reading matter and other resources in your area. Local units of national volunteer groups may also be able to offer useful ideas for patients who want help with handling their emotions.

Nutrition During Therapy

What Extra Nutrition is Required?

The importance of maintaining your weight during RT cannot be stressed enough. A number of side effects can cause problems with eating and digesting food, but you should always try to consume enough calories and protein to help damaged tissues rebuild themselves.

One rule of thumb says that during cancer therapy people may need extra protein and more calories. It is important to check your weight during treatment. Your doctor or RT nurse can tell you whether your treatment calls for special attention to diet.

If your appetite is poor, you may have to try new ways to spark it. When you do feel like eating, it's easy to pack in extra nutrients. A varied diet in ample amounts is your best defense against the nutritional problems that can result from RT.

What if Eating is Difficult?

Coping with short-term diet problems may be easier than you expect. There are a number of diet guides and recipe booklets available for patients who need help with nourishment. One NCI booklet, *Eating Hints*, describes how to build your intake of nutrients without eating more food. The recipes it contains can be used for the whole family, and they are marked for people with special concerns such as salt restriction.

If you're troubled by poor appetite or have pain when you chew and swallow, your doctor might advise you to use a powdered or liquid diet supplement. Many of these products, which you buy at the drug store without prescription, are made in variety of flavors. They are tasty when used alone and can be combined with other foods such as pureed fruit or added to milk shakes.

Some of the companies that make diet supplements have produced recipe booklets to help you increase your nutrient intake. Ask your dietitian or pharmacist for further information or contact the Cancer Information Service.

The American Cancer Society offers diet advice and recipes for patients. You can also ask your hospital's RT department and dietitian's office if they have any materials you could use.

The dietary needs of people having radiation treatments will vary as much as their other responses to therapy. If food problems persist, get help from a trained dietitian, who can study your particular needs and suggest a personal diet plan.

Followup Care

What Does "Followup" Mean?

The need for health care related to your cancer will not end when your course of RT is over. No matter what type of cancer you've had, you will need regular checkups and, perhaps, lab tests and X-rays. The radiation therapist will want to see you at least once more after your treatments. The doctor who referred you will schedule followup visits as needed.

Followup care, in addition to checking on the results of your radiation therapy, might include further cancer treatment,

rehabilitation, and counseling. Taking good care of yourself is also a part of following through after radiation treatments.

Who Provides Care After Therapy?

Some patients return to the radiation therapist for followup visits. Others are referred back to their original doctor, to a surgeon, or to a doctor who is trained to give chemotherapy (treatment with anticancer drugs). The next steps in followup care depend on the type and stage of your disease and on other treatments that you had or expect to have.

If you are having surgery as well as RT, you may need some type of rehabilitative care, such as physical therapy or speech training. You might consult with a plastic surgeon or arrange to be fitted with a prosthesis (an artificial body part). The doctor who handles most of your followup care will advise you about the best time to take these steps and will refer you to suitable sources of further health care.

What Other Care Might Be Needed?

Individual needs vary, and your doctor will prescribe and schedule the types of followup care that best suit your case. Don't hesitate to ask about the tests or treatments that your doctor recommends. Try to learn all the things you should do to care for yourself as best you can.

Following are some of the questions that you may want to ask after you have finished a course of radiation therapy.

- How often do I need to return for checkups?

- Why do I need more X-rays (scans, blood tests, and so on)? What will these tests tell you?

- Will I need chemotherapy (surgery, other treatments)?
- How will you know if I'm cured of cancer? What are the chances that it will come back?

- How soon can I go back to my regular activities—
   —work?
   —sexual activity?
   —sports?

- Do I need to take any special precautions?

- Do I need a special diet?

- Should I be on an exercise program?

- Can I wear a prosthesis?

- How soon can I have reconstructive surgery?

What if Pain is a Problem?

A small percentage of patients will need help to manage pain if it continues after radiation therapy, Some people need only a light medication. You should not use a heating pad or warm compress to relieve pain in the area treated with radiation.

If you have severe pain, ask the doctor about prescribed drugs or other methods of relief. Be as specific as possible when telling the doctor about your pain so you can get the best treatment for it.

Because pain can be worse when you are afraid or worried, it may help to try relaxation exercises. Other methods, such as hypnosis, biofeedback, and acupuncture, are under study to find out whether they can be useful for cancer patients. *Questions and Answers About Pain Control* is a free booklet that may help you to understand more about cancer pain (see "Resources").

How Can I Help Myself After RT?

Patients who have had RT need to continue, at least for a short while, some of the special care used during treatment. For instance, you could have skin problems for several weeks after your treatments end. You should continue to be gentle with skin in the treatment area until all signs of irritation are gone. Don't try to scrub the inked lines that mark your treatment area. They will fade and wear away soon.

You may find that you still need extra rest while your healthy tissues are rebuilding. Keep taking naps as needed and try to get some more sleep at night. You'll need some time to test your strength, little by little, so don't plan to resume a full schedule of activities right away.

After treatment for cancer, you're likely to be more aware of your body and to notice even slight changes in how you feel from day to day. The doctor will want you to report any unusual symptoms. If you have any of the problems listed below, tell your doctor at once:

■ A pain that persists, especially if it's always in the same place;

■ Lumps, bumps, or swelling;

■ Nausea, vomiting, diarrhea, loss of appetite;

■ Unexplained weight loss;

■ A fever or cough that persists;

■ Unusual rashes or bleeding;

■ Any other signs mentioned by your doctor or nurse.

Glossary

adjuvant therapy: A treatment method used in addition to the primary therapy. Radiation therapy is often used as an adjuvant to surgery.

alopecia: Hair loss.

anesthesia: A procedure in which a patient receives medications that block out pain.

anorexia: Absence or loss of appetite for food.

antiemetic: A medicine to prevent or relieve nausea and vomiting.

benign tumor: A growth that is not a cancer and does not spread to other parts of the body.

betatron: A machine that uses electrons to create and deliver radiation for the treatment of cancer; useful for tumors deep in the body.

biopsy: The removal and microscopic examination of living tissue for purposes of diagnosis.

brachytherapy: Treatment with radiation applied at or very near the surface of the body.

cancer: A general term for more than 100 diseases characterized by uncontrolled, abnormal growth of cells that can invade and destroy healthy tissues.

chemotherapy: Treatment with anticancer drugs.

cobalt 60: A radioactive substance used to treat cancer.

dosimetrist: A person who plans and calculates the proper radiation dose for treatment.

external radiation: Radiation therapy using a machine that focuses on the cancer site. (See also brachytherapy and teletherapy.)

fluoride therapy: Application of fluoride gel to prevent tooth decay; can be done by the patient, using a custom-fitted mouthpiece.

gamma rays: A form of radiation used to treat cancer.

immunotherapy: Treatment by stimulation of the body's immune defense system. Doctors are doing research on immunotherapy as a possible treatment for cancer.

implant: A small container of radioactive material placed in or near a cancer.

internal radiation: A type of therapy in which a radioactive substance is implanted in the body close to the area needing treatment. (See also interstitial implant and intracavitary implant.)

interstitial implant: A radioactive source placed directly into the tissue (not in a body cavity).

intracavitary implant: A radioactive source implanted in a body cavity such as the chest cavity or the vagina.

intraoperative radiation: A large dose of radiation therapy to the tumor bed and surrounding tissue at the time of surgery; an experimental technique being done only at selected institutions.

linear accelerator: A machine that creates and uses high-energy X-rays to treat cancers.

malignant: Cancerous (see cancer).

metastasis: The spread of a cancer from one part of the body to another. Cells in the new cancer are like those in the original site.

oncologist: A doctor who is a specialist in the treatment of tumors, especially cancers.

palliative therapy: A treatment that may relieve symptoms without curing the disease.

physical therapist: A professional trained in the use of physical methods of treatment (such as exercise and massage).

rad: Short form for "radiation absorbed dose"; the amount of radiation absorbed by tissues.

radiation physicist: A person trained in computing proper radiation treatment doses.

radiation therapist: A doctor who specializes in using radiation to treat disease.

radiation therapy: The use of high-energy penetrating rays to treat disease. Sources of radiation include X-ray, cobalt, and radium. (See also gamma rays, brachytherapy, teletherapy, and X-ray.)

radiologist: A physician with special training in reading diagnostic X-rays.

radiotherapy: See radiation therapy.

registered dietitian: A professional who arranges diet programs for the purposes of proper nutrition of the well or therapeutic nutrition of the sick.

teletherapy: Treatment in which the radiation is at a distance from the body (opposite of brachytherapy).

tumor: An abnormal mass of tissue that results from excessive cell division and performs no useful body function. Tumors are either benign or malignant.

X-ray: A type of radiation that can be used at low levels to diagnose disease or in its high-energy form to treat cancer.

Chapter 27

Chemotherapy and You

A Guide to Self-Help During Treatment

Introduction

Chemotherapy and You was written to help cancer patients, their families, and their friends understand chemotherapy. Basic information on cancer chemotherapy is divided into sections that cover how the treatment works, how it is given, the importance of diet during therapy, and management of some of the more common side effects. Another section lists the anticancer drugs that are used most often and describes many of their possible effects.

What is Chemotherapy and How Does it Work?

Chemotherapy is the use of drugs or medications to treat disease. The term comes from two words that mean "chemical" and "treatment." Most people have had some type of chemotherapy for illness during their lives, for example, taking penicillin for an infection. Today, the word "chemotherapy" is used most often to describe a method of cancer treatment.

Cancer chemotherapy can consist of one drug or a group of drugs that work together (*combination chemotherapy*). A treatment plan that also includes surgery and/or radiation therapy is called *combined modality treatment*. In *adjuvant chemotherapy*, anticancer drugs are used after another treatment, to destroy any cancer cells that may remain after surgery or radiation therapy.

Chemotherapy has proven very effective in cancer treatment. In 1980, over 46,000 cancer patients were cured with the use of anticancer drugs, either alone or combined with radiation therapy and/or surgery.

How Do Anticancer Drugs Work?

Cancer cells grow in an uncontrolled manner, and they may break away from their original site and spread to other parts of the body. Anticancer drugs disrupt the cancer cells' ability to grow and multiply.

Chemotherapy may be given in several ways. Sometimes the drugs are used to obtain a local effect (for instance, in treating skin cancer). In other cases, chemotherapy is given to achieve a total-body (systemic) effect. This chapter, for the most part, describes systemic chemotherapy.

The best way to get the drug to the cancer site depends on the particular type of cancer and the drug or combination of drugs used. The medicine may be taken by mouth or injected into a muscle, or it may be given through a vein. Once in the blood, an anticancer drug is carried through the body to reach as many cancer cells as possible. How fast the cells are destroyed may vary with different medicines and different types of cancer.

Anticancer drugs can affect normal tissues also, because they act on any rapidly dividing cells in the body. The normal cells most likely to be affected are those in the bone marrow, gastrointestinal (GI) tract, reproductive system, and hair follicles. Most normal cells are able to recover quickly when the treatment is over.

Chemotherapy and You

How Are Anticancer Drugs Prescribed?

The choice of anticancer drugs for each patient depends on the type and location of the cancer, its stage of development, how it affects normal body functions, and the general health of the patient. You may be treated with one drug or several. A combination may be used because cancer cells that are not affected by one anticancer drug may be destroyed by others. Also, drugs sometimes work better together than they can alone. The most commonly used combinations are described in the section called "Anticancer Drugs and Combinations."

How Is Chemotherapy Given?

Most anticancer drugs are given by one of three routes, as described below:

• *Oral.* When drugs are given by mouth, they get into the bloodstream through the lining of the stomach or upper intestines. Some medicines cannot be given in oral doses because they are not readily absorbed, or they may damage the stomach lining.

• *Intramuscular.* Anticancer drugs given by injection into a muscle (IM) are those that work best when they are slowly absorbed into the bloodstream.

• *Intravenous.* When drugs are injected or infused into a vein (IV), they get to work in the blood very rapidly. Drugs

that can irritate healthy tissue may best be given in IV doses because the flow of blood helps to dilute the chemicals in the drugs.

Is Chemotherapy Painful?

Taking anticancer drugs usually doesn't cause pain. If you take them by mouth, it's the same as taking any other medicine in a liquid, capsule, or tablet. When the medicine is injected into a muscle, it feels much like a flu shot. An IV injection usually feels like having a blood sample drawn for lab tests. Some patients having chemotherapy by IV say that there is sometimes a slight burning feeling in the area of the needle.

Some drugs may cause you discomfort while others cause none at all. Any unpleasant sensation, however, will be temporary in most cases. Certain drugs, if they seep out of the vein, may cause redness and scarring of the tissue. If you feel any pain with an IV treatment, report it to your doctor or nurse right away.

Where Will I Have My Treatments?

Chemotherapy can be given in a doctor's office, a hospital, or a clinic. Some patients take their anticancer drugs at home. Where you are treated will depend on your treatment program, your doctor's policy, hospital rules, and your convenience. When you first start treatment, you may need a short stay in the hospital so that the doctor can closely watch the medicine's effects and adjust the dose if necessary.

Is Chemotherapy Expensive?

The cost of chemotherapy varies with the kinds of drugs used, where the treatments are given, and the length and frequency of treatment. Most health insurance policies, including Medicare Part B, cover at least part of the cost of cancer treatments.

Be sure to discuss your expected costs and health care coverage with your doctor's office staff or the hospital business office. Your pharmacist can tell you about the cost of drugs prescribed for you to take at home.

If you need help to pay for treatments, get in touch with a hospital social worker, the Cancer Information Service, or a local unit of the American Cancer Society. These people may be able to direct you to sources of financial aid.

How Long and How Often Will I Receive Treatments?

The length and frequency of your chemotherapy depend on the kind of cancer you have, the drugs being used, and how your body responds to them. Chemotherapy may be given daily,

weekly, or monthly. Sometimes treatment is given in an on-and-off cycle that includes rest periods so that your body has a chance to build healthy new cells and regain strength.

Your doctor should be able to estimate how long you will be receiving chemotherapy. The planned schedule may be adjusted, as time goes by, to suit your individual responses and treatment needs.

What If I'm Taking Other Medications

Some other medicines may interact with the anticancer drugs you are taking; that is, the use of one kind of drug may change the effects of another. Before you start chemotherapy, it's a good idea to take all your medicines, or a written list of them, to the doctor or nurse. Your list should include the name of each drug, the strength of each dose, how often you take it, and the reason for taking it. Remember to include any over-the-counter (nonprescription) medicines you use, such as laxatives, cold pills, aspirin, and vitamins. After you begin chemotherapy, be sure to check with your doctor, nurse, or pharmacist before taking any other medication or stopping the ones you already take.

How Will I Know If the Chemotherapy is Working?

Your nurse and doctor will use several methods to measure how well your treatments are working. You will have frequent physical examinations, blood tests, scans, and X-rays. Do not hesitate to ask the doctor if you want to know about test results and what they show about your progress.

Sometimes patients think that the absence of side effects means that their drugs aren't working, or that if they have side effects, the drugs are working well. Since side effects vary so much from one patient to another, and from one drug to another, their occurrence is usually not a good indicator of the therapy's effectiveness.

Why Do Some People Have Side Effects From Chemotherapy?

To understand why side effects occur, you need to recall how chemotherapy works. Cancer cells divide and reproduce rapidly, so the drugs chosen for chemotherapy are those most likely to stop fast-growing cells. Since some normal cells also grow quickly, they can be likewise affected by some of the anticancer drugs, and unwanted side effects may result. The side effects reported most often are nausea and vomiting, fatigue, and hair loss.

Whether you have side effects depends on the particular drug used and your individual response to it. There are more than 50 drugs used alone and in various combinations to treat the more than 100 types of cancer. Therefore, it is hard to predict whether a particular patient will have a specific side effect. In fact, you could notice a certain side effect after one treatment and not see the same effect the next time.

You should discuss possible side effects with your doctor, nurse, or pharmacist. You need to know what to expect from treatment and which side effects may need medical attention. Selected side effects for individual drugs are listed under "Anticancer Drugs and Combinations." The "Coping with Side Effects" section gives tips to help you deal with the reactions that occur most often.

How Long Do Side Effects Last?

Some side effects of chemotherapy (for instance, fatigue and hair loss) may start in the early weeks of treatment and continue through its end. Others, such as nausea and vomiting, may occur for just a few hours right after a treatment. Most side effects of chemotherapy will gradually disappear once treatment is stopped and the healthy cells have a chance to grow normally. The unwanted effects of treatment can be unpleasant, but they must be measured against the medicine's ability to destroy the cancer.

People having chemotherapy can become discouraged because of the length of the treatment or the side effects that occur. If you begin to feel unhappy about your therapy or how it's progressing, talk to your doctor or nurse. It may be that your medication or the treatment schedule can be altered. Remember, though, that your doctor will not ask you to continue treatments unless the expected benefits outweigh the problems you may have.

460

Some side effects can decrease during treatment, as your body adjusts to the therapy. However, you should remember that the time it takes to get over some of the troublesome side effects and regain energy varies from person to person. How soon you will feel better depends on many factors, including your condition and the kinds of medicines you've been taking. Talk to your doctor or nurse if you have any questions about the way you feel in the weeks after chemotherapy.

461

Eating and Chemotherapy

Why Is Eating Well So Important?

By eating well, you give yourself the best possible chance at coping with both the disease and your therapy. Doctors, nurses, and researchers are finding that patients who have a balanced diet during treatment are better able to withstand its side effects.

Eating well means choosing a variety of foods that contain vitamins, minerals, protein, and other elements needed to keep the body working normally. It means having a diet that is high enough in calories to keep weight up and eating foods high in protein to build and repair the skin, hair, muscles, and organs.

Protein is used to repair body tissues that may be injured during therapy, but only if you are getting enough calories. When your intake of calories is too low, the body must use protein for energy first, and there may not be enough to repair the body tissues. Some nutrition experts believe that during chemotherapy you may need as much as 50 percent more protein than usual and 20 percent more calories.

How Can I Improve My Eating Habits?

To achieve and maintain a well-balanced diet, try to include the following four groups of foods in your daily meal planning:

- *Fruit and vegetable group.* Include salads, cooked vegetables, raw or cooked fruits, and juices. These foods supply some of the important vitamins and minerals your body needs.

- *Poultry, fish, and meat group.* By including fish, poultry, eggs, and meat (or—if you are vegetarian—beans, peas, and nuts), you will be getting protein as well as many vitamins and minerals.

- *Cereal and bread group.* Foods in this group supply some proteins and a variety of vitamins, minerals, and carbohydrates. Your diet should include cereals from corn, wheat, rice, and oats, or whole grain breads, muffins, and macaroni.

- *Milk group.* Milk and other dairy products, such as ice cream and cheese, supply protein, calcium, and a number of vitamins.

What If I Don't Feel Like Eating?

Chemotherapy may cause changes in your eating habits. People who have always been light eaters may find their appetites increased. The reverse may be more of a problem: People who have always had a good appetite may find that they don't feel like eating.

Even when you know that eating properly is important, there may be days when you cannot eat as much as you think you should. If you don't have much appetite, or find you are losing weight, try eating frequent small meals throughout the day. You also can try taking a walk before meals to help increase your appetite. Make the most of days when you do feel like eating to help catch up on food intake. Generally it's best not to try to lose weight while you're having chemotherapy.

Many people lose their appetite for red meats during chemotherapy because changes in the taste buds can cause meat to taste bitter. If this is a problem, try soaking or cooking meats in soy sauce, fruit juice, or wine. Some patients have found that using plastic forks, knives, and spoons rather than metal ones helps to reduce the bitter taste.

Other common diet-related problems are nausea, a feeling of fullness, and difficulty in chewing or swallowing. In the section called "Coping with Side Effects," you'll find ideas to help you maintain good nutrition in spite of these problems.

If you are unable to eat very much food, it is important that what you *do* eat is highly nutritious. In the booklet titled *Eating Hints*, you'll find both tips to help you enjoy eating and recipes designed to increase your protein and calorie intake. For a free copy of *Eating Hints*, call the Cancer Information Service or write to the National Cancer Institute.*

What About the Need for Fluids?

Some anticancer drugs can affect the bladder or kidneys. Check with your doctor, nurse, or pharmacist to see if this is the case with your medicines, and ask how much fluid you should drink each day. You may need to take in extra fluids to keep your kidneys working well. Water, juice, tea, soft drinks, broth, ice cream, soup, ice sticks, and gelatin are all considered fluids.

Drinks that contain alcohol must be considered separately. Alcohol can interact with some medicines, causing them to not work as well or to produce more severe side effects. For this reason, some people need to limit their alcohol intake during chemotherapy. Check with your doctor, nurse, or pharmacist before drinking any beer, wine, or liquor.

---

* For NCI publications write, National Cancer Institute, Office of Cancer Communications, Building 31, Room 10A24, Bethesda, MD 20892.

Coping With Side Effects

On the pages that follow you will find suggestions for dealing with some of the more common side effects of chemotherapy. You may have none of these side effects, or you could have several. It depends on the drugs you are taking and your particular reaction to them. Refer to "Anticancer Drugs and Combinations," later in this chapter, for details on your specific drugs.

What Can I Do About Problems With Digestion?

Nausea and vomiting—Some anticancer drugs cause nausea and vomiting because they affect the stomach lining and the part of the brain that controls vomiting. Your doctor may give you a medicine to help prevent stomach upset. There are also a number of ways you can adjust your diet to reduce nausea and vomiting. Try any of the ideas below that appeal to you, and keep testing until you find the ones that work best for you.

• Eat small meals throughout the day so your stomach won't feel too full.

• Avoid liquids at mealtime to prevent filling your stomach with fluid. Instead, have liquids at least an hour before or after eating.

• Avoid sweets and fried or other fatty foods.

• Eat foods at room temperature rather than very hot or chilled.

• Eat slowly so that only small amounts of food enter your stomach at one time.

• Chew your food well so you can digest it more easily.

• Eat dry foods like toast, dry cereal, or crackers. They often help to ease an upset stomach.

• Avoid eating a heavy meal immediately before your treatment.

• Drink cool, clear, unsweetened beverages such as apple juice, or light sodas such as ginger ale (after letting it go flat).

• Avoid any odors that offend you (e.g., food odors, smoke, perfumes).

• If the smell of food makes you feel sick, try to stay away from the kitchen while meals are being prepared.

• On days that you feel well, prepare several meal-size dishes and freeze them for days when you don't want to cook.

• It may be helpful to rest after eating, since activity can slow your digestion and increase any discomfort. Try to rest in a chair; avoid lying flat for at least 2 hours after meals.

• Remove dentures or partial dentures on days you receive drug treatments, since objects in the mouth often tend to promote vomiting.

• Try breathing through your mouth when you feel nauseated.

Some people have nausea when they just think about having their drug treatment. If you feel queasy before treatments, try the coping techniques discussed under "Chemotherapy and Your Emotions."

Diarrhea—If you are having diarrhea and it continues for more than 24 hours, or if you have pain or cramping

464

along with it, call your doctor. In severe cases, an antidiarrhea medicine may be prescribed.

Some of the ways you can help to control diarrhea are listed below.

• Try a clear liquid diet to allow your bowels time to rest.

• Drink plenty of fluids to replace those you have lost, especially mild, clear liquids such as apple juice, water, weak tea, or clear broth. Liquids should be taken warm or at room temperature; they should never be iced or very hot. Let carbonated drinks lose their fizz before you drink them.

• Eat smaller amounts of food, but eat more often.

• Avoid foods that can cause cramps (e.g., coffee, beans, nuts, cabbage, broccoli, cauliflower, highly spiced foods, and sweets).

• When you feel better, gradually add foods that are low in fiber, such as rice, cream of rice cereal, bananas, applesauce, mashed potatoes, dry toast, and crackers.

• When you have diarrhea, you may lose potassium (a mineral that is very important to your body's functioning). Unless your doctor has told you otherwise, try to increase the amount of high-potassium foods in your diet. Bananas, oranges, and potatoes are good sources.

• Avoid milk and milk products if they seem to make the diarrhea worse.

Constipation—Some anticancer drugs cause constipation. Ask your doctor, nurse, or pharmacist whether your medicine is one that does. The suggestions below may help to prevent or relieve constipation:

• Drink plenty of fluids to help loosen the bowels.

• Include high-fiber foods (for instance, bran, raw fruits and vegetables, whole grain breads, and nuts) in your diet.

• Keep up a normal level of activity or exercise if you can. Notify your doctor or nurse if bowel movements are off-schedule for more than a day or two. You may need to take a laxative or stool softener.

How Are Mouth and Throat Problems Managed?

Some anticancer drugs can cause dryness or soreness of the mouth and throat. Your doctor might suggest that you use artificial saliva if dryness is a serious problem for you.

Chewing and swallowing can be difficult when you have dryness or discomfort in your mouth or throat. Try the following steps to help increase moisture and make eating easier:

• Drink lots of liquids.

• Suck on ice chips.

• Use sugarless hard candy or sugarless gum to increase moisture.

• Eat moist foods such as fruit and ice cream.

• Moisten dry foods with butter, margarine, gravy, sauces, or broth.

• Try dunking dry, crisp foods in coffee, tea, milk, etc.

• Put cooked foods in the blender so they will be smooth and easier to swallow.

• Try eating soft, cold foods, such as ice cream, pudding, ice sticks, watermelon, baby food, or gelatin. (Soft, sweet foods can promote tooth decay, so be sure to brush your teeth with a soft brush right after eating.)

Mouth sores (stomatitis) can result when chemotherapy affects the rapidly growing cells of the lining of the mouth. Your doctor may prescribe a medicine to reduce pain while the lining of your mouth heals. You can also help to prevent mouth pain in the following ways:

• Avoid food and juices with a high acid content, such as tomato, orange, and grapefruit. Foods that will not sting your mouth include apricot and pear nectars, squash, beans, and peas.

• Avoid salt and spicy foods if they sting.

• Keep your mouth and gums clean to prevent infection.

If you develop sores in your mouth, contact your doctor or nurse for advice. Sometimes mouth sores indicate a serious problem, and your doctor may have to provide further treatment.

Do I Need Special Care for My Mouth?

Good mouth care during chemotherapy is very important because the mouth tissues may become more susceptible to infection. Some simple precautions will help you prevent infection:

• Use a soft toothbrush and a gentle touch when cleaning your teeth. Brushing too hard can damage soft mouth tissues.

• Make a soothing, effective mouthrinse with one teaspoon of baking soda in one cup of warm water. Hold the rinse in your mouth for about a minute.

• Avoid mouthwash products that contain a large amount of salt or alcohol.

• If your mouth becomes painful, eat soft, unseasoned foods such as soft-boiled eggs and oatmeal.

• Use lip balm if your lips become dry.

Ask your dentist to show you the best techniques for brushing and flossing your teeth during chemotherapy. Because your cancer treatments could make you more prone to develop cavities, the dentist may suggest that you apply fluoride to your teeth each day to help prevent decay. Ask your doctor whether you should have any needed dental work before you start your chemotherapy.

Why is Infection More Likely?

Most anticancer drugs affect the bone marrow, decreasing its ability to produce blood cells. The white blood cells produced in the bone marrow help to protect your body by fighting bacteria that cause infection. If the number of white cells in your blood is reduced, there is a higher risk of your getting an infection.

During the course of your therapy, the doctor will closely watch your blood cell count. If the white cell count becomes too low, your doctor may want to postpone treatment or give a lower dose of anticancer drugs for a while. If you have a reduced white cell count, it is very important that you try to prevent infection by taking the steps listed below.

• Wash your hands often during the day; be sure to wash them well before eating and after using the bathroom.

• Avoid crowds as well as people who have contagious illnesses such as chicken pox or flu.

• Do not tear or cut your nail cuticles. Use cuticle cream and remover instead.

• To prevent breaks in your mouth, avoid using a hard toothbrush or dental floss. Your doctor, nurse, or dentist can suggest ways to clean your mouth gently.

• To prevent breaks in your skin, use an electric shaver rather than a razor.

• Do not squeeze or scratch pimples.

• Take a warm shower every day, and lightly pat your skin dry rather than rubbing briskly.

• If your skin becomes dry and cracked, use lotion or oil to soften and heal it.

• If you do cut or scrape your skin, clean the area at once with warm water and soap.

• After each bowel movement, clean the rectal area gently but thoroughly. If there is irritation or if hemorrhoids are a problem, ask your doctor or nurse for advice.

What Are the Signs of Infection?

Even if you take extra care, it is possible to get an infection, and you could have some of the following symptoms:

• A fever (over 100° F).

• Chills.

• Sweating, especially at night.

• Loose bowels.

• A burning feeling when urinating.

• A severe cough or sore throat.

If any symptoms of infection appear, report them to your doctor or nurse right away. Do not use aspirin or any other medicine to reduce fever unless you first check with your doctor, nurse, or pharmacist.

Are All Blood Cells Affected by Chemotherapy?

Anticancer drugs may affect any of the blood cells that bone marrow produces—red blood cells and platelets as well as the white blood cells that fight infection. Each type of blood cell plays an important role in your body's normal functions.

Red blood cells—The red blood cells carry oxygen to all parts of the body. When your red blood cell count is low (a problem called "anemia"), your body tissues do not get enough oxygen to do their work. With anemia, you may feel tired, dizzy, or chilly or become short of breath. Be sure to report any of these symptoms to your doctor.

If you become anemic, there are several things you can do to help yourself feel better:

• Get plenty of rest; conserve your energy.

• Add more green, leafy vegetables,

liver, and red meats (if you can) to your diet.

• Move slowly to avoid getting dizzy. For example, when you wake up, instead of getting out of bed quickly, sit on the side of the bed for a while before standing. If you still feel dizzy, talk to your doctor or nurse about what you should do.

Your doctor may want you to have blood transfusions to build up the red cell count if it gets too low.

Platelets—Platelets help to make your blood clot to stop the bleeding when you hurt yourself. If there are not enough platelets in your blood, you may bleed or bruise more easily than usual, even from a minor injury. Here are some ways to avoid problems when your platelet count is low:

• Do not take any medication (not even aspirin or aspirin-free pain relievers) without first checking with your doctor, nurse, or pharmacist.

• Do not have any alcoholic drinks unless your doctor says it's all right.

• Use cotton swabs, rather than a toothbrush, to clean your mouth.

• Clean your nose by blowing gently, never use fingers.

• Be extra careful when using knives or tools.

• Be very careful not to burn yourself, especially when ironing or cooking. Use a padded glove when you reach into the oven.

• Avoid contact sports and other activities that might result in injury.

• Wear heavy gloves for digging in the garden or working near plants with thorns.

If your platelet count gets too low, you may need a transfusion of platelets. Be sure to tell your doctor if you are bruising easily or if you have red spots under the skin. Also, report any unusual bleeding, such as from the gums or nose. The doctor can tell you what signs you should look for to detect blood in your urine or stools.

Do People in Chemotherapy Always Lose Their Hair?

The hair follicles of the head and body are made up of cells that grow and divide rapidly, so they can react to some anticancer drugs. Your medicines may or may not affect hair growth. No one can predict exactly how your hair will be affected, but your doctor, nurse, or pharmacist can give you some idea of what to expect. If there is a change, it will most likely be temporary.

When hair is damaged by chemotherapy, it breaks at or near the skin. Your scalp may become tender, and hair that is still growing may become dull and dry. You could lose body hair as well as scalp and facial hair.

Severe hair loss can begin within a few days or weeks of treatment. You may first notice a greater than normal amount of hair loss when brushing, combing, or washing your hair. Loss of hair may stop at severe thinning or may continue to total baldness.

What Can I Do About Hair Loss?

For some patients, loss of hair from the head can be decreased or prevented by

468

scalp hypothermia (chilling) before and during treatment sessions. This technique has been helpful for patients taking certain drugs, but it is not recommended for all patients. Your doctor can tell you about scalp hypothermia and whether it would be right for you.

Some people who have severe hair loss choose to cover their heads, while others prefer not to. If you would feel better with your head covered, you could wear a cap, scarf, or turban. You might want to buy a wig or toupee before you begin treatment or early in your chemotherapy program. That way you'll have the option of matching your natural hair color and usual style.

Losing hair from your head, face, or body isn't easy to accept and may take some emotional adjustment. At times you may feel angry or depressed about losing your hair. Such emotions are neither unusual nor wrong, and you might feel better by talking about them. Remember that your hair will grow back when your chemotherapy is over. In fact, it may begin to return during treatment. Some people will find that their new hair is slightly different in color or texture.

How Are Sexual Organs Affected?

Chemotherapy may—but does not always—affect sexual organs and function in both men and women. The side effects that might occur depend on the type of anticancer drugs used and the patient's age and general health.

Drug treatments for cancer generally do not affect the ability or the desire to have sex. Some people, though, find that the stress of their illness or their treatment schedule makes them feel more tired than usual. If fatigue is a problem, you may want to set aside time for physical intimacy after a period of rest.

The many drugs used in chemotherapy act differently, and patients have different reactions and personal needs. If you have any concerns about your medicine's effects on sexual functioning, try to discuss them with your doctor or nurse before treatment is started. You will want to know what to expect and how to handle any problems that occur.

For women—Women having some types of chemotherapy may notice changes in their menstrual cycles. Menstrual periods may become irregular, or they may stop during the course of treatment. You could have "hot flashes" and other symptoms of menopause. Hormone changes caused by chemotherapy can also result in itching, burning, or dryness of vaginal tissue. Your doctor or nurse may suggest a cream or ointment to help ease the problem.

Some anticancer drugs can cause infertility, which may be temporary or permanent, depending on your age and the type of treatments you receive. While it may be possible to become pregnant during chemotherapy, it is not advisable because some anticancer drugs may cause birth defects. Women of childbearing age (from the teens through the end of menopause) are strongly urged to use birth control throughout their course of treatment.

Talk to your doctor or nurse about birth control methods you might consider.

Certain drugs are not recommended for pregnant women because of their possible effects on the unborn child. If a woman is pregnant when her cancer is discovered, it may be possible to delay treatment until after delivery. For the woman who needs therapy sooner, the doctor may suggest starting chemotherapy after the 12th week of pregnancy (when the fetus is beyond the stage of greatest risk). In some cases, termination of the pregnancy may also be considered.

For men—Men may become infertile as a result of chemotherapy. Anticancer drugs may lower the number of sperm cells, reduce their mobility, or cause other cell abnormalities. Infertility may continue through the course of chemotherapy. After treatment, some men remain infertile, while others find that their sperm count returns to normal. Because permanent sterility is possible, you should talk to your doctor about this side effect before you begin treatment. You may want to find out about sperm banking (having sperm frozen to allow artificial insemination at a future date).

What Can I Do About Skin Problems?

You may have one or more minor skin problems while you are having chemotherapy. Possible side effects include redness, itching, peeling, dryness, and acne. In most cases, you can treat these problems by yourself.

If you develop acne, try to keep your face clean and dry, and use over-the-counter medicated creams or soaps. For itching, apply cornstarch as you would a dusting powder. Use creams or lotions on dry skin areas. If skin problems don't respond to these measures, get further advice from your doctor.

When anticancer drugs are given through a vein, they may cause irritation and produce a dark area along the vein. This dark pathway often can be covered by makeup. The darkened areas, in most cases, will fade a few weeks after treatment ends.

Certain medicines, if they seep out of the vein, may cause permanent tissue damage and scarring. Tell the doctor or nurse right away if you have any pain, burning, or swelling at the injection site during or after your treatment.

Exposure to the sun may increase the skin side effects of some anticancer drugs. Your skin may become more likely to burn from the sun or a sunlamp. Check with your doctor, nurse, or pharmacist to find out if either type of sensitivity might be a problem for you. A PABA sunscreen lotion (protection factor 15) may help to prevent burning if you have to be outdoors. In some cases, a product that fully blocks out the sun (for instance, zinc oxide) may be needed.

Although most skin problems are not serious, certain symptoms may mean that you are having an adverse reaction to your medicine. Contact your doctor *at once* if you have sudden or severe rash, hives, or itching, especially if you also have trouble breathing.

What Can I Do About Other Side Effects?

Muscle and nerve effects—Weak, tired, or sore muscles may result from a low level of red blood cells, or they could be a direct effect of some drugs. You might have a tingling or burning feeling in your hands or feet, like when they "fall asleep." You could become somewhat clumsy in your movements or feel a loss of balance.

If you have minor problems with muscles and nerves, you can protect yourself by using caution and common sense. For example, if your fingers are numb, you need to be very careful when grasping objects that are sharp, hot, or otherwise hazardous. If your sense of balance or muscle strength is affected, move slowly, and use handrails when you have to go up and down stairs.

With some medicines, these effects may be temporary and will not need medical attention. In other cases, though, muscle and nerve symptoms may indicate serious problems and you might need medical help. Ask your doctor, nurse, or pharmacist for information about your medicines and whether these side effects should be reported.

Effects on the urinary tract—Some anticancer drugs cause urine to change color. Don't be alarmed if your urine is red while you're taking doxorubicin (Adriamycin®) or daunorubicin, or bright yellow if you take methotrexate. Your urine could also take on a strong or medicine-like odor from certain drugs. The color and odor of semen also may be affected.

In general, it is a good idea to drink plenty of fluids to ensure good urine flow and help prevent problems. Your doctor should advise you if your anticancer drugs are among those that can damage the kidney and bladder. Ask about signs you should watch for and what to do if problems occur.

Fluid retention—When people tend to retain excess fluid in their bodies, it may be because of their disease, the drugs they're taking, or hormone changes that can occur during treatment. If you notice swelling or puffiness in your face, hands, feet, or abdomen, check with your doctor or nurse for advice. You may need to limit your intake of salt and foods with a high sodium content. If the problem is severe, your doctor can prescribe a medicine to help your body rid itself of excess fluids.

Flu-like syndrome—Some patients report feeling like they have the flu a few hours to a day after treatments. Flu-like symptoms—muscle aches, headache, tiredness, nausea, slight fever, chills, and loss of appetite—may last from 1 to 3 days. These symptoms could be caused by your disease, the medicines you are taking, or an infection. If you get flu symptoms, check with your doctor for instructions.

Chemotherapy and Your Emotions

The need for chemotherapy and its effect on your life can prompt a range of negative feelings. Fear, anxiety, and depression are common to many cancer patients.

When you start chemotherapy, your lifestyle may change; you may have to adjust your routine to fit treatment schedules; and your overall health may suffer from treatment side effects. These kinds of changes are not pleasant, but you can handle most of them by adjusting your own attitudes and behavior. It is important to remember that you are not alone and that many other cancer patients have successfully dealt with similar feelings and problems.

During your treatment, you may wonder what is happening to you, whether the drugs are working, and how you can deal with your stress and anxiety. If you don't understand what is happening to you physically, ask questions; and if you don't understand the way it is explained, keep asking until you do. Be aware of your emotional well-being also, and remember that it is as important as your physical health. If you feel frightened or discouraged, seek out help.

Talking with an understanding friend or family member or with another patient may be helpful. You may wish to talk things over with a member of the clergy or a health professional with whom you feel comfortable. Talk with your doctor, nurse, or social worker, or ask about seeing a mental health professional. Everyone needs some support during difficult times, and you should not hesitate to ask for help while you're being treated for cancer.

How Can I Make My Daily Life Easier?

There are things you can do to help smooth the course of your chemotherapy. Some suggestions are the following:

• Remember that eating well is very important. Your body needs food to maintain itself, to rebuild body tissues, and to regain strength.

• Keep your treatment goals in mind to help maintain a positive attitude.

• Find out as much as you want to know about your disease and its treatment. This can lessen your fear of the unknown.

• Keep a journal or diary while you're in treatment. A record of your activities and thoughts can help you learn about the feelings you have as you go through treatment. It may also clarify what questions you need to ask your doctor or nurse.

• Learn the skills you need to take care of yourself. Whatever you can do for yourself will help you feel more in control of the events that make up your life.

• Limit your activities if you tire quickly. Try doing only the things that mean the most to you. Don't let chemotherapy or its side effects rob you of your social life.

- Explore new methods to help you cope with your illness. Some chemotherapy patients have found meditation and relaxation exercises helpful.

- Set realistic goals for yourself. Trying to complete tasks too quickly can be discouraging. Don't be too hard on yourself.

- Plan activities for those days when you feel the best.

- Try new hobbies and learn new skills.

- Exercise if you can. Using your body can promote self-esteem, help you get rid of tension or anger, and build your appetite. Ask your doctor, nurse, or physical therapist for advice about a practical exercise program.

- Ask your doctor or nurse about cancer patient support groups. You may want to talk to other cancer patients who are going through the same kind of adjustments you are having to make.

Can My Family and Friends Help?

You may need to rely more on the people closest to you to help during your cancer treatment, but this may be difficult at first. Many people do not understand cancer, and they may avoid you because they're afraid of your illness. Others may worry that they will upset you by saying the wrong thing.

At a time when you might expect others to rush to your aid, you may have to make the first moves. Try to be open in talking with others about your illness, your treatment, your needs, and your feelings. Once people know that you can discuss these things, they may

be more willing to open up and lend their support.

By keeping the lines of communication open, you can help to correct mistaken ideas, and you and your loved ones will be better able to help each other through a difficult time. Another booklet from the National Cancer Institute, *Taking Time*,*offers more useful advice to help cancer patients and their families

How Can I Cope With Stress?

There are a number of methods you can use to cope with the stresses of cancer and its treatment side effects. The techniques presented here have proven useful in relieving the nausea and vomiting that may occur *before* drug treatments, and have helped patients to relax at any time during therapy. These methods may or may not work for you, but they have worked for others with cancer, so they may be worth a try.

Control of nausea and vomiting—Some patients suffer nausea and vomiting just at the thought of having their drug treatments. The problem (known as "anticipatory nausea and vomiting") results from anxiety about receiving the treatments and the expectation of being sick afterward. You might find it helpful to lie down in a quiet place for 15 to 40 minutes before chemotherapy. Just before you receive the medicines, place a cool washcloth over your eyes. If you feel like talking to someone while you rest, do so. A conversation that keeps your mind occupied with other thoughts can often help to relieve feelings of nausea.

* *The mentioned publication is reprinted within this book. See CONTENTS for chapter entitled, **Emotional Support**.*

Relaxation techniques—Basic relaxation can help you fall asleep, give you more energy, and reduce your anxiety. You can help yourself relax while sitting up or lying down. Choose a quiet place, if you can, and be sure you are comfortable. To keep your circulation free, wear loose-fitting clothes and do not cross your arms or legs. Begin the relaxation technique by staring at an object, or closing your eyes and thinking of a peaceful scene, or concentrating on your breathing for a minute or two.

There are many ways to practice basic relaxation. Some require deep breathing, and people with lung problems should check with the doctor before they try any deep-breathing exercise. Here are some methods that have helped other cancer patients to cope with stress and discomfort:

- *Tension relaxation technique.* Take a slow, deep breath, and as you breathe in, tense a particular muscle or group of muscles. For example, you can squeeze your eyes shut, frown, clench your teeth, make a fist, or stiffen your arms or legs. Hold your breath and keep your muscles tense for a second or two. Then, let go! Breathe out and let your body go limp while you feel the tension draining. Relax.

- *Rhythm technique.* Take deep breaths, keeping a slow rhythm. Keep saying to yourself, "In, one, two; Out, one, two." Each time you breathe out, feel yourself relax and go limp. Continue this for just a few seconds or up to 10 minutes. To end your rhythmic breathing, count silently and slowly from one to three.

You may want to listen to slow, familiar music through an earphone or a headset while trying these relaxation methods.

- *Imagery.* Imagery is sort of a daydream that uses all of your senses, although it is usually done with the eyes closed. To begin, breathe slowly and feel yourself relax. Concentrate on breathing comfortably from your abdomen. Imagine a ball of healing energy—perhaps a white light—forming somewhere in your body.

When you can "see" the ball of energy, imagine that the air you breathe in blows it to any part of the body where you feel pain or discomfort such as nausea. When you breathe out, picture the air moving the ball away from the body, taking with it the pain or discomfort and tension. (Be careful not to blow as you breathe out; breathe naturally.)

Continue to picture the ball moving toward you and away each time you breathe in and out. You may see the ball getting bigger as it takes more and more discomfort and tension away. To end the imagery, count slowly to three, breathe in deeply, open your eyes, and say to yourself, "I feel alert and relaxed." Begin moving about slowly.

- *Distraction.* Many people use distraction, without realizing it, when they watch television or listen to the radio to take their minds off their worries or discomfort. Any activity that holds your attention can be used for distraction. Working with your hands—doing needlework, building models, or painting—may be helpful. Losing yourself in a good book is another way to keep from thinking about pain or other problems.

• *Biofeedback.* Special machines are used in biofeedback to help you control certain body functions such as heart rate, blood pressure, and muscle tension. This method can also be used to help you relax. Cancer patients have used biofeedback to reduce anxiety and to help them handle treatments. Your doctor or nurse can refer you to someone trained in teaching bio-feedback if you want to know more.

• *Hypnosis.* A trance-like state can be either self-induced or induced by a person trained in the technique. Self-hypnosis is a skill that can be mastered by many patients and can be a benefit in reducing anxiety. If you are interested in hypnosis, ask your doctor or nurse to refer you to someone trained in this method.

Does Chemotherapy Affect Sexuality?

The feelings we have about our maleness or femaleness affect the way we relate and respond to others. These feelings of sexuality are often expressed in close physical and intimate relation-ships. Changes in sexuality are often related to the way we think we look to others, changes in tolerance for physical activity, level of fatigue, and anxiety about survival, family, or finances. These very natural feelings sometimes place a strain on normal expressions of sexuality and can create concerns about sexual desirability.

The effects of chemotherapy on sexuality are diverse. Some people go through their treatments unaffected, while others have changes in their desires or desired levels of activity. Some find that the experience draws them closer to their partner and increases their desire for sexual activity. Others may consider sexual activity less important during their illness. There are no typical responses.

If you were comfortable with and enjoyed sexual relations before starting therapy, chances are you will still find pleasure in such intimacy during your treatment as well. Feel free to discuss with your doctor and nurse any matters relating to your sexuality and sexual relationships. If they cannot answer your questions, they will be able to refer you to a counselor or other health professionals who can help.

Although your sexual needs and desires are highly individual concerns, many people have found the following advice helpful:

• *Seek information.* Some patients are concerned about the safety of resuming sexual activity both for themselves and their partners. Ask your doctor or nurse about any health implications of having sexual relations.

• *Open the lines of communication.* Share your feelings, desires, and worries with people who care for you. They cannot help unless they know your needs.

• *Explore new forms of expression.* Your sexuality may be expressed in many ways other than those you're used to. Expressions can take the form of new ways of touching, changes in attitudes, new ways of showing affection, and special times for closeness.

- *Recognize that you are not alone.* Don't hesitate to seek information or counseling if problems arise. Help is available from a number of resources. If you are having difficulties, ask those who are providing care for you—doctors, nurses, pharmacists, social workers, physical therapists, and clergy.

Questions to Ask About Chemotherapy

A written list of questions to ask the doctor, nurse, or pharmacist can help you recall what you would like to know about your treatment. You are likely at some point to have questions other than the ones listed below. It's a good idea to write your questions in at the end of the list; then take this list with you when you visit the doctor before your therapy, go for a treatment visit, or pick up medicines to take home.

- Why do I need chemotherapy?
- What are the pros and cons (benefits and risks) of chemotherapy?
- How successful is this treatment for the type of cancer I have?
- Are there other treatments for my type of cancer?
- When will my chemotherapy begin?
- Who will be giving me the treatments?
- Where will I receive my treatments?
- How often will I receive treatments?
- How long will I need chemotherapy?
- What drug or drugs will I be taking?
- What are the medicines supposed to do?
- How will the medicines be given?
- Can I go back to work while I'm having chemotherapy?

- What kinds of tests will I need?
- What if I miss a dose or several doses?
- What are the possible side effects?
- Are there any long-term side effects?
- What should I do if I have side effects?
- Are there any side effects that I should report right away?
- Will the medicine affect any future children I may have?
- May I take other medicines while I'm having chemotherapy?
- May I drink alcohol (beer, wine, cocktails)?
- Are there any special foods I should or shouldn't eat?
- Is there anything that I should not try to do during chemotherapy?
- How much will the treatment cost?
- Other questions:

_____

_____

_____

_____

_____

Anticancer Drugs and Combinations

This section will acquaint you with the anticancer drugs you are taking. All drugs are listed alphabetically by their generic rather than brand names. For example, cyclophosphamide is the generic name for Cytoxan®. To help you find your medicines, the index at the end of this chapter lists both generic and brand names.

For each drug listed in this section, there is a brief discussion of possible side effects as well as other useful information. The listed side effects are those that *could* occur, not necessarily those that you are most likely to have. Many of the problems described in this section are very rare.

Because much of what you should know about your medicine is common to most anticancer drugs, a section headed "General Information" precedes the listing of specific drugs. Please read that section first. Your doctor, nurse, and pharmacist are good sources for additional information or to answer questions.

Other Information

Before receiving any medicine: Tell your doctor, nurse, and pharmacist if you. . .

• Are allergic to any medicine;

• Are pregnant or intend to have children (some medicines may cause birth defects or affect your ability to have children in the future);

• Are breast-feeding an infant (some medicines may pass into the breast milk

and affect the child);

• Are taking any other prescription or nonprescription (OTC) medicine; using certain medicines together may cause problems;

• Have any other medical problems; certain medical problems may affect your therapy.

Remember—It is important to keep the following points in mind about the use of any medicine.

• If any of the information you learn about your medicines causes you special concern or if you want additional information about your medicines and their use, check with your doctor, nurse, or pharmacist.

• Your medicine has been prescribed for your current medical problem only. It must not be given to other people or used for other problems unless you are otherwise directed by your doctor.

• In order for your medicine to work, it must be taken as directed.

• Keep all medicines out of the reach of children.

Combination chemotherapy—In some cases, several different medicines used in the treatment of cancer are given together. This may allow for more effective treatment.

If you are using a combination of medicines, it is important that you receive each medicine at the proper time. If you are taking some of these medicines by mouth, ask your doctor, nurse, or pharmacist to help you plan a way to remember to take them at the right time.

477

Remember that if you are receiving more than one medicine, each will have different effects. Read the specific information for each one.

Oral medication—If you are taking some of your anticancer medicines by mouth, take them only as directed. The exact amount of medicine you need has been determined by your doctor. If you change the amount you are taking, it may not work as well or it may cause serious side effects. Ask your doctor, nurse, or pharmacist about what to do if you miss a dose of the medicine.

Checkups—It is very important that your doctor check your progress at regular visits in order to make sure that your medicine is working properly and to check for unwanted effects.

Side effects—Side effects may occur with any medicine. These can differ for each medicine and for each patient. Some side effects may be serious and should be reported to your doctor. Others may be simply bothersome. It is important that you know what side effects to expect with the medicines you are receiving and whether they should be reported to your doctor.

Ask the doctor to explain *when* side effects might be expected. Some side effects begin right after a treatment is given, but others may not be noticed until days or weeks later. You will also want to know which side effects are likely to pass quickly and which may be more long-lasting.

Many cancer medicines can cause nausea, vomiting, and loss of appetite. However, it is very important that you continue to have the medicine even if you begin to feel ill. If nausea and vomiting are severe, keep taking the medicine and check with your doctor or nurse for ways to reduce these problems. You may also want to refer to other sections in this booklet that discuss ways to control nausea and vomiting.

Some cancer medicines may cause a temporary loss of hair in some people.

After treatment has ended, normal hair growth should return, although the new hair may be a slightly different color or texture. Refer to the "Coping with Side Effects" section of this chapter for more information on hair loss.

Unexpected side effects may also occur. If you notice any unusual symptoms, check with your doctor or pharmacist.

Most chemotherapy side effects begin to lessen when the therapy is stopped. However, remember that each individual is different and the length of time this takes will vary. It will also depend on your condition and the kinds of drugs you have received. Talk to your doctor, nurse, or pharmacist if you have any questions about the way you feel after your therapy has been completed.

On the pages that follow, the anticancer drugs and drug combinations most often used for cancer chemotherapy in the United States are listed.

Information on the drugs has been taken from *USP DI Advice for the-Patient*, published by the United States Pharmacopeial Convention. Should you wish additional details, this reference book is available at most hospital libraries and many community-pharmacies.

Anticancer Drugs

Asparaginase

Pronunciation:
A-SPARE-a-gin-ase

Brand names:
A commonly used brand name is Elspar®.

How given:
Asparaginase is given by injection.

Special precautions: While you are using asparaginase, your doctor may want you to drink extra fluids so that you will pass more urine. This will help prevent kidney and bladder problems and keep your kidneys working well.

Side effects needing immediate medical attention: Difficulty in breathing; joint pain; puffy face; skin rash or itching; stomach pain with nausea and vomiting (severe).

Other side effects needing medical attention as soon as possible: Yellowing of eyes and skin; confusion; drowsiness; fever, chills, or sore throat; flank or stomach pain; hallucinations (seeing, hearing, or feeling things that are not there); mental depression; nervousness;

sores in mouth or on lips; swelling of feet or lower legs; tiredness; unusually frequent urination; unusual thirst; convulsions (seizures); headache (severe).

After you stop receiving this medicine, it may still produce some side effects that need attention. During this time, check with your doctor immediately if you have severe stomach pain with nausea and vomiting.

Side effects that usually do not require medical attention (unless prolonged or severe): Headache; loss of appetite; nausea and vomiting; stomach cramps; weight loss.

Bleomycin

Pronunciation:
Blee-oh-MY-sin

Brand names:
A commonly used brand name is Blenoxane®.

How given:
Bleomycin is given by IV or IM injection.

Side effects needing immediate attention: Fever and chills (occurring within 3 to 6 hours after a dose is given); faintness; confusion; sweating; wheezing.

Other side effects needing medical attention as soon as possible: Cough; shortness of breath; sores in mouth and on lips.

Side effects that affect the lungs (for example, cough and shortness of breath) may be more likely if you smoke. Lung problems are also more likely to occur in older patients (over age 70).

Side effects needing immediate attention after you stop using this medicine: Cough; shortness of breath.

Side effects that usually do not require medical attention: Darkening or thickening of the skin; itching of skin; skin rash or colored bumps on fingertips, elbows, or palms; skin redness or tenderness; swelling of the fingers; vomiting and loss of appetite.

Busulfan

Pronunciation:
Byoo-SUL-fan

Brand names:
A commonly used brand name is Myleran®.

How given:
Busulfan is taken by mouth.

Special precautions: While you are using busulfan, your doctor may want you to drink extra fluids so that you will pass more urine. This will help prevent kidney and bladder problems and keep your kidneys working well.

Side effects needing medical attention as soon as possible: Fever, chills, or sore throat; unusual bleeding or bruising; cough; side or stomach pain; joint pain; shortness of breath; swelling of feet or lower legs.

Side effects needing attention after you stop using this medicine: Fever, cough,

or shortness of breath; unusual bleeding or bruising.

Side effects that usually do not require medical attention: Darkening of the skin; confusion; diarrhea; dizziness; loss of appetite; nausea and vomiting; unusual tiredness.

Carmustine

Pronunciation:
Kar-MUS-teen

Commonly referred to as:
BCNU

Brand names:
A commonly used brand
name is BiCNU®.

How given:
Carmustine is given by
IV injection.

Side effects needing immediate medical attention: If carmustine accidentally seeps out of the vein, it may damage some tissues and cause scarring. Tell the doctor or nurse right away if you notice redness, pain, or swelling at the IV site.

Other side effects needing medical attention as soon as possible: Cough; fever, chills, or sore throat; shortness of breath; unusual bleeding or bruising; flushing of face; sores in mouth and on lips; unusual tiredness or weakness; swelling of feet or lower legs; unusual decrease in urination.

Side effects that affect the lungs (for example, cough and shortness of breath) may be more likely if you smoke.

Side effects needing attention after you stop using this medicine: Cough; fever, chills, or sore throat; shortness of breath; unusual bleeding or bruising.

Side effects that usually do not require medical attention: Nausea and vomiting (usually lasting no longer than 4 to 6 hours); discoloration of skin along the vein of injection; diarrhea; difficulty in swallowing; difficulty in walking; dizziness; loss of appetite; loss of hair; skin rash and itching.

Chlorambucil

Pronunciation:
Klor-AM-byoo-sill

Brand names:
A commonly used brand
name is Leukeran®.

How given:
Chlorambucil is taken by
mouth.

Special precautions: While you are using chlorambucil, your doctor may want you to drink extra fluids so that you will pass more urine. This will help prevent kidney and bladder problems and keep your kidneys working well.

Side effects needing medical attention as soon as possible: Fever, chills, or sore throat; sores in mouth and on lips; unusual bleeding or bruising; side or stomach pain; joint pain; skin rash;

swelling of feet or lower legs; convulsions; cough; shortness of breath; yellowing of eyes and skin.

Side effects needing attention after you stop using this medicine: Cough; fever, chills, or sore throat; shortness of breath, unusual bleeding or bruising.

Cisplatin

Pronunciation:
SIS-pla-tin

Commonly referred to as:
Cis-platinum

Brand names:
A commonly used brand
name is Platinol®.

How given:
Cisplatin is given by IV
injection.

Special precautions: While you are receiving cisplatin, your doctor may want you to drink extra fluids so that you will pass more urine. This will help prevent kidney and bladder problems and keep your kidneys working well.

Side effects needing immediate medical attention: Swelling of face; unusually fast heartbeat; wheezing.

If cisplatin accidently seeps out of the vein, it may damage some tissues and cause scarring. Tell the doctor or nurse right away if you notice redness, pain, or swelling at the IV site.

Other side effects needing medical attention as soon as possible: Difficulty in

hearing; fever, chills, or sore throat; side or stomach pain; joint pain; ringing in ears; swelling of feet or lower legs; unusual bleeding or bruising; loss of taste; unusual tiredness or weakness; numbness or tingling in the fingers, toes or face; blurred vision.

Hearing problems are more likely to occur in children.

Side effects needing attention after you stop using this medicine: Difficulty in hearing; fever, chills, or sore throat; ringing in ears; swelling of feet or lower legs; unusual bleeding or bruising; unusual decrease in urination.

Side effects that usually do not require medical attention (unless prolonged or severe): Nausea and vomiting.

Cyclophosphamide

Pronunciation:
sye-kloe-FOSS-fa-mide

Brand names:
A commonly used brand name is Cytoxan®.

How given:
Cyclophosphamide may be given by mouth or by injection.

Special precautions: While you are taking cyclophosphamide, it is important that you drink extra fluids so that you will pass more urine. This will help prevent kidney and bladder problems and keep your kidneys working well.

Side effects needing immediate medical attention: Blood in urine; painful urination.

Other side effects needing medical attention as soon as possible: Dizziness, confusion, or agitation; fever, chills, or sore throat, missed menstrual periods; tiredness; cough, side or stomach pain; joint pain; shortness of breath; swelling of feet or lower legs; unusual bleeding or bruising; unusually fast heartbeat; black, tarry stools; sores in mouth and on lips; unusually frequent urination; unusual thirst; yellow eyes and skin.

If you are receiving this medicine by injection, also check with your doctor if you notice redness, swelling, or pain at the place of injection.

Check with your doctor immediately if you notice blood in your urine after you have stopped taking this medicine.

Side effects that usually do not require medical attention: Darkening of skin and fingernails; loss of appetite (unless severe); loss of hair; nausea or vomiting (unless severe).

Cytarabine

Pronunciation:
sye-TARE-a-been

Commonly referred to as:
Ara-C

Brand names:
A commonly used brand name is Cytosar-U®.

How given:
Cytarabine is given by injection.

Special precautions: While you are using cytarabine, your doctor may want you to drink extra fluids so that you will pass more urine. This will help prevent kidney and bladder problems and keep your kidneys working well.

Side effects needing medical attention as soon as possible: Fever, chills, and sore throat; unusual bleeding or bruising; side or stomach pain; joint pain; numbness or tingling in fingers, toes, or face; sores in mouth and on lips; swelling of feet and lower legs; tiredness; black, tarry stools; bone or muscle pain; chest pain; cough; difficulty in swallowing; fainting spells; general feeling of body discomfort or weakness; heartburn; irregular heartbeat; pain at place of injection; reddened eyes; shortness of breath; skin rash; unusual decrease in urination; weakness; yellowing of eyes and skin.

Side effects needing attention after you stop using this medicine: Fever and chills; sore throat; unusual bleeding or bruising.

Side effects that usually do not require medical attention (unless prolonged or severe): Loss of appetite; nausea and vomiting.

Dacarbazine

Pronunciation:
Da-KAR-ba-zeen

Brand names:
A commonly used brand name is DTIC-Dome®.

How given:
Dacarbazine is given by IV injection.

Side effects needing immediate medical attention: If dacarbazine accidentally seeps out of the vein, it may damage some tissues and cause scarring. Tell the doctor or nurse right away if you notice redness, pain, or swelling at the IV site.

Other side effects needing medical attention as soon as possible: Fever, chills, or sore throat; unusual bleeding or bruising; sores in mouth and on lips.

Side effects needing attention after you stop using this medicine: Fever, chills, or sore throat; unusual bleeding or bruising.

Side effects that usually do not require medical attention: Loss of appetite; nausea or vomiting (should lessen after 1 or 2 days).

Dactinomycin

Pronunciation:
Dak-ti-noe-MYE-sin

Brand names:
A commonly used brand name is Cosmegen®.

How given:
Dactinomycin is given by IV injection.

Side effects needing immediate medical attention: Fever, chills, or sore throat: unusual bleeding or bruising; wheezing.

If dactinomycin accidentally seeps out of the vein, it may severely damage some tissues and cause scarring. Tell the doctor or nurse right away if you notice redness, pain, or swelling at the IV site.

Other side effects needing medical attention as soon as possible: Black, tarry stools; continuing diarrhea; continuing stomach pain; difficulty in swallowing; heartburn; sores in mouth and on lips; joint pain; swelling of feet or lower legs; yellowing of eyes and skin.

Side effects needing attention after you stop using this medicine: Black, tarry stools; diarrhea; fever, chills, or sore throat; sores in mouth and on lips; stomach pain; unusual bleeding or bruising; yellowing of eyes and skin.

Side effects that usually do not require medical attention: Darkening of skin; loss of hair (may include eyebrows); nausea and vomiting (unless severe); reddening of the skin; skin rash or acne; tiredness.

Daunorubicin

Pronunciation:
Daw-noe-ROO-bi-sin

Brand names:
A commonly used brand name is Cerubidine®.

How given:
Daunorubicin is given by IV injection.

Special precautions: While you are using daunorubicin, your doctor may want you to drink extra fluids so that you will pass more urine. This will help prevent kidney and bladder problems and keep your kidneys working well.

Daunorubicin causes urine to turn reddish in color, which may stain clothes. This is not blood. It is perfectly normal and lasts for only 1 or 2 days after each dose is given.

Side effects needing immediate medical attention: Irregular heartbeat; pain at the place of injection; shortness of breath; swelling of feet and lower legs.

If daunorubicin accidentally seeps out of the vein, it may damage some tissues and cause scarring. Tell the doctor or nurse right away if you notice redness, pain, or swelling at the IV site.

Other side effects needing medical attention as soon as possible: Fever, chills, or sore throat; sores in mouth and on lips; side or stomach pains; joint pain; unusual bleeding or bruising; skin rash or itching.

Heart problems are more likely to occur in children under 2 years of age and in adults over age 70; older patients may also be more likely to have blood problems.

Side effects needing immediate attention after you stop using this medicine: Irregular heartbeat; shortness of breath; swelling of feet and lower legs.

Side effects that usually do not require medical attention; Loss of hair; nausea and vomiting (mild); darkening or redness of the skin; diarrhea.

482

oxorubicin

onunciation:
x-oh-ROO-bi-sin
and names:
commonly used brand
me is Adriamycin®.
ow given:
xorubicin is given by
injection.

Special precautions: While you are taking doxorubicin, your doctor may want you to drink extra fluids so that you will pass more urine. This will help prevent kidney and bladder problems and keep your kidneys working well.

Doxorubicin causes the urine to turn reddish in color, which may stain clothes. This is not blood. It is perfectly normal and lasts for only 1 or 2 days after each dose is given.

Side effects needing immediate medical attention: Unusually fast or irregular heartbeat; pain at place of injection; shortness of breath; swelling of feet and lower legs; wheezing.

If doxorubicin accidentally seeps out of the vein, it may damage some tissues and cause scarring. Tell the doctor or nurse right away if you notice redness, pain, or swelling at the IV site.

Other side effects needing medical attention as soon as possible: Fever, chills, or sore throat; sores in mouth and on lips; side or stomach pain; joint pain; unusual bleeding or bruising; skin rash or itching.

Side effects needing immediate attention after you stop using this medicine: Irregular heartbeat; shortness of breath; swelling of feet and lower legs.

Side effects that usually do not require medical attention: Loss of hair; nausea or vomiting (unless severe); reddish urine; darkening of soles, palms, or nails.

tramustine

onunciation:
s-tra-MUSS-teen
and names:
commonly used brand
me is Emcyt®.
ow given:
tramustine is taken by
uth.

Side effects needing immediate medical attention: Headaches (severe or sudden); loss of coordination (sudden); pains in chest, groin, or legs (especially calves); shortness of breath (sudden, for no apparent reason); skin rash or fever; slurred speech (sudden); vision changes (sudden).

Other side effects needing medical attention as soon as possible include: Fever, chills, or sore throat; skin rash or fever; unusual bleeding or bruising; unusual tiredness or weakness.

Side effects that usually do not require medical attention (unless prolonged or severe): Breast tenderness or enlargement; nausea; diarrhea; swelling of feet or lower legs.

toposide

onunciation:
TOE-poe-side
and names:
me commonly used
and names or other
mes are VePesid and
>-16.
ow given:
oposide is given by injection.

Side effects needing medical attention as soon as possible: Fever, chills, or sore throat; sores in mouth or on lips; unusual bleeding or bruising; difficulty in walking; numbness or tingling in fingers and toes; pain at the site of injection; rapid heartbeat; shortness of breath or wheezing; weakness.

Side effects that usually do not require medical attention: Loss of appetite; loss of hair; nausea and vomiting; diarrhea; unusual tiredness.

Floxuridine

Pronunciation:
Flox-YOOR-i-deen

Brand names:
A commonly used brand
name is FUDR®.

How given:
Floxuridine is given by
injection.

Special precautions: Floxuridine
sometimes causes nausea and vomiting.
Tell your doctor if this occurs, especially if you have stomach pain.

Side effects needing immediate medical
attention: Diarrhea; sores in mouth and
on lips; stomach pain or cramps; black,
tarry stools; heartburn; fever, chills, or
sore throat; nausea and vomiting;
swelling or soreness of tongue; difficulty in walking; unusual bleeding or
bruising; yellowing of eyes and skin.

Fluorouracil

Pronunciation:
Floor-oh-YOOR-a-sill
Commonly referred to as:
5-FU.

Brand names:
A commonly used brand
name is Adrucil®.

How given:
Fluorouracil is given by
injection.

Side effects needing immediate medical
attention: Diarrhea; fever, chills, or
sore throat; heartburn; sores in mouth
and on lips; black, tarry stools; nausea
and vomiting (severe); stomach cramps;
unusual bleeding or bruising.

Side effects needing medical attention
as soon as possible: Chest pain; cough;
difficulty with balance; shortness of
breath.

Side effects needing immediate attention after you stop using this medicine:
Fever, chills, or sore throat; unusual
bleeding or bruising.

Side effects that usually do not require
medical attention (unless prolonged or
severe): Loss of appetite; loss of hair;
nausea and vomiting; skin rash and
itching; weakness.

Hydroxyurea

Pronunciation:
Hye-DROX-ee-yoo-REE-
ah

Brand names:
A commonly used brand
name is Hydrea®.

How given:
Hydroxyurea is taken by
mouth.

Special precautions: While you are using hydroxyurea, your doctor may
want you to drink extra fluids so that
you will pass more urine. This will help
prevent kidney and bladder problems
and keep your kidneys working well.

Side effects needing medical attention
as soon as possible: Fever, chills, or
sore throat; sores in mouth and on lips;
unusual bleeding or bruising; convulsions; dizziness; side or stomach pain;
hallucinations (seeing, hearing, or feeling things that are not there); headache; joint pain; confusion; swelling of
feet or lower legs.

The above side effects are more likely
to occur in children and in elderly
patients.

Side effects needing attention after you
stop using this medicine: Fever, chills,
or sore throat; unusual bleeding or
bruising.

Side effects that usually do not require
medical attention (unless prolonged or
severe): Diarrhea; drowsiness; loss of
appetite; nausea; vomiting.

omustine

ronunciation:
>e-MUS-teen

>mmonly referred to as:
CNU

rand names:
commonly used brand
ame is CeeNU®.

ow given:
>mustine is taken by
>uth.

Special precautions: In order that you receive the proper dose of lomustine, there may be two or more different types of capsules in the container. This is not an error. It is important that you take all of the capsules in the container as one dose so that you receive the right amount of medicine.

Side effects needing medical attention as soon as possible: Fever, chills, or sore throat; unusual bleeding or bruising; awkwardness; confusion; slurred speech; sores in mouth and on lips; swelling of feet or lower legs; unusual

decrease in urination; unusual tiredness or weakness; yellowing of eyes and skin; cough or shortness of breath.

Side effects needing attention after you stop using this medicine: Fever, chills, or sore throat; unusual bleeding or bruising.

Side effects that usually do not require medical attention: Loss of appetite; nausea and vomiting (usually lasts less than 24 hours); darkening of skin; diarrhea; loss of hair; skin rash and itching.

Iechlorethamine

ronunciation:
.e-klor-ETH-a-meen

>mmonly referred to as:
itrogen Mustard

rand names:
commonly used brand
ame is Mustargen®.

ow given:
.echlorethamine is given
/ IV injection.

Special precautions: While you are using mechlorethamine, your doctor may want you to drink extra fluids so that you will pass more urine. This will help prevent kidney and bladder problems and keep your kidneys working well.

Side effect needing immediate medical attention: Wheezing.

If mechlorethamine accidentally seeps out of the vein, it may damage some tissues and cause scarring. Tell the doctor or nurse right away if you notice redness, pain, or swelling at the IV site.

Other side effects needing medical attention as soon as possible: Fever, chills, or sore throat; missed menstrual periods; painful rash; unusual bleeding or bruising; dizziness; side and stomach

pain; joint pain; loss of hearing; ringing in ears; swelling of feet or lower legs; black, tarry stools; itching; numbness, tingling, or burning of fingers, toes, or face; shortness of breath; yellowing of eyes and skin.

Side effects needing attention after you stop using this medicine: Fever, chills, or sore throat; unusual bleeding or bruising.

Side effects that usually do not require medical attention: Nausea and vomiting (usually lasts about 8 to 24 hours).

Ielphalan

ronunciation:
IEL-fa-lan

rand names:
commonly used brand
ame is Alkeran®.

'ow given:
Ielphalan is taken by
>outh.

Special precautions: While you are using melphalan, your doctor may want you to drink extra fluids so that you will pass more urine. This will help prevent kidney and bladder problems and keep your kidneys working well.

Side effects needing immediate medical attention: Sudden skin rash and itching.

Side effects needing medical attention as soon as possible: Black, tarry stools; fever, chills, or sore throat; unusual bleeding or bruising; side or stomach

pain; joint pain; sores in mouth and on lips; swelling of feet or lower legs.

Side effects needing attention after you stop using this medicine: Fever, chills, or sore throat; unusual bleeding or bruising.

Side effects that usually do not require medical attention (unless prolonged or severe): Nausea and vomiting.

Mercaptopurine

Pronunciation:
Mer-kap-toe-PYOOR-een

Brand names:
A commonly used brand name is Purinethol₄.

How given:
Mercaptopurine is taken by mouth.

Special precautions: While you are using mercaptopurine, your doctor may want you to drink extra fluids so that you will pass more urine. This will help prevent kidney and bladder problems and keep your kidneys working well.

Avoid alcoholic beverages until you have discussed their use with your doctor. Alcohol may increase the harmful effects of this medicine.

Side effects needing medical attention as soon as possible: Fever, chills, or sore throat; unusual bleeding or bruising; unusual tiredness or weakness; yellowing of eyes and skin; loss of appetite; side or stomach pain; joint pain; nausea and vomiting; swelling of feet or lower legs; black, tarry stools; sores in mouth and on lips.

Side effects needing attention after you stop using this medicine: Fever, chills, or sore throat; unusual bleeding or bruising; yellowing of eyes and skin.

Methotrexate

Pronunciation:
Meth-o-TREX-ate

Brand names:
A commonly used brand name is Mexate®.

How given:
Methotrexate is given by mouth or by injection.

Special precautions: While you are using methotrexate, your doctor may want you to drink extra fluids so that you will pass more urine. This will help prevent kidney and bladder problems and keep your kidneys working well.

Do not drink alcohol while using this medicine. Alcohol can increase the risk of liver problems. If you have any questions about this, check with your doctor.

When you begin to take methotrexate, avoid too much sun or use of a sunlamp because you may become more sensitive to sunlight than usual. In case of a severe burn, check with your doctor.

Do not take aspirin or any other preparations containing aspirin or salicylate compounds without first checking with your doctor. These medicines may increase the effects of methotrexate.

Side effects needing immediate medical attention: Black, tarry stools; bloody vomit; diarrhea; sores in mouth and on lips; stomach pain.

Side effects needing medical attention as soon as possible: Fever, chills, or sore throat; usual bleeding or bruising; blood in urine; blurred vision; confusion; convulsions or seizures; cough; dark urine; dizziness; drowsiness; headache; joint pain; shortness of breath; swelling of feet or lower legs; unusual tiredness or weakness; yellowing of eyes and skin.

Side effects needing attention after you stop using this medicine: Blurred vision; convulsions or seizures; dizziness; drowsiness; headache; confusion; unusual tiredness or weakness.

Side effects that usually do not require medical attention (unless prolonged or severe): Loss of appetite; nausea or vomiting.

The above side effects may be more likely to occur in very young and very old patients.

Mitomycin

Pronunciation:
mye-toe-MYE-sin

Brand names:
commonly used brand name is Mutamycin®.

How given:
Mitomycin is given by IV.

Side effects needing immediate medical attention: Blood in urine.

If mitomycin accidentally seeps out of the vein, it may damage the skin and cause scarring. Tell the doctor or nurse right away if you notice redness, pain, or swelling at the IV site.

Other side effects needing medical attention as soon as possible: Fever, chills, or sore throat; unusual bleeding or bruising; cough; decreased urination; shortness of breath; sores in mouth and on lips; swelling of feet or lower legs; bloody vomit.

Side effects needing attention after you stop using this medication: Blood in urine, fever, chills, or sore throat; unusual bleeding or bruising; decreased urination; shortness of breath; swelling of feet or lower legs.

Side effects that usually do not require medical attention (unless prolonged or severe): Loss of appetite; nausea and vomiting.

Mitotane

Pronunciation:
MYE-toe-tane

Brand names:
commonly used brand name is Lysodren®.

How given:
Mitotane is taken by mouth.

Special precautions: Mitotane may cause some people to become dizzy, drowsy, or less alert than they are normally. Make sure you know how you react to this medicine before you drive, use machines, or do other jobs that require you to be alert.

Mitotane will add to the effects of alcohol and other central nervous system (CNS) depressants (medicines that slow down the nervous system, possibly causing drowsiness). Check with your doctor before using alcohol or other CNS depressants while you are using this medicine.

Check with your doctor right away if you get an injury, infection, or illness of any kind.

Stop taking this medicine and check with your doctor immediately if the following side effects occur: Darkening of skin; diarrhea; dizziness; drowsiness; loss of appetite; mental depression; nausea and vomiting; skin rash, tiredness.

Other side effects needing medical attention as soon as possible: Blood in urine; blurred or double vision; shortness of breath; wheezing.

Plicamycin

Pronunciation:
plye-ka-MYE-sin

Brand names:
some commonly used brand names or other names are Mithracin® and Mithramycin®.

How given:
Plicamycin is given by injection.

Special precautions: Do not take aspirin (ASA) or any other preparations containing aspirin or salicylate compounds without first consulting your doctor.

Side effects needing immediate medical attention: Bloody or black, tarry stools; flushing, redness, or swelling of face; skin rash or small red spots on skin; sore throat and fever; unexplained nosebleed; unusual bleeding or bruising; vomiting of blood.

Side effects that usually do not require medical attention (unless prolonged or severe): Diarrhea; irritation or soreness of mouth; loss of appetite.

Other side effects needing attention and which may occur 1 to 2 hours after the injection is started and continue for 12 to 24 hours: Nausea or vomiting; drowsiness; fever; headache; mental depression; pain, redness, soreness, or swelling at place of injection; unusual tiredness or weakness.

Side effects needing attention after you stop using this medicine: Bloody or black, tarry stools; small red spots on skin; sore throat and fever; unexplained nosebleed; unusual bleeding or bruising; vomiting of blood.

Prednisone

Pronunciation:
PRED-ni-sone

Brand names:
Commonly used brand names are Deltasone®, Meticorten®, and Orasone®.

How given:
Prednisone is taken by mouth.

Special precautions: If you will be using prednisone for a long time, your doctor may want you to follow a low-salt diet and/or a potassium-rich diet.

Stomach problems are more likely to occur if you drink alcoholic beverages while taking this medicine. Do not drink alcoholic beverages unless you have first checked with your doctor.

Before having any kind of surgery (including dental surgery) or emergency treatment, tell the doctor in charge that you are taking prednisone.

Diabetic patients—This medicine may affect blood sugar levels. If you notice a change in the results of your urine sugar test, or if you have any questions about this, check with your doctor.

Side effects needing medical attention as soon as possible: Decreased or blurred vision; frequent urination; increased thirst; skin rash, acne, or other skin problems; back or rib pain; bloody or black, tarry stools; filling or rounding out of the face; irregular heartbeats; menstrual problems; depression;

mood or mental changes; muscle cramps or pains; muscle weakness; nausea or vomiting; seeing halos around lights; sore throat and fever; stomach pain or burning (continuing); swelling of feet or lower legs; unusual tiredness or weakness; wounds that do not heal.

After you stop using this medicine, your body may need time to adjust.

Side effects needing immediate medical attention after you stop using this medicine: Pain in abdomen, stomach, or back; dizziness or fainting; fever; loss of appetite (continuing); muscle or joint pain; nausea or vomiting; shortness of breath; frequent or continuing headaches; unusual tiredness or weakness; unusual weight loss.

Side effects that usually do not require medical attention (unless prolonged or severe): Indigestion; false sense of well-being; increase in appetite; nervousness or restlessness; trouble in sleeping; weight gain.

Procarbazine

Pronunciation:
Pro-KAR-ba-zeen

Brand names:
Some commonly used brand names are Matulane® and Natulan®.

How given:
Procarbazine is taken by mouth.

Special precautions: Check with your doctor or hospital emergency room immediately if severe headache, stiff neck, chest pains, or rapid heartbeat, with nausea and vomiting, occur while you are taking this medicine. These may be symptoms of a serious high blood pressure reaction, which should have a doctor's attention.

When taken with certain foods, drinks, or other medicines, procarbazine can cause very dangerous reactions. To avoid such reactions:

—Do not eat foods that have a high tyramine content (most common in foods that are aged to increase their flavor), such as cheeses, sour cream, yogurt, pickled herring, chicken liver, canned figs, raisins, bananas, avocados, soy sauce, broad bean pods (fava beans), yeast extracts, or meats prepared with tenderizers.

--Do not drink alcoholic beverages, including beer and wines (especially Chianti and other hearty red wines.).

—Do not take any other medicine unless prescribed by your doctor. This especially applies to over-the-counter medicine such as that for colds (including nose drops), cough, asthma, hay fever, and appetite control or stay-awake products.

After you stop this medicine you must continue to obey the rules of caution concerning food, drink, and other medication for at least 2 weeks, since procarbazine may continue to react with certain foods or other medicines for up to 14 days after you stop taking it.

This medicine may cause some people to become drowsy or less alert than they are normally. Make sure you know how you react to this medicine before you drive or do other jobs that require you to be alert.

Stop taking this medicine and check with your doctor immediately if the following side effects occur: Chest pains; rapid or irregular heartbeat; severe headache; stiff neck.

Other side effects needing medical attention as soon as possible: Black, tarry stools; bloody vomit; convulsions; cough; fever, chills, or sore throat; hallucinations (seeing, hearing, or feeling things that are not there); missed menstrual periods; shortness of breath; thickening of bronchial secretions; continuing tiredness or weakness; unusual bleeding or bruising; diarrhea; sores in mouth and on lips; tingling or numbness of the fingers or toes; unsteadiness or awkwardness; yellowing of eyes and skin; fainting; skin rash, hives, or itching; wheezing.

Side effects that usually do not require medical attention (unless prolonged or severe): Drowsiness; muscle or joint pain; muscle twitching; nervousness; nightmares; nausea and vomiting; sleeplessness; sweating; tiredness, weakness; darkening of skin; dizziness or lightheadedness when getting up from a lying or sitting position; feeling of warmth and redness in face.

Streptozocin

Pronunciation:
Strep-toe-ZOE-sin

Brand names:
A commonly used brand name is Zanosar® .

How given:
Streptozocin is given by IV injection.

Special precautions: While you are receiving streptozocin, your doctor may want you to drink extra fluids so that you will pass more urine. This will help prevent kidney and bladder problems and keep your kidneys working well.

If streptozocin accidentally seeps out of the vein, it may damage some tissues and cause scarring. Tell the doctor or nurse right away if you notice redness, pain, or swelling at the IV site.

Side effects needing immediate medical attention if they occur shortly after the medicine is given: Anxiety, nervousness, or shakiness; chills, cold sweats, or cool, pale skin; drowsiness or unusual tiredness or weakness; headache; pain or redness at place of injection; unusual hunger; unusually fast pulse.

Other side effects needing medical attention as soon as possible: Swelling of feet or lower legs; unusual decrease in urination; fever, chills, or sore throat; unusual bleeding or bruising; yellowing of eyes or skin.

Side effects needing attention after you stop using this medicine: Swelling of feet or lower legs; unusual decrease in urination.

Side effects that usually do not require medical attention: Nausea and vomiting (usually occurs within 2 to 4 hours after receiving dose); diarrhea.

Tamoxifen

Pronunciation:
Ta-MOX-i-fen

Brand names:
A commonly used brand name is Nolvadex® .

How given:
Tamoxifen is given by mouth.

Special precautions: Tamoxifen may make you more fertile. It is best to use some type of birth control while you are taking it; however, do not use an oral contraceptive (the "Pill"), since it may change the effects of tamoxifen. Tell your doctor right away if you think you have become pregnant while taking this medicine.

Side effects needing medical attention as soon as possible: Blurred vision; confusion; pain or swelling in legs; shortness of breath; unusual weakness or sleepiness.

Side effects that usually do not require medical attention (unless prolonged or severe): Hot flashes; nausea or vomiting; weight gain; bone pain; changes in menstrual period; headache; genital itching; skin rash or dryness; vaginal bleeding or discharge.

490

nblastine

onunciation:
1-BLAS-teen

and names:
commonly used brand
me is Velban®.

w given:
nblastine is given by
injection.

Special precautions: While you are using vinblastine, your doctor may want you to drink extra fluids so that you will pass more urine. This will hlep prevent kidney and bladder problems and keep your kidneys working well.

Side effects needing immediate medical attention: If vinblastine accidentally seeps out of the vein, it may damage the skin and cause some scarring. Tell the doctor or nurse right away if you notice redness, pain, or swelling at the IV site.

Other side effects needing medical attention as soon as possible: Fever,

chills, or sore throat; side or stomach pain; joint pain; swelling of feet and lower legs; unusual bleeding or bruising; black, tarry stools; difficulty in walking; dizziness; double vision; drooping eyelids; headache; jaw pain; mental depression; numbness or tingling in fingers and toes; pain in fingers and toes; pain in testicles; sores in mouth and on lips; weakness.

Side effects that usually do not require medical attention: Loss of hair; muscle pain; nausea and vomiting.

ncristine

onunciation:
n-KRIS-teen

and names:
commonly used brand
me is Oncovin®.

w given:
ncristine is
ven by IV
ection.

Special precautions: Vincristine frequently causes constipation and stomach cramps. Your doctor may want you to take a laxative or stool softener; however, do not decide to take these medicines on your own without first checking with your doctor.

While you are using vincristine, it may be necessary to drink extra fluids so that you will pass more urine. This will help prevent kidney and bladder problems and keep your kidneys working well. Ask your doctor if this is necessary for you.

Side effects needing immediate medical attention: If vincristine accidentally seeps out of the vein, it may damage some tissues and cause scarring. Tell the doctor or nurse right away if you notice redness, pain, or swelling at the IV site.

Other side effects needing medical attention as soon as possible: Blurred or double vision; constipation; difficulty in walking; drooping eyelids; side or stomach pain; headache; jaw pain; joint pain; numbness or tingling in fingers

and toes; pain in fingers and toes; pain in testicles; stomach cramps; swelling of feet or lower legs; weakness; agitation; bed-wetting; confusion; convulsions; dizziness or lightheadedness when getting up from a lying or sitting position; hallucinations (seeing, hearing, or feeling things that are not there); lack of sweating; loss of appetite; mental depression; painful or difficult urination; seizures; trouble in sleeping; unconsciousness; unusual decrease or increase in urination; cough; fever, chills, or sore throat; shortness of breath; sores in mouth and on lips; unusual bleeding or bruising.

Nervous system effects may be more likely to occur in older patients.

Side effects that usually do not require medical attention: Loss of hair; bloating, diarrhea, weight loss; nausea and vomiting; skin rash.

Anticancer Drugs Combinations

Refer to the individual drug listing for information on each medicine in these drug combinations.

ABVD	A combination of doxorubicin + bleomycin + vinblastine + dacarbazine
CHOP	A combination of cyclosphosphamide + doxorubicin + vincristine + prednisone.
CMF	A combination of cyclophosphamide + methotrexate + fluorouracil.
COPP	A combination of cyclophosphamide + vincristine + procarbazine + prednisone.
CVP	A combination of cyclophosphamide + vincristine + prednisone.
CY-VA-DIC	A combination of cyclophosphamide + vincristine + doxorubicin + dacarbazine.
FAC	A combination of fluorouracil + doxorubicin + cyclophosphamide.
FAM	A combination of fluorouracil + doxorubicin + mitomycin.
MOPP	A combination of mechlorethamine + vincristine + procarbazine + prednisone.
MPL + PRED	A combination of melphalan + prednisone.
MTX + MP + CTX	A combination of methotrexate + mercaptopurine + cyclophosphamide.
PVB (See VBP)	
VAC	A combination of vincristine + dactinomycin + cyclophosphamide.
VBP	A combination of vinblastine + bleomycin + cisplatin.
VP-L-Asparaginase	A combination of vincristine + prednisone + asparaginase.

Glossary

Adjuvant chemotherapy: The use of drugs in addition to surgery and/or radiation to treat cancer.

Alopecia: The loss of hair from the body and/or the scalp.

Anemia: Low red blood cell count; symptoms include shortness of breath, lack of energy, and fatigue.

Anorexia: Absence or loss of appetite for food.

Antiemetic: A medicine that prevents or controls vomiting.

Benign: Used to describe a tumor that is not cancerous.

Blood count: The number of red blood cells, white cells, and platelets in a given sample of blood.

Bone marrow: The inner spongy tissue of a bone where red blood cells, white cells, and platelets are formed.

Cancer: A general name for over 100 diseases in which abnormal cells grow out of control; a malignant tumor.

Catheter: A tube used for injection or withdrawal of fluid.

Cell: The basic structure of living tissues; all plants and animals are made up of one or more cells.

Chemotherapy: The treatment of disease with drugs.

Combination chemotherapy: The use of several drugs at the same time or in a particular order to treat cancer.

Gastrointestinal (GI): Having to do with the digestive tract, which includes the stomach and the intestines.

Infusion: The process of putting fluids into the vein by letting them drip slowly through a tube.

Injection: The use of a syringe to "push" fluids into the body; often called a "shot."

Intramuscular (IM): Into a muscle; some anticancer drugs are given by IM injection.

Intravenous (IV): Into a vein; anticancer drugs are often given by IV injection or infusion.

Malignant: Used to describe a tumor made up of cancerous cells.

Metastasis: Action during which cancer cells break from their original site and spread through the body.

Oncologist: A physician trained to treat patients who have cancer.

Pathologist: A doctor who studies cells and tissues to determine if a disease is present.

Radiation therapy: Cancer treatment with radiation (high-energy X-rays).

Red blood cells: Cells that supply oxygen to tissues throughout the body.

Remission: The disappearance of signs and symptoms of disease.

Stomatitis: Sores on the inside lining of the mouth.

Tumor: An abnormal growth of cells or tissues; tumors may be benign (non-cancerous) or malignant (cancerous).

White blood cells: The blood cells responsible for fighting infection.

Chapter 28

Bone Marrow Transplantation

A Type of Treatment

Introduction

Recent advances in scientific knowledge and technology have made bone marrow transplantation a viable treatment for some patients with leukemia, lymphoma, aplastic anemia, severe combined immunodeficiency syndrome, and certain inherited blood disorders such as thalassemia. A bone marrow transplant replaces a patient's abnormal or diseased marrow with healthy marrow from a donor.

This *Research Report* discusses the bone marrow transplantation procedure and possible complications, current research in the field, and diseases that can be treated with bone marrow transplants.

Description and Function of the Bone Marrow

The large human bones are made up of hard, dense, bony tissue around a core of spongy tissue. Spongy bone contains many large spaces filled with marrow. This bone marrow produces three types of bloods cells: leukocytes (white blood cells); erythrocytes (red blood cells); and platelets (clotting cells).

Leukocytes help defend the body against infection. Leuko-

cytes are made up of three lines of white blood cells: granulocytes, lymphocytes, and a cell line that includes monocytes and macrophages. Neutrophils are the most common type of granulocyte and play a major role in fighting infections by engulfing and digesting bacteria. Lymphocytes are further divided into B cells, which produce antibodies, and T cells, which attack virus-infected cells, foreign tissue, and cancer cells.

Erythrocytes carry oxygen from the lungs to all tissues of the body, and then pick up carbon dioxide as a waste product to be carried back to the lungs and breathed out. This function is made possible by iron-rich hemoglobin in the red blood cells.

Platelets (also called thrombocytes) prevent bleeding by initiating a chain of reactions that form blood clots. Platelets are small cell fragments derived from a larger cell called a megakaryocyte.

Diseases Treated with Bone Marrow Transplants

Bone marrow transplantation may be part of the treatment for several kinds of leukemia and lymphoma, which are types of cancer. Marrow transplants also can help patients with several noncancerous disorders: aplastic anemia, severe combined immunodeficiency disease, and thalassemia.

Leukemia

Leukemia is a cancer that arises in the blood-forming cells. Immature, abnormal white blood cells, unable to perform their infection-fighting roles, begin filling the bone marrow and spilling into the bloodstream. Leukemia cells cannot do the work of normal cells. These abnormal cells also reduce the production of normal red blood cells and platelets. As a result, patients with leukemia are often anemic and prone to bleeding. Other symptoms may include easy bruising, fever, weakness, chronic fatigue, recurrent infections, and pain in joints and bones.

A diagnosis of leukemia is made by blood tests and a bone marrow biopsy. Treatment usually starts immediately, and usually involves chemotherapy designed to destroy leukemia cells directly or to block their ability to reproduce. Supportive therapy may include antibiotics, radiation therapy, and transfusions of granulocytes and platelets.

Additional information on leukemia is available in publications listed in "Suggestions for Additional Reading" at the end of this *Report*.

Bone marrow transplants can be part of the treatment for several types of leukemia: acute lymphocytic leukemia (ALL), acute nonlymphocytic leukemia (ANLL), and chronic myelocytic leukemia (CML). Lymphocytic leukemia affects the lymphocytes, and nonlymphocytic leukemia affects other cell lines, like the neutrophils or monocytes. Chronic myelocytic leukemia affects the granulocytes. Many successful transplants have been performed on patients with each of these types of leukemia. Generally, transplants performed in the earlier phases of leukemia have a higher success rate than those performed in patients with advanced disease that has become resistant to anticancer drugs.

Lymphoma

Lymphoma is a term used for any cancer that develops in the lymphoid tissue, which includes lymph nodes, lymph vessels, the spleen and the thymus. There are several types of lymphomas, including Hodgkin's disease and a number of non-Hodgkin's lymphomas. A diagnosis of lymphoma is usually established by the surgical removal and microscopic examination of lymphoid tissue. Hodgkin's disease and several other types of lymphoma can be treated successfully with radiation or combinations of anticancer drugs. In certain cases where large doses of radiation offer increased chances for effective therapy, bone marrow transplants make the high-dose treatment possible by replacing marrow destroyed by the radiation.

Additional information on lymphoma is available in publications listed in the "Suggestions for Additional Reading" at the end of this *Report.*

Aplastic Anemia

In aplastic anemia, the bone marrow is unable to produce all the necessary blood cells. The disease is often fatal despite conventional treatments. Bone marrow transplantation thus offers a way to treat this otherwise incurable condition.

Immunological Diseases

Severe combined immunodeficiency disease (SCID) is the deadliest of the immunodeficiency diseases. SCID patients lack all of the body's natural immune defenses and are thus unable to ward off diseases. These patients are often placed in a germ-free protective environment. Bone marrow transplantation has cured SCID in some patients, and is the only known cure for SCID at present. The procedure is not possible with all patients, however, and is not always successful.

Thalassemia

Thalassemia is an inherited blood disorder characterized by abnormal hemoglobin in the red blood cells. As a result, the red blood cells are stunted and do not carry oxygen efficiently. Symptoms include shortness of breath, severe pallor, and chronic fatigue. The disease is fatal in 2 to 3 years if untreated. Although other treatments can extend a patient's life by many years, bone marrow transplantation has cured the disorder in some of the patients where the technique has been possible.

Bone Marrow Transplantation Procedure

The steps involved in a bone marrow transplant may vary from one medical center to another. Various details also may change as research continues. A transplant will generally include the following steps:

Patient Selection and Consent

When patients and physicians consider bone marrow transplantation as a treatment option, they must evaluate factors such as the patient's specific illness, age, and medical history; other treatments that might have been tried earlier; and the possible risks and benefits of a transplant in the patient's particular case. Some types of leukemia and lymphoma, for example, are curable in many cases with anticancer drugs (chemotherapy) and/or radiation therapy. These treatments would be tried before bone marrow transplantation is considered.

The complications and risks of marrow transplantation are discussed later in this *Report,* and should be given serious consideration. Some complications, particularly infections and graft-versus-host disease, can be life-threatening. Physicians discuss these matters with patients and marrow donors before consent is given to go ahead with the procedure.

Selection of the Donor

Ideal donors are identical twins, because the identity includes the immune system's signals for recognizing a graft as being "self" or "foreign." When an identical twin is the donor, there is no risk that the patient will reject the graft or that the leukocytes of the donated marrow will react against the patient. Because most patients do not have identical twins, however, transplants usually have been performed with other family members. Studies with animals have shown that a graft is more likely to "take" if certain proteins on the surface of white blood cells are the same with both the donor and the recipient. In humans, these proteins are called HLA antigens. HLA antigens are inherited from the parents, one set from the mother and one from the father. There is thus a 25 percent chance that any one brother or sister will be HLA-identical to the patient.

There are three different kinds of grafts, depending on the

source of the marrow. An *autologous* graft is the patient's own marrow, removed before the patient is given treatment with chemotherapy and/or radiation that may destroy the remaining marrow. The removed marrow also may be treated before being retransplanted in the patient. A *syngeneic* graft comes from an identical twin and is genetically identical to the patient. To date, syngeneic grafts have been the most successful. An *allogeneic* graft comes from a sibling or parent. These grafts, which are the most common type, have the greatest chance of success when the donor and recipient are HLA-identical.

Preparation of the Patient

Unless the patient totally lacks a functioning immune system, the patient must be given some type of immunosuppressive treatment before the donor marrow can be infused. The treatment is intended to keep the patient's immune system from rejecting the "foreign" marrow. Radiation and a high dose of cyclophosphamide (Cytoxan) are commonly used. If the patient has leukemia or other types of cancer, high-dose chemotherapy will be given to destroy cancer cells in the marrow and elsewhere. This is usually followed by a total of 1,000 to 1,500 rad of radiation over the entire body, to penetrate the bones and kill leukemia cells in the marrow. The radiation treatment is often given in smaller doses over the course of several days to minimize the risk of side effects.

For patients with aplastic anemia, large doses of cyclophosphamide commonly are given before the transplant to suppress the immune response. If the aplastic anemia patient has had many blood transfusions, other procedures may be added.

Infusion of the Marrow

The bone marrow transplant procedure begins with aspiration of the marrow from the donor. In an operating room with the donor under general or spinal anesthesia, marrow is taken from the pelvic bone with a needle and syringe. A number of aspirations are taken to avoid dilution of the marrow with blood. From 500 to 800 milliliters of marrow and blood cells are usually obtained. After the aspirations, a unit of blood, which had been taken from the donor a week before, is returned to the donor to prevent anemia. The donor may feel some pain and stiffness at the aspiration site for a few days.

The marrow is passed through stainless steel screens to break up particles. It is then injected into the patient intravenously. The marrow cells enter the general circulation and migrate through the blood to marrow cavities in the patient's bones. The cells begin to grow in the marrow and produce new white blood cells, red blood cells, and platelets.

Supportive Care

Because 2 to 4 weeks or longer may pass before the marrow begins producing new blood cells, the patient needs intensive supportive care. Infections must be prevented. Patients and visitors use face masks and hand-washing to minimize exposure to bacteria. The patient is given antibiotics and sometimes is placed in the sterile environment of a laminar air-flow room.

Transplant patients may receive granulocyte transfusions to help prevent infection when their granulocyte level falls below 200 cells per cubic millimeter of blood. The granulocyte donor is usually the marrow donor or another closely matched family member. At any sign of infection by viruses, fungi or bacteria,

granulocytes may be given until the patient's own marrow can begin to produce enough of these white blood cells.

The patient receives red blood cells to prevent anemia. If the hematocrit (a measure of the concentration of red cells in the blood) falls below a certain level, whole blood transfusions are given.

Transfusions of platelets help keep the platelet level above 20,000 per cubic millimeter and thus prevent uncontrolled internal or external bleeding. Some patients do not respond to platelets donated from random donors. When this occurs, family members donate platelets.

All blood products given to transplant patients are treated with approximately 1,500 rad of radiation. This inactivates lymphocytes from the donor, which could cause an immune reaction against the patient.

Adequate nutrition is another important supportive measure. Preparation for the transplant often causes nausea, vomiting, and irritation of the linings of the mouth and the gastrointestinal tract. The patient thus may have trouble eating for several weeks. As an alternative method of nutritional support, the patient can be given a complete diet in the form of nutrients dissolved in intravenous fluids given through a Hickman catheter that was inserted in a large vein when the patient was admitted for the transplant. This is called "total parenteral nutrition." The catheter also can be used for giving blood products, antibiotics, and other drugs, as well as for withdrawing blood samples. Use of the catheter avoids the multiple needle pricks associated with lengthy treatment. Although some catheters eventually have to be removed due to infection, most can be kept in place for up to 3 months.

A rise in the number of granulocytes and platelets is usually a sign that the graft has "taken." Gene markers in the blood and cytogenetic studies are among tests used to confirm that the donor marrow is growing.

Possible Complications

Infection

Because the patient's white blood cell count is low and defenses against infection are poor during the first 2 to 4 weeks after transplant, he or she is at high risk for viral, fungal, and bacterial infections. Mucositis, herpes simplex, and herpes

zoster are common problems. With current antibacterial therapy and granulocyte transfusions, bacterial infections account for fewer than 10 percent of deaths associated with bone marrow transplantation. Despite the use of antifungal drugs like amphotericin, fungal infections have caused a high rate of illness and about 15 percent of deaths.

Interstitial pneumonia is another major cause of illness and death. About half the pneumonias are caused by cytomegalovirus infections, which have been fatal in about 80 percent of the cases. This is the most common cause of death in transplant patients.

Bleeding

When the patient's platelet count is low, nosebleeds and bleeding gums can be frequent. More serious bleeding can also occur. Treatment is with platelet transfusions.

Liver Disease

Liver disease is another problem that may occur in the months following a bone marrow transplant. Possible causes include toxic effects of drugs and radiation, obstructed veins in the liver, viral hepatitis, fungal and bacterial infections, and graft-versus-host disease. Many of these conditions are reversible and treatable.

Rejection

Although rejection of a marrow graft is relatively rare in leukemia patients, it occasionally occurs in patients with aplastic anemia who have been treated previously with blood transfusions. The transfusions appear to make the patient's immune system unusually reactive against antigens of the donated marrow that are not involved in the matching of HLA antigens. For this reason, marrow transplants should be carried out before blood transfusions have been given.

Relapse

For acute nonlymphocytic leukemia patients who receive transplants while they are in first remission, the rate of leukemia recurrence has been 10 to 15 percent. Patients with all other types of leukemia who have relapsed at least once before the transplant have had a recurrence rate of 50 to 65 percent.

Graft-Versus-Host Disease

Graft-versus-host disease (GVHD) is the reaction of the donor marrow against the tissue of the host patient. It occurs because the transplanted white blood cells recognize the host organs as "foreign," even though the white blood cell types are the same. GVHD chiefly affects the skin, liver, and gastrointestinal tract. Symptoms can range from mild to severe, and GVHD can be fatal. The most common symptoms are skin rashes, jaundice, liver disease, and diarrhea.

Chronic GVHD has occurred in about one-fourth of all long-term survivors. It is associated with abnormal pigmentation of the skin, and a hardening and thickening of patches of skin and the layers of tissue under the skin. The mouth and surface of the eye may dry out. Occasionally the esophagus, gut, or liver is affected. Bacterial infections and weight loss are common. Early and prolonged treatment with corticosteroids and other drugs is effective in a majority of patients.

To reduce the chances that GVHD will occur, patients routinely receive a drug called methotrexate after transplant.

Still, about 50 percent of the patients have developed GVHD. About 30 percent get it in a severe form, and it is life-threatening in about 20 percent of these severe cases. Other steps taken to prevent or treat the severe form of GVHD may include high-dose steroids such as prednisone, antithymocyte globulin, and cyclosporine. About one-third of the patients respond, but not always to the same treatment. Of those patients who get acute GVHD, about half will improve after treatment.

Older patients and patients who receive transplants from donors who are not HLA-matched are more likely to develop GVHD.

Current Research and Advances

In recent years significant advances have been made in marrow transplantation, and many transplant teams around the world are investigating new techniques to improve results even more.

Several discoveries may make possible the use of an unrelated donor or a partially HLA-matched donor. The implications of this are immense, because 60 to 70 percent of patients with leukemia or other blood and im-

mune diseases do not have relatives whose tissues are HLA-identical to theirs. One approach uses lectins, substances found in soybeans, which clump together with mature T cells when the two are mixed. T cells are the white blood cells that are mainly responsible for GVHD. Marrow is aspirated from the donor, mixed with lectins, and then placed on top of a thick substance, such as albumin, in a test tube. The aggregates of T cells and lectins sink to the bottom because they are heavier. Although the remaining marrow cells are almost entirely free of T cells, they are purified again by mixing them with red blood cells of sheep, which bind with any remaining T cells. The purified marrow is then given to the patient.

Another technique uses specially prepared antibodies, called monoclonal antibodies, to attack mature T cells and eliminate them from a marrow sample. If T cells remain, investigators may try to destroy them by giving the monoclonal antibodies directly to the patient.

Autologous transplants are another highly experimental procedure. Use of the patient's own marrow carries with it the risk that the marrow may be con-

505

taminated with cancer cells. Therefore, techniques to "cleanse" the removed marrow of cancer cells are under study. These include the use of:

- monoclonal antibodies prepared against cancer cells, either alone or with added complement, a complex of proteins that are part of the body's normal immune response;

- monoclonal antibodies combined with cell-destroying toxins such as ricin or linked with magnetic particles that permit the removal of cancer cells with a magnet;

- centrifugation to remove cancer cells by spinning at ultra-high speeds;

- anticancer drugs.

After the patient is treated with intensive chemotherapy and radiotherapy in an effort to kill all cancer cells in the patient's body, the purified marrow can be returned to the patient.

Studies are also examining the possibility of establishing a donor bank to collect marrow samples from donors in the general population. Tissue typing would match this donated marrow with unrelated recipients who need marrow transplants.

It may be possible to expand the application of bone marrow transplants to other disorders such as small cell cancer of the lung, testicular cancer, breast and ovarian cancers, and inherited marrow and blood disorders like sickle cell disease.

Conclusion

Although bone marrow transplantation has become the treatment of choice for certain stages of some diseases, it is still a complex procedure and should only be undertaken in medical centers with experienced staff and adequate resources. Research is needed to understand more about the complications of bone marrow transplants, the possibilities for marrow transplants from unrelated donors, and the uses of transplantation in other diseases. Bone marrow transplantation has been shown to improve long-term survival for patients with diseases such as acute leukemia and aplastic anemia. It offers the hope of saving lives of other patients with life-threatening disorders.

Questions To Ask Your Doctor

Answers to the following questions might help patients who are considering having a bone marrow transplant.

Is a bone marrow transplant the best option for treatment of my condition?

What are the chances that the donated marrow will not grow in me?

With my condition, what are my chances of becoming completely cured?

What are the risks and possible side effects of a bone marrow transplant?

What is the cost of a marrow transplant, and how does it compare with the cost of other possible therapy?

How long will I have to stay in the hospital? How long will I be treated as an outpatient?

What are some of the risks and side effects of the radiation and chemotherapy used to prepare me for transplantation?

Will I be able to resume normal activities after transplantation?

If a transplant is done, will I need other treatment?

After the transplant, how often will I need medical checkups?

Because of the risk of infection, will I be able to have friends and family visit me in the hospital?

Glossary of Terms

Allogeneic—Genetically different, as in distinguishing a patient from a relative.

Anemia—A condition in which there is a decreased number of red cells, which results in weakness and fatigue.

Antithymocyte globulin (ATG)—A protein preparation used to treat and prevent graft-versus-host disease.

Aspiration—The removal of the marrow from the marrow cavities by suction.

Autologous—A graft or tissue from the same source; that is, taken from the patient and then returned to the patient.

Chemotherapy—Treatment with anticancer drugs.

Cyclophosphamide—A drug used for immunosuppression and destruction of leukemia cells. A commonly used brand name is Cytoxan.

Cyclosporine—A drug used to treat and prevent graft-versus-host disease.

Cytogenetics—The study of the origin, structure, and function of the chromosomes in the blood cells.

Cytomegalovirus—A viral infection that can cause serious illness in immunosuppressed patients.

Dyspigmentation—Abnormal coloration of the skin.

Engraftment—The successful implantation of donor marrow in the patient's marrow cavities.

Genetic markers—Various characteristics linked with a person's genes, which help to determine if blood cells produced by the marrow are coming from the donor's marrow.

Granulocyte—One of the major groups of white blood cells. They are also called polymorphonuclear cells or myeloid cells. Granulocytes include neutrophils, eosinophils, and basophils.

Herpes simplex—A viral infection that usually produces small, temporary, irritating and sometimes painful fluid-filled blisters on the skin and mucous membranes.

Herpes zoster—A viral infection that produces shingles, painful skin eruptions that follow the underlying route of nerves inflamed by the virus.

Hickman catheter—A catheter designed for long-term use in giving drugs and total parenteral nutrition, and in withdrawing blood samples.

Histocompatibility—The state of similarity between tissues of the donor and the recipient.

Immunosuppression—Reduction of the functions of the immune system to prevent a reaction against donor marrow cells and to prevent graft-versus-host disease.

Interstitial pneumonia— Inflammation of the lung tissue, often caused by a virus.

Laminar air-flow room—A room with one-way air flow from a sterile source, which helps prevent the spread of air-borne bacteria and viruses.

Leukocyte—The term for all the types of white blood cells.

Lymphocyte—One of the major groups of white blood cells. B lymphocytes make antibodies against bacteria and other foreign substances in the body; T lymphocytes attack virus-infected cells and other foreign cells directly.

Methotrexate—A drug used to treat and prevent graft-versus-host disease.

Mucositis—Inflammation of the mucous membranes.

Neutrophil—The most common type of white blood cell in the bloodstream.

Prednisone—A hormone-like drug used to treat and prevent graft-versus-host disease.

Steroids—Drugs used to treat and prevent graft-versus-host disease.

Subcutaneous tissue—Tissue beneath the skin.

Syngeneic—Genetically identical, as from an identical twin.

Veno-occlusive disease—Disease caused by blocked veins.

Suggestions for Additional Reading

Except as noted, the following materials are not available from the National Cancer Institute. They can be found in medical libraries, many college and university libraries, and some public libraries.

Beatty, P.G., Clift, R.A. et al. "Marrow Transplantation from Related Donors other than HLA-Identical Siblings," *New England Journal of Medicine,* Sept. 26, 1985, pp. 765-771.

Bone Marrow Transplantation Questions and Answers, prepared by the Public Education and Information Department, Leukemia Society of America, 1984.

Champlin, R.E. and Gale R.P. "Role of Bone Marrow Transplantation in the Treatment of Hematologic Malignancies and Solid Tumors: Critical Review of Syngeneic, Autologous, and Allogeneic Transplants," *Cancer Treatment Reports* 68:145-161, 1984.

Chemotherapy and You: * *A Guide to Self-Help During Treatment,* prepared by the Office of Cancer Communications, National Cancer Institute. NIH Publication No. 85-1136, Revised August 1985.

Radiation Therapy and You: * *A Guide to Self-Help During Treatment,* prepared by the Office of Cancer Communications, National Cancer Institute. NIH Publication No. 85-2227, Revised January 1985.

Ramsey, N.R. et al. "A Randomized Study of the Prevention of Acute Graft-Versus-Host Disease," *New England Journal of Medicine,* vol. 306, 1982, pp. 392-397.

Research Report: Hodgkin's Disease and the Non-Hodgkin's Lymphomas, * prepared by the Office of Cancer Communications, National Cancer Institute. NIH Publication No. 85-172.

Research Report: Leukemia, * prepared by the Office of Cancer Communications, National Cancer Institute. NIH Publication No. 85-329.

Thomas, E.D. (interview). "Bone Marrow Transplantation: A Lifesaving Applied Art," *Journal of the American Medical Association,* vol. 249, 1983, pp. 2528-2536.

Thomas, E.D. "Bone Marrow Transplantation: Present Status and Future Expectations," *Principles of Internal Medicine,* 1982, pp. 135-152.

Thomas, E.D. "Marrow Transplantation for Malignant Diseases," *Journal of Clinical Oncology,* vol. 1, 1983, pp. 517-531.

What Are Clinical Trials All About?, * prepared by the Office of Cancer Communications, National Cancer Institute, NIH Publication No. 86-2706.

Zimmerman, S. et al. "Bone Marrow Transplantation," *American Journal of Nursing,* August 1977, pp. 1311-1317.

---

* *The mentioned text is reprinted within this book. See CONTENTS for location.*

Chapter 29

Clinical Trials:
What Are They All About?

*Information for
Patients With Cancer*

Foreword

Research studies conducted with patients are called clinical trials. As a cancer patient, you may take part in a clinical trial. This text is written for you, your family, and friends, to explain what clinical trials are and to help you make a decision about entering the trial.

The time when cancer is diagnosed or when treatment decisions are being made is very difficult. It is often hard to understand or remember complex medical explanations. The information in this material is meant to supplement what your doctors tell you. It provides answers to questions asked most often about clinical trials. (You may not want to read the whole book at one time. It is broken down into questions and answers that you can read now or later.)

As you read this chapter you may wish to make notes, and write down questions to ask your doctor or nurse. Also there is a glossary of words that relate to clinical trials and cancer care. This is a quick way to look up terms that you may hear or read. More information on many cancer-related topics is available at no cost in other publications from the National Cancer Institute.

We hope this text will help to explain how clinical studies are designed and carried out. Of course, there are good treatments and good care for cancer patients if they take part in clinical trials or if they receive standard treatments. You may decide not to take part in a trial, and you can still receive good medical care. The decision to enter a clinical trial or not is always up to you.

What Is A Clinical Trial?

In cancer research, a clinical trial is a study conducted with cancer patients, usually to evaluate a new treatment. Each study is designed to answer scientific questions and to find new and better ways to help cancer patients.

The search for good cancer treatments begins with basic research in laboratory and animal studies. The best results of that research are tried in patient studies, hopefully leading to findings that may help many people.

Before a new treatment is tried with patients, it is carefully studied in the laboratory. This research points out the new methods most likely to succeed, and, as much as possible, shows how to use them safely and effectively. But this early research cannot predict exactly how a new treatment will work with patients. With any new treatment there may be risks as well as possible benefits. There may also be some risks that are not yet known. Clinical trials help us find out if a promising new treatment is safe and effective for patients. During a trial, more and more information is gained about a new treatment, its risks, and how well it may or may not work.

Standard treatments, the ones now being used, are often the base for building new, hopefully better treatments. Many new treatments are designed on the basis of what has worked in the past, in efforts to improve on this.

Only patients who wish to, take part in a clinical trial. You may be interested in or asked to enter a trial. Learn as much as you can about the trial, before you make up your mind.

Why Are Clinical Trials Important?

Advances in medicine and science are the results of new ideas and approaches developed through research. New cancer treatments must prove to be safe and effective in scientific studies with a certain number of patients before they can be made widely available.

Through clinical trials, researchers learn which approaches are more effective than others. This is the best way to test a new treatment. A number of standard treatments were first shown to be effective in clinical trials. These trials help us find new and better treatments.

Why Would a Patient Be Interested In a Clinical Trial?

Patients take part in clinical trials for many reasons. Usually, they hope for benefits for themselves. They may hope for a cure of disease, a longer time to live, a way to feel better. Often they want to contribute to a research effort that may help others.

Based on what researchers learn from laboratory studies, and sometimes earlier clinical studies and standard treatments as well, they design a trial to see if a new treatment will improve on current treatments. The hope is that it will. Often researchers use standard treatments as the building blocks to try to design better treatments.

Many trials have turned out to be better than standard treatments; others have either been not as good as or no better than the treatments already being used. Although there is always a chance that a new treatment will be disappointing, the researchers involved in a study have reason to believe that it will be as good as, or better than, current treatments.

The patients in a clinical trial are among the first to receive new research treatments before they are widely available. How a treatment will work for a patient in a trial can't be known ahead of time. Even standard treatments, although effective in many patients, do not carry sure benefits for everyone. But, patients should choose if they want to take part in a study or not, only after they understand both the possible risks and benefits.

The patients who take part in clinical trials that do prove to be better treatments, have the first chance to benefit from them. All patients in clinical trials are carefully monitored during a trial and followed up afterwards. They become part of a network of clinical trials carried out around the country. In this network, doctors and researchers pool their ideas and experience to design and monitor clinical studies. They share their knowledge from many specialties about cancer treatment and care. Patients in these studies receive the benefit of their expertise. At cancer centers, patients receive care from a special research team. Through new programs, community hospitals and doctors are also coming more and more into the research network.

Are There Risks or Side Effects in Clinical Trials?

Yes. The treatments used in clinical trials can cause side effects and risks depending on the type of treatment and the patient's condition. Side effects vary from patient to patient.

Because clinical trials are research into new areas of treatment, the risks involved are not always known ahead of time, though efforts have been made to find out what they might be. For this reason, trials can carry unknown dangers and side effects as well as hoped-for benefits. Patients need to know what is involved in a study—what side effects may be expected—and, as much as possible, what "unknowns" or uncertainties they may be facing.

You will be told about the treatments being tested and will be given a form to read that discusses the risks and hoped-for benefits. If you agree to take part, you will be asked to sign a form, called the informed consent form. Before you sign, be sure you understand what risks you face. Ask the doctor or nurse to explain any parts of the form or the trial that are not clear. If you do not want to be in the trial, you may refuse. Even if you sign the form, you are free to leave the trial at any time and can receive other available medical care.

In clinical trials, most side effects are temporary and will gradually go away once treatment is stopped. For example, some anticancer drugs cause hair loss and nausea and some do not.

516

They can also affect the bone marrow which produces blood cells. During treatment, the number of blood cells, called blood counts, may fall too low. Since this could lead to possible infection or other problems, patients have their blood counts checked often. Luckily, bone marrow has a great ability to replace blood cells, so that blood counts can usually return to normal.

Some side effects in clinical trials can be permanent and serious, even life-threatening. Also, certain side effects may not appear until later, after the treatment itself is over. (These "late" effects may include damage to a major organ like the heart, lungs, or kidneys; sterility; or a second cancer.) Many cancer patients are now living longer, largely because of better treatments. Researchers are concerned and trying to prevent late complications of treatments.

As a patient, it can be hard to decide about your treatment. There are a number of things to consider. Cancer is a life-threatening disease which causes symptoms of its own that are not related to treatment. In each case, the unavoidable risks of the cancer itself, and your condition, should be weighed against the potential risks and benefits of a new research treatment.

Standard treatments, as well as treatments in clinical trials, can also cause side effects and risks.

Why Does Cancer Treatment Have Side Effects?

Any medical treatment can carry the potential for side effects in some patients. Cancer treatment is particularly powerful, because it is designed to destroy constantly dividing cancer cells. It can also affect healthy dividing cells and this can cause side effects. The challenge to researchers has been to develop treatments that destroy cancer cells but do not harm healthy cells.

What Is Being Done to Lessen Side Effects of Treatment?

Cancer researchers are trying to make cancer treatment more effective and lessen its side effects for the cancer patient. Results of such efforts include:

• new anticancer drugs with less side effects;

• better antinausea medicine;

• some shorter periods of time on anticancer drugs;

• special ways to protect normal tissues during radiation therapy;

• new methods of surgery that are less extensive and less damaging to the body; and

• psychological support programs and information on ways to cope during difficult times. How patients feel during and after treatment is important.

If You Are Thinking of Entering A Clinical Trial...

Are You Eligible for a Clinical Trial?

Every clinical trial is designed to answer a set of research questions. If you fit the guidelines for a trial, you may be eligible to take part. Each study enrolls patients with certain types and stages of cancer and certain health status. A study that involves two or more treatments can yield reliable answers only if all the patient cases are the same so they can be compared with each other.

Before a decision is made about your treatment

(whether it is in a clinical trial or not), your type of cancer will be diagnosed and "staged." Staging tells how far the disease has spread. Deciding on treatment depends on many things, including the stage of the disease and your general condition. You would most likely be referred to a trial by your own doctor or by a doctor who knows your case. Some patients find out about trials from other sources. In any case, you must have a reasonable understanding of your role in a research study and be freely willing to take part in it. Ask what you can expect if you take part in a trial.

What Trials Are Available for Your Type of Cancer?

There are many ways to find out what your treatment choices are. Talk with your doctors and get the opinion of cancer specialists (oncologists). You should not be afraid to ask for a second opinion. A helpful, new computer information system called PDQ, is supported by the National Cancer Institute. PDQ can give your doctor the latest information on clinical trials being offered around the country for each type and stage of cancer. This ready reference is kept up to date. Your doctor can check it from a library or personal computer.

The Cancer Information Service (CIS) is another source of information. This program, also sponsored by the National Cancer Institute, answers cancer-related questions from the public, cancer patients and their families, and health professionals. If you have questions, call the toll-free number: 1-800-4-CANCER , and you will be connected to the CIS office serving your area.

What is Best for You?

This is a big question. Finding answers and

519

making decisions are often hard for a cancer patient. The diagnosis of cancer and deciding what to do about it can be overwhelming, and you may be confused and upset. It is important to discuss your options with medical experts—including your own doctor—and with those close to you. Your personal doctor, who may be your family doctor, and cancer specialists can counsel you about your choices for standard treatment or clinical trials.

Talk to them and ask questions about the problems you are facing. If you understand what is going on, you can help your doctor work with you more effectively. You may want to take a friend or relative along with you when you talk to your doctor about your case.

Take time to ask your questions and to discuss what you want to know. It may help you and your doctor if you plan what to ask and write questions down ahead of time. No question is foolish. Learn what is available to you. Find out your choices and the risks and benefits of each. Each patient is different. You are an individual with individual needs, and your health is important. If you are a parent of a child with cancer, of course, you have great concerns about making the best decision for your child's care.

As you decide about treatment, if it is in a clinical trial or not, remember that you are not alone. There are many people to help you—doctors, nurses, social workers, clergy, your family, friends, and other patients. Although it is YOUR decision, they can help you think about it and decide what is best for you.

What Are Important Questions to Ask About a Clinical Trial?

If you are thinking about taking part in a clinical trial, here are some important questions to ask:

• What is the purpose of the study?

- What does the study involve? What kinds of tests and treatments? (Find out what is done and how it is done.)

- What is likely to happen in my case with, or without, this new research treatment? (What may the cancer do and what may this treatment do?)

- What are other choices and their advantages and disadvantages? (Are there standard treatments for my case and how does the study compare with them?)

- How could the study affect my daily life?

- What side effects could I expect from the study? (There can also be side effects from standard treatments and from the disease itself.)

- How long will the study last? (Will it require an extra time commitment on my part?)

- Will I have to be hospitalized? If so, how often and for how long?

- Will I have any costs? Will any of the treatment be free?*

- If I am harmed as a result of the research, what treatment would I be entitled to?

- What type of long-term followup care is part of the study?

What is Informed Consent?

Informed consent, a key part of a good trial, is required in studies that are federally regulated or funded as well as by many state laws. Informed consent means that as a patient, you are given information so you can understand what is involved in a trial, including its potential benefits

---

*Costs are a major concern of patients and families. Different arrangements and policies exist at different institutions and, of course, insurance coverage varies. Patients should freely discuss what costs are involved in their cases ahead of time. If you need financial aid, contact the hospital social services office, the Cancer Information Service, or the local American Cancer Society Chapter. They may be able to direct you to a source of help.

and risks, and then decide freely to take part in it or not. The nature of the treatment is explained by the doctors and nurses in the trial. You are given an informed consent form to read and consider carefully. Ask any questions you may have. Then, if you agree to take part, you can sign the form. Of course, you may also refuse.

The informed consent process is an ongoing process. If you enter a trial, you will continue to receive any new information about your treatment that may affect your willingness to stay in the trial. Signing a consent form does not bind you to the study. You can still leave at any time.

What Is It Like to be a Patient in a Clinical Trial?

Whether cancer patients are in a research study or not, they face a new world of medical terms and procedures. For some people, myths and fears of "experimentation" or of being a "guinea pig" come with the idea of clinical trials. And, surely, there are fears of the unknown. Understanding what is involved can ease some of your anxieties. Patients in a clinical trial, for example, receive their care in the same places that standard treatments are given—at cancer centers, hospitals, clinics, or doctors' offices.

Because a growing number of cancer specialists are now in private practice in the community, most cancer care can be given in an area near your home. Doctors, nurses, social workers and other health professionals from many different specialties may help care for you. They are working together for your good. There is consideration for your privacy and well-being.

If you join a research study, you will be watched closely and data on your case will be carefully recorded. You may receive more examinations and tests than are usually given. (These are to follow your progress as well as to collect study data.) Of course, tests can carry certain risks and benefits or discomforts of their own. Although they can be inconvenient, these tests can assure an extra ounce of observation along the way.

During the course of a study, if it is clear that a treatment is not in your best interest, you will be removed from the study and you can discuss other options.

Can You Leave at Any Time?

Yes. Just as you can refuse to join a study, you may leave a study at any time. Your rights as an individual do not change because you are a patient in a clinical trial. You may choose to take part or not, and you can always change your mind later, even after you enter a trial.

You may also refuse to take part in any aspect of the research. If you have questions at any time about any part of the study, be sure to ask your doctors. If you are not satisfied with the answers, you may consider leaving the study. If you decide to leave, it will not be held against you. Don't be afraid that you will receive no further care. You can freely discuss other possible treatments and care with your doctors and nurses.

What Protection Do You Have as a Patient in a Clinical Trial?

The ethical and legal codes that govern medical practice apply to clinical trials. In addition, most clinical research is federally regulated or federally funded (at least in part), with built-in safeguards to protect patients. These safeguards include regular review of the protocol (the study plans) and the progress of each study by researchers at other places.

For example, federally funded and federally regulated clinical trials must first be approved by an Institutional Review Board (IRB) located at the institution where the study is to take place. IRBs, designed to protect patients, are made up of scientists, doctors, clergy and other people from the local community. An IRB reviews a study to see that it is well designed with safeguards for patients, and that the risks are reasonable in relation to the potential benefits.

Federally supported or regulated studies also go through reviews by a government agency, such as the National Cancer Institute,* which sponsors and monitors many trials around the country.

Any well-run clinical trial, whether federally supported or not, is carefully reviewed for medical ethics, patient safety, and scientific merit by the research institution. Every study should provide for monitoring the data and the safety of patients on an ongoing basis.

As discussed earlier, informed consent is also an important process that helps to protect patients.

After patients join a clinical trial and it progresses, the doctors report the results of the trial to scientific meetings, to medical journals whose articles are approved by experts, and to various government agencies.

What Can Help You Learn If a Trial is Sound and Well Run?

Things that make a sound, well-run trial to safeguard patients include the items discussed in the previous section of this booklet. Keeping these items in mind, here are some important questions for you to ask to find out if a study is well run:

• What is its purpose?

---

*The National Cancer Institute (NCI) is the Federal Government's chief agency for cancer research. Located at the National Institutes of Health (NIH) in Bethesda, Maryland, the Institute funds cancer research across the country and conducts research at its own facilities. For information about NCI trials, call: 800-638-6694 (in Maryland, call 800-492-6600).

- Who has reviewed and approved the study?
- Who is sponsoring the study?
- How are the study data and patient safety being checked?
- Where will information from the study go? (In government-related research, for example, reports might go to the National Cancer Institute and/or the Food and Drug Administration.)

For your own protection, be sure to get satisfactory answers to these questions before you agree to take part.

What Kinds of Clinical Trials Are There?

There are many kinds of clinical trials. They range from studies of ways to prevent, detect and diagnose, control and treat cancer, to studies of the psychological impact of the disease and ways to improve the patient's comfort and quality of life (including pain control).

Most cancer clinical trials deal with new treatments. These treatments often involve surgery, radiation therapy (the use of X-rays, neutrons or other types of cell-destroying radiation), and chemotherapy (the use of anticancer drugs). Alone, or in combination, these types of treatments can cure many cancer patients and prolong the lives of many others. A fairly new area of cancer treatment is biological therapy —the use of biologicals (substances produced by the body's own cells) and biological response modifiers (substances that affect the body's natural defense systems against disease).

How Are Trials Divided Into Phases?

Clinical trials are carried out in phases, each designed to find out certain information. Patients may be eligible for studies in different phases depending on their general condition and the type and stage of their cancer. More patients take part in the later phases of studies than in the earlier ones.

In a Phase I study, a new research treatment is given to a small number of patients. The researchers must find the best way to give a new treatment and how much of it can be given safely. They watch carefully for any harmful side effects. The research treatment has been well tested in laboratory and animal studies but no one knows how patients will react. Phase I studies may involve significant risks for this reason. They are offered only to patients whose cancer has spread and who would not be helped by other known treatments. Phase I treatments may produce anticancer effects, and some patients have been helped by these treatments.

Phase II studies determine the effect of a research treatment on various types of cancer. Each new phase of a clinical trial depends on and builds on information from an earlier phase. If a treatment has shown activity against cancer in Phase II, it moves to Phase III. Here it is compared with standard treatment to see which is more effective. Often researchers use standard therapy as the base to design new, hopefully better treatments. Then in Phase III, the new treatment is directly compared to the old one. In Phase IV studies, the new research treatment becomes part of standard treatment in patient care. For example, a new drug that has been found effective in a clinical trial may then be used together with other effective drugs, or with surgery, and/or radiation therapy.

How Are Clinical Trials Conducted?

The doctors who conduct a clinical trial follow a carefully designed treatment plan called a "protocol." This spells out what will be done and why. Studies are planned to safeguard the medical and psychological health of patients as well as to answer research questions.

Some clinical trials test one research treatment in one group of patients. Other trials compare two or more treatments in separate groups of patients who are similar in certain ways, such as the extent of their disease. This way, the treatment groups are alike and the results from each can validly be compared.

One of the groups may receive standard (the most accepted) treatment so the new treatments can be directly compared to it. The group receiving the standard treatment is called the "control" group. For example, one group of patients (the control group) may receive the usual surgical treatment for a certain cancer, while another patient group with the same type of cancer may receive surgery plus radiation therapy to see if this improves disease control.

Sometimes, no standard treatment yet exists for certain cancer patients. In drug studies for such cases, one group of patients might receive a new drug and the control group, none. But no patient is placed in a control group without treatment if there is any known treatment that would benefit that patient. The control group is followed as often and carefully as the "treatment" group.

One of the ways to prevent the bias of a patient or doctor from influencing study results is "randomization." If a patient agrees to be randomized, this means he or she is selected by chance to be in one group or another. The researchers do not know which treatment is best. From what is known at the time, any one of the treatments chosen could be of equal benefit to the patient.

If the treatment in a trial is not helping the patient, the patient's doctor can decide to take him or her out of the study. Of course, the patient can decide to leave, as well, and still receive other available care. There are regular reviews of the results of a trial and the information is shared. This is important, because if a treatment is found to be too harmful or not effective, it is stopped. Also, when there is firm evidence that one method is better than the others in a study, the trial is stopped and all patients in the trial are given the benefit of the new information. Such information may help present and future patients.

Throughout a clinical study, a patient's personal doctor will be kept informed of the patient's progress. Patients are encouraged to maintain contact with their referring doctors.

The National Cancer Program and Clinical Trials

A nationwide effort to conquer cancer intensified with the National Cancer Act of 1971. As a result of the National Cancer Program, created by that legislation, more cancer patients are being cured today than ever before, and many others are living longer with improved quality of life.

The National Cancer Program brings together a network of researchers at many public and private institutions around the country. These include the National Cancer Institute, cancer centers, universities, community hospitals and private industry. Groups involving hundreds of researchers are working to discover and put to use new knowledge to benefit the cancer patients of today and tomorrow.

Knowledge gained from research studies with patients—clinical trials—has been essential to overall progress. Such studies have led to increased survival for childhood cancers, Hodgkin's disease, breast, uterine, testicular and bladder cancers, as well as others. These studies continue to play a key role in progress against cancer.

Today, major scientific discoveries in the laboratory are part of a revolution in biology. New tools to unravel the process of cancer are leading to exciting new approaches against cancer. Clinical trials continue to be the link between such basic research and patients. The goal is to translate the best of that research into findings that directly help people.

Glossary

Adjuvant Chemotherapy (ad'ju-vant kee-mo-ther'a-pee)—One or more anticancer drugs used in combination with surgery or radiation therapy as part of the treatment of cancer. Adjuvant usually means "in addition to" initial treatment.

Antibody (an'ti-bod-ee)—A protein produced by a plasma cell in the lymphatic system or bone marrow. An antibody binds to the specific antigen that has stimulated the immune system. Once bound, the antigen can be destroyed by other cells of the immune system. See **Immune System.**

Antigen (an'ti-jen)—A substance, foreign to the body, that stimulates the production of antibodies by the immune system. Antigens include foreign proteins, bacteria, viruses, pollen and other materials.

Biological Therapy—Use of biologicals (substances produced by our own cells) or biological response modifiers (substances that affect the patient's defense systems) in the treatment of cancer.

Blood Count—Measurement of the number of red cells, white cells, and platelets in a sample of blood.

Bone Marrow (mair'oh)—The inner, spongy core of bone that produces blood cells.

Cancer (kan'ser)—A general term for more than 100 diseases characterized by abnormal and uncontrolled growth of cells. The resulting mass, or tumor, can invade and destroy surrounding normal tissues. Cancer cells from the tumor can spread through the blood or lymph to start new cancers in other parts of the body.

CCOP (Community Clinical Oncology Program)—This new program links community physicians with NCI clinical research programs, so that more cancer patients can participate in clinical trials in their own communities. NCI has funded 62 CCOPs affiliated with over 200 hospitals in 34 states.

Chemotherapy (kee-mo-ther'a-pee)—Treatment with anticancer drugs.

Clinical Trial—The systematic investigation of the effects of materials or methods, according to a formal study plan and generally in a human population with a particular disease or class of diseases. In cancer research, a clinical trial generally refers to the evaluation of treatment methods such as surgery, drugs or radiation techniques, although methods of prevention, detection or diagnosis also may be the subject of such studies.

Combination Chemotherapy (kee-mo-ther'a-pee)—Use of two or more anticancer drugs.

Combination Therapy (ther'a-pee)—The use of two or more modes of treatment—surgery, radiotherapy, chemotherapy, immunother-apy—in combination, alternately or together, to achieve optimum results against cancer.

Control Group—In clinical studies this is a group of patients which receives *standard treatment,* a treatment or intervention currently being used and considered to be of proved effective-ness on the basis of past studies. Results in patients receiving newly developed treatments may then be compared to the control group. In cases where no standard treatment yet exists for a particular condition, the control group would receive no treatment. No patient is placed in a control group without treatment if there is any beneficial treatment known for that patient.

Double-blind—Characteristic of a controlled experiment in which neither the patient nor the attending physician knows whether the patient is getting one or another drug or dose. In *single-blind* studies, patients do not know which of several treatments they are receiving, thus pre-venting personal bias from influencing their reac-tions and study results. In either case, the treat-ment can be quickly identified, if necessary, by a special code.

Hormone—Chemical product of the endocrine glands of the body, which, when secreted into body fluids, has a specific effect on other organs.

Immune System—A complex network of organs, cells and specialized substances distributed throughout the body and defending it from foreign invaders that cause infection or disease.

Immunotherapy (im-mew-no-ther'a-pee)—A form of biological therapy. An experimental method of treating cancer, using substances which stimulate the body's immune defense system.

Informed Consent—The process in which a patient learns about and understands the purpose and aspects of a clinical trial and then agrees to participate. Of course, a patient may decline to participate. This process includes a document defining how much a patient must know about the potential benefits and risks of therapy before being able to agree to undergo it knowledgeably. (Informed consent is required in federally conducted, funded or regulated studies as well as by many state laws.) If a patient signs an informed consent form and enters a trial, he or she is still free to leave the trial at any time, and can receive other available medical care.

Interferon (in-tur-feer'on)—A protein substance produced by white blood cells and other types of cells that have been exposed to certain viruses. In test animals, interferon has shown some activity against tumors. Studies of its usefulness in treating some types of human cancer are under way. One of a number of new agents available as biological therapy.

Investigational New Drug—A drug allowed by the Food and Drug Administration (FDA) to be used in clinical trials but not approved by the FDA for commercial marketing.

Investigator—An investigator is the experienced clinical researcher who prepares a protocol or treatment plan and implements it with patients.

531

Metastasis (me-tas'ta-sis)—The transfer of disease from one part of the body to another. In cancer, metastasis is the migration of cancer cells from the original tumor site through the blood and lymph vessels to produce cancers in other tissues. Metastasis also is the term used for a secondary cancer growing at a distant site.

Metastatic Cancer (met-a-stat'ik)—Cancer that has spread from its original site to one or more additional body sites.

Monoclonal Antibodies (mon-o-klone'al an'ti-bod-eez)—One of several new substances used in biological therapy. These antibodies, all exactly alike, are mass-produced and designed to home in on target cancer cells. Monoclonal antibodies are products of new scientific techniques and may prove useful in both cancer diagnosis and treatment.

Multimodality Therapy (mul'ti-mo-dal'i-tee ther' a-pee)—The combined use of more than one method of treatment, for example, surgery and chemotherapy.

Oncologist (on-kol'o-jist)—A physician who is a cancer specialist.

PDQ—PDQ, supported by NCI, is a computerized database available to physicians nationwide. Geographically matrixed, it offers the latest information on standard treatments and ongoing clinical trials for each type and stage of cancer. The information is easily accessible for physicians via libraries and personal computers.

Placebo (pla-see'bo)—An inactive substance resembling a medication, given for psychological effect or as a control in evaluating a medicine believed to be active. It is usually a tablet, capsule, or injection that contains a harmless substance but appears to be the same as the medicine being tested. A placebo may be compared with a new drug when no one knows if any drug or treatment will be effective.

Protocol (pro'to-kol)—The outline or plan for use of an experimental procedure or experimental treatment.

Radiation Therapy, also called Radiotherapy—
Treatment using X-rays, cobalt-60, radium, neutrons, or other types of cell-destroying radiation.

Radiosensitizers (ray'dee-o-sen-si-ty'zers)—
Drugs being studied to try to boost the effect of radiation therapy.

Randomized Clinical Trials (ran-duh'mized)—A study in which patients with similar traits, such as extent of disease, are chosen or selected by chance to be placed in separate groups that are comparing different treatments. Because irrelevant factors or preferences do not influence the distribution of patients, the treatment groups can be considered comparable and results of the different treatments used in different groups can be compared. (There is no way at the time for the researchers to know which of the treatments is best.) See also **Clinical Trials.** (It is the patient's choice to be in a randomized trial or not.)

Regression (ree-gresh'un)—The state of growing smaller or disappearing; used to describe the shrinkage or disappearance of a cancer.

Remission (ree-mish'un)—The decrease or disappearance of evidence of a disease; also the period during which this occurs.

Risk/Benefit Ratio—The relation between the risks and benefits of a given treatment or procedure. Institutional Review Boards (IRBs) (located where the study is to take place) determine that the risks in a study are reasonable with respect to the potential benefits. It is also up to the patient to decide if it is reasonable for him or her to take part in a study.

Side Effect—A secondary and usually adverse effect, as from a drug or other treatment. For example, nausea is a side effect of some anti-cancer drugs.

Single Blind—(See **Double Blind**)

Staging—Methods used to establish the extent of a patient's disease.

Standard Treatment—A treatment or other intervention currently being used and considered to be of proved effectiveness on the basis of past studies.

Study Arm—Patients in clinical trials are assigned to one part or segment of a study—a study "arm." One arm receives a different treatment from another.

Therapeutic (ther'a-pew'tik)—Pertaining to treatment.

Chapter 30

When Cancer Recurs

Meeting the Challenge Again

When Cancer Recurs: Meeting the Challenge Again

In the back of every cancer patient's mind is the possibility that the disease may return. And yet, when it does, the first reaction often is "How can this be happening again?"

The shock is back. The fears are back—of telling your family and friends, of more treatment, and possibly of death. The anger is there too—after all you've been through, it should have been enough. And the unanswered question is "Will the treatment really work this time?"

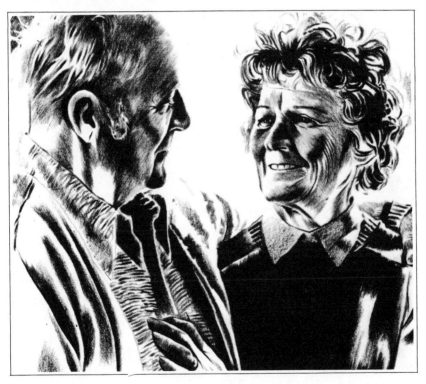

Even though you may feel some of the same things you felt when you were first diagnosed, now there's a difference. You've been through this before, faced cancer and its treatment and the changes that came to your life. You know that medical and emotional support is available to you. Facing cancer again is a difficult challenge but one you can handle.

This is about cancer that has returned—its diagnosis and treatment, suggestions for coping, and where to get help. The glossary at the end explains some of the terms that you will read here or that you may hear in talking with your treatment team.

As you read this, remember that there are more than 100 different types of cancer. Each person's cancer is different, and each person responds to treatment differently. No single book can cover every situation for every person. As a result, the information given here is general, and some of it will not apply to you. Still, a lot of people have handled recurring cancer in similar ways, and their experiences may help you.

Many people who have faced cancer's return say that knowledge and understanding help. By learning more about your illness and treatment, you give yourself the option of participating in your care. By maintaining a positive attitude toward treatment, you may be able to control some of your emotional and physical reactions to it. By drawing on your own strengths and borrowing support from the people and resources around you, you can meet this challenge again.

Why Cancer Can Recur

"Recur" means "to happen again." When cancer recurs, it means that the disease that was thought to be cured, or was at least inactive (in remission), has become active again. Cancer may recur after several months or years.

Cancer that has recurred is very much like the first cancer in the way that it starts: An abnormal cell begins growing and multiplying quickly. If not stopped, cancer cells can eventually replace normal cells.

Recurrent cancer gets its start from cells that broke away from the original tumor and traveled through the lymph system or bloodstream to start new cancer growths. Your previous treatment was meant to destroy the original cancer and many of the cells that may have become detached from it. However, sometimes a small number of undetectable cancer cells may survive and be found later after they have multiplied.

In recurrent disease, the cancer that reappears is the same type as the original cancer—no matter where it appears. This means, for example, that if breast cancer recurs in the lung, it is not lung cancer; it is breast cancer that has spread to the lung.

Where Cancers Can Recur

Not every cancer cell that breaks away is able to start a new growth elsewhere. Most are stopped by the body's natural defenses or destroyed by treatment with radiation or anticancer drugs. Just as different cancers vary in their response to treatment, they also differ in their ability to recur and the places where they may recur. For this reason, recurrent cancers are classified by location: local, regional, or metastatic.

Local recurrence means that the cancer has come back in the same place as the original cancer. The term "local" also means that there is no sign of cancer in nearby lymph nodes or other tissues. For instance, a woman who has had a mastectomy could later have a local recurrence of breast cancer in or around the area of the surgery.

A *regional* recurrence involves growth of a new tumor in lymph nodes or tissues near the original site, but with no evidence of growth at distant sites. A woman who has been treated for breast cancer, for instance, might have a regional recurrence in the lymph nodes under her arm.

In *metastatic* recurrence, cancer has spread to organs or other tissues at some distance from the original site. For example, a woman with breast cancer could have metastasis to the bone.

Diagnosing Recurrent Cancer

Over the last several months or years, you may have had a number of tests and checkups to see that your treatment was effective. Most likely, you were told to watch for changes in your body and to report any unusual symptoms to your doctor.

Perhaps you noticed a weight change, bleeding, or continuing pain, or the doctor may have found signs of further illness while examining you. In either case, several kinds of tests are used to find out the exact cause of the problem and the best treatment.

Specific procedures and tests (some of which are described below) help your doctor answer these questions:

- Are the signs and symptoms caused by cancer or by some other medical problem?

- If there is cancer, is it a recurrence or is it a different type?

- Is cancer present in more than one site?

Because certain types of cancer tend to recur in certain parts of the body, your doctor is likely to test those locations. How often a test is done is based on the type of cancer you had and the way it spreads. Each piece of information from exams and tests helps the doctor make an accurate diagnosis so that your treatment is the best one for your problem.

Physical Exams

In addition to a manual exam (feeling for lumps, swelling, and so on), your doctor may need to use instruments to look at certain internal organs. Depending on the type of cancer you originally had, you may be examined through various special "scopes" that provide a direct view of the lower colon, upper digestive tract, breathing passages, bladder, or cervix. In some cases, the doctor may even take a tissue sample through the scope that will be looked at under a microscope.

Laboratory Tests

A number of lab tests are used to help diagnose recurrent cancer. Many of these same tests are also used to detect other conditions. For example, blood samples can be tested to check the levels of certain proteins or enzymes that may change when cancer recurs. Using other fluid samples, doctors can look for signs of cancer cells in the tissues that produce the fluids. A Pap smear to test for cancer of the cervix is an example of this kind of test.

Another test is used to detect internal bleeding that may be too slight for you to notice. A stool smear or sample of fluid from the stomach may show whether blood vessels have been broken. If any blood cells are found in the sample, a series of X-rays or another type of test would be needed to find out whether the bleeding is caused by cancer or by some other problem, such as an ulcer.

X-Rays and Scans

To learn the location and size of suspected cancer, the doctor can use X-rays, CT scans, nuclear scans, or ultrasound.

These advanced tests use radiation, computers, magnets, and other very sophisticated equipment. If you have questions about how they are used, their risks or benefits, or what you should expect during the procedure, be sure to discuss your concerns with your doctor, nurse, or technician.

X-Rays. Tumors that are fairly large and more dense than the normal tissue around them can often be seen with the standard X-ray (the chest X-ray, for example) that most people have had. Other tests combine X-rays with a barium solution, dye, or air to give sharp pictures of organs that cannot be seen clearly with X-rays alone, such as the stomach, kidney, and colon. Many people are familiar with the "GI series" (upper gastrointestinal X-ray and barium enema), an example of this kind of study.

CT Scans. A newer type of X-ray study, the CT (computed tomography) scan, takes a series of pictures from several directions. The CT scan gives pictures that are more detailed than standard X-rays for certain parts of the body and is often used for soft tissues such as the liver and brain.

Nuclear Medicine Scans. Nuclear medicine scans are often used to see the brain, liver, bone, spleen, and thyroid. A weak radioactive substance is swallowed or injected into the bloodstream, and then the scanner takes pictures of the areas to which the substance is attracted. A cancer can show up in the pictures as an area of higher or lower radioactivity than the tissue around it.

Ultra Sonic Scans. An ultrasound scan uses a microphone-like device that is passed over the patient's skin and sends out sound waves that bounce off internal organs. The sound-wave echoes form a picture that shows whether a tumor is present and whether it is solid or filled with fluid.

Biopsy

A biopsy is often the best way to tell if cancer is present. Even though a tumor can frequently be seen through scopes or on X-ray films, a biopsy shows whether or not it is made up of cancer cells.

For some cancers, the doctor can do a needle biopsy to withdraw fluid or remove small tissue samples. When a surgical biopsy is needed, the entire tumor or a piece of it is removed. Surgical biopsies are done under local or general anesthesia.

After either biopsy procedure, the sample of cells or tissues that was removed is examined under the microscope. The doctor can tell whether the sample contains cancer cells and, if it does, what type of cancer it is.

If your cancer has recurred, an accurate diagnosis is the first step in getting the disease under control again.

Treatment Methods

In planning treatment for recurrent cancer, many of the same factors that affected treatment choices for the original cancer will be taken into account. The type of cancer, its size and location, your general health, and other treatments you've had are all considered before a treatment decision can be made.

In many cases, doctors are able to treat recurrent cancer with more intensive use of the therapies that were used during the first series of treatments. Your doctor may recommend further surgery, radiation to new sites, or more anticancer drugs. For certain cancers, such as those in the reproductive organs, the doctor may suggest hormone therapy to limit tumor growth.

Discussing treatment goals, methods, and effects with your doctor will help determine which treatment will be best for you. It is important that you take an active part in the decision by asking questions and expressing your feelings about specific treatments.

The following paragraphs describe the most common treatments, some of the newer methods that are now under study, and "unproven" treatments that you may have heard about. You will also find a list of questions that patients often ask about the various treatment.

Surgery

Surgery is often the treatment of choice when cancer first occurs, but it is used less often in recurrent disease. For many sites of recurrence, other methods have been shown to be more effective. The doctor may recommend an operation to remove a local or a single metastatic recurrence that appears on the skin or in the lung, liver, bone, brain, or lymph nodes. In some cases, the surgery may be followed by radiation therapy or chemotherapy.

When a patient has metastatic cancer in a weight-bearing bone (such as in the leg), there may be a threat of fracture caused by the growing tumor. In such a case, the doctor may suggest an operation to support the bone and prevent a break. This can help to relieve pain and keep the patient active while going through other forms of treatment to control the cancer.

Radiation Therapy

Radiation treatment—the use of high levels of radiation (tens of thousands of times the amount used, for instance, to produce a chest X-ray) directed at a cancerous tumor—destroys the ability of cells to grow and divide. Both normal and diseased cells are affected by radiation, but many normal cells can replace themselves quickly.

Doctors are using radiation to treat cancer in almost every part of the body. Sometimes radiation therapy is used before surgery, to shrink a cancerous tumor. After surgery, it may be used to stop the growth of any cancer cells that remain. In some cases, doctors prefer to use radiation and anticancer drugs, rather than surgery, to destroy a cancerous growth and prevent it reappearance.

The type of cancer, location, stage, and other factors will determine whether radiation therapy is right for a patient. Metastatic sites that may be treated with radiation include the brain, lung, and bone. For most patients with metastatic recurrence in the brain, radiation therapy is the treatment of choice.

Radiation treatment can cause side effects, but most are not serious. They usually disappear within a few weeks after treatment ends, although some are more lasting. The type of side effects you may have often depends on the part of the body that is being treated. Nausea is one common side effect. Diet changes and medicine can help control it. Fatigue is another common side effect. Many patients have no side effects at all. If radiation therapy is prescribed for you, ask your doctor to explain the side effects that might occur and how you can best manage them. *Radiation Therapy and You**is a booklet available from the National Cancer Institute that answers many questions about radiation treatment.

Chemotherapy

Chemotherapy is the treatment of cancer with anticancer drugs. Drugs can be very effective in the treatment of some cancers. They may be used alone or in a treatment plan that also includes radiation therapy and/or surgery.

Chemotherapy may be given by mouth or by injection into the veins or muscles. The drugs reach and destroy cancer cells in nearly every part of the body. The speed with which the cells are destroyed varies with different types of cancer and different drugs. As a result, the length of treatment varies among patients. Treatment may consist of a single drug or a combination of two or more.

Because anticancer drugs can reach sites that are far away from the original cancer and can destroy cancer cells circulating

---

* See chapter entitled, **Radiation Therapy and You.** Consult CONTENTS for page location.

in the body, chemotherapy is the primary treatment for many kinds of recurrent cancers. It is often the treatment of choice for metastases in the lung and liver. When combined with radiation treatment, chemotherapy has also been useful in the control of brain metastases.

Side effects may occur during chemotherapy because the drugs can affect *any* rapidly growing cells in the body—normal cells as well as cancer cells. The normal cells most likely to be affected are those in the bone marrow, digestive tract, reproductive organs, and hair follicles. However, many normal cells are able to replace themselves quickly.

Every person reacts differently to chemotherapy. Some people have few or no side effects; others say their side effects were less severe than they expected; others have a more difficult time. Ask your doctor, nurse, or pharmacist about side effects that could occur with the specific anticancer drugs prescribed for you. They can give you suggestions to help manage problems that may occur during treatment. Most side effects gradually stop before or shortly after treatment ends. However, the fatigue that some patients experience during chemotherapy sometimes lingers for a while.

The National Cancer Institute's booklet *Chemotherapy and You*[*] provides further information about this type of cancer treatment.

Hormone Therapy

Some cancers are sensitive to changes in hormone levels. By adding, removing, or limiting the activity of a given hormone, doctors can influence the growth or activity of cells affected by that hormone. For example, if a breast cancer is the kind that is stimulated by the female hormone estrogen, an antiestrogen medicine that helps to limit the tumor's growth may be given.

Sometimes surgery or radiation treatment is used to stop the body from producing a specific hormone. Other hormones or drugs that keep hormones from being produced may be given along with other anticancer drugs. A treatment plan that includes hormone therapy may be used for cancers of the breast, uterus, and prostate, and for some types of lymphoma and leukemia.

---

[*] *See chapter entitled, **Chemotherapy and You**. Consult CONTENTS for page location.*

Supportive Therapy

When you were first treated for cancer, you may have had physical therapy or used the services of a psychological counselor or social worker. Consider seeking those kinds of help again. Two other types of supportive therapy that could also be important to you now—nutritional support and pain management—are discussed below.

Nutrition. Maintaining good nutrition during cancer therapy is very important. Studies have shown that patients who eat well may be able to cope with the effects of cancer and its treatment more successfully.

Eating well means choosing foods that have the vitamins, minerals, and other elements needed to keep the body working normally. It also means getting enough calories to avoid weight loss and enough protein to rebuild damaged tissues. Dieting during treatment is not advised because it deprives the body of needed calories and nutrients.

You could have problems with eating and digesting food because of treatment side effects, but coping with diet problems may be easier than you expect. The National Cancer Institute's publication *Eating Hints* has many suggestions on healthy eating habits during treatment, as do the booklets *Chemotherapy and You*[*] and *Radiation Therapy and You*,[*] which discuss specific nutrition problems for those treatments.

If keeping up your food intake and maintaining normal weight continue to be a problem in spite of your efforts, ask a dietitian on your treatment team to suggest a diet plan to help you. For severe nutrition problems, special treatments can be given at home or in the hospital.

Pain Control. Although many people with cancer do not have serious problems with pain, others need help with pain management. Pain from cancer or its treatment may need only a light medication—such as aspirin—to relieve it. If the pain is not helped by light pain relievers, talk to your doctor about prescription medicines or other nonmedical methods of pain relief. If you're having radiation therapy or chemotherapy, be sure to check with your doctor before taking *any* medicines.

***

* The mentioned text is reprinted within this book. See CONTENTS for location.

When describing a pain to your doctor, be as specific as you can. To recommend the best pain treatment for you, your doctor will want to know the following things:

- Where *exactly* is your pain? Does it ever move from one spot to another?
- How does the pain feel (dull, sharp, burning, etc.)?
- How often does it occur?
- How long does the pain last?
- Does it start at a specific time (before or after meals, after certain activities, etc.)?
- Does anything (lying down, sitting, eating, etc.) seem to relieve the pain?

Because pain can be worse when you are frightened or worried, you may find some relief by using relaxation exercises or meditation. These activities, which usually involve deep, rhythmic breathing and quiet concentration, can be done almost anywhere.

A number of other ways to reduce pain have been gaining attention in recent years. Hypnosis and biofeedback have been helpful for some people with serious illness. These and other methods are being studied to see if they can help cancer patients. If you want to learn about them, ask your doctor or nurse to refer you to a health professional who is trained to teach these methods. You may also want to read the American Cancer Society/National Cancer Institute publication *Questions & Answers About Pain Control.*

Experimental and Unproven Treatments

The words "experimental" and "unproven" are very similar in meaning, but there are important differences when they are used to describe cancer treatments. Understanding the difference can help you when discussing and choosing among your treatment options.

Experimental Methods. Experimental (or investigational) treatments are given under strict scientific conditions. These methods have been tested on animals, and they have shown

---

* Text of the named publication appears in this book, beginning on page 561.

promise for treating cancers in humans. Examples of experimen tal treatments under study at this time include new combinations of drugs, hyperthermia (heat treatments), and drugs that make radiation treatments more effective. If proven effective, the experimental treatments of today could become standard treatments in the future.

For most cancer patients, standard treatments offer the best hope for control of cancer. Sometimes, however, your cancer might be more effectively treated with an experimental method and you might want to consider entering a clinical trial, which is a scientific study using new types of cancer treatments.

Clinical trials involve the use of new substances (such as new anticancer drugs), a new way of using a treatment, or a new combination of anticancer drugs and other forms of treatment. All treatment methods, drugs, and devices in a clinical trial are under strict regulation by the Federal Government. The doctors who are approved to conduct clinical trials follow detailed guidelines for treating patients. The National Cancer Institute sponsors clinical trials of cancer therapies to be sure that the treatments are safe and effective before they are put into widespread use.

Participation in a clinical trial is always voluntary. The doctor handling your experimental treatment will explain to you which parts of the therapy are experimental and which are standard, what risks are involved, and what side effects might occur. The treatment cannot begin without your consent.

Information on current clinical trials is available to you and your doctor through the National Cancer Institute's Cancer Information Service. See the chapter on clinical trials, beginning on page 511.

Unproven Methods. A treatment method described as "unproven" is one for which the substance used (a vitamin, food, etc.) or the way it is given has not been shown, by accepted scientific methods, to be effective. Perhaps the most widely known unproven cancer treatment involves Laetrile, a product made from apricot pits. Other unproven methods you may have heard about use various diets, vitamins, herb mixtures, and serums.

The American Cancer Society has developed a list of clues to help you know whether a new treatment is "experimental" or "unproven." One way is looking at how results of treatment are reported. Findings from experimental treatments are usually first reported in medical and scientific journals and may later be reported in newspapers and magazines directed to the general public. Unproven methods are usually reported only in newspapers and magazines. They generally rely on first person accounts by patients and do not discuss scientific data. Use of these unproven treatments may actually be harmful because it may delay or interfere with treatments of proven benefit. Some of them may even cause dangerous reactions themselves.

Call the Cancer Information Service if you want to learn more about unproven methods. The booklet *Unproven Methods of Cancer Management*, available from the American Cancer Society, provides information on many of these treatments. Be sure to consider carefully the list of suggested questions below if you are considering either experimental therapies or unproven methods among your treatment options.

Questions To Ask the Doctor

Before you and your doctor agree on a treatment plan, you should understand why one treatment is recommended over others. You should also be aware of how the treatment compares to others in terms of possible benefits, risks, side effects, and impact on your lifestyle.

The questions listed below are examples of what patients often want to know about their treatment. You may want to add your own questions to the list to discuss with your doctor, nurse, or social worker. Family members or others close to you may have questions too.

● Questions to ask about any recommended treatment:

— Why do you think this treatment is the best one for me?
— Is this the standard treatment for my type of cancer?
— Are there other treatments? What are they?
— What benefits do you expect from the treatment?

— Are there side effects with this treatment? Are they temporary or permanent?

— Is there any way to prevent or relieve the side effects?

— How safe is this treatment? What are the risks?

— How will you know if the treatment is working?

— Will I need to be in the hospital?

— What will happen if I don't have the treatment?

— What does my family need to know about the treatment? Can they help?

— How long will I be on this treatment?

— How much will the treatment cost?

• About radiation therapy:

— What benefits do you expect from this therapy?

— What type of radiation treatment will I be getting?

— How long do the treatments take? How many will I need? How often?

— Can I schedule treatments at a certain time of day?

— What if I have to miss a treatment?

— What risks are involved?

— What side effects should I expect? What can I do about them?

— Who will give me the treatments? Where are they given?

— Will I need a special diet?

— Will my activities be limited?

• About chemotherapy and hormone drug therapy:

— What do you expect the drugs to do for me?

— Which drugs will I be getting? How is each one given?

— Where are the treatments given?

— How long do the treatments take? How many will I need?

— What happens if I miss a dose?

— What risks are involved?

— What side effects should I expect? What can I do about them?

— Will I need a special diet or other restrictions?

— Can I take other medicines during treatment?

— Can I drink alcoholic beverages during treatment?

- About experimental treatments or unproven methods:
  — What benefits can I expect from the treatment?
  — What can you learn from it?
  — Is there scientific evidence that the treatment can help?
  — What are the known or potential risks? Possible side effects?
  — Can I continue my regular treatments while I'm trying the new one?
  — Will I have to get the new treatment from a different doctor?
  — Will my insurance cover the costs of treatment?
  — Will I have to travel to get the treatment? How often?

Helping Yourself

From your own experience, you may remember that much of the fear and anxiety that you felt the first time cancer appeared in your life was "fear of the unknown." Once you had the tests and went through the treatments, you knew what to expect. This knowledge may have helped you cope. Important ways that you can help yourself again are to gather information, to participate in your treatment as much as possible, and to learn to deal with your feelings about your cancer's recurring.

Gathering Information

If you know how your illness can affect your body and if you stay informed about the progress of your treatment, you have a better chance to take part in your care. Some people prefer to leave treatment decisions entirely to their doctor; this is not unusual. However, it may still help you to know the reasons behind your doctor's decisions.

Learn as much as you can about what is happening to you and around you. If you have questions, ask your doctor and other members of your treatment team. Your pharmacist is another good person to talk to if you have questions about your medicines. If you don't understand the answer to a question, ask it again.

Some patients hesitate to ask their doctors about treatment options for recurrent cancer. They may think that doctors resent having their recommendations questioned, or that they may be unwilling to discuss experimental treatments or unproven treatments they may have heard about. Many doctors, however, believe that the best patient is an informed patient. They understand that coping with treatment is easier when patients understand as much as possible, and they encourage patients to discuss their concerns.

When you see the doctor to talk about possible treatments or to get help for problems that come up during treatment, take along your list of questions and ask a friend or relative to go with you. You'll get the most useful advice if you and your companion speak openly to the doctor about your needs, expectations, wishes, and concerns.

Participating in Your Treatment

Taking an active part in your care can help you maintain a sense of well-being. There are many ways you can contribute. One is to follow the care measures recommended for you, such as a special diet or exercise program or avoiding tight clothing or too much sun.

Another way you can help is to keep your doctor informed. port honestly how you feel, and if problems arise, be as specific as possible when describing them. Don't ever hesitate to report symptoms to your doctor or to request advice on what to do

about them. Although many health-related signs and symptoms may seem unimportant to you, they could provide valuable information to your doctor. Know what signs you should look for, and if any of them appear, tell your doctor as soon as possible.

Remember the difference between "doing" and "overdoing." Rest is very important to you now—both physically and emotionally. Some things you can do to keep up your strength are to:

- *Eat well*—This may be one of the most important things you can do to improve your body's response to treatment.
- *Get extra rest*—Your body will use a lot of extra energy during treatment. Get more sleep at night and take naps whenever you feel the need.
- *Adjust activities*—Try not to demand too much of yourself. Ask other people to take over some of your tasks if necessary. If your energy level becomes low, do the things that are most important to you and cut back on the others.

If you find your strength limited by your illness or the side effects of treatment, you may want to seek out less tiring activities. You can try things that you may not have taken time to enjoy before. Plan a reading program—perhaps a friend likes the same books and you could read them together. Writing a journal each day has been a valuable activity for many cancer patients. You can also take time for letter-writing, phone calls, and visits, if you want.

Managing Your Emotions

The diagnosis of cancer, whether for the first time or when it recurs, can threaten anyone's sense of well-being. Some people, when they first find out that cancer has returned, feel shock and denial. Many had put their experience with cancer completely behind them, and the new diagnosis hits them as hard as—or even harder than—it did the first time. Others are not surprised, as if they had been expecting it all along.

There may be times when you'll feel overcome by fear, anxiety, depression, or even rage. These emotions are common ways to cope with a difficult situation, and many people with recurrent cancer experience them. Feel free to express these feelings if they occur. None of them are "wrong" reactions, and letting them out will help you deal with them.

Starting cancer treatments again can place demands on your spirits as well as your body. Your attitudes and actions really can make a difference. Remember that you have coped with this situation before. Keeping your treatment goals in mind may help you keep your spirits up during therapy and see you through "down" spells that may occur.

As you go through treatment, you're bound to feel better about yourself on some days than on others. The uncertainty of living with recurrent cancer can sometimes contribute to ups and downs. When a bad day comes along, try to remember that there have been good days and there will be more. Feeling low today does not mean you will feel that way tomorrow or that you are giving up. At these times, try distracting yourself with a book, a hobby, or plans for a new garden. Many people say it helps to have something to look forward to—even simple things like a drive, a visit with a friend, or a phone call. Sometimes, however, you may just want to cry—this is okay too.

You may need to rely more on the people closest to you to help during your treatment, but this may be difficult at first. Many people do not understand cancer, and they may avoid you because they're afraid of your illness. Others may worry that they will upset you by saying the wrong thing.

At a time when you might expect others to rush to your aid, you may have to make the first moves. Try to be open in talking with others about your illness, your treatment, your needs, and your feelings. Once people know that you can discuss these things, they may be more willing to open up and lend their support.

By keeping the lines of communication open, you can help to correct mistaken ideas, and you and your loved ones will be better able to help each other through a difficult time. Another booklet from the National Cancer Institute, *Taking Time,* offers more useful advice to help cancer patients and their families.

At times you may want a listener who's more objective than your family or friends. Try talking to someone on your treatment team with whom you feel comfortable. The health professionals caring for you have your overall well-being as their primary goal. When they know about your personal concerns, how your household has been affected, and what changes in your situation you'd like to see, they will be better able to provide the best types of physical and emotional support for you.

At times you are likely to feel stressed by the continuing changes in your life. Some stress can help because it may prompt you to take action. Too much stress, though, can harm

---

* *The text, TAKING TIME, appears in this book under the title, EMOTIONAL SUPPORT. See CONTENTS for location.*

554

your health and emotional well-being. You may not be able to remove all the stress around you, but you can try to limit it. Relaxation techniques can be used to reduce stress and improve your sense of well-being. Rhythmic breathing, imagery, and distraction are among the techniques that are easy to learn and use whenever you need them. If you are interested, ask your doctor or nurse to refer you to someone trained to teach these techniques. The local library also has useful books on relieving stress.

There are many reasons for the emotional problems cancer patients experience. You can probably manage a number of these problems on your own or with the help of family, friends, or clergy, but for others you may want professional help. A counselor trained to help cancer patients deal with their emotions may be a valuable addition to your health care team. These counselors understand the special problems that go along with serious illness, as well as the various ways of coping that others have found useful. If you think this kind of professional support could help you, ask your doctor or nurse for the name of an appropriate counselor.

Support Programs and Organizations

Doctors and patients alike have learned the value of mutual support among patients. When someone with a serious illness feels frightened or depressed, it often helps to discuss those feelings with another person who has been through the same experience. This can help patients get practical information, understand their feelings, and develop their own ways of handling their problems. Families and other people who are close to someone with a serious illness can also use this type of help.

Make Today Count has self-help programs in more than 100 chapters around the country. The American Cancer Society (ACS) also offers programs to help cancer patients and those close to them. Among the ACS programs that may be helpful when cancer recurs are CanSurmount and I Can Cope.

The ACS and several other organizations also offer education materials, in-home services, equipment loans, and referral to other sources to help. The addresses and phone numbers listed

555

at the end of this section are for the national headquarters of major organizations. To contact local ACS chapters or units, look in your telephone book or call the Cancer Information Service.

Home Health Care Services

Some patients will need help caring for themselves during or after their cancer treatments. Many state and county health departments have programs that provide instruction in caring for the cancer patient at home. Such knowledge may be very useful after surgery or during bouts of illness. Commercial services, such as visiting nurses, may be listed under "home health agencies" in your telephone book.

The American Red Cross also provides instruction in first aid and home nursing. Your local chapter may be able to help you locate someone to assist with activities such as personal care, housework, and shopping if you need this type of help.

Other Organizations

American Cancer Society
90 Park Avenue
New York, NY 10016
212-736-3030

A voluntary organization offering a variety of patient services. ACS is also involved in cancer education and research.

American Red Cross
17th and D Streets, N.W.
Washington, DC 20006
202-737-8300

A network of local chapters provides various community services, including nursing health programs and a large portion of the voluntary blood donations made in this country.

Leukemia Society of America, Inc.
733 Third Avenue
New York, NY 10017
212-573-8484

Supplemental financial assistance and consultation services are offered to cancer patients with leukemia and related disorders.

Make Today Count
P.O. Box 222
Osage Beach, MO 65065
314-348-1619

This organization helps patients with cancer and other diseases and their families cope with illness and improve their quality of life.

United Cancer Council
Suite 340
650 East Carmel Drive
Carmel, IN 46032

Federation of independent cancer agencies with programs of education, research, and service to cancer patients and their families.

United Ostomy Association
2001 W. Beverly Boulevard
Los Angeles, CA 90057
213-413-5510
(local chapters listed under "Ostomy")

A network of local chapters offers emotional support, aid, and education to those who have had colostomy, ileostomy, or urostomy surgery.

Glossary

Adjuvant therapy—a treatment method used in addition to the primary therapy; radiation therapy and chemotherapy are often used as adjuvants to surgery.

Alopecia—hair loss.

Anesthesia—a procedure in which a patient receives medications that block out pain.

Antiemetic—a medicine to prevent or relieve nausea and vomiting.

Benign tumor—a growth that is not a cancer and does not spread to other parts of the body.

Biopsy—the removal and microscopic examination of tissue for diagnosis.

Cancer—a general term for more than 100 diseases characterized by uncontrolled, abnormal growth of cells that can invade and destroy healthy tissues.

Chemotherapy—treatment with anticancer drugs.

Dietitian—a professional who arranges diet programs for proper nutrition of the well or therapeutic nutrition of the sick.

Hormones—substances made by the body that regulate the activity of certain cells or organs. They are largely responsible for sexual function and the aspects of appearance (such as facial hair) that distinguish the sexes.

Immunotherapy—treatment by stimulation of the body's immune defense system; immunotherapy is an experimental treatment that is being investigated.

Linear accelerator—a machine that creates and uses high-energy X-rays to treat cancers.

Lymph nodes—part of the lymphatic system that removes wastes from body tissues and carries fluids that help the body fight infection.

Malignant—cancerous (see *cancer*).

Metastasis—the spread of a cancer from one part of the body to another; cells in the new cancer are like those in the original site.

Oncologist—a doctor who is a specialist in the treatment of cancers.

Palliative therapy—a treatment that may relieve symptoms without curing the disease.

Pathologist—a doctor specially trained to examine cells and tissues to find changes caused by disease.

Radiation oncologist—a doctor who specializes in using radiation to treat cancer.

Radiation therapy—the use of high-energy penetrating rays to treat disease; sources of radiation include X-ray, cobalt, and radium.

Radiologist—a physician with special training in the diagnostic and/or therapeutic use of X-rays and other forms of radiant energy.

Recurrence—reappearance of cancer at the same site (local), near the initial site (regional), or in other areas of the body (metastatic).

Tumor—an abnormal mass of tissue that results from excessive cell division and performs no useful body function; tumors are either *benign* or *malignant*.

X-ray—a type of radiation that can be used at low levels to diagnose disease or in its high-energy form to treat cancer.

Chapter 31

Control of Cancer Pain

The Patient Has a Key Role in Reducing Pain

Control of Cancer Pain

Efforts to relieve pain have been going on for thousands of years. Although many drugs prescribed by modern doctors are based on plants and herbs that were used by ancient peoples to ease pain, a wide variety of pain relief medications is now available. Techniques such as hypnosis and distraction, once used as religious rituals in primitive cultures to exorcise the "evil spirits" that were believed to cause pain, have been refined and improved. Today, major research efforts are continuing to look into the causes of pain and treatments to reduce it.

Cancer is not always accompanied by pain. It is rarely a symptom of early cancer, and advanced cancer patients do not always have pain. But if pain does occur, there are many ways to relieve or reduce it.

What Causes Pain in People With Cancer?

Cancer patients may have pain for a number of reasons, depending on the type of cancer, stage of the disease, and pain threshold (resistance to pain). Cancer pain that lasts a few days or longer may result from:

- Pressure on a nerve by the tumor.

- Infection or inflammation.

- Poor blood circulation because of blocked blood vessels.

- Blockage of an organ or tube in the body.

- Bone fractures caused by cancer cells that have spread to the bone.

- After effects of surgery, stiffness from inactivity, or side effects from medications, such as constipation or mouth sores.

- Nonphysical responses to illness, such as tension, depression, or anxiety.

What Can Be Done for Such Pain?

Whenever possible the cause of the pain is treated by removing the tumor or decreasing its size. In order to do this, the doctor may recommend surgery, radiation therapy, or chemotherapy. Or, the pain itself can be treated without affecting the cancer. Methods for treating pain include medicines, operations on nerves, nerve blocks, and techniques such as relaxation, distraction, and imagery.

What Medicines Are Used to Relieve Pain?

Medicines that relieve pain are called analgesics. Analgesics act on the nervous system to relieve pain without causing loss of consciousness. They provide only temporary pain relief because they do not cure the cause of the pain. Analgesics simply suppress pain to a more tolerable level.

Nonprescription pain relievers are used for mild and moderate pain. These analgesics can be bought without a doctor's prescription. Sometimes they are called "over-the-counter" pain remedies. The most common nonprescription pain relievers are aspirin, acetaminophen (Tylenol, Datril), and ibuprofen (Advil, Nuprin). Ibuprofen is one of a new group of pain relievers that has been developed for the treatment of mild to severe pain. These drugs are known as nonsteroidal anti-inflammatory agents. The 200 mg. strength of ibuprofen is available without a prescription. Larger doses of this drug as well as most other nonsteroidal antiinflammatory drugs (Motrin, Dolobid, Nalfon, Anaprox, Feldene, Clinorial) must be ordered by your doctor. Because these drugs are not narcotics, their use does not result in drug tolerance or physical dependence. Other non-narcotic prescription drugs are effective for relieving muscle pain in cancer patients.

Most prescription pain relievers are narcotics, drugs that have the ability to relieve pain and cause drowsiness or sleep. All narcotics have similar side effects and may be habit forming.

Narcotic pain relievers include:

codeine
morphine

hydromorphone (Dilaudid)
oxycodone (in Percodan)
levorphanol (Levo-Dromoran)
oxymorphone (Numorphan)
meperidine (Demerol)
pentazocine (Talwin)
methadone (Dolophine)
propoxyphene (Darvon)

These pain relievers can be obtained only with a doctor's written prescription. They may be taken by mouth (orally, PO), by injection (intramuscularly, IM), through the vein (intravenously, IV), or by rectal suppository, although not all narcotics come in all these forms.

These drugs are used alone or with nonprescription pain relievers to treat moderate to severe pain.

Does the Use of Narcotics Cause Addiction?

Fear of addiction is very common among people who must take narcotics for pain relief. Many people use the term "addiction" without understanding exactly what it means—the compulsive use of habit-forming drugs to satisfy physical, emotional, and psychological needs rather than for medical reasons. Drug addiction in patients with cancer pain can occur, but it is not a major problem. As long as narcotics are used under proper medical supervision, the chance of addiction is small. Most patients who take narcotics for pain relief can stop taking these drugs if their pain can be controlled by other means. If narcotics are the only effective way

564

to relieve pain, the patient's comfort is more important than the possibility of addiction.

What Is Drug Tolerance?

Persons who take narcotics for pain control sometimes find they have to take gradually larger doses over a period of time to relieve their pain. This may be due to an increase in the pain or to the development of drug tolerance. When narcotics are taken regularly, the body doesn't respond to them as well as it once did, and these drugs become less effective. Larger or more frequent doses must be taken to obtain the effect that was achieved with the original dose. Increasing the doses of narcotics to relieve increasing pain or to overcome drug tolerance is *not* addiction, although it may lead to physical dependence on the drugs.

How Are Medicines Best Used to Relieve Pain?

A preventive approach-staying "on top" of the pain-is the best way to control pain and may actually require lower doses of pain reliever. For pain present to some degree throughout the day, medicine should be taken on a scheduled basis to prevent the pain from getting worse. Taking a mild pain reliever three to four times a day on a regular schedule, rather than waiting for the pain to return, may be enough to control pain.

What Are Some Nonmedical Ways to Treat Pain?

Some ways to relieve pain without using medicine include relaxation, imagery, distraction, and skin stimulation.

Relaxation has been found to relieve pain or keep it from getting worse by reducing the tension in the muscles. It can promote sleep, give more energy, combat fatigue, reduce anxiety, and make other pain relief methods work better.

Imagery is using imagination to create mental pictures or situations. When used to relieve pain, imagery can be thought of as a deliberate daydream or self-hypnosis.

Distraction means turning one's attention to something other than the pain. Many people use this method without knowing it when they watch television or listen to the radio to "take their mind off" the pain. Any activity that occupies attention can be used for distraction.

Skin stimulation is the use of pressure, friction, temperature changes, chemical substances, or mild electrical current to excite the nerve endings in the skin. Scientists believe that the same nerve pathways transmit the feelings of pain, heat, cold, and pressure to the brain. When the skin is stimulated so that pressure, warmth, or cold is felt, pain sensation is lessened or blocked.

Are There Any Other Pain Relief Methods?

Other medicines: Other types of drugs can be taken with analgesics to help control pain, though not all patients will benefit from them. Antidepressants, tranquilizers, cortisone, and alcohol are some of the drugs that might be useful.

Surgical methods: Pain cannot be felt if the nerve pathways that relay pain impulses to the brain are blocked. To block these pathways, a neurosurgeon may cut a nerve close to the spinal cord (rhizotomy) or cut bundles of nerves in the spinal cord itself (cordotomy).

Nerve blocks: When certain substances are injected into or around a nerve, that nerve is no longer able to transmit pain. A local anesthetic, which may be combined with cortisone, provides temporary pain relief. For longer-lasting pain relief, phenol or alcohol can be injected. Loss of all feeling in the affected area is a frequent side effect of a nerve block.

Transcutaneous electric nerve stimulation (TENS or TNS): This is a technique of skin stimulation in which mild electric currents are applied to certain areas of the skin by a small power pack attached to two electrodes. The sensation is described as a buzzing, tingling, or tapping feeling: it does not feel like a shock. The small electric impulses seem to block incoming pain sensations.

Biofeedback: With the help of special machines, people can learn to control certain body functions such as heart rate, blood pressure, and muscle tension. Biofeedback is sometimes used to help people learn to relax. Cancer patients can use biofeedback techniques to reduce anxiety in order to help them cope with their pain. Biofeedback may be used along with other pain-relief methods.

Acupuncture: In acupuncture, special needles are inserted into the body at certain points and at various depths and angles. Particular groups of acupuncture points are believed to control specific areas of pain sensation. The procedure has been used in China and elsewhere to treat many types of pain and as an anesthetic, but its usefulness for cancer patients has not been proven.

Hypnosis: No one knows how hypnosis works to control pain. Hypnosis is a trance-like state that can be induced by a person trained in special techniques. During hypnosis a person is open to suggestions made by the hypnotist. To relieve pain, the hypnotist may suggest that when the person "wakes up", pain will be gone. Some cancer patients have learned methods of self-hypnosis that they use to control pain. However, the effectiveness of hypnosis for pain relief is unpredictable.

What If Pain Is Not Relieved and the Doctor Says Nothing More Can Be Done?

No one doctor can be expected to know everything about all medical problems. Pain management for cancer is a rather new field. New techniques have been developed in the last few years. Pain specialists such as oncologists, anesthesiologists, other doctors, nurses, and pharmacists are available for consultation. Below is a list of sources that can provide names of specialists or pain programs in local areas.

- American Pain Society,
  Suite 925,
  1615 L Street NW.,
  Washington, D.C. 20036

- International Association for the Study of Pain,
  Suite 306,
  909 Northeast 43rd Street,
  Seattle, Washington 98105

- National Hospice Organization,
  Suite 307,
  1901 North Fort Meyer Drive,
  Arlington, Virginia 22209

- The oncology department in a hospital or medical center.

- The local unit of the American Cancer Society listed in your telephone directory. The American Cancer Society can also provide more information about pain control in a booklet called *Questions and Answers about Pain Control.*

For additional information on this subject and for other NCI publications, write to the Office of Cancer Communications, National Cancer Institute, Bethesda, Maryland 20892, or call the Cancer Information Service at 1-800-4-CANCER.

In Alaska call 1-800-638-6070: in Hawaii, on Oahu call 524-1234 (call collect from neighbor islands). Spanish-speaking staff members are available to callers from the following areas (daytime hours only): California, Florida, Georgia, Illinois, New Jersey (area code 201), New York, and Texas.

Chapter 32

PART III—
COPING

Emotional Support

*A Text For
People With Cancer
and For People Who
Care About Them*

Introduction

EDITOR'S NOTE: Unlike other chapters of this book, the text that follows was not created by a medical reporter. It is the collective effort of many people—everyday people—who have been affected by cancer. Some experienced it personally, some were close to a loved one who did. That point of view is a very useful one—it gives a certain "I've been there" confirmation to the gentle advice which it dispenses.

" A diagnosis of cancer . . . is a powerful stimulus against procrastinating on warm and kindly or beautiful things . . . a reminder that many of the material things aren't all that urgent after all . . . Take time to watch the sunset with someone you love; there may not be another as lovely for the two of you."

These are the thoughts of a woman with cancer who needed to share her feelings with someone who would care and who could understand.

This book is written for those affected by cancer: you, someone in your family or someone very close to you. We wrote this book because, as another person described it, we often feel that "we share a common bond that only victims of cancer know, the feelings of anguish and the loneliness no one else can share."

We've used letters, conversations, books and articles from, with and by cancer patients, families and friends. The observations of professionals who work with cancer patients as expressed in conferences, seminars and journals certainly have been explored. Our main emphasis, though, is on what the people who live with cancer in their own lives and their own homes think, feel and do to cope with the disease.

No two people with cancer are alike as are no two relatives or friends of people with cancer. Although the material in this book is intended to be helpful, some sections may not apply to certain circumstances; a few might suggest responses that make you feel uncomfortable. Each person has to cope with cancer in an individual way. What follows is intended as a guide: a brief look at how some people with cancer and their loved ones feel and the ways they found to deal with those feelings.

Perhaps, if we explore together our emotions—a side of cancer that neither surgery, drugs nor radiation can treat—we can help each other dispel some of those feelings.

People with cancer, dear friends and family members face intense fears, anxieties and frustrations that are new to many of us, although others have taken the journey we now begin. We travel a road paved with an awesome mingling of hope and despair, courage and fear, humor and anger and constant uncertainty. Perhaps, sharing the experiences of those who have walked the road before will help us define our own feelings and find our own ways of coping.

Our bodies and minds are not completely separate. It will help us keep our bodies strong if we also deal successfully with the emotional turmoil of cancer. We shall talk about some of the emotional problems we might face and some possible adjustments. We'll explore learning to express and share our feelings about cancer; dealing with new responsibilities; coping with rejection by others, finding new meaning in our days and using each day to its fullest measure.

There is another good reason for learning to define and live with our feelings about cancer. They may be with us for a long time. Cancer is undeniably a major illness; it is not necessarily fatal. Today, nearly two million Americans are alive and considered cured of cancer. That means that 5 years or more after their initial diagnosis and treatment they are free of evidence of disease.

For them cancer has become a chronic condition, somewhat like hypertension, diabetes or a mild heart condition. As is true for others with chronic conditions, periodic health checkups will be part of their lifelong routine. They will, undeniably, be more sensitive to and anxious about minor signs of illness or discomfort. Unlike others with chronic disease, they most likely will not need lifelong medication or special diets to remind them daily that they once were ill. Many will live for years, grow old and die much as they had expected to do before cancer was diagnosed.

It is hard not to think about dying, but it's important to concentrate on living. Remember, a diagnosis is not a death sentence; 1 of 3 people with cancer is saved. For some forms of the disease, 9 of 10 people diagnosed can be considered cured. Of the others, many will live a long time before dying with the disease. Indeed, there are sunrises as well as sunsets to be enjoyed. So let us take a look at living—living with cancer and its treatment, but living nonetheless.

—The Authors

Sharing the Diagnosis

- Cancer can be unutterably lonely. No one should try to bear it alone.

- Patient, family and friends usually learn the diagnosis sooner or later. Most people find it easier for all if everybody can share their feelings instead of hiding them. This frees people to offer each other support.

- Patients usually agree that hiding the diagnosis from them denies them the right to make important choices about their life and their treatment.

- Families say patients who try to keep the diagnosis secret rob loved ones of the chance to express that love and to offer help and support.

- Family members and intimate friends also bear great emotional burdens and should be able to share them openly with each other and the patient.

- Even children should be told. They sense when something is amiss, and they may imagine a situation worse than it really is.

- The patient might want to tell the children directly; or it may be easier to have a close friend or loving relative do so.

- The children's ages and emotional maturity should be a guide in deciding how much to tell. The goal is to let children express their feelings and ask questions about the cancer.

- By sharing the diagnosis, patient, family and friends build foundations of mutual understanding and trust.

One question many people ask after diagnosis is, "Should I tell?" Perhaps not. A family member could be too old, too young or too emotionally fragile to accept the diagnosis, but people are surprisingly resilient. Most find ways to deal with the reality of illness and the possibility of death—even when it involves those they love most. They find the strength to bounce back from situations that seem to cause unbearable grief.

The way in which people differ is in the speed with which they bounce back. The diagnosis of cancer hits most of us with a wave of shock, of fright, of denial. Each person needs a different amount of time to pull himself or herself together and to deal with the reality of cancer. In reading the sections that follow, you should remember that only you really know your emotional timetable. Think about sharing at a time when you are ready to do so.

Should You Tell?

Usually, family and close friends learn sooner or later that you have cancer. Most people with cancer have found the best choice is to share the diagnosis and to give those closest to them the opportunity to offer their support. They have found it easier, in the long run, to confide their fears and hopes rather than trying to hide them. Of course, you must use the words and timing that you find comfortable to tell family and friends that you have cancer. We will talk more about that in the next chapter.

If you have no family, it is especially true that the road appears less lonely when shared with a few close friends. You might lose one or two. Some people will find it too difficult to talk with you or to be around you, and they will slip away. On the other hand, you may discover hidden strengths and compassion in the least likely of companions.

A woman with cancer wrote, "As for whether or not people should keep their illness a secret, I think they will learn whom they can talk to. Some people make themselves scarce if cancer is mentioned. But, cancer patients soon learn who their trusted friends are."

Another person said, "I don't think a cancer patient should keep it to himself. If it isn't revealed, family and friends are robbed of the opportunity to share the feelings and anxieties that arise from having the disease. At most, life is very short for everyone. Since there are no guarantees, we should make the most of each day."

On a practical level, trying to hide the diagnosis is usually fruitless. As you move from hope to despair and back again, family and close friends will sense something is deeply troubling you, even

576

before they learn the facts. When you feel ready, try to share your news with them.

As you ponder whether you can share the diagnosis of cancer with others, it might help to remember the following. In telling the people you love that you have cancer, you give them the opportunity to express their feelings, to voice their fears and hopes and to offer their hand in support. Then, each can give and take strength as they are able.

When Family Must Decide

Sometimes family members are the first to learn the diagnosis. If, as a family member, the decision falls to you, should you tell the patient? Some might think not, but most people with cancer disagree. "I think a cancer patient should be told the truth," one wrote. "Time is so valuable, and there may be things the person would like to accomplish. There are decisions to be made . . ."

All of us have important life choices to make. People with cancer often find these choices become crystal clear when they feel their life span could be cut short. They might outlive any one of us, but people with cancer have the right to know and to decide how they will spend their remaining days. There are exceptions to any generalization, but most people relate that "Mom took the news much better than we thought she would."

A woman who herself has cancer recalled how things have changed since her mother was diagnosed in 1930. "My relatives never told my mother that she had cancer. Of course, then, they didn't have the treatment they have available now. Looking back I realize no one fooled her. In not telling her, though, she was deprived of a very valuable outlet for her emotions."

Family members also bear great emotional burdens during the period of diagnosis. They, too, need the comfort of sharing their feelings. Yet, it is almost impossible to support the rest of the family if you are hiding the diagnosis from the person with cancer. He or she inevitably learns the truth. The consequences can be deep anger, hurt or bitterness. The patient might believe that no one is being honest about the diagnosis because the cancer is terminal. On the other hand, while you are trying to "spare the patient," the person with cancer might be trying to protect family and friends from learning the truth.

Then each ends up suffering alone, with thoughts and feelings locked within.

Somehow Children Know

Even children sense the truth. Some parents who tried to "spare" their children from knowing later voiced regret at not discussing the truth during the course of the disease. Children have amazing capabilities when they understand a situation. However, when their normal world is turned upside down and whispered conversations go on behind closed doors, they often imagine situations that are worse than reality. Young children dwell on "terrible" things *they* have done or said that place responsibility for the upheaval in the household on themselves. This is especially true if the child is going through a period of testing parental authority or in some other way is in disagreement with family members. Children—especially young ones—tend to view themselves as the center of the universe and see many situations only in direct relationship to themselves.

The children's ages and emotional maturity should suggest what and how much to disclose. It might help to realize that including the children among those who know comforts them by confirming their belief that something is amiss within the family.

A parent with cancer might want to tell the children directly. "I've been sick a lot lately, haven't I? I have a disease called cancer. The doctors are doing everything they can to make me well. I can't spend so much time with you as I want to; it's going to be hard on all of us, but I still love you very much."

Perhaps this is too painful. A close and loving aunt or uncle or friend might be able to explain things more comfortably. "Your daddy is ill. The doctors are almost sure they can make him well, but sometimes his treatments make him feel sad or grouchy. It's nothing you kids have done, but he needs your patience and understanding."

The goal in telling the children that someone in the family has cancer is to give them opportunities to ask questions about the disease and to express their feelings about it. Of course, all of us want to shield our children from pain, but pain they understand is easier for them to cope with than hurts that they imagine. Some adults tell us that they still remember the feelings of rejection they suffered as children of cancer patients. As children they were aware of great disruption within the family, but at the time they were denied knowledge of the cause. They were hurt and confused by what seemed to be lack of attention and unreasonable demands or expectations.

Sharing Mutual Support

We begin to see that the most compelling reason for sharing the diagnosis with adults and children alike is that cancer can be so terribly lonely. No one need try to bear it alone. At times you will feel totally without ally or solace, regardless of supports. There is no need to increase these moments with poses meant to convince others close to you that you do not need their help. At a time when each of us who is trying to cope with cancer is in need of mutual support, we should not shut each other out. Through sharing we can build foundations of mutual understanding to sustain us through the long period ahead. We can share anxiety and sorrow, but we also can share love and joy and express our appreciation for each other in ways we ordinarily might find difficult or embarrassing.

Sharing Feelings

- Some in the family are able to absorb the impact of diagnosis sooner than others. This can create clashing needs as some wish to talk and some need to be private and introspective.

- Verbal and nonverbal clues help determine when is a good time to discuss the illness and how each will learn to live with it.

- If family members cannot help each other, other emotional support systems are available in the form of groups or professional counselors.

- The person with cancer has the primary right to set the timetable for when he or she is ready to talk. Others can encourage that readiness through their love and continued presence.

- Talking may include expressing anger, fear and inner confusion.

- False cheeriness—the "everything will be all right" routine—denies the person with cancer the opportunity to discuss fears and anxieties.

- Emphasizing the uniqueness of each person, positive test results or good response to treatment is true support, both valid and valuable.

- The person with cancer needs family or friends as a constant in a changing world. "I'm here," offers great reserves of support.

S ometimes, the whole family suspects the truth before the diagnosis is made. Someone recognizes the symptoms, or the family doctor seems overly concerned. Nonetheless, hearing those words—tumor . . . cancer . . . leukemia—we are stunned as we never may have been in our lives. It is often impossible to take in the diagnosis immediately. We hear it, but somehow we don't believe it. This is normal. People's minds have a wonderful capacity for absorbing information only as they are ready to accept it.

Emotional Timetables

All of us may not operate on the same emotional timetable. One of the family might feel the need to talk about the cancer before the others come to grips with it. Each of us has to decide when we are ready to talk; none should feel forced to do so.

This sometimes creates clashing needs—some need to talk; others need to be private and introspective or even to shut the whole subject out of their minds for a while. The desire to respect privacy may be pitted against an equal need to get the whole thing out in the open.

In some families everyone becomes overly considerate of everyone else's needs for time to adjust. Instead of meeting anyone's needs, everyone avoids one another, building walls just when they ought to be opening doors to communication.

It is important to let the person who has cancer call the signals for when it's time to talk. But, it is always helpful to look for clues to determine when might be a good time to discuss the cancer and how to live with it.

Signs such as apparently idle conversation, more time than usual spent with other family members, or even unusual nervousness might indicate that a person wants to talk but doesn't know where to begin. Yet, facing cancer together makes it easier. It eliminates the need for pretense when there are so many important matters to get on with. As you talk, you should try to be sensitive to what family members or friends say, how they position their bodies, and whether or not they make eye contact. These clues suggest whether the conversation is serving a purpose or driving someone you care about into hiding.

Some people cannot adjust their feelings and cannot help each other. Not all families can be open and sharing, and a crisis is a difficult time to be adjusting family patterns. Nonetheless, the situation may not eliminate the need to air feelings. This is the time to turn to one of several sources outside the family for emotional support. These are described in the chapter "When You Need Assistance."

Consider Your Needs

When cancer is first diagnosed, some people can absorb only the most basic information, and even that might need to be repeated. That's normal. We each have the right to digest information and to determine when we are ready for more, when we are ready to talk about what we know or want to know.

If others in the family want to talk about cancer before you are ready, try to postpone the discussion without rejecting the person. "I appreciate your concern but not yet. I can't talk yet," for example, suggests that the day will come when you will be ready to talk. Taking care of your own needs, which are great, while trying to recognize the fears and anxieties of those you love is not easy, it's true.

The period right after diagnosis is often a time of anger, fear and inner confusion. You might need to sort out conflicting emotions before you can express them. Or, you might find yourself lashing out, wishing to find a target for anger and frustration. Often it is those closest who bear the brunt of these outbursts. You don't want to hurt them, but you may be angry that they will live and you might die. Perhaps you assume that they will understand and endure the rage.

Family members have feelings, too. They may lash back, express-ing their own anger and hurt at your outbursts, at the possibility of losing you, at the burden of new responsibilities or at their powerless-ness to change the reality of the disease. As you express your own feelings, try to remember that others need the same release.

The Family Adjusts

The period following diagnosis is a difficult time of adjustment for family members. Each has to deal with individual feelings, while trying to be sensitive to those of the person who has cancer. Being part of the family doesn't mean you can make people talk about their feelings before they are ready, but you need outlets, too. There are ways to encourage openness. Be ready to listen when others are ready to talk, and let your continued presence show your support. But re-member, the person with cancer gets to set the timetable.

If the decision is to talk, you may find yourself the target for a lot of anger and frustration. It is easier to *tell* yourself that you are not the cause of this hostility than it is to *accept* this. You know you should respond with patience and compassion, but sometimes you answer anger with anger. Even these exchanges can have value if everyone learns through them to share feelings.

The opposite of anger may be false cheer. In trying to bolster the person with cancer, you may actually cut off his or her attempts to express feelings. Remember that lifting the spirit doesn't mean hiding from the truth. Sensing despondency, some people rush in with assurances that "everything will be all right." But everything is not "all right." If you insist it is, you deny the reality of the patient's world. In response, he or she may withdraw, feeling deserted and left to face an uncertain world alone. Without meaning to, you've abandoned the one you hoped to help and set up patterns that can be difficult to change just when support is so important. Although the cancer may be controlled, the gulf between you may endure.

It may help the one with cancer to know that you share the same fears and anxieties about the uncertainty of the future. People who honestly share these feelings find they can hold them to the light, better accept that the future may be questionable, and turn more readily to fulfilling the present. This is a very difficult period, but if you can share the difficulties, you will find there are more good days to enjoy together. And you are less likely to be devastated by truly difficult ones.

Finding Hope

There are ways to find hope during periods of despondency or despair. We all need to remember the individuality of each case. We tend to get caught up in statistics and averages, but no two cancers ever behave exactly the same way. Each individual has different genes and an immune system, a distinctive will to live and an urge to fight. These cannot be measured on charts or graphs. No one can offer any of us "forever," but there are good prognoses; with an increasing number of cancers, the outlook is good for a lifetime free of disease. You can look to promising test results and to treatments that have been effective in many people before. Even if the future is guarded, there may be another remission, good days, comfortable nights and shared experiences. These are real beyond any statistics. The enjoyment of life's gifts constitutes living, not the number of days we are given in which to enjoy them.

There are safeguards against hopelessness even if there is no real cause for hope. You can still provide reassurance of continuing love and comfort. At times, "I'm here" may be the two most supportive words you can say.

Listening, Sharing, Being Yourself

There are different ways in which you can be important as a family member or friend. You can listen to expressions of feeling or act as a sounding board for a discussion of future plans. You can help focus anger or anxiety by helping to explore the specific causes—drug reactions, the job situation, finances and so forth. This may be what is needed—someone to listen, to react and absorb the patient's outpourings, not necessarily to "do" anything. It is a difficult role, but it can be immensely rewarding.

There is a more passive but equally difficult role. Some cancer patients view theirs as a private battle to be fought alone with only their physicians as allies, and they prefer to fight their emotional battles alone as well. But they need family and friends for silent support, as respite, shelter or an island of normality. It can be draining to provide "safe harbor" from a day in the clinic or nights of sleepless panic. It can be a struggle to be forced to plan an evening out, to ask friends in or simply to stand by with wordless support. However, there may be times when this is what is needed most.

Many people think they don't know "how to act" with people with cancer. The best you can offer is to be natural, to be yourself. Let your intuition guide you. Do what you comfortably can do; don't try to be someone you are not. This in itself is comforting. Dealing with cancer entails enough mystifying changes without having to adapt to a new you.

Coping Within the Family

• Cancer is a blow to every family it touches. How it is handled is determined to a great extent by how the family has functioned as a unit in the past.

• Problems within the family can be the most difficult to handle; you cannot go home to escape them.

• Adjusting to role changes can cause great upheavals in the way family members interact.

• Performing too many roles at once endangers anyone's emotional well-being and ability to cope. Examine what tasks are necessary and let others slide.

• Consider hiring professional nurses or homemakers. Financial costs need to be weighed against the physical and emotional cost of shouldering the load alone.

• Children may need special attention. They need comfort, reassurance, affection, guidance and discipline at times of disruption in their routine.

Although cancer has "come out of the closet," much of what we read in newspapers and magazines is about the disease itself—its probable causes or new methods of treatment. There is little information about how families deal with cancer on a day-to-day basis. This gap reinforces feelings that families coping with cancer are isolated from the rest of the world: that everyone else is managing nicely while you flounder with your feelings, hide from your spouse and are incapable of talking to the children.

Cancer is a blow to every family it touches. How you handle it is determined to a great extent by how you have functioned as a family in the past. Families who are used to sharing their feelings with each other usually are able to talk about the disease and the changes it brings. Families in which each member solves problems alone or in which one person has played the major role in making decisions might have more difficulty coping.

Not Everyone Can

Problems within the family can be the most difficult to handle simply because you cannot go home to escape them. Some family members deny the reality of cancer or refuse to discuss it.

It is not uncommon to feel deserted or to feel unable to face cancer openly. "My brother-in-law is suffering from cancer," one man confided. "The entire situation is depressing, and my reaction has been one of running and hiding. I have not visited them for I feel I have nothing to offer."

A woman with cancer found none of her family could help her. "My two wonderful sons tolerated their dad's heart surgeries very well, but now I have cancer, and they don't know how to act. Phone calls and letters expressing sympathy are not what I need. I've tried since last November to express my thoughts to my husband, but he shuts out what I'm saying. I know that he's uncertain about our future, but I can't seem to get through to him; I've learned it's a common complaint."

In these situations individual counseling or cancer patient groups can provide needed support and reinforcement. Moreover, these resources provide an outlet for the frustrations you are facing within the family.

Changing Roles

Families may have difficulty adjusting to the role changes that are sometimes necessary. One husband found it overwhelming to come home from work, prepare dinner, oversee the children's homework, change bedding and dressings and still try to provide companionship

586

and emotional support for his children and ill wife.

In addition to roles as wife, mother and nurse, a woman might have to add a job outside the home for the first time. A spouse who was sharing the load sometimes becomes the sole breadwinner and homemaker. The usual head of the household might now be its most dependent member.

These changes can cause great upheavals in the ways members of the family interact. The usual patterns are gone. Parents might look to children for emotional support at a time when the children themselves need it most. Teenagers might have to take over major household responsibilities. Young children can revert to infantile behavior as a way of dealing with the impact of cancer on the family as a unit and on themselves as individuals. The sheer weight of responsibility can become insurmountable, destroying normal family associations, devouring time needed for rest and recreation, and depriving family members of wholesome opportunities for expressing anxiety and resentment.

The Health of the Family

Performing too many roles at once can endanger emotional well-being and the ability to cope. Examining what's important can solve the problem. For example, you can relax housekeeping standards or learn to prepare simpler meals. Perhaps the children can take on a few more household chores than they have been handling.

If a simple solution is not enough, consider getting outside help. Licensed practical nurses can help with the patient; county or private agencies might provide trained homemakers. If outreach is an important part of your church, feel free to ask for help with cooking, shopping, transportation and other homemaking tasks. One family was adopted by the daughter's Scout troop when the girls learned of the extra responsibility she had assumed. Everyone benefited from the relationship.

Let someone who can be objective help you sort out necessary tasks from those that can go undone. The financial cost of professional services needs to be weighed against the emotional and physical cost of shouldering the load alone. It is important to remember that the family is still a unit. If the family strength is sapped, the patient suffers, too.

The San Diego chapter of Make Today Count, a mutual support group for patients and families, compiled a "Bill of Rights for the Friends and Relatives of Cancer Patients." Several items address the problems of family burdens:

o *The relative of a cancer patient has the right and obligation to take care of his own needs. Even though he may be accused of being selfish, he must do what he has to do to keep his own peace of mind, so that he can better minister to the needs of the patient.*

o *Each person will have different needs . . . These needs must be satisfied. The patient will benefit, too, by having a more cheerful person to care for him.*

o *The relative may need help from outsiders in caring for the patient. Although the patient may object to this, the relative has the right to assess his own limitations of strength and endurance and to obtain assistance when required.*

o *. . . When the relative knows that he is already doing all that can reasonably be expected of anyone in caring for the patient, he can have a clear conscience in maintaining contacts with the rest of the world.*

o *If the patient attempts to use his illness as a weapon, the relative has the right to reject that and to do only what can reasonably be expected of him.*

o *If the cancer patient's relative responds only to the genuine needs of the moment—both his own needs and those of the patient—the stress associated with the illness can be minimized.*

o Increased burdens and shifting responsibilities can occur whether the patient in the household is a spouse, a child or an elderly parent. Each family member must take care to meet his or her own needs and those of the other healthy members of the family as well as those of the patient.

Help for the Children

Children might have difficulty coping with cancer in a parent. Mother or Dad may be gone from the house—in a hospital that may be hundreds of miles from home—or home in bed, in obvious discomfort, and perhaps visibly altered in appearance.

In the face of this upheaval, children often are asked also to behave exceptionally well: to "play quietly," to perform extra tasks or to be understanding of others' moods beyond the maturity of their years. The children may resent lost attention. Some fear the loss of their parent or begin to imagine their own death. Some children, formerly independent, now become anxious about leaving home and parents. Discipline problems can arise if children attempt to command the attention they feel they are missing.

It may help if a favorite relative or family friend can devote extra time and attention to the children, who do need comfort and reassurance, affection, guidance and discipline. Trips to the zoo are important, but so is regular help with homework and someone to attend the basketball awards banquet. If your efforts to provide support and security fail, professional counseling for child, or child and parent together, may be necessary and should not be overlooked.

When You Need Assistance

- When cancer develops, many people need to learn to ask for and accept outside help for the first time. These are good ways to begin:

- Don't be afraid to ask medical questions of your doctor, nurse specialists, therapists and technologists.

- Make lists of questions. Write out or tape-record the answers. Take someone else along as a second listener.

- Ask your physician about unorthodox treatments if you have questions about them.

- Physicians wait for clues from their patients to determine how much to say. Let your doctor know whether you want to know everything at once or in easy stages.

- Remember that there is a difference between a physician who does not know that cancer need not be fatal and one who will not promise you a miracle.

- Trust and rapport between patient and physician are important; you must be able to work together to treat the cancer most effectively.

- Your physician, hospital, library, local chapters of the American Cancer Society, American Lung Association, Leukemia Society of America, the National Cancer Institute or affiliated Cancer Information Service offices are good sources of facts about cancer. Many also can provide the names of local support and service organizations established to help you cope with the emotional stresses of the disease.

- Emotional assistance takes many forms. Counseling or psychiatric therapy for individuals, for groups of patients and for families often is available through the hospital or within the community.

- Many groups have been established by patients and their families to share practical tips and coping skills. One may be right for you.

- Your minister or rabbi, a sympathetic member of the congregation or a specially trained pastoral counselor may be able to help you find spiritual support.

Which one of us did not feel that the world had stopped turning when cancer struck us? But somehow each day goes on. During the period of active treatment a pressing number of decisions need to be made, questions must be answered and arrangements handled.

There are medical questions. There might be confusion or disagreement over the diagnosis—what did the doctor say; what do various terms mean; what is the outlook for recovery?

Financial burdens can be crushing. Transportation to and from treatment can seem a major, frustrating obstacle. Where does one get a hospital bed, a night nurse, a person to look after the children?

The stress of handling such responsibilities can be enormous. A new kind of communication and acceptance becomes necessary: asking for and accepting outside help, which is an entirely new role for some. People who were raised to believe that "going it alone" indicated maturity and strength now might have to overcome their distaste for appearing to be in anything less than total control.

Some simply do not know where to turn. You might feel uncomfortable asking for help—even from those agencies that were designed precisely for emergencies such as you now face. So, where do you turn?

The Health Care Team

Physicians or nurses are good sources of answers to medical questions. It's helpful to write down on a sheet of paper all questions you have about cancer, its treatment, any side effects from it or any limitations treatment may place on your activities. (Incidentally, there may be surprisingly few limitations other than those caused by changes in physical capability.) Other members of your treatment team—physical therapists, nutritionists, radiation technologists and such can explain the "Whys" of these aspects of your therapy.

Writing questions down makes them easier to remember at the next doctor's appointment. It's also helpful to call the office beforehand to alert the receptionist that you will need extra time for your appointment. This time around you can be better prepared to retain the answers. Some people take notes, some a tape recorder, some a clear thinking friend or relative. The point is to depend on something more reliable than your own memory at a time when emotions are likely to overwhelm intellect.

Asking Important Questions

Fear of being thought ignorant or pushy has kept many people

from asking their doctors about a most important topic—the unorthodox treatments they read about in the tabloids or hear about from
friends. You may be urged by well-meaning people to try methods
that will "spare you any pain or discomfort." Yet they are never available through your cancer specialist. If you are being pressured to aban-
don the care you are now getting, but haven't discussed it with your
doctor because you think you will insult "establishment medicine,"
you might try this approach. "I keep hearing about the bubblegum
treatment for cancer. Can you tell me why it isn't accepted by most
American doctors? Why do some people think it works, and why do
you believe it won't?"

What you have asked for is information. You haven't attacked
the treatment you are getting now or the professionals who are giving
it to you. And if you are comfortable with the answers you get, it will
help you respond when you are urged to try these methods.

Too many fail to ask the medical questions most important to
their physical and emotional well-being through a fear of "taking up
the doctor's valuable time." Some say, "I'm sure he told me all this
once before." Of course, you want to be a "good" patient or a
"cooperative" family member! But it's also true: It's your body. It's
your life. It's also true that a well-informed patient is better able to
understand his or her therapy, its possible side effects or any unusual
signs that should be reported to the doctor.

A good approach can be simply to admit that you are asking for
a repeat performance. "I'm pretty sure you told me some of this before, but I couldn't remember anything; I was so shocked. Now, I
think I'd feel less anxious if we talked about it."

Some are ready to hold this conversation sooner than others.
Some ask a few questions at a time, absorbing each piece of information before they are ready to go on. Some never ask directly. (If so,
someone in the family should speak with the doctor to learn the extent of disease and the outlook for the future.) But sooner or later, in
whatever way you find comfortable, it's important to let the doctor
know that you understand you have cancer and want to talk about it.

In an ideal world, physicians all would be patient, understanding
and able to sense your every mood. They would know when to bring
out all the X-ray films and lab tests and when to draw only the sketch-
iest picture of your case. They would have unlimited time to wait
until *you* were ready to ask questions, and then they would gently help
you to phrase them in just the right way.

As a matter of fact, books for cancer specialists—physicians, nurses, therapists—and courses in the health professional schools are beginning to emphasize the importance of recognizing the feelings of the person with cancer. Nonetheless, each person is different, and no textbook can describe your unique needs.

In the real world physicians admit that they wait for clues from you, the person with cancer. *They* need to know what the patient wants to know. Physicians are not mind readers. Whether you like it or not, it is usually up to you to take the first steps toward open communication with your doctor.

Changing Doctors

Some physicians have never learned to speak comfortably with patients or families who are facing what might be a life-threatening illness. These physicians may appear to be abrupt, aloof and uncaring, although they are not. Nonetheless, if their discomfort creates a barrier, you might be wise to seek referral to someone else. When fighting cancer you have to work as a team. Lack of trust is fair neither to you nor to the doctor. It is fair, however, to let the doctor know you wish to see someone else—even to ask him or her for a referral. The physician probably is as aware as you that a relationship based on trust and open communication has not been established.

It is also appropriate to ask your physician to suggest other doctors if you wish a second opinion on the diagnosis before deciding on treatment.

There still might be a physician here or there who believes that all cancer is fatal and that "nothing can be done." In such a case it is only common sense to ask for referral to a cancer specialist.

Most family physicians practicing now know that nearly half the patients who get cancer today will live out their lives free of further disease, and others can be provided an extended time of reasonable comfort and activity. While continuing as the personal physician, they usually will refer their patients to cancer specialists—surgeons, radiologists or medical oncologists—for active treatment. (It's something like an orchestra conductor calling on the soloists while keeping the whole orchestra playing together.)

You need to be honest with yourself and recognize the difference between a physician who believes all cancer is fatal and one who believes the outlook for a particular case is not good. Refusing to promise complete cure is not the same as forsaking the patient.

A physician who uses all available methods to treat the disease, to minimize its effects, and to keep you comfortable and functioning as long as possible is doing everything he or she can to care for your physical needs. How frustrating it is, then, when you seek to relieve your emotional aches and pains, to be rebuffed by the same otherwise excellent specialist. As one man put it, "I found it impossible to discuss the nitty-gritty facts with my doctors and the radiation therapist. I felt that if I told the radiologist how fearful I was, I would be considered childish." Nonetheless, a decision to change physicians should be based on reality and not on a quest to find a doctor who will promise a cure and guarantee to relieve all your fears.

Information Resources

It's easier to come to grips with the reality of any crisis if we replace ignorance with information. There is much to learn about each form of cancer, its treatment, the possibility for recovery and methods of rehabilitation. Well-versed in the facts, you are less likely to fall prey to old wives' tales, to quacks touting worthless "cures" or to depressing stories of what happened to "poor old Harry" when he got cancer. Often, the more you know, the less you have to fear.

Local libraries, local divisions of voluntary agencies such as the American Cancer Society or the Leukemia Society of America, and major cancer research and treatment institutions are sources of information about cancer and its treatment. Depending on the degree of your desire for information and your ability to understand scientific terms, you can get everything from short, concise pamphlets to scientific papers. It's a good idea to share the fruits of your research with your own doctor. Cancer is a complex set of diseases; the treatment and its side effects may differ slightly for each person.

On a national level, the National Cancer Institute (NCI), which is part of the National Institutes of Health, operates an information office for the public. Its information specialists can answer many general questions about cancer, its diagnosis and treatment. In addition, the NCI coordinates a network of information offices among the nation's top cancer research and treatment centers. Cancer Information Service (CIS) counselors can provide the names of facilities that are most appropriate in terms of both geography and specialization. They also have written materials and information about local self-help and service organizations for cancer patients and their families.

The NCI specialists also maintain lists of excellent cancer hospitals outside the CIS network that are conducting federally funded research in new methods of cancer treatment. They can suggest not only institutions but also specialists with whom your own physician might wish to consult. However, information staff members cannot offer medical advice or arrange for referral to a specific physician or institution.

The names, addresses and phone numbers of the sources of information described in this section can be found in the appendix at the end of this book.

Emotional Assistance

It is said that we cope with cancer much as we cope with other problems that confront us. Many do come to terms with the reality of cancer. After initial treatment, they find somehow they are able to continue their normal working and social relationships. Or, as one psychologist put it, they learn to get up in the morning and pour the coffee, even knowing that they have cancer. They find, sometimes to their amazement, that they can laugh at bad jokes, can become totally absorbed in a good movie or a hard-fought football game.

At other times, strength deserts them. They feel overwhelmed by this new world of uncertainties. Some lose interest in favorite hobbies or activities, viewing them as painful reminders of what will be lost if treatment is unsuccessful. They want to cope, but they need help, some support systems beyond their own. Where does one look for such support?

At the Hospital

It was not very long ago that emotional assistance for the cancer patient or family was impossible to find. Attention to emotional needs is a relatively recent addition to standard cancer treatment. Growing numbers of hospitals routinely include a mental health professional as a member of the cancer treatment team or offer group counseling programs. This is a hopeful sign; it says, "This diagnosis does not mean imminent death. We have a whole person to treat here, one with a future and a life to live. This person should be able to live as normally as possible. We must provide the emotional tools to get the job done."

Counseling also is now available for health professionals to help them face feelings of frustration and uncertainty in their work. They have recognized the awesome degree of stress that cancer can create in those it touches. You should have no feelings of shame or hesitancy, then, if you feel the need to seek professional help.

Some hospitals consider some form of **group counseling** as part of the standard treatment—as necessary as an exercise class, for example. Programs are organized in a variety of ways. Many begin within days of surgery. Some groups meet only for the length of the hospital stay; others are long-term to enable members to work through problems in the everyday world. Some are composed of people with the same disease site (breast or colon cancer patients); some by type of treatment (in-hospital surgery or outpatient radiation therapy); and some by patient age. Some are just for patients; others include spouses, family or other special people.

Groups can incorporate music, poetry or role-playing in attempts to help members explore their feelings. Some are action-oriented with "veteran" patients helping others now facing the same problem. All counseling groups should be run by trained professionals so that the direction of exploration is truly helpful to each participant.

In the Community

If you want to explore your feelings in **individual therapy,** you will find a growing number of psychologists, psychiatrists or psychiatric social workers specializing in counseling people affected by cancer. Many find it helpful to explore feelings—especially those they don't want to accept, such as guilt, resentment and intense anger—with a person who, without judgment, will help them understand these feelings and find ways to channel them constructively.

Often the problem is not an individual one. The family is a unit, and each member is affected when any one member is. **Family counseling** can help absorb the shock and deal with the stresses of cancer.

It can be difficult for persons with cancer and their family members to discuss their emotions. Cancer patients themselves have tagged the absence of open communication within their families as a major problem. People are particularly hesitant to express negative feelings when no one is "at fault." Yet major shifts in responsibilities such as those cancer brings to a family can cause great resentment by those shouldering (or incapable of shouldering) extra burdens. A loss of accustomed responsibility or authority also can cause resentment mingled with anxiety over a loss of power.

Children, especially, find that their usual roles no longer are defined clearly. Parents may not have the emotional energy to provide the usual support, love and authority. Teenagers can feel torn between expressing independence and a need to remain close to the sick parent.

These problems become less difficult to face if the family can discuss them. Some can do this without outside help. Those who cannot should feel comfortable in seeking professional assistance.

Your physician, a hospital social worker or hospital psychologist are good sources for referrals to psychologists, psychiatrists or other mental health professionals trained to counsel individuals and families affected by cancer. Many county health departments include psychological services, and neighborhood or community mental health clinics are becoming common in increasing numbers of cities. Community service organizations such as the United Way usually support mental health facilities. County government listings in the telephone book may include an "Information and Referral" listing, one more resource for counseling services.

Helping Each Other

There are numerous **self-help** groups organized by people like you and designed to help you overcome both the practical problems of cancer and the feelings these changes cause. Some groups are local chapters of national organizations; others are strictly "grass roots." Some are only for patients; others include family members.

These organizations shun a "pity me" approach. They exist to help you work through your feelings and frustrations. Whether you accept them or change them, you can do so within the framework of a supportive group of people who know firsthand the problems you are wrestling with.

Some offer family members an opportunity to share feelings, fears and anxieties with others bearing similar burdens. Some provide patients a place to express negative feelings which they don't want to unload on their families. Patients without families can speak openly and release their pent-up emotions without fear of taxing existing friendships.

Some support groups provide skills training and helpful tips for special sets of patients such as those who have had a laryngectomy, ostomy or mastectomy. Organizations designed to offer emotional support nonetheless can provide opportunities to exchange practical information, such as how to control nausea from chemotherapy or how to talk to an employer about cancer.

A self-help group can give those recovered from cancer an opportunity to aid those who follow. With training, some become group counselors or discussion leaders. Many former cancer patients have found that helping others gives a marvelous and oft-needed boost to their own self-esteem. (That can be so important after a long stretch of feeling dependent on and at the mercy of physicians and hospital staff.)

Mutual assistance groups sometimes work with health professionals and the clergy to help them understand the special emotional needs of people with cancer.

The names of mutual support or rehabilitation groups with a national office are listed in the appendix.

Spiritual Support

Religion is a source of strength for some people. Some find new faith in their divine being and new hope from their sacred writings when cancer enters their lives. Others find the ordeal of disease strengthens their faith, or that faith gives them new-found strength. Others never have had strong religious beliefs and feel no urge to turn to religion at such a time.

Members of the clergy in increasing numbers are completing programs to help them minister more effectively to people with cancer and their families.

Individual pastors can provide hope and solace, but they vary, as do physicians and lay people, in their capacity to cope with life-threatening illnesses and the possibility of death. A religious leader untrained in illness counseling nonetheless may refer you to an associate trained to work with people with cancer. He or she also might introduce you to another member of the congregation who can provide comfort and, perhaps, more time on a regular basis than the leader of a congregation can spare.

Selves and Self-Images

- Cancer treatment can extend over weeks or months; side effects may come and go.

- Side effects can make you feel rotten, even make you think the cancer has returned.

- The known is less frightening than the unknown. Learn about your cancer, its treatment, any possible side effects and how to treat them.

- Fears and anxieties caused by cancer can affect a sexual relationship. Remember: Cancer is not catching. Remember, also, cancer or other chronic illnesses are rarely the cause for infidelity in a good relationship.

- Treatment might make you feel uncomfortable about your body and sexually unattractive. Open discussion of these feelings with your mate is very important.

- Intangible personal qualities make up a great part of your attraction for your mate. These have not changed with treatment.

- Spouses sometimes hesitate to initiate physical contact. Support, love and affection do include hugs and caresses. These may lead the partner with cancer to feel more comfortable about sexual intimacy.

- Physical exercise improves bodily self-image and feelings of well-being.

- Taking on new hobbies and learning new skills can bolster your good feelings about yourself.

- Reconstructive surgery and well-made prostheses help some people overcome physical disabilities and emotional distress.

- If you cannot seem to regain good feelings about yourself, do seek professional counseling or therapy.

- If your relationship is endangered by the stress of cancer, get professional help. You need each other at this time.

When Treatment Brings You Down

Cancer treatment is nearly always aggressive. Surgery can be disfiguring. Radiation or drug treatment may be prescribed following surgery to ensure that no hidden, microscopic cancer cells are left to travel to other parts of the body. Treatment can extend over weeks or months, and its side-effects can include nausea, hair loss, fatigue, cramps, skin burns or weight changes. It is not unusual for the treatment to cause more illness or discomfort than the initial disease. The cancer patient has to contend with emotional reactions to such treatment and side-effects.

It is difficult to convince yourself that you are recovering when you feel absolutely rotten. It is hard to be optimistic when you feel worse now than at the time of diagnosis. The schedule of radiation or drug treatments may seem endless. You are convinced that there never was a day when you didn't feel awful; there never will be one when you will feel normal—if only you could remember how normal feels.

Some even interpret these physical reactions to treatment as signs that the cancer is returning. This is rarely the case, although it may be necessary to remind yourself of this fact again and again. Feel comfortable in sharing such anxieties with your doctor.

A return to the hospital setting for outpatient treatment causes anxiety for some. Researchers studied a group of women undergoing radiation therapy following breast cancer surgery. They found that the women felt better psychologically immediately after leaving the hospital after surgery than they did once followup treatment began. It can be unsettling, indeed, to return again and again to the hospital or physician's office, places which may have come to represent the most frightening aspects of cancer.

You can try to plan special activities for the days when you feel well and brace yourself for the days when you feel awful. It's helpful to others and easier for you if you inform people that treatment may cause shifts in moods. You can let them know matter-of-factly that you will have up days and down days.

The known is usually easier to cope with than the unknown. It is important to be familiar with each treatment's side-effects and its causes. Not only does knowledge reduce fear, but some side-effects can be eliminated (or at least eased) through treatment changes, medication or changes in diet. There is no need to be more uncomfortable than is absolutely necessary. Written materials with information on what to expect in the way of side-effects from treatment usually are available from your physician or treatment center. However, the best way to obtain accurate information about your own situation is through a frank and thorough discussion with the nurse or physician administering treatment.

This brings us back to the problem of busy, unresponsive health professionals. If your physician has been less than helpful, try one of the information resources or special support groups referred to in the previous chapter. Ask one more nurse, one more oncology resident. As one of our "expert patients" wrote, "Look for assistance wherever you have to when you need it. It's a mistake to give up when rebuffed or disregarded by any one individual. There is always a source of comfort somewhere. One has only to look for it." Comfort and, we might add, information.

What About Sex?

The problems and emotional stresses of cancer might follow you into the bedroom. Some couples arrange the financial matters and handle the day-to-day tasks, only to find that sexual problems threaten their relationship. There are a variety of reasons for such problems.

A few people still have the mistaken belief that cancer is contagious. One man complained, "My wife won't kiss me anymore. She thinks cancer is catching." Fact: Cancer is not catching. If your mate believes it is, call your physician. You may feel embarrassed discussing sex, but this is too important a problem to let modesty stand in the way of a solution.

Infidelity, or more likely fear of it, can present a problem. Exploring these fears with your mate is probably the best way to deal with them. If you admit that you are plagued by uncertainty and insecurity, you probably will receive the needed support and affection and can lay your doubts to rest.

Some cancer patients cite disfiguring treatment as a cause of sexual problems. You need to deal not only with discomfort or disability but also with what this change in your body has done to your feelings about yourself. As awkward as it may seem, you need to find ways to communicate those feelings to your partner. An inability to express them may complicate an already difficult period.

Body Images

Each of us develops over the years an image in our mind about our body. We may not be completely satisfied with that image, but usually we are comfortable with it when with someone we love. This helps us feel sexually attractive to our mate. Disfigurement, hair loss, nausea, radiation burns—even fatigue—can destroy your good feelings about your physical appeal. If you now believe you are unattractive, you might anticipate rejection and avoid physical contact with your partner. It is well to remember that in most cases your partner is more concerned about your well-being than his or her own. The overriding reactions probably begin with, "Will treatment succeed?" "How can I show my love and support?" . . . and, only finally, "What about sex?"

In reality, your partner may be afraid to appear overeager and therefore insensitive. So it may be up to you to show a desire for physical contact and to let it be known whether you are interested in sexual intercourse as well as other expressions of affection—hugging, caressing and kissing.

It might help to keep in mind that it's not only your body that makes you "sexy." There are also intangible qualities that your mate finds attractive. A sense of humor, intellect, a certain sweetness or great common sense, special talents, loving devotion—each of us knows what makes us special; and it's more than anatomy. If you feel you have lost those special qualities along with a breast or leg or prostate gland, counseling may help you change that perspective.

Rebuilding Mind and Body

Time, along with demonstrations of love, understanding and affection by your partner and family should help you work through feelings about your changed body image. In addition, some find that physical activities—sports, dancing classes, exercise or judo—improve their sense of being in touch with their bodies. A ballet teacher who has had a mastectomy is teaching other women the feeling of grace and balance that comes from dance.

"After I took up yoga," another woman exclaimed with some surprise, "I achieved a sense of wholeness about my body—even without one breast—that I had never had before."

People who take on a challenging activity that moves them beyond a disability—skiing for amputees for example—find it can provide a whole new sense of self-worth. "Can you believe, I have more pride in this ragged body than I did when it was all there?" asked a tennis ace, who took up the game after his colostomy.

Poetry, music, painting, furniture building, sewing and reading provide creative growth of which you can be equally proud. If anything needs strengthening it is our personal self image. Acquiring new interests and talents can help develop that strength.

Physical Restoration

Reconstructive surgery or cosmetic and functional prostheses (artificial devices) help some people with cancer overcome both physical disabilities and emotional distress from disfiguring surgery. A small but growing body of skilled craftsmen build prostheses for people who have had radical oral and facial surgery. These lifelike pieces enable people to go out in public again with some degree of emotional comfort. For some, they are the difference between silence and the ability to speak. For others, they put eating solid food back into the realm of possibility.

Breast implants are being improved continuously in comfort, fit and natural appearance. Breast reconstruction is becoming an accepted surgical option for women who have had mastectomies. It is not without problems, but surgeons are working to improve the procedure.

Insurance companies are beginning to cover restorative or cosmetic surgery and various prosthetic devices as a necessary part of the rehabilitation process. This is good news, for it is further recognition that cancer patients are entitled to as close to normal a life as possible. No longer are they asked to be grateful and satisfied just to be alive.

What Spouses Can Do

Disfigurement or debilitation caused by treatment can affect reactions to a partner with cancer. You expect to see beyond these physical changes to the person within, the one who more than ever needs your love and physical reassurance of that love. Nonetheless, you might find yourself responding negatively, unable to provide that support. You might feel awkward about physical contact because you think your partner is not ready for it and that you will be judged insensitive.

It helps to remember that touching, holding, hugging and caressing are ways to express the acceptance and caring that is so important to the person with cancer. More than words, they show love and express your belief in the patient's continued desirability as a physical being.

Admittedly it is a difficult time. Beset by treatment reactions, anxiety, self-doubt or a mistaken notion of what your feelings are, your spouse might withdraw from you. Together, try to prevent a cycle of misunderstanding from developing. As the well partner, try to feel sure in your love and reach out gently and repeatedly, if necessary, to provide the reassurance that cancer cannot destroy love.

If barriers begin to grow, perhaps a professional counselor can help you work out your reactions toward the patient, the disease or your feelings that too much of the responsibility has been placed upon your shoulders. Make sure you are doing whatever you can to re-establish bonds of closeness and caring.

Together As a Couple

Essentially, each of us must deal with heartrending problems in ways that are compatible with our relationship. Facing this battle can strengthen everything that is good in it. Sometimes, it shows us how minor are problems once considered so important. However, cancer also can strain a relationship already stressed by other serious problems.

Sometimes the sexual relationship becomes the barometer of a marriage. In a mature relationship, sex is an expression of love, affection and respect—not the basis for it. As one woman put it, "If a husband and wife had a good relationship before mutilating surgery, there is little basis for new problems. I contend this is an excuse not to have sexual relations or to seek a new, more exciting partner. The real reasons for problems were there before the surgery, just as the cancer was there before the diagnosis."

Most people find ways to face and overcome the stresses cancer places on their relationship. They find strength in each other, and they work together to establish a new and comfortable routine. Sharing their feelings with each other usually has been their first step toward finding effective solutions.

Sometimes a trained counselor can help you understand ways in which you can begin helping each other. Family therapists or psychiatric social workers sometimes should be included in the personal cancer treatment team. Support groups of other couples dealing with cancer can be helpful, even in dealing with intimate problems. The usual personal barriers often fall when you know you have sympathetic and experienced confidants who may be able to offer practical (and tested) guidance. Those who have found ways to maintain or recapture closeness and intimacy throughout this ordeal might be able to help others in a group setting.

The World Outside

- Some friends will deal well with your illness and provide gratifying support.

- Some will be unable to cope with the possibility of death and will disappear from your life.

- Most will want to help but may be uncomfortable and unsure of how to go about it. Help your friends support you:

- Ask yourself, "Have friends deserted me or have I withdrawn from them?"

- Telephone those who don't call you.

- Ask for simple assistance—to run an errand, prepare a meal, come and visit. These small acts bring friends back into contact and help them feel useful and needed.

- If you are alone, ask your physician, social worker or pastor to "match" you with another patient. Someone else needs friendships, too.

- Groups of other cancer patients can offer new friendships, understanding, support and companionship.

- When you return to work, coworkers, like others, may shun you, support you or wait for your cues on how to respond.

- There are laws to protect you against job discrimination.

Anyone who has been affected intimately by cancer knows that it can change the pattern of our relationships outside the family as well as those within. Friends react as they do to other difficult situations. Some handle it well; others are unable to maintain any association at all. Casual acquaintances, and even strangers, can cause unintended pain by asking thoughtless questions about visible scars, artificial devices or other noticeable changes in appearance.

One or two people within your circle may be gratifying in their devotion and in the sensitivity they show toward your needs. One woman said her mother-in-law found one or two close friends with whom she felt truly relaxed. They were not startled when she laughed nor ill at ease when she cried. With others she maintained an outward calm.

"I have three really good friends with whom I can talk about my cancer," explained another. "I have talked about dying with my sister, and she does understand a lot more than I thought a person without cancer could."

When Friends Don't Call

Lost friendships are one of the real heartbreaks people with cancer face. Friends do not call for a variety of reasons. They might not know how to respond to a change in your appearance. They might be avoiding you in order to avoid facing the possibility of your death and the eventuality of their own. Their absence does not necessarily mean they no longer care about you. Still, it is little comfort to know that "out there" you have friends if they have so little confidence in their worth as companions that they would rather say nothing than risk saying the wrong thing.

"I see that my friends don't know how to talk to me, and they shy away from me," wrote one person with cancer. "Most people are very ignorant on the subject of cancer."

If you believe discomfort rather than fear is keeping a particular friend from visiting, you might try a phone call to dissolve the barrier. Yet you cannot combat all the reasons why people avoid you; some still believe that cancer is contagious. Certainly, you cannot call them up and say, "Hey, get out of the Dark Ages. It's not catching!"

Knowing that others are ignorant does little to lessen the hurt and frustration of being needlessly isolated. You only can change the attitudes of others if you are among them. Examine carefully whether friends shun you or whether you have withdrawn from your usual social contacts to protect your own feelings. You can neither enlighten nor draw comfort from an empty room. If possible, the best place to be is out in the world with other people.

Easing the Way for Others

Most people fall into a middle group, somewhere between the

staunch friends and the "avoiders." They are groping for an approach to cancer with which they can be comfortable. These people may say things which sound inane, insincere or hurtful. You have to keep reminding yourself that they are trying their best. If you are open about cancer, they may relax, too.

A perceptive high school student explained, "I guess what I'm trying to say boils down to this. One of these days people may not feel so uneasy around a disabled person. I'm not bitter with people; I'm really quite at ease with them and strive to make them feel at ease with me. They feel afraid of me, and consequently trip over their tongues. I have learned a lot by living in a handicap's world and am quite willing to share it. One of these days, I may be given the chance."

A woman who had had extensive surgery for oral cancer explained how she tried to lessen the discomfort of others without causing discomfort for herself. She focused on her disability rather than its cause.

"I am determined to put people at ease, so when I speak on the telephone, or to someone for the first time, I immediately say, 'I have a speech defect, so please don't hesitate to tell me if you don't understand me.' I also carry a pencil and paper and offer to write what can't be understood. I find it much more frustrating to have people try to save my feelings by pretending to understand me when they don't."

A man we know startled his fishing buddies, who were paying a group visit to his hospital room. He positively threw open the door to honest communication when he boomed out, "You know, I've learned one hell of a lot about cancer since I became a member of the club."

We can't all be that direct. He had been a straightforward man all his life. But he had let his friends know that he preferred talking about his cancer to pussyfooting around it.

Helping Friends Help

Many times friends are waiting for some clue as to what behavior is appropriate. They might not be sure you want company. They might call to "see how things are going," then add as they hang up the phone, "Let me know if there's anything I can do to help."

These friends are asking for more than a job to do. They are asking for direction, giving you clues that they will not desert you if only they have some guidance on how to proceed. The next time friends or

607

relatives offer assistance, try to look at the offer in that light. If you can think of one specific errand they can run, one chore they can take off your hands, you have done them and yourself a favor.

"Mother hasn't been out since Dad became ill. I think a Saturday afternoon at the shopping center would do wonders for her."

"We'll be at the hospital all day Thursday for chemotherapy. It would be such a help to me if you could whip up a casserole for our dinner."

"I don't feel much like talking these days, but if you'd bring your needlepoint and come sit with me, it would be pleasant to have your company."

Most people are grateful if there is something concrete they can do to show their continuing friendship. If such tasks bring them into your home, it gives them a chance to see that you are still living and functioning—not a funeral waiting to happen. Their next visit might be easier, and then they may be able to stop by without a "reason."

Choosing to help friends in this way is no easy undertaking. When you feel stretched to breaking just keeping your own life going, it is difficult to extend your energies further to make others feel at ease. It can be a new and difficult experience for some, this reaching out, but the rewards can be exhilarating. We all feel better giving than receiving, so it might be easier if you think of your requests for assistance as letting others feel useful, rather than as petitions for help.

Fighting Loneliness

Regardless of what you do, your friends might desert you. Circumstances might have left you alone before cancer struck. This is a special, awful loneliness for any human being to endure. There are no easy answers, no pat solutions. The mutual support of other people with cancer might provide some solace and comfort. (See the appendix for suggestions.) There probably are others in your community who need your companionship as much as you need theirs. Being housebound need not deprive you of visits from others who would like to share some quiet moments or some deeply felt sorrow with someone who will understand. A physician, social worker, visiting nurse or member of the clergy should be able to help you contact another cancer patient or shut-in who could use company.

On the Job

For many of us, work forms a cornerstone of life. In addition to income, it provides satisfaction and a chance to interact with peers. Returning to work as soon as you are physically able is one way to return stability to your life. If treatment has made it impossible to return to a former line of work, investigate the availability of rehabilitation and retraining programs within the community to prepare you for another occupation.

You might find on returning to your job that relationships with co-workers have changed. One person with cancer found his associates had requested separate restroom facilities for him—that old "cancer is catching" bugaboo again!

More people face an "If we pretend Jane never had cancer, it will go away" approach by co-workers, and that can be most demoralizing. Some have found that if you look well and are able to function, people tend to underestimate the seriousness of your condition. They might mumble something like, "Glad you're back; you look great," and never ask how you really feel. In turn, you might find you resent their good health and nonchalance as you wonder what happened to the companionship you had looked forward to in returning to work.

The best you can do is assume that your co-workers, like so many others, are unsure of what to say or are trying to protect your feelings —or their own.

Others returning to work might be perfectly delighted with a rather cavalier attitude toward their condition. "Glad you're back," might be all you want to hear before plunging into your old routine. If you are being coddled at home, returning to a situation where others do not think of you as sick might be the greatest therapy yet devised.

Some people believe it eases relationships with co-workers if they are quite open about their condition. One young woman described in a speech to other cancer patients why she decided to tell about the cancer.

"Since my bones don't cooperate, it's hard for me to appear graceful, but I have a choice in this situation," she said. "I can either move as though nothing is bothering me (while gritting my teeth and giving my contact lenses a salty bath), or I can move awkwardly in reasonable comfort. I think this is one of the reasons I don't mind people knowing I have multiple myeloma. I keep having this flash of having died and having someone who just found out about the myeloma saying, 'So that's why she kept falling over.' "

If cancer treatment meant leaving your old job, discrimination may be a hurdle to returning to work. Even the person who is completely recovered may find it difficult to obtain employment. The rationale, one hears from indirect sources, is that people who have had cancer take too many sick days, are a poor insurance risk or will make co-workers uncomfortable.

How does one cope? You might begin with this information: The Rehabilitation Act of 1973, a Federal statute, includes persons who have been treated for cancer among the handicapped, and thus covered by the Act. You may not think of yourself as handicapped, but it is indeed a handicap if misconceptions about cancer have limited your chances of finding a job.

In substance, the Act requires firms with contracts or subcontracts to the Federal government of $50,000 or more and with 50 or more employees to prepare and maintain an affirmative action program for the handicapped—and that means you. (Such a program might include rehabilitation training.) In addition, the Act makes illegal discrimination against a handicapped individual by any entity, regardless of size, if it receives money, regardless of amount, from the Department of Health and Human Services (formerly the Department of Health, Education, and Welfare).

Today, many firms, local governments and educational and health institutions do business or receive funding from the Federal government. You might want to target your job hunting in their direction.

If you apply for a job with a firm with government contracts and believe you did not get the job because of your cancer, you can file a complaint under Section 503 of the Act with the Office of Federal Contract Compliance Programs of the U.S. Department of Labor. If your complaint is against an agency receiving money from Health and Human Services, file your action with the DHHS Office of Civil Rights. For reference, your complaint falls under Section 504 of the Act.

A number of states also have passed statutes prohibiting discrimination against cancer patients. Your State Department of Labor or Office of Civil Rights can advise you on the law. (The Labor Department also may know of rehabilitation and retraining programs.) In addition, you may be able to obtain information and assistance from union representatives, regional or national offices of the Rehabilitation Services Administration, the Equal Employment Opportunities Commission, the National Labor Relations Board or the American Civil Liberties Union.

Living Each Day

- Each person must work through, in his or her own way, feelings of possible death, fear and isolation. Returning to normal routines as much as possible often helps.

- Give the pleasures and responsibilities of each day the attention they deserve.

- Responsible pursuits keep life meaningful; recreation keeps it zesty. Fill your life with both.

- Remember the difference between "doing" and "overdoing." Rest is important to both physical and emotional strength.

- It's harder to bolster one's will to live if you are alone. Yet many have acted as their own cheering squad and have found ways to lead meaningful lives.

- Family members must not make an invalid of a person with cancer who is fully capable of physical activity and responsible participation in the family.

- Family members should not equate physical incapability with mental failing. It is especially important that an ill patient feel a necessary part of the family.

- Families must guard against "rehearsing" how they will act if the patient dies by excluding him or her from family affairs now.

Whether the outlook for recovery is good or poor, the days go by, one at a time, and patient and family must learn to live each one. It's not always easy. On learning the diagnosis, some decide that death is inevitable, and there is nothing to do but give up and wait. They are not the first to feel that way.

Orville Kelly, a newspaperman, described his initial battle with the specter of death. "I began to isolate myself from the rest of the world. I spent much time in bed, even though I was physically able to walk and drive. I thought about my own impending funeral and it made me very sad."

These feelings continued from his first hospitalization through the first outpatient chemotherapy treatment. On the way home from that treatment, he was haunted by memories of the happy past, when "everything was all right." Then it occurred to Kelly, "I wasn't dead yet. I was able to drive my automobile. Why couldn't I return home to barbecue ribs?"

He did, that very night. He began to talk to his wife and children about his fears and anxieties. And he became so frustrated at the feelings he had kept locked up inside himself that he wrote the newspaper article that led to the founding of Make Today Count, the mutual help group that now includes several hundred local chapters.

Each person must work through individual feelings of possible death, fear and isolation in his or her own good time. It is hard to overcome these feelings if they are never confronted head on, but it is an ongoing struggle. One day brings feelings of confidence, the next day despair. Many people find it helps considerably if they strive to return, both as individuals and as a family, to their normal lives.

Each day brings pleasures and responsibilities totally outside the realm of cancer. We should try to give each the attention it deserves. These are the threads of the fabric that enfolds our lives. They give it color and meaning.

The days can be more valuable if you can learn to enjoy common moments as well as memorable occasions. This is true whether you have weeks or years left. It is true, in fact, whether you have a life-threatening disease or not. Physical well-being is closely tied to emotional well-being. The time you take out from attending to cancer strengthens you for the time you must devote to it.

Staying Involved

When you have cancer, you need responsibilities, diversions, outings and companionship just as before. As long as you are able, you should go to work, take the kids to the zoo, play cards with friends, go on a trip. Try to remember that responsible pursuits keep life meaningful, and recreation keeps it zesty. You need activities that give you a sense of purpose and those that provide enjoyment.

Some people find cancer is a spur to do the fun, adventurous or zany things they've always wanted to do but have put off as being not quite responsible. That's a great idea. It helps ward off two overreactions—one is giving up, and the other is trying to cram a life's worth of responsible accomplishment into a very short time.

A young woman with cancer put it this way: "Too often we patients fill up our lives with meaningful activities and neglect the frivolous outlets that keep us sane. And we tend to forget how important our sense of humor is." She quotes Betty Rollin, author of *First You Cry,* as saying that cancer won't bestow a sense of humor on someone who doesn't have it, but a sense of humor can sure get you through the experience.

There is no scientific or medical proof for it, but cancer patients who have "places to go and things to do" seem to live longer—or at least they feel that life still stretches before them. "I'm in my own real estate business, started a year ago, and serve as an officer in eight civic organizations," a woman wrote. "Life has never been fuller, and for a 47-year-old grandmother, I've never felt stronger or better." Seven years earlier, her family had been told she had six months to live.

Others have combined humor with too much interest in life to let go of it. "Mine has been a long battle, but I'm not ready to call it quits yet," one such person declared. "I'm just too busy to schedule my demise, or maybe I just haven't the good sense to lie down and let it happen!" Many have found they cannot retire from living. It's much like employment—every day you show up, you may as well give it your best!

"Doing," it might be pointed out, is not the same as overdoing. Try to recognize your limitations as well as your capabilities. Fatigue can bring on crushing despair, and many people have found that as simple a safeguard as adequate rest fends off depression. Exhaustion weakens our physical and emotional defenses.

Pain also can make a mockery of attempts to function normally. Physicians are learning much about controlling pain without drugging the patient, so pain, especially if it is prolonged, should be discussed with your physician.

"Putting one's house in order" is a desire that strikes many who learn they have cancer. This is not the same as giving up. In fact, everyone needs to review insurance policies, update wills and clean out the closets and drawers from time to time—and that gives you something constructive to do.

Going It Alone

It is obvious that many of these remarks have been directed toward the person with cancer who is part of a family. Some live alone, however, and some feel they have no one to "live for." This increases loneliness and can make the will to live seem a bitter irony. They may want to pull the covers over their head and "get it over with." If you have no one else to provide encouragement, you have to act as your own cheering squad. It is hard, but it's not impossible.

An amazing gentleman of 73, who had been treated on and off for 8 years for Hodgkin's disease, described how he coped. "I kept on fighting. This is what you must do. Positive thinking and an active life are two things which will do a great deal to relieve the tension." In order to stay involved with life and mentally active, he enrolled in the university where he had received his bachelor of arts degree and began work on his master's degree. "Some people think I'm crazy," he admits. "Maybe I am, but it is a nice crazy anyway. At least, I have achieved happiness."

An elderly woman decided to "start a new life, make what's left of this one count." She started helping a state school for the retarded, and her home became "a depot for people with used clothing and toys. Now I have branched out to helping with nursing homes. I am so busy and happy; I have no worries."

Not everyone can go beyond themselves and give to others to this extent. You might not have the physical or emotional strength. It may not be natural to your personality, and you are still the same person you were. But many find cancer is easier to live with if they choose constructive ways to fill their time—to make part of each day count for what they can put into it.

Support From the Family

The desire to "do something" is common among nearly everyone with a family member or dear friend who has cancer. There is nothing you can do to change the course of cancer, so you do everything you can for the person. Sometimes, doing everything is the worst course to follow.

People with cancer still have the same needs and often the same capabilities as they did before. If they are physically able, they need to participate in their normal range of activities and responsibilities—

right down to taking out the garbage. Helplessness, or worse, an unnecessary feeling of helplessness, is one of the great woes of the person with cancer. In the words of one:

"I am deeply angry over the way patients (not only cancer patients but any patient with a life-threatening diagnosis) are automatically treated as if we were mentally incompetent. Our relatives have RIGHTS: we have none. This is by a sort of mutual consent, an unconscious conspiracy which seems to be part of our culture. Let an individual become a patient . . . and he is treated, without any 'competency hearing,' as if he had been found in a court of law to be incompetent. Only the relatives are consulted or empowered to make decisions . . ."

There is great bitterness in this woman's words, and they can stand as a lesson to all. Although bedridden, a patient probably still is able to discuss treatment options, financial arrangements and the children's school problems. The rest of the family must make every effort to preserve as much as possible the patient's usual role within the family.

The least you can do is to keep the patient informed of necessary decisions. You can help the seriously ill patient ward off feelings of helplessness or abandonment if you continue to share your activities, goals and dreams as before.

Few of us who are well know what it is like to be placed in a position of dependency. Cancer attacks one's self concept as a whole person as well as threatening one's life. Feelings of helplessness are real enough when one is flat on one's back. Make every effort not to compound them by ignoring the wishes of the patient, or worse, by trying to make an invalid of a person who is up and around. Pulling one's weight is good exercise.

How the Family Copes

The needs of the family as a unit are important, too. Maintain normal living patterns within the family as well as possible. This is important for long-range as well as day-to-day coping. Sometimes, when the patient is in active treatment, family life becomes totally disrupted. If that happens, it is harder to resume functioning as a unit during periods of extended remission or permanent control.

"My worst emotional problem," one patient said, "was finding

615

that my improved health posed inconveniences and threw my family's plans all out of line."

Understanding such a situation might help prevent it. There are many ways we cope with fear, anxiety and the threat of loss or death. One way is to begin preparing ourselves for an event by thinking about it, without being aware that we are doing so, as if it had already happened. Thus, we "rehearse" life as it will be so that we can assume our new roles more easily when the time comes. People do this throughout their lives, although usually they are unaware of it. For example, teenagers spend increasing amounts of time with friends rather than with family, "rehearsing" for the time when they will go out on their own.

When a family member has cancer, you may be "rehearsing" the future in your own mind. You might begin to "practice" how the family will function if that person dies. Watch for signs that you are excluding the patient and turn the routine back toward normal if you are. Knowing that these things happen, however, try not to feel guilty if you find yourself emotionally out of step with remission or recovery.

The Years After

C ancer is not something anyone forgets. Anxieties remain as active treatment ceases and the waiting stage begins. A cold or a cramp may be cause for panic. As 6-month or annual check-ups approach, you swing between hope and anxiety. As you wait for the mystical 5-year or 10-year point, you might feel more anxious rather than more secure.

These are feelings we all share. No one expects you to forget that you have had cancer or that it might recur. Each must seek individual ways of coping with the underlying insecurity of not knowing the true state of his or her health. The best prescription seems to lie in a combination of one part challenging responsibilities that command a full range of skills, a dose of activities that seek to fill the needs of others and a generous dash of frivolity and laughter.

You still might have moments when you feel as if you lived perched on the edge of a cliff. They will sneak up unbidden. But they will be fewer and farther between if you have filled your mind with other thoughts than cancer.

Cancer might rob you of that blissful ignorance that once led you to believe that tomorrow stretched forever. In exchange, you are granted the vision to see each today as precious, a gift to be used wisely and richly. No one can take that away.

Appendix

Information Services and Resources

You may want more information for yourself, your family, and your doctor. The services explained below will help you obtain what you need.

Cancer Information Service

The National Cancer Institute sponsors a toll-free Cancer Information Service, open 7 days a week to help you. By dialing 1-800-4-CANCER (1-800-422-6237),* you will be connected to a Cancer Information Service office, where a trained staff member can answer your questions and listen to your concerns.

PDQ Service

The National Cancer Institute has developed PDQ (Physician Data Query), a computerized data base designed to give doctors quick and easy access to:
- The latest treatment information for most types of cancer.
- Descriptions of clinical trials that are open for patient entry.
- Names of organizations and physicians involved in cancer care.

To get access to PDQ, a doctor can use an office computer with a telephone hookup and a PDQ access code or the services of a medical library with online searching capability. Most Cancer Information Service offices (1-800-4-CANCER) provide a physician with one free PDQ search and can tell doctors how to get regular access to the data base. Patients may ask their doctor to use PDQ or may call 1-800-4-CANCER themselves. Information specialists at this toll-free number use a variety of sources, including PDQ, to answer questions about cancer prevention, diagnosis, and treatment.

*In Alaska, call 1-800-638-6070; in Hawaii, on Oahu, call 524-1234 (on neighboring islands, call collect).
Spanish-speaking staff members are available to callers from the following areas (daytime hours only): California, Florida, Georgia, Illinois, northern New Jersey, New York, and Texas.

For additional written resources about cancer, information about particular forms of the disease, its treatment, and possible side effects, and nutritional information and recipes for the cancer patient, ask the Cancer Information Service to send you information or write:

Office of Cancer Communications
National Cancer Institute
Building 31, Room 10A24
Bethesda, Maryland 20892

Support and Service Organizations

The following organizations offer information, assistance, and emotional support to patients and families on a national basis through local chapters.

American Cancer Society, Inc.
90 Park Avenue
New York, New York 10016
(212) 736-3030

The American Cancer Society is a national voluntary organization whose programs include education, patient services, and rehabilitation. Local ACS units conduct such service programs for cancer patients and their families as information, counseling, and guidance; referral to community health services and other resources; equipment loans for care of the homebound patient; surgical dressings; transportation to and from treatment, and rehabilitation programs.

The National ACS provides local units with resource materials for setting up a variety of self-help groups. Services may be more or less extensive, depending on facilities and resources of the local unit. Before contacting national headquarters, check your local telephone directory for an ACS unit in your community.

Two rehabilitation and education programs sponsored nationally by the American Cancer Society are:

International Association of Laryngectomees

The Association is an umbrella group for 225 local clubs, such as the Lost Chords, that promote and support the total rehabilitation of people with laryngectomies. When requested by a physician, members—who are themselves laryngectomees—call on hospitalized patients to offer moral support and encouragement. Preoperative visits may be made as well, and help can extend to the patient's family. The association also conducts education and information programs.

Reach to Recovery

Through a corps of carefully trained volunteers who have successfully adjusted to their own surgery, Reach to Recovery is designed to meet the physicial, psychological, and cosmetic needs of women who have had mastectomies. On referral from the patient's physician, the volunteers make hospital visits a few days after surgery, bringing information about rehabilitation exercises and a temporary breast form (prosthesis).

Reach to Recovery also distributes educational materials for health professionals and provides lectures and demonstrations at health institutions.

Two mutual support programs, which began as grassroots efforts, recently have been designated as national programs of the American Cancer Society. They are:

CanSurmount

CanSurmount brings together the patient, family member, the CanSurmount volunteer and the health professional. On physician referral, a trained CanSurmount volunteer, who is also a cancer patient, meets with patient and family in the hospital or home. The goal of the program is to improve mutual help and understanding through continuing education and support for volunteers, patients, families, health professionals, and the community.

I Can Cope

This program addresses the educational and psychological needs of people with cancer and their families. It is a series of eight classes covering learning about the disease, learning to cope with daily health problems, learning to express feelings, learning to live with limitations, and learning about local resources. Through lectures, group discussions, and study assignments, the course helps people with cancer regain a sense of self-control over their lives.

Cancer Care, Inc.
1180 Avenue of the Americas
New York, New York 10036
(212) 302-2400

This service arm of the National Cancer Foundation helps patients and families cope with the emotional, psychological, and financial consequences of cancer at all stages of illness through home visits by trained volunteers, individual, family, and group counseling, and literature, information referrals to local and regional resources, and assistance for nonmedical expenses.

Candelighters Childhood Cancer Foundation, Inc.
Suite 1011
2025 I Street, N.W.
Washington, D.C. 20006
(202) 659-5136

An international organization of parents whose children have or have had cancer, this foundation provides guidance and emotional support as well as referral services for families through self-help and support groups, including adolescent support groups and a youth newsletter. Logistical support—crisis intervention, babysitting, transportation—is available, and some groups provide financial assistance.

CHUMS (Cancer Hopefuls United for Mutual Support)
3310 Rochambeau Avenue
Bronx, New York 10467
(212) 655-7566

This organization of cancer survivors offers hope and emotional support for cancer patients and their families through self-help, crisis intervention, information, referrals, and peer support. Support is provided by cancer survivors who contact patients who have diagnoses similar to theirs.

The Concern for Dying
250 West 57th Street
New York, New York 10107
(212) 246-6962

The Concern for Dying is a nonprofit educational organization that distributes information on "the living will," a document that records patient wishes concerning treatment, euthanasia, and death and dying. Psychological and legal counseling are provided, as is referral to local organizations.

Corporate Angel Network
Westchester County Airport
Building 1
White Plains, New York 10604
(914) 328-1313
    This organization alleviates costs for cancer patients who are receiving special tretment in NCI-approved treatment centers by arranging for ambulatory patients and one attendant/family member to fly free on corporate aircraft when seats are available.

Leukemia Society of American, Inc.
733 Third Avenue
New York, New York 10017
(212) 573-8484
    Chapters of the Leukemia Society offer patients with leukemia and allied disorders financial assistance, transportation, and consultation services for referrals to other means of local support.

Make-a-Wish Foundation of America
Suite 205
4601 North 16th Street
Phoenix, Arizona 85016
(602) 234-0960
    Works closely with families that have terminally ill children (up to age 18) to cover expenses and arrange details necessary for granting a child's "special wish" that will provide encouragement, respite from the current situation, and special memories.

Make Today Count
P.O. Box 222
Osage Beach, Missouri 65065
(314) 348-1619
    Cancer patients and other people with life-threatening diseases, their families, nurses, physicians, other health professionals, and interested community members have formed more than 200 chapters of Make Today Count. Its goal is to help

patient and family "live each day as fully and completely as possible." The organization is for emotional self-help only, and chapters are organized informally with meetings held monthly or semimonthly.

National Hospice Organization
Suite 902
1901 North Fort Myer Drive
Arlington, Virginia 22209
(703) 243-5900
    The nonprofit membership organization consists of groups and institutions concerned with or providing care for the terminally ill and their families. The organization furnishes literature, information, and referrals to local hospice programs and to regional and other national resoures.

United Cancer Council, Inc.
Suite 340
650 East Carmel Drive
Carmel, Indiana 46032
(317) 844-6627
    The United Cancer Council is a federation of voluntary cancer agencies funded through the United Way of Giving in most communities where they are located. Services include nursing, homemaking, housekeeping, medications, prostheses, and rehabilitation.

United Ostomy Association, Inc.
2001 West Beverly Boulevard
Los Angeles, California 90057
(213) 413-5510
    The United Ostomy Association offers emotional support from others with common problems, although not all members are cancer patients. More than 500 chapters are made up of ostomates whose goal is to provide mutual aid, moral support, and education to those who have had colostomy, ileostomy, or urostomy surgery.
    The following organizations offer information, assistance, and emotional support to patients and families on a regional basis:

TOUCH
513 Tinsley Harrison Tower
University Station
Birmingham, Alabama 35294
(205) 934-3814

Support groups provide assistance to cancer patients and their families in forming realistic, positive attitudes toward cancer and its treatment. Counselors guide peer emotional support groups for both inpatients and outpatients and assist with continuing education programs on treatment methods.

We Can Do!
P.O. Box 723
Arcadia, California 91006
(818) 357-7517

This support program addresses the long-term psychological and education needs of cancer patients and family members through group meetings, educational programs, referrals to local resources, and classes for spouses of cancer patients.

Chapter 33

When Someone in Your Family Has Cancer

From the Perspective of the Young Person

When Someone in Your Family Has Cancer

Editor's Note: The text which follows was written from the young person's perspective. The point of view as well as the modes of expression assume that the reader is a young boy or girl seeking adjustment to the shifts in family life, and in his or her own feelings when a sibling or a parent is a cancer patient.

Introduction

When someone in your family has cancer things can change for everyone — sometimes a little, sometimes a lot. What having a parent or a brother or sister (sibling) with cancer is like depends on a lot of things, such as:

• Who in your family has cancer

• What type of cancer the person has and how it's treated

• How old you are

• If you have relatives or close friends nearby who can help

• Whether you live with two parents or with one

• If you have brothers and sisters at home and how old they are

• How far the person with cancer goes for treatment — across town or to another city or state — and if you can visit or call them

• How long the person has to stay in the hospital

• How well or sick the person with cancer feels

• Whether your parents know the answers to your questions about cancer

• How easy it is for your parents to talk with you about cancer

• How comfortable you feel talking about cancer

• Whether your friends understand what's going on and how they treat you

Any of these can make a difference, and only you know how cancer has affected your life. No book can answer all your questions. This one was written to help you understand more about cancer, how it's treated, and the changes that may be happening in your life. It also may help you understand and deal with feelings you have about cancer and about the person in your family who has it.

Cancer and the Family

Any illness changes family life for a while. A parent or a brother or sister who is home sick with the flu can't spend as much time with the family as usual. The sick person may get special attention and you may need to help around the house. But most illnesses don't last long and family life soon goes back to normal.

When someone has cancer, however, it is different. He or she needs special medical treatment and may go to the hospital or clinic often. Everyone in the family may worry, both for the person who has cancer and for themselves. Cancer is a serious illness, and it is scary if you don't know for sure whether the person will get well or not.

Every member of your family may react differently. They may be afraid or angry that their life has changed, or tired, or nervous about the future. They may be tense, and not as easy to talk to as before because they're worried. Some people may go on just as if nothing has happened and they may not seem different at all. If you're upset, this may make you wonder if they care about the family member who has cancer. It's important to remember that everyone reacts in their own way. You may get mad at other members of your family for the way they're acting. If you do, talking with them so you can better understand each other is better than just staying mad.

Some Things You Should Know

- More people are living with cancer now than ever before, and new ways to treat cancer are being discovered
- Having cancer doesn't necessarily mean a person will die from it
- Nothing you did or didn't do caused your family member to get cancer
- Nothing you thought or said caused your family member to get cancer
- Cancer is *not* contagious — you *can't* catch it from someone else
- You or your parents could not have protected your brother or sister from getting cancer
- If one of your parents has cancer, that doesn't mean that someone else in your family will get it too
- If you have a sibling with cancer, that doesn't mean that you or someone else in your family will get it too
- There's no answer to any questions you may have about why your parent or sibling is sick and you're healthy
- The way you behave cannot change the fact that someone has cancer or that your family is upset
- If you are sick that doesn't mean you have cancer too
- It is good for you to continue with school and outside activities

Cancer: Can It Be Cured?

Some people think that because a person has cancer he or she is going to die. Although some people do die from cancer, many do not. More people are living with cancer today than ever before. In many cases, cancer treatment can cause a remission (ree-MISH-un),* which means there are no more signs or symptoms of the cancer. A remission can last for months or years, and sometimes lasts so long that the person is said to be cured. Sometimes, however, the cancer comes back. If this happens, it is called a relapse (REE-laps) or recurrence (re-KUR-unce), and treatment aimed at another remission usually starts.

Whether the person in your family can be cured of cancer depends on many things, and no booklet can tell you exactly what to expect. If you wonder how your parent or sibling is doing, ask an adult who you think will know — someone in your family or someone who works with people who have cancer. If your parents agree, you may want to talk to the doctor, nurse, or social worker at the hospital where your family member goes for treatment. Nobody can tell you why someone in your family has cancer or exactly what will happen in the future, but you can get help to better understand and to live with what is happening today.

Some people with family members who have cancer have found that it helps to hope for the best. A lot of cancer research is being done and progress is always being made in treating cancer.

One Way to Help Yourself: Learn About Cancer

One thing that has helped other young people to understand what is happening to their family member is learning about the type of cancer that person has and

---

*Groups of letters surrounded by ( ) are here to help you pronounce words that might be new to you.

the treatment being used for it. Both of these are important to know about because there are more than 100 different types of cancer and the treatment for each type is different. In addition, there may be more than one way of treating a type of cancer, so people who have the same type of cancer may not even get the same type of treatment. Treatment will depend on how old the patient is, if the cancer has spread to other places in the body, and what the doctors believe is best for each patient.

Treatment will usually follow a protocol (PRO-to-kol), which is a plan for treating cancer. However, even if two people have the same type of cancer and the same treatment, the treatment may not work the same way for both of them. Therefore, if you know or hear of someone who has had the same type of cancer and treatment as your family member and that person didn't do well, it doesn't mean that your family member isn't going to get well. It is important to remember that each person is different and can react to treatment differently.

What is Cancer?

Cancer is a word used to describe a group of diseases. Each has its own name (such as lung cancer, breast cancer, leukemia), its own treatment, and its own chances of being cured. Although each type of cancer is different from the others in many ways, every cancer, whatever it's called or whatever part of the body it's in, is a disease of the body's cells.

The millions of tiny cells that make up the human body are so small that they can be seen only by looking through a microscope. There are different kinds of cells — some are hair cells, some skin cells, some blood cells — but they each make new cells by dividing into two. This is how worn-out old cells are replaced with strong new ones.

What happens when someone has cancer is that a cell changes and doesn't do the job it is supposed to do for the body. When it divides, it makes more cells like itself, cells that are not normal. These cells keep dividing into more cells and eventually they crowd out and destroy the normal healthy cells and tissues the body needs.

A group of runaway cells is called a tumor (TOO-mur). There are two kinds of tumors. A benign (bee-NINE) tumor is not a cancer. The cells of a benign tumor can crowd out healthy cells but they cannot spread to other parts of the body. A malignant (ma-LIG-nunt) tumor is a cancer. Like a benign tumor, it can take over other healthy cells around it, but it can also spread to other parts of the body.

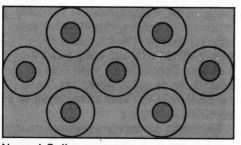

Normal Cells

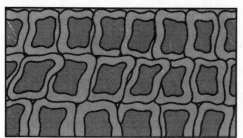

Cancer Cells

To do this, a cell or group of cells from the tumor separates and moves, usually through the bloodstream, to other parts of the body. There they divide and grow and start tumors made up of malignant cells like those from the original tumor. When this happens it is called a metastasis (me-TAS-ta-sis).

Cancer: It's Not Contagious

Scientists know that you can't "catch" cancer from someone who has it. It is not a contagious disease like chicken pox or the flu, and you can't catch it from being with someone who has cancer or by drinking from the same glass of that person.

You may know that cancer isn't contagious, but you may wonder if having someone in your family who has cancer means that you are going to get cancer yourself. Instead of worrying, it is best to talk with your parents and the doctor about this. They can tell you that cancer usually doesn't run in families, and you can talk about your fears.

Cancer Treatment

There are three major kinds of treatment for cancer — surgery, chemotherapy, and radiation therapy. These are used to destroy cancer cells and bring about a remission. Depending on what type of cancer your parent or sibling has, he or she could have one kind of treatment or a combination of them.

Treatments for cancer sometimes cause unwanted side effects. Side effects are problems caused by the treatment, not the cancer itself. This happens because when cancer treatment aims at cancer cells, it can affect some normal cells too.

Surgery

Surgery (SIR-ja-ree) is an operation. In cancer surgery, all or part of the cancer, or tumor, may be cut out. Sometimes healthy tissue around the tumor is also removed. When people have major surgery, they often have to stay in the hospital until they are strong enough to come home. When they do come home, they may still be weak from the surgery. There may be some things they shouldn't do for awhile, such as lifting heavy things or climbing stairs, because the body needs time to heal after surgery.

Chemotherapy

Chemotherapy (kee-mo-THER-a-pee) is the treatment of cancer with special drugs that destroy cancer cells. These drugs go into the bloodstream and move through it to cancer cells anywhere in the body. Chemotherapy is usually given repeatedly for several months. Even after the person is in remission, the treatments may continue in order to destroy any scattered cancer cells that may still be in the body.

Chemotherapy is most often taken through a needle inserted into a vein, called an intravenous (in-tra-VEE-nus) or IV for short; or into a muscle (a shot); or by mouth (liquids or pills). Many different drugs are used in chemotherapy. Doctors decide which drug or combinations of drugs to use depending on what type of cancer the person has. The names of some of these drugs — vincristine (vin-KRIS-teen), Adriamycin (A-dree-a-MY-sin), methotrexate (meth-o-TREKS-ate), Cytoxan (sy-TOK-sin), or many others — may become common words around your house.

Chemotherapy works mainly on the rapidly dividing cancer cells. But healthy cells, especially those that also divide rapidly, can be harmed as well. This can cause unwanted side effects, and almost all people taking chemotherapy will have side effects. Most side effects are temporary and will gradually go away after treatment is stopped. The doctor can tell your parents or the person with cancer which side effects their chemotherapy is most likely to cause.

Side Effects of Chemotherapy

When chemotherapy acts on normal cells in the stomach and the rest of the digestive tract, from the mouth on down, it can cause nausea and vomiting and sometimes make people lose their appetites. If they have mouth sores on the tongue, gums, or inside of the cheeks, that also makes it hard to eat, especially if the food is too hot, cold, or spicy. People often lose some weight from these side effects.

Nausea and vomiting will usually stop within a day or two after the drug is taken. Mouth sores may last longer and may not even start until 1 or 2 weeks after taking certain drugs. Many people with mouth sores use special mouthrinses to ease the pain.

Temporary hair loss is another common side effect of chemotherapy. Sometimes the hair falls out all at once, and other times it slowly thins out. There's no way to know whether all the hair will come out or not. Even if it does, it will grow back after treatment has stopped. Some people wear a wig, cap, or scarf until their hair grows back.

The bone marrow, the inner core of the bone, makes new blood cells. If chemotherapy affects the bone marrow, it cannot produce as many blood cells as usual. There may be a temporary decrease in the red blood cells, white blood cells, or platelets (PLAYT-lets), which are different kinds of cells in the blood.

Red blood cells carry needed oxygen to the tissues. When red blood cells are low, the person may be more tired, pale, or cranky than usual.

White blood cells fight infection. When they are low the person is more likely to get sick and may need to stay out of crowded places or away from people who have something they could catch—like a cold, the flu, or chicken pox. Because of this, you may need to stay away from them if you get sick. If you are exposed to something contagious at school or a friend's house, tell your parents so they will know to watch for signs of you getting sick.

Platelets help stop bleeding. People who don't have enough platelets may bruise or bleed more easily. They may have to stay away from rough play. If they get a nosebleed while their platelets are low, don't panic. They may bleed a little more than someone else would, but it will stop.

You may notice changes in how the person who is getting chemotherapy acts sometimes. Everyone has ups and downs, but these may be more extreme in a person taking some kinds of chemotherapy. People may feel depressed or nervous or especially hungry because of the chemotherapy. Of course, every change like this isn't due to chemotherapy. Just like others in the family, the person with cancer may be sad or worried about the changes it is bringing to his or her life.

The side effects people have depend on the drugs they take. They may have some or none of the side effects mentioned here, or they may have others. Young people who have had a parent or sibling with cancer have found that it is best to find out what to expect by talking to your parents or the person with cancer.

Side effects of chemotherapy are not pleasant, but they don't last forever. The drugs do not destroy all of the normal cells. Once chemotherapy is over the hair grows back and the bone marrow produces the normal amount of new blood cells. People with cancer begin to feel and act like themselves again.

Radiation Therapy

In radiation therapy (ray-dee-AY-shun THER-a-pee), high energy X-rays or rays from radioactive substances are aimed at malignant tumor to damage the ability of the cancer cells to divide. Some normal cells close to the tumor also will be damaged. But most healthy cells are protected by placing special lead shields over them.

To be sure the radiation is aimed right at the cancer, dye or felt tip markers are used to mark the target area on the skin. These marks stay on until treatments are finished.

If you've ever had an X-ray, you know something about what radiation therapy is like and that it does not hurt. Any X-rays taken to look at teeth or for broken bone are not as strong as the X-rays used to treat cancer. The treatments take only a few minutes and often are given over a period of several weeks.

In some cases, radiation is not beamed through a machine but instead comes from a source implanted or placed in the tumor. Surgery is used to insert radiation implants in the tumor so cancer cells will be destroyed from inside the body.

The person who gets radiation therapy is not radioactive during or after radiation therapy, and none of the treatments he or she is getting will hurt other people. When people have an implant in place, however, you will not be allowed to get too close to them until it is removed. They will be in the hospital during this short period of time.

632

Side Effects of Radiation Therapy

Although radiation therapy isn't painful, it can cause unwanted side effects. The person may be more tired than usual. Cells on the skin where radiation is aimed may feel like they would when sunburned and need to be protected from the sun. Hair may also fall out, but only in the area receiving radiation. If the radiation therapy aims at the stomach or head, the person may have nausea or vomiting, headaches, diarrhea, or a sore mouth.

Side Effects: What You Can Do To Help

There's nothing you can do to prevent side effects from cancer. But you can help to make them a little easier to live with. Just knowing that your parent or sibling may feel cross or tired or sick from side effects may help you to be more patient if this happens. And if the person with cancer is tired or sick but wants company, you can spend time with them doing quiet things — talking, reading, watching TV, or playing games like checkers.

The most important thing you can do, however, is to remember that your parent or brother or sister is still the same person as before, even if he or she looks different or can't do what they used to. It is important to treat your parent or sibling as you did before.

Learning More On Your Own

Now you know something about cancer, how it's treated, and about side effects from treatment. You may want to know more about your family member's cancer — like what kind it is, its treatment, and what that means for all of you. If you want to know more, ask someone who knows answers to such questions as:

• What kind of cancer is it? What is it called?

• Where is the cancer?

• Are they going to get better?

• What kind of treatment are they having? Will the treatment hurt? Will they have other kinds?

• How do they feel when they get the treatment?

• Will the treatment change the way they look?

• Will the treatment or cancer change how they feel and act — will they be weaker or grouchy or the same as before?

• How often will they go back for treatment? How long will treatment for the cancer last?

• How long will they have to stay to have each treatment — a morning, a week? Can I come and visit?

• What is it like where they go to have treatment? Can I come?

• What will happen to me while they're gone?

• Will they be able to go back to school or work while they're having treatment? Will they be at home?

• Will they be able to eat the same foods as the rest of the family?

• What can I do to help?

Sometimes people who have a parent or brother or sister (sibling) with cancer can go to see the cancer treatment center instead of imagining what it's like. They can see the building and equipment and meet the people who work there, and sometimes other cancer patients. If the hospital your parent or sibling goes to is too far away or has rules against your visiting, you could ask the person with cancer and others who have gone to the hospital to tell you what it's like. They can tell you about the people they know — the doctors, nurses, social workers, and patients — and describe a typical day. They can draw you pictures and take photographs. This way they can share their experiences with you, and you can learn a little about what it's like for them.

Reading About Cancer

Reading about cancer may also be useful. If you decide to read about cancer, be sure that what you read is up-to-date. Cancer treatment is improving so fast that even good information may be out of date in less than 5 years.

And remember that, just as you're an individual, so is the person in your family who has cancer. His or her experiences will not be exactly like those you read about. If you read something or see something on TV or in the movies, don't assume that what happens to the cancer patient in the story will happen to the person in your family.

If you read something or see something on TV or in the movies that you don't understand or you want to talk about, you may want to share it with your parents or another adult you trust. Pick someone who knows you and what your family is going through. Give them the book or article to read or tell them about what you saw. It may help to talk it over and share how you feel.

Cancer in the Family: What It's Like for You

When someone in your family has cancer, it may mean many things to you. Other people who have been through it say it can be a lot of things: confusing, scary, lonely, and much more. You may find that you have feelings that are hard to understand and sometimes hard to talk about.

The next part of this booklet shares the experiences of others who've had a family member with cancer. Some of what you read, especially about feelings, may not make sense or seem right to you. It may even seem silly. Or it may seem pretty close to what you've felt and what's happened to you.

Remember, feelings aren't "good" or "bad." They are just feelings, and are usually perfectly normal and shared by many others. And even if you try to wish them away, to ignore them, or if you feel guilty or ashamed of them, they'll still be there.

A good way to handle feelings is to admit you have them and talk about them. Talk to your parents or other adults or with your friends or others who have been through what you're going through. You'll be surprised how much better you feel once you've gotten your feelings off your chest.

It May Be Hard To Talk About Cancer

Sometimes it's not easy to talk about what you feel or about problems. Not only is it hard to say what you feel, but other people may not be ready or able to listen or to be helpful. Some of your questions may upset your parents because they don't know how to answer or because your worries remind them of their own. It's possible that your parents may not be ready to talk when you are.

They may need more time to sort things out in their own minds before they can talk with you. Some parents, no matter how much they love their children, don't know how to talk about upsetting things with them. If your parents aren't able to talk with you about your feelings, they may be able to help you find someone you can talk to, such as someone at the hospital, a relative or friend, or a teacher or school counselor.

Here is what some others who've had a parent or brother or sister with cancer have said about what they felt.

Being Scared

"I really didn't understand much at first. Mostly, I was afraid that she might die, because my sister and I are pretty close. I was really scared and I also thought it might be catching or something."
— Laura, age 13

The girl who said this had a sister with cancer, but it can be just as scary for people who have a parent with cancer. When someone is first diagnosed with cancer it may seem as though your whole world has fallen apart. You may not know much about it, so you may remember what you've heard about cancer before. Being afraid someone might die from cancer is normal, especially if the only people you've heard of who have had cancer did die. And being afraid that you or another person in the family might catch it is normal, too. Why? Because there are so many things you can catch from someone else — like a cold or the flu. It's easy to think cancer may be the same, but it's not. Learning about cancer can help you. You will feel better knowing about it than being afraid of what you don't know.

Hearing about the treatment and the tests can be hard. Some people find it's scary just to think about the needles and blood tests and radiation treatments. Sometimes learning about these things and talking to the person with cancer or someone else about what it's really like is the best way to deal with these fears. If a trip to the hospital is possible it might help.

"One day I went to the clinic with my brother for his treatment. I saw the machine that he gets radiation from and how IVs work, and I met his doctor and the nurses. I saw lots of other kids who didn't have any more hair than he does. Now when he goes to the clinic I don't have to wonder what he's going through. I know what it's like. It's no fun for a little kid like him, but it's not as bad as I thought."
— Matthew, age 14

When one parent has cancer, sometimes the other one spends a lot of time at the hospital and away from the rest of the family. Having their parents at the hospital instead of at home can be scary to some young people. They may worry about their parents and need to have some special contact to feel that things are all right.

"When Dad's in the hospital Mom goes too and I stay with my Aunt Emily. She's nice, but sometimes I get scared because I don't know how Dad is, or I miss them. So now Mom and Dad call me every night before dinner and they tell me what's happening and I can tell them about my day, and I know they're all right."
— Erin, age 9

Feeling Guilty

"I got really mad at Chrissy one day. She wouldn't let me go bike riding with her and my cousin and I got mad and said

'I wish you were dead.' Now she has leukemia and she could die and I think maybe it's my fault. I was scared to tell anyone because then they'd all know what I did and be mad. But my dad heard me crying one night and he got me to tell him why. He says it isn't my fault or anybody else's that Chrissy has cancer, and you can't make somebody get cancer just by what you say."

— Katy, age 10

Until you understand what does and doesn't cause cancer, it's easy to think that anything could have done it — even words or a fall.

"I left my junk all over the floor one night instead of putting it away and the next morning Mom fell over it. She was mad and had a lot of bruises. A little later the doctor told her she had cancer. She's in the hospital now. Maybe if she hadn't fallen down because of me she'd be okay."

— Tom, age 11

Just as words can't cause cancer, neither can bruises or bumps, or even broken bones.

Some people are afraid to tell anyone what they are thinking and may feel guilty for a long time. Even if your parents can see that something is worrying you, they may not be able to guess what it is. It's hard to talk about, especially if you think you've done something wrong and everyone will be mad at you. But it's best to get it out in the open so you and your parents or someone at the hospital can talk it over.

People sometimes feel guilty because they're well and their parent or sibling is sick. Young people may feel that it's not right for them to enjoy things they like to do when the person with cancer can't do what he or she likes. These feelings show that you care about your family, but it's important to care not only for the person with cancer, but for yourself, too. It's best for everyone if you keep being you and doing things that are important to you as long as they don't hurt anyone else. You may have to find ways to do them.

"Last year, Mom and Dad always drove me to play softball, but now Dad's sick and Mom's always at the hospital or busy at work or home. I didn't think I'd be able to play this year, and I wasn't sure I should with my dad so sick. I told my grandmom and she said I should play and she'd take me. She likes to come and she tells my folks all about the game and how I played. Next year, maybe they'll all be able to come."

— Dave, age 11

Getting Mad

"Sometimes I feel mad at my brother for having cancer. I know that's not right and he can't help it. But it's changed everything. My mom and dad don't talk about anything but him and neither does anyone else. It's just not fair."

— Sharon, age 13

People who have a brother or sister or a parent with cancer can feel angry at that person for getting sick and changing their lives. This may seem wrong, and people sometimes feel guilty about getting mad. But, if having someone with cancer in your family means you can't be with

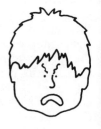

your parents as much or have to stay somewhere else or give up things you like, it can be hard. Even if you understand why it's happening, you don't have to like it. Others who have been through it say it's important to remember that things won't always be this way. And when you get mad, remember that it doesn't mean you're a bad person or don't love the person with cancer. It just means you're mad.

Feeling Neglected

One of the things that young people get mad about is feeling left out or neglected. Some feel that they don't get as much attention as they used to, and often they are right. Family members, including your parents, all have a lot on their minds and they may have to put all their energy into helping the person with cancer. This may not leave much time for you, especially if they are going back and forth to the clinic or hospital.

Siblings of people with cancer often feel that the brother or sister with cancer gets more attention from their parents.

"At night my parents go in and turn on my sister's light and kiss her good night and they don't come in my room — well, sometimes Mom will. She tells me, 'Don't think we are partial to her.' "
— Maria, age 15

And they may feel that the sibling with cancer gets away with a lot of things they don't.

"If I do something wrong, Mom yells. If my brother does, they let it pass."
— Dennis, age 13

Why do some parents do this? It's not because they don't love all their children. This is a confusing time for them, just as it is for you. They have to learn a lot about cancer and hospitals very fast. They are tired and worried. They see one of their children sick and may try to make

up for it by giving him or her a little more attention. Parents know, as you do, that some people die from cancer and they could be afraid of that and want to do all they can for your brother or sister who has cancer. Sometimes they give a young person with cancer special treatment that he or she doesn't want.

"I have a sister who has cancer. She gets upset because she's treated differently now. She doesn't want to be babied, just treated normally like she was before. She and Mom always used to fight and now Mom is really sweet all the time and it's weird. Not that my sister likes to fight, but it's just not normal."
— Peggy, age 15

For whatever reason, and whether your brother or sister likes it or not, your parents may give special treatment to the one who has cancer. At times like this, it's normal to feel jealous, even if people tell you that you shouldn't because you don't have cancer and your brother or sister does. It's hard not to want time with your parents and some special attention, too.

Young people who have a parent with cancer also may feel neglected.

"Now that Mom's sick everything at our house is different. We hardly ever eat together as a family anymore and there's never anyone to help me with my homework or listen to what's been happening to me. Mom used to do that. I feel like it's sort of being left up to me to take care of myself."
— Martha, age 13

When one parent has cancer, the other one may be so busy that neither one of them can spend much time with the rest of the family.

"Sometimes my father feels like he is neglecting us because he is with Mom so much. And in a way it's true. I know he

can't help it, he has to work and wants to see Mom, but he's not around like he used to be and he doesn't do things with us like he did. He's just too busy."

— Barry, age 16

If you feel like you're not getting much attention, whether you have a parent or a sibling with cancer, remember this: The person with cancer is getting more attention because they need special care, not because you are loved less.

Feeling Lonely

"I was really surprised, but a lot of my friends don't want to be with me anymore now that Mom has cancer. They act like it's some real freak thing or they're going to catch cancer from me. My dad says if they act like that they're not real friends anyway. But they were my friends and I miss them."

— Cheryl, age 15

You may be lucky and have a special friend or friends who treat you the same as before your family member was diagnosed with cancer. But many young people with cancer in their families have found that they've lost a few friends. Sometimes this happens because friends may not know much about cancer and be afraid of catching it from you. Or they may not know what to say and find it easier to stay away than to be embarrassed. Having cancer in your family may make you act a little differently because you're upset or scared or embarrassed, or because you want to be with your family.

"Sometimes my friends wonder why I act strange. I wish they understood that sometimes I don't want to do what they're doing, I really want to be with my sick sister."

— Nan, age 12

But your friends may not understand and think that you don't want to see them anymore. It can be a hard time for all of you.

What can you do? You may need to reach out to your friends, even if that's hard to do. Not everyone may respond as you'd like, but it helps if you give them a chance. Often friends just don't know how to act and need you to tell them how you want to be treated. They may also need you to show that you still need them, even if you seem a little different because you're upset.

If this is a hard time for you, remember that it won't last forever. Old friends may become close to you again. And people who have lost friends have found that they also made new ones. There may be someone at school who has had a sick person in the family and will understand how you feel. That person could be a special new friend.

Answering Questions

When your friends do talk to you, some of them may not say what you want to hear. Sometimes, especially in the beginning, people ask a lot of questions that are hard to answer.

"People asked me questions all the time. They'd say things like 'I heard Jean is in coma' or 'I heard you were hysterical.' Whenever I told them the truth, they didn't believe me. And they'd ask dumb questions like 'Can Jean walk, can she write?' They didn't know what was going on and I didn't know how to answer them. I got sick of it."

— John, age 1

One way to get answers to your classmates' questions is for you and your parents to talk to your teacher and see if the teacher or someone who knows about cancer and its treatment can talk to your class. Then your friends can ask their

638

questions and be sure they're getting the right answers — not about your family member, but about cancer in general.

Other people ask questions, too, and they may not know that some of them are hard for you to answer or make you feel bad. If you want to answer their questions, it's a good idea to think of what people might ask and have an answer ready. People may ask you how the person with cancer is feeling or how long they'll be in the hospital. And they can also ask questions like these: "Are you going to get cancer from your mother?" "Why does your brother always wear that cap — did his hair really fall out?" "Is your dad going to die?" "What did your sister do to get cancer?" You may want to get help when it comes to finding an answer to questions like these. Remember, you can always tell people that you don't want to talk about something. You don't have to answer their questions.

Feeling Embarrassed

"Since my brother lost his hair and got so pale and thin, I don't want to bring my friends home anymore. I don't want them to see how different Tim looks now, and I don't think he likes to see them. Besides, it's not easy to laugh and giggle at home when someone is sick."
— Caroline, age 12

Sometimes people who have a person with cancer in their family may feel embarrassed because now their family is different. It is different from what it used to be and it is different from their friends' families. And people who ask them questions they can't answer just embarrass them more. So sometimes they want to try to leave the cancer at home and hope that none of their friends learn about it. Of course, you can't really do that because when someone you love is sick you need people you can talk to and who

understand if you're upset. If you feel a little embarrassed around people because someone in your family has cancer, remember that others have felt this way too, and that this feeling often goes away once everyone has gotten used to what is happening.

Even though others feel all right about asking a lot of questions, some people with a family member who has cancer find that it embarrasses them to ask questions.

"At first I didn't ask any questions, although I had a lot of them. I thought people would think I was really dumb. But now I know it really helps to ask."
— Brad, age 14

Dealing With the Side Effects

"Diane had all this hair and some nights it would fall out and be all over her pillow when she woke up, or fall out in her comb or when she washed her hair. It really kind of scared me to see that happen at first, but she took it pretty well."
— Lois, age 16

When someone you love has side effects from cancer treatments, you have to learn to live with these changes, too. It may seem a little strange at first, or scary, but other people have found that they soon got used to it. Some people outside the family may not understand, and they may hurt the feelings of the person with cancer.

"When my little brother James went back to school he was still on chemo and had lost all his hair, so he wore a baseball cap. One day a kid pulled the cap off and teased him. James said everybody stared at him. Mom says we should feel sorry for that kid because he doesn't know any better. But I don't, I feel sorry for James."
— Amy, age 12

It's hard to imagine why anyone would want to tease James, but it's not as important to know why someone did it as it is to know that these things may happen, and you can't always protect your brother or sister. What you can do for people with cancer is try to understand how they feel and help them see that they still have friends. And, if you tease them from time to time like you did before they had cancer, it's not a bad thing as long as you don't keep it up for long or keep doing it when you see that it really hurts their feelings. Brothers and sisters all tease each other, and it's important that, even when your brother or sister has cancer, you treat each other as much like before as you can.

You may be shocked if the person in your family who has cancer comes home from the hospital looking and acting very differently from when they left.

"My dad has cancer and he was in the hospital for a long time. When he finally got to come home, he was still really sick. I had to help him up the stairs because he was so weak. It was strange, because he had been so big and always strong and now he was weak. It bothered me."
— Richard, age 16

Even if someone tells you that your family member won't look the same, you may not be prepared for the changes. It may be hard for you, but it's important to remember that, even if they look different, they're still the same person you love.

Changing

Some young people who have a family member with cancer may change a little themselves. Sometimes they're not aware of it or don't know why. But, given all the new and different experiences and feelings,

it's not surprising that people change. They may have trouble at school or be unable to concentrate or to get along with other people as well as they used to.

They may start to be a little less careful or to do things that are dangerous, maybe getting hurt more often. They may worry a lot about getting sick themselves and even get sick more often. Their school grades may fall or they may become more involved in school than they were before and make better grades.

Any of these changes can happen because young people are scared or worried, because their lives may have changed, or even because they need more attention at home. Just as with other problems or worries, talking with people who care and understand what's happening helps.

If you haven't noticed that you've changed, someone else may have, and they may want to talk to you about it. If they do, it's because they want to help. Your parents or teachers and guidance counselors or social workers at the hospital or clinic may all be able to help if you've changed in a way that isn't good for you or that makes you sad and uncomfortable.

Not all of the changes are bad; there is a good side to it too. Many young people who have had cancer in the family feel it has helped them to grow up and that it brought the family closer together.

"My brother is in remission now. Things were pretty bad at first. Then, after a while, things sort of settled down and got back to the way they were before. I think Billy's having cancer brought us all closer together. I get along better with him and my sister and even my older brother now. I'm closer to Mom and Dad. And I think we all grew up a lot while he was sick."
— Alice, age 15

How Your Parents Feel

Young people who have a person with cancer in the family often wonder how their parents feel. There's no one answer to this question. Just as with everyone else, parents may feel many different things when they have cancer themselves or when another member of their family does. They may be worried, scared, tired, or a little confused by all the decisions they need to make and all the changes that cancer can bring. Along with this, parents feel a responsibility to keep the family together during this time. They may feel that they don't have enough energy to do all the things they'd like to do or share all they'd like to with other family members. This section shares some things parents have said about how they feel.

A parent who has cancer may worry that their being sick is upsetting the family's life.

"I feel bad because now that I'm sick my husband tries to be with me a lot. I think my children's feelings are hurt but they won't say so. I just wish we could talk about it as a family."

Or they may know that being sick means that they can't do some things with their children that other parents do. They may wish they could.

"I feel like I'm letting my son down, like I'm not being a real father because I can't run around with him the way other fathers do."

When this happens, parents find they need to look for something they can do with their children that they'll all enjoy.

A parent whose husband or wife has cancer often finds that he or she needs to learn to do new things for their family and may be concerned about how well they'll do.

"Now that my wife is sick I need to be both mother and father while she's in the hospital. I'm afraid I don't do as good a job at some things as she does. The other day, our youngest son said 'Mommy never scrambled eggs like that.' I don't blame him, I'd rather eat her cooking too. I asked her how she scrambles eggs and now at least breakfast tastes a little better."

Parents don't expect their children to pretend that everything is all right or tastes great when it doesn't. Even if they get mad for a little while, most parents would rather hear what other family members feel than not know when others are upset.

Parents may know when they've been treating a child with cancer differently than the others, or when they've been short-tempered. They may feel like they can't help it, but still wish it didn't happen.

"After I spend a day in the pediatrics clinic with Lisa I'm so drained when I get home that I yell at my other kids over the least little thing. Then they get upset and I get more upset because I know that I shouldn't have done that."

Some parents worry that their children are upset and even though they want to help their children they don't know what to do. Sometimes this is because young people don't want to talk to their parents about cancer. They may be afraid that their parents will worry or won't understand. In fact, most parents worry more if they feel you are upset but they don't know why or you won't discuss it with them.

"Since I've been sick my kids have changed. I know something is bothering them, but when I ask what it is they say it's nothing. I just wish they would talk about it. I want to help them."

Often, one thing young people can do to help is to talk about how they feel and give their parents a chance to say how they feel too.

Parents say that they want their children to know that the family is there to help even when one of its members has cancer. Your family life may change when someone has cancer. The important thing, however, is that you're a family and families solve problems together. Even if life is a little different, you're still a family and your parents are still there for you.

Putting It All Together

There are many different ways to think and feel about having a person with cancer in your family. It's important to remember that people can learn to adjust to changes in their lives. Sometimes it takes a little work, but you can almost always find something or someone who can help you when you need it. Keep on trying and don't be afraid to ask for help.

• Don't be ashamed or afraid of the way you feel. Others in your situation have felt the same way.

• Sometimes things are better if you talk about them. Share your feelings with your parents or another adult or a friend you can trust.

• Learn about cancer and the way it is treated. What we first imagine about cancer is often far worse than what is really happening.

• Try to find other people your age who have a person in their family with cancer or a serious illness. You may be able to share your feelings with them.

• If you overhear someone talking and what you hear scares you, ask them to explain what they said. Don't assume that you heard everything and understood

what it meant; ask about it.

• Don't forget the adults other than your parents who can help you.

Other Sources of Information

Toll-Free Telephone Answers

If you have any questions about cancer that haven't been answered here, call the Cancer Information Service (CIS). The CIS is a group of offices around the country where people are specially trained to answer questions about cancer Your call won't cost anything—it's free. Call 1-800-4-CANCER (1-800-422-6237). If you live in Alaska, call 1-800-638-1234 (call collect from neighboring islands).

Spanish-speaking staff members are available to callers from the following areas (daytime only): California, Florida, Georgia, Illinois, New Jersey (area code 201), New York, and Texas.

National Cancer Institute Booklets

The National Cancer Institute (NCI) has a variety of free booklets available. Two of them might be of special interest to you. These are **Young People With Cancer: A Handbook for Parents,***and **Help Yourself: Tips for Teenagers With Cancer** (booklet and tape). If you would like to receive one of these booklets or a listing of other NCI publications that you may order, write to:

National Cancer Institute
Building 31, Room 10A24
Bethesda, Maryland 20892

To find other books about cancer, check with your local or hospital library or bookstores. In addition, you may want to call the American Cancer Society, the Leukemia Society, or the Candlelighters Childhood Cancer Foundation. Look in your telephone book for local offices of these organizations.

---

* The mentioned text is reprinted within this book. See CONTENTS for location.

Chapter 34

Young People With Cancer

A Parent's Guide

Foreword

The outlook for the survival of children with cancer has improved dramatically in recent years. Childhood cancer was once considered a swift and certain killer. Today, treatment techniques capable of producing disease-free states(remissions) have increased the length of survival and, in some cases, brought about apparent cures.

Although childhood cancer in general can be viewed as a chronic, treatable illness, it is life-threatening. Treatment efforts are not always successful, and children with cancer and their families may live with uncertainty and the fear of death.

Treatment for childhood cancers is aggressive and demands much of patients and those who provide them with support and comfort. These demands are both physical and emotional and are disruptive on many levels. For the parents of young people with cancer it is necessary to face their own fears while providing support to their sick child and to their healthy brothers and sisters. They must strive to continue life in as normal a manner as possible in an abnormal situation. In their efforts, they are aided by the staff at treatment centers, by other parents, and by family members and friends, but still the primary responsibility is theirs as parents.

The text which follows on the next few pages attempts to provide parents with information on the most common types of cancer, on treatments and side effects, and on the common issues that arise when a child is diagnosed with cancer. It contains medical information and practical tips gathered from the experience of others. Our aim is that this book will be of use to you and other family members in understanding the medical side of cancer and its treatment and in coping with the changes this brings to your daily life.

Vincent T. De Vita, Jr, M.D.
Director
National Cancer Institute

Introduction

The text on the next few pages was written for you--a parent of a young person with cancer. It addresses some of the most common questions about cancer in the young, combining medical information with practical suggestions. Special consideration is given to the emotional impact of cancer on patients and family members. This information is designed to help you cope with the stress of a chronic disease that entails rigorous treatment, frequent visits to the doctor and hospital, interruptions in schooling and social activities, physical change, and perhaps most frightening of all, uncertainty about the future.

Because cancer in adults and children actually involves over 100 distinct diseases and no two patients or families are alike, this text cannot address every issue or situation that will arise. Instead, it provides a general guide to childhood cancer: what to expect from it and how to deal with it.

Direct specific questions to your family physician and/or other members of the treatment team. If you want more information in special interest areas, you may be interested in obtaining a book or pamphlet mentioned in the list of additional reading materials which occurs near the end of this text.

The terms used here are those used by treatment team members when talking about your child's disease or treatment. Some of these at first may be unfamiliar to you. The glossary defines terms used in the text and others that might be used by your doctor or others involved in your child's care.

The Disease

Cancer is actually a group of diseases, each with its own name, its own treatment, and its own chances of control or cure. It occurs when a particular cell or group of cells begins to multiply and grow uncontrollably, crowding out the normal cells. Cancer may take the form of leukemia, which develops from the white blood cells, or solid tumors, found in any part of the body.

Despite considerable and continuing research, no one knows why children get cancer. Some common misconceptions about cancer are addressed below:

1. So far as scientists have been able to determine, nothing you or your child did or didn't do caused the disease. Cancer in children is still a largely unexplained disease, and there is no evidence that you could have prevented it.

2. Few cases of childhood cancer are due to genetic (inherited) factors.

3. In almost all cases of childhood cancer, its appearance in one child does not mean that a brother or sister is more likely to develop it.

4. Cancer is not contagious. It cannot be spread from person to person like a cold, or from an animal to a person.

5. No food or food additive has been implicated as a cause of any childhood cancer.

Leukemia

Leukemia is a cancer of the blood and develops in the bone marrow, the body tissue that produces blood cells.

The bone marrow is a jelly-like substance that fills the inside of the bones.

The bone marrow makes three kinds of cells:

1. *Red blood cells (erethrocytes)*,
   They give the blood its red color. These cells pick up oxygen and carry it to the tissues. They are also known as RBCs.

2. *Platelets (thrombocytes)*,
   They help stop bleeding if there is injury.

3. *White blood cells (leukocytes)*,
   They fight infections. They are also known as WBCs. Leukemia develops from these blood cells. In leukemia, certain white blood cells escape the normal control mechanisms that direct their maturing. Instead of aging so they are able to assume certain functions, they remain young and continue to multiply. This can happen to any of the three main kinds of while blood cells:

   a. Neutrophils, which eat bacteria

   b. Lymphocytes, which make substances to fight bacteria

   c. Monocytes, which destroy foreign materials

What Is a Blast?

In speaking about leukemia, "blast" is the short name used for lympho-blasts, the immature white blood cells. There are normal blasts and leukemic blasts. Normally, blasts compose less than 5 percent of the cells made by the bone marrow and grow to form mature white blood cells with certain typical features visible under the microscope. Leukemic blasts are abnormal because they remain immature and do not function like mature white blood cells. In many cases, they look different from normal blasts when viewed under a microscope.

What Happens in Leukemia?

When a large number of blasts (leukemic cells) appear in the bone marrow, several things happen. As the leukemic blast cells accumulate in the bone marrow, they begin to crowd out the normal blood cells that develop there. Eventually, they take up so much room that red blood cells, platelets, and normal white blood cells cannot be produced. When that happens, the young person develops symptoms indicating that normal blood cells are not being manufactured in adequate numbers:

- If red blood cells are crowded out by leukemic cells, the blood will look thin, which makes the patient look pale. The young person also may be tired, because the thin blood cannot carry enough oxygen to the heart, lungs, and muscles.

- If blood platelets are crowded out in the bone marrow, the young person may have bleeding problems and unusual bruising.

- If the normal, mature kind of white cells known as neutrophils are crowded out by the blasts, there will be no cells to combat bacteria, and infections may occur.

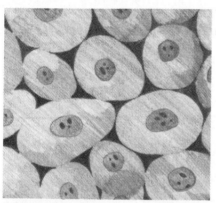

Normal cells

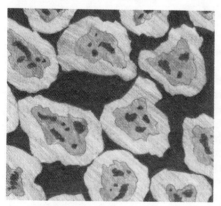

Cancer cells

In some cases, leukemic blasts may spill over from the bone marrow into the blood, where they can be seen by microscopic examination. This may cause a rise in the number of white cells in the blood (the white blood cell count). In other cases, only a few blasts appear in the blood, and the white cell count does not change much. When leukemic blasts are present in the blood, they may be carried to other places in the body and enter various body organs. Sometimes they grow in these organs as well as in the bone marrow.

Kinds of Leukemia in Young People

Leukemia is not just one disease. There is actually a type of leukemia for each of the three major kinds of white blood cells – neutrophils, lymphocytes, and monocytes.

Leukemia in any one person can affect only one kind of blood cell. The most common kinds of leukemia are lymphocytic (also called lymphoblastic or lymphoid) and myelogenous (also called granulocytic, myelocytic, myeloblastic, or myeloid). Other types (monocytic, myelomonocytic, progranulocytic, or erythroleukemia) are very rare, but still act much like the more common kinds.

If leukemia affects a young person quickly, it is called "acute" because it comes on suddenly and progresses rapidly without treatment. Almost all childhood leukemias are acute, but the disease is sometimes of the "chronic" type. In chronic leukemia, the bone marrow is able to produce a good number of normal cells as well as leukemic cells so that, compared to acute leukemia, the actual disease course is milder for a period of time.

Even without treatment, the disease usually progresses more slowly.

Acute Lymphocytic Leukemia

Acute lymphocytic leukemia (ALL for short) is commonly known as "childhood leukemia." It is the most common leukemia among the young and is the most commonly occurring cancer in children. As its name suggests, it affects the lymphocytes. Most children are between 2 and 8 years old when diagnosed, but the disease can occur in people in their twenties and thirties as well. For reasons yet to be understood, slightly more boys get ALL than girls, and it occurs more frequently among white children than black children.

Acute Myelogenous Leukemia

Acute myelogenous leukemia (AML) is also called acute granulocytic leukemia. It usually occurs in people over 25, but sometimes is found in teenagers and children. In AML, the leukemic blasts develop from the stem cells that would normally give rise to neutrophils. The characteristics of the blasts in AML are generally similar to those of acute lymphocytic leukemia, but special tests can be done to help determine whether a leukemia is myelogenous or lymphocytic.

Chronic Myelogenous Leukemia

Chronic myelogenous leukemia (CML) is not common in children. CML's distinguishing feature is the presence of very large numbers of immature neutrophil cells, which seem to mature more efficiently than blast cells. The progression of CML varies greatly, sometimes changing to a type of acute myelogenous leukemia.

Diagnosis and Treatment

Diagnosis of leukemia requires blood tests and examination of the cells in the bone marrow, because early symptoms can mimic many other diseases including mononucleosis, anemia arising from other causes, tonsillitis, rheumatic conditions, meningitis, mumps, and other kinds of cancer.

In any acute leukemia, it is necessary to determine which type of white blood cell has become leukemic, because treatment and response to it are different for each kind. Usually the type of leukemic cell involved can be determined from its appearance under the microscope, but sometimes special tests of the chromosomes and cell chemistry are needed for complete certainty. In rare instances, the cells are too young to be classified. Such cases are called acute stem cell leukemia or acute undifferentiated leukemia (AUL). Other tests such as X-rays and lumbar puncture may also be undertaken to determine if areas other than the bone marrow are involved.

The primary treatment for leukemia is combination chemotherapy, where two or more anticancer medications are used to control or eradicate the disease. Radiation, platelet and red cell transfusions, antibiotic therapy, and occasionally surgery (for unusual complications) are also a part of many treatment programs. In some forms of leukemia, bone marrow transplantation is attempted.

Solid Tumors

What Is a Solid Tumor?

The word tumor does not always imply cancer. Some tumors (collections of abnormally growing cells) are benign (not cancerous). In discussing tumors that are malignant (cancerous), how-ever, the term solid tumor is used to distinguish between a localized mass of tissue and leukemia. (Leukemia is actually a type of tumor that takes on the fluid properties of the organ it affects – the blood.)

Different kinds of solid tumors are named for the type of cells of which they are composed:

Sarcomas
Cancers arising from connective or supportive tissues, such as bone or muscle.

Carcinomas
Cancers arising from the body's glandular cells and epithelial cells, which line body tissues.

Lymphomas
Cancers of the lymphoid organs, such as the lymph nodes, spleen, and thymus, which produce and store infection-fighting cells. These cells also occur in almost all tissues of the body, and lymphomas therefore may develop in a wide variety of organs.

Kinds of Solid Tumors in Young People

Lymphomas

Lymphomas are cancers of the lymphatic tissues, which make up the body's lymphatic system. This system is a circulatory network of:

• vessels carrying lymph (an almost colorless fluid that arises from many body tissues).

• lymphoid organs such as the lymph nodes, spleen, and thymus that produce and store infection-fighting cells.

• certain parts of other organs such as the tonsils, stomach, small intestine, and skin.

Lymphomas have been broadly divided into Hodgkin's disease and non-Hodgkin's lymphomas, which include a number of diseases. Hodgkin's disease tends to involve peripheral lymph nodes (those near the surface of the body), where the first sign of disease may be a painless swelling in the neck, armpit, or groin. Hodgkin's disease occurs most commonly in patients in their twenties and thirties and occasionally in adolescents; it is rare in younger children.

In children, non-Hodgkin's lymphomas most frequently occur in the bowel, particularly in the region adjacent to the appendix, and in the upper midsection of the chest, a site where Hodgkin's disease may also occur. An initial sign of disease in these cases may be abdominal pain or swelling, breathing difficulties and sometimes difficulty in swallowing, or swelling of the face and neck. Non-Hodgkin's lymphomas may also occur in other organs, including the liver, spleen, bone marrow, lymph nodes, central nervous system, and bones. Lymphomas can be definitively diagnosed only through a biopsy, where a piece of tumor tissue is obtained surgically and examined under a microscope. Once the diagnosis is made, many tests must be done to determine the extent of the tumor, including special X-rays, CAT scans, isotope scans, and ultrasound. Blood tests are also necessary.

In the case of Hodgkin's disease, radiation therapy is highly effective for localized disease and has been the main form of treatment. However, it is believed that most lymphomas in young people are spread throughout the body, even though tumors may be detected in only one region. Because chemotherapy acts on cells throughout the body, it is the most important aspect of treatment. Surgery and radiation therapy are sometimes valuable in particular circumstances. Except in Hodgkin's disease, treatment is usually given to prevent the spread of disease to the brain and spinal column.

Brain Tumors

As a group, brain tumors are the second most common cancers of childhood. They may occur at any age, including early infancy and in adolescence, but are seen most often in children 5 to 10 years old.

Symptoms include seizures, morning headaches, vomiting, irritability, behavior problems, changes in eating or sleeping habits, lethargy, or clumsiness. Diagnosis is often difficult, because these symptoms can and frequently do indicate any number of other problems, either physical or emotional. If a brain tumor is suspected, diagnostic tests usually include skull X-rays, a brain scan, and CAT scans.

Treatment depends on the type of brain tumor involved. For the most part, surgery, radiation, or both are used. Recently anticancer drugs that can be given intravenously or orally and penetrate the brain and central nervous system have been used to treat brain tumors.

Neuroblastomas

Neuroblastoma arises from very young nerve cells that for unknown reasons, develop abnormally. More than half of these tumors occur in the adrenal glands, which are located in the abdominal area near the kidneys. Neuroblastoma is found in children only, with one-fourth of those affected showing initial symptoms during the first year of life, and three-fourths before age 5.

Symptoms include a mass, listlessness, persistent diarrhea, and pain in the abdomen or elsewhere. Again, these symptoms can point to other conditions. Diagnostic tests include an intravenous pyelogram (IVP), blood tests, ultrasound echo studies, and other procedures, depending on the site of the cancer. Because most children with this particular cancer secrete a substance that can be detected in the urine, urine tests may also be performed. The diagnosis may be further established by a biopsy for examination under an electron microscope.

Surgery is performed to remove as much of the cancerous growth as possible. If some remains after surgery, radiation is frequently used. Chemotherapy alone or combined with radiation can also be effective in treating the remaining tumor or in preventing metastases, the spread of the disease to another site.

Wilms' Tumor

Wilms' tumor is a cancer that originates in the cells of the kidney. It occurs in children from infancy to age 15, is rare in older patients, and is very different from adult kidney cancers. It may rarely be hereditary, and about 5 percent of the cases involve both kidneys.

Parents frequently bring Wilms' tumor to the attention of the doctor after they have noticed a slight swelling or a lump in their child's abdomen. Symptoms such as blood in the urine, weakness, fever, loss of appetite, or abdominal pain may or may not be present.

Diagnosis begins with a physical examination and review of the child's medical history. An IVP is the X-ray method most often used. A special X-ray tomogram of the kidney (nephrotomography), CAT scan, or other specialized diagnostic X-ray tests may also be ordered. Ultrasound pictures and other types of examination may be ordered as needed.

Wilms' tumor is one of several cancers for which treatments have been developed combining surgery, radiation therapy, and chemotherapy. The way in which these three methods will be used depends upon the child's medical history and general health and, above all, on the stage of the disease. Radiation therapy, for example, is not often used in children under the age of 2 when their disease is localized. Surgical treatment of Wilms' tumor (radical nephrectomy) involves removal of the diseased kidney and neighboring tissue and lymph nodes. When radiation therapy is used after surgery, its purpose is to guard against recurrence of the cancer where the tumor has been removed. Chemotherapy is used to treat virtually all cases of Wilms' tumor.

Retinoblastomas

Retinoblastoma is a relatively rare cancer of the eye. It may be hereditary, and one-third of the cases involve both eyes. Retinoblastoma can be seen by looking at the young person's eye, but is usually diagnosed by an examination under general anesthesia using an ophthalmoscope, an instrument used in examining the interior of the eye. The disease tends to remain localized for long periods, but in advanced stages, it can metastasize, or spread to other parts of the body. X-rays, bone marrow examination, spinal fluid examination, and a bone scan can be done to check for metastases.

If diagnosed early, it is possible to destroy the tumor with radiation therapy and preserve normal vision. If the tumor is so large that there is no hope of maintaining useful vision through radiation, the eye is removed. In cases where both eyes are involved, an attempt is made to preserve vision in both eyes through treatment with radiation. When advanced disease is found in both eyes, an attempt is made to preserve vision in *at least* one eye. If there is any possibility of useful vision, all efforts are made to preserve it. Chemotherapy, radiation, or both may also be used to treat metastases.

Rhabdomyosarcoma

Rhabdomyosarcoma, also called rhabdosarcoma, is a type of soft tissue sarcoma arising from muscle cells. It occurs slightly more frequently in males and usually affects children between the ages of 2 and 6. Although it can occur in any muscle tissue, it is generally found in the head and neck area, the pelvis, or in the extremities.

Although rhabdomyosarcoma tends to grow and spread very rapidly, fortunately its symptoms are quite obvious compared to those of other forms of childhood cancer. A noticeable lump or swelling is present in almost all cases. Other symptoms depend on the location: if the growth is near the eyes, for example, a vision problem may develop. If the neck is involved, there may be hoarseness or difficulty in swallowing. Definite diagnosis relies on biopsy. Evidence of tumor spread is sought with X-rays, tomograms, gallium scan, bone scan, liver scan, and bone marrow examination. Other procedures, such as lymphangiography, brain scan, and spinal fluid examination, may also be done, depending on the tumor's location.

Traditionally, surgery has been the primary treatment, followed by intensive chemotherapy and radiation. However, if the tumor is so large that surgery presents a major risk to the patient or would result in serious disfigurement or physical impairment, then chemotherapy, radiation, or both are used to reduce the tumor's size until it can be removed more safely. In some cases, the cancer can be treated effectively with chemotherapy and radiation alone.

Osteogenic Sarcoma

Osteogenic sarcoma, also called osteosarcoma, is the most common type of bone cancer in children. It arises in the ends of the bones. The bones most frequently involved are the large bones of the upper arm (humerus) and the leg (femur and tibia). Osteogenic sarcoma usually occurs between the ages of 10 and 25 and is more common among males than females.

Young people with this type of cancer generally complain of pain and swelling, which they sometimes blame on an injury. Diagnosis can be difficult, because the disease is easily confused with local infection, effects of injury, glandular deficiencies, arthritis, vitamin deficiencies, and benign tumors. Although osteogenic sarcoma may be suspected by the way the bone looks on X-rays, diagnosis can be confirmed only by biopsy. Because the disease commonly spreads

(metastasizes) to other parts of the body, especially the lungs, chest X-rays, lung tomograms, CAT scans of the chest, and an X-ray skeletal survey or bone scan may also be done before treatment.

Treatment usually involves amputation of the affected limb, followed by a course of chemotherapy using one or more anticancer drug. A prosthesis (artificial limb) and physical rehabilitation are important parts of therapy.

The use of implants and limb preservation as opposed to amputation is still experimental. In this process, the portion of the bone that is cancerous is removed and replaced with a special implant. For more information on this technique and whether its use is appropriate for your child, ask your physician.

Ewing's Sarcoma

Ewing's sarcoma differs from osteosarcoma in that it affects a different part of the bone – the bone shaft – and tends to be found in bones other than the long bones of the arm and leg, such as the ribs. Like osteogenic sarcoma, it usually occurs between the ages of 10 and 25, is seen more often in males, and frequently spreads to other bones and the lungs.

Young people with this type of cancer usually have more general signs – fever, chills, and weakness – than are present in osteogenic sarcoma. Because the symptoms can point to other conditions, definitive diagnosis depends on biopsy. A bone survey, bone scans, chest X-rays, lung tomograms, liver scans, and brain scans may be done as well to look for evidence of metastases.

Treatment involves use of a combination of intensive radiation therapy and chemotherapy.

Treatment

When a diagnosis of cancer is confirmed, it is best for your child to begin treatment at a treatment center that has an experienced staff and the resources to apply the most effective form(s) of treatment right from the beginning. Your family physician or pediatrician can help you find such a center where specialists in childhood cancer will be in charge of your child's care.

Your child's treatment will be based on medical advances learned from treating many other young people. For some types of cancer, treatment programs may be well established. However, research for effective treatments is constantly under way, and your child may be treated under a research protocol (or regimen), which is a general treatment plan that several hospitals use for treatment of one type of cancer. The protocol is carefully designed to establish the ideal type, frequency, and duration of treatment.

Still, because children's reactions to therapy vary, the treatments may need to be modified to allow for individual differences. If a child is unable to tolerate a treatment plan or protocol, and minor adjustments do not correct this, another treatment plan may be begun or a specially designed program created. Before any therapy begins, the doctor should discuss the treatment program with you, including benefits and risks, and obtain your consent. Depending on the hospital's policy on the age at which a patient's agreement is necessary to undertake therapy, your child may also be required to approve it.

The treatment plan may look complicated at first, but each of the steps will be carefully explained, and you will soon become familiar with the routine.

At the treatment center, your child may be seen by different physicians from time to time, all of whom will follow the basic treatment plan. Your child may also be examined by resident physicians, fellows, and medical students who are working in the center as part of the educational program in cancer medicine and pediatrics. All residents and fellows are experienced physicians who are near the end of their training period, and their work is supervised by a senior physician.

In addition to these physicians at the treatment center, your family physician or pediatrician may continue to play an active role in the care of your child. With current information on the therapy prescribed for your child, your doctor can remain a source of advice and treatment for routine medical care and problems. Especially if distance between your home and the treatment center is a factor, your local physician may be called on to do blood tests or administer chemotherapy prescribed by the center physicians, thus reducing the number of visits to the center. If that is the case, your child's initial hospitalization or outpatient treatment will usually take place at the center, and you will return there for periodic checkups.

The exact type of treatment your child will receive depends on the type of cancer. Most patients receive surgery, radiation therapy, chemotherapy, or a combination of these. These treatments aim at bringing about a remission, the decrease or disappearance of symptoms of the cancer. There are two major phases of treatment: remission induction and remission maintenance. Remission induction attempts to establish a "clinical" remission, in which detectable cancer has been eliminated. If this phase is successful, maintenance therapy aims at reaching undetectable cancer cells, which experience has shown may remain in the body. Remission induction may be accomplished through surgery, radiation, or chemotherapy. Maintenance therapy involves the use of chemotherapy and may last only a few months or go on for several years.

Hospitalization

With admission to the hospital, the child enters a new world, with new people and strange machines, procedures, and routines. The child sees other patients, observes their conditions, and strives to achieve some kind of order out of the surrounding confusion. From the beginning, it is important to encourage your child to ask any and all questions, express all concerns, and seek answers to what may not be understood in the hospital environment.

Hospitalization can be a traumatic experience for any child. This is especially true when treatment requires removal from parents, on whom the child depends for emotional and social support. More and more hospitals have unrestricted visiting hours for parents. Beds in the child's room or bedrooms adjacent to the area are sometimes made available to parents so they can be with their child during extended hospital stays. If that is not the case in your hospital, you might want to ask if you can sleep in a chair near your child's bed during crucial times, such as the days before and after surgery, or the first night in the hospital.

Experiencing difficult medical procedures and continually meeting new people who do all sorts of things to the child build up tension. The young patient may become nervous, anxious, and unruly. For the hospitalized child, some form of outlet in play is essential.

Most hospitals have playrooms for patients. These offer children an opportunity to interact with one another in a way similar to their play with friends at home. In hospital playrooms, children may relax and become less fearful and better able to cope with their feelings about hospital equipment, medical procedures, and medical personnel. They may act out their concerns in play and thus deal with them in their own way.

Playroom personnel are often trained professionals with backgrounds in psychology, special education, childhood development, social work, nursing, or recreational therapy. As part of the treatment team, they are in a position to alert other caregivers and parents about concerns the child may be able to express only through play.

If the child is confined to bed and unable to go to the playroom, recreational therapists or child life workers may pay bedside visits. A child life worker is a new category of professional who is responsible for making the hospital and treatment experience less intimidating for the child by coordinating play therapy, schoolwork, and other activities.

Playrooms may also be equipped to provide outlets for the energies of older children and adolescents, who may enjoy taking part in crafts or playing games appropriate to their ages. Record and tape players for use in the playroom or loan for their own rooms are popular with teens.

Hospitalization threatens the growing sense of independence in older children. The young person is taken to the doctor, taken to the hospital, given treatment. This role is passive rather than active. The lack of independence resulting from hospitalization and cancer treatment is particularly displeasing to the adolescent, who may frequently and loudly protest the forced dependence. It is not uncommon for adolescents to refuse treatment, break hospital rules, miss outpatient appointments, or undertake activities against the doctor's orders. Besides rebelling against the feelings of dependence, teenagers may be acting on the normal adolescent resistance to authority figures and reluctance to appear different from peers outside the hospital. Some hospitals have responded by relaxing certain rules so teenagers can dress in street clothes whenever possible and have visits from their friends. Hospitals may also fill the oncology ward's refrigerator with their patients' favorite foods. Parents can help by allowing the adolescent a share of the responsibility for his or her own care and by respecting the need for independence and privacy, hard as that may be under the circumstances. But more than anything else, your teenager needs to know that you are there if you are needed and that you can be relied on for honest, dependable answers.

Surgery

For many solid tumors, surgery is the primary and most effective treatment. For very large tumors, radiation or chemotherapy is often used before surgery to reduce the size of the tumor, make surgery safer for the patient, and lessen any physical or functional defects.

The young person facing surgery is likely to be afraid. To counter some of that fear, many hospitals prepare patients for surgery by letting them visit the operating and recovery rooms, where they can meet and talk with the people who will be present during the operation. These people explain what they will be doing and how they will look. They might, for instance, bring along a surgical mask and put it on for the younger child. This advance preparation can at least ease the shock and accompanying fear of the sterile operating room, strange equipment, and uniformed, masked personnel.

In addition, the patients should be encouraged to discuss their feelings and fears concerning surgery. Young people commonly worry about the anesthesia, whether there will be a lot of pain, how their bodies will be changed, and whether their parents will be there when they wake up. If an internal organ has been removed, some children feel a lack of wholeness afterward. Amputations for bone cancer, primarily osteosarcoma, may produce similar feelings. Amputation also means the young person must accept and learn to use an artificial limb.

Your child will have questions about the surgery, and these must be answered as honestly as possible, because the child may feel betrayed if what you said does not match up with what actually happened. You will want to learn as much about the operation as possible. The surgeon and other members of the treatment team can help you. If you wish, they may be able to arrange for your child to see and talk with another young person who has had the same type of surgery and is doing well. If a limb must be removed, the center's staff might show the child a prosthesis. If appropriate, your child may begin to practice walking with crutches even before amputation of the leg makes crutches temporarily necessary.

Chemotherapy*

Chemotherapy is treatment with anticancer drugs. These drugs may be taken by mouth (pills or liquids) or given by injection into a muscle (intramuscularly or IM), a vein (intravenously or IV), or just below the skin (subcutaneously or SC). These are different ways of getting the medication into the bloodstream so that it can be distributed throughout the body. Another method, used for treatment of brain tumors and prevention of central nervous system disease in leukemia, is to inject the anticancer drug into the spinal fluid (intrathecally or IT).

Insertion of the IV needle may be painful and, once in the vein, the drugs may cause an uncomfortable burning sensation. If the drug leaks from the vein, it may severely burn the skin, so care must be taken to make sure the IV line is securely in place, and the nurse or doctor must act immediately if the needle comes out of the vein.

Injections are generally given by physicians or nurses, but pills may be given at home. Taking chemotherapy pills can sometimes be a problem with younger children, but the tablets can be broken into smaller pieces for swallowing or powdered and mixed with apple sauce, jam, custard, etc. Older children, particularly adolescents, may wish to be responsible for taking and keeping track of their oral medication(s). However, it is still important for parents to be familiar with the medications

and check to be sure they are being taken correctly.

Whether you or your child is responsible, you may want to develop a system for keeping track of when medications are taken. Marking a special calendar when medications are taken is one way of doing this.

Chemotherapy and Its Side Effects

Once in the bloodstream, chemotherapeutic drugs are taken up by cells that divide rapidly, such as cancer cells. In the cancer cell, the drugs act by interfering with the duplication and growth of the cell, primarily by preventing it from dividing or depriving it of a substance it requires to function, and the cell is eventually destroyed. Anticancer drugs can affect not only cancer cells, but also other rapidly dividing normal cells such as those in the gastrointestinal tract, bone marrow, hair follicles, and reproductive system. Because of this, unwanted side effects of the treatment can and often do occur in normal tissues. Almost all side effects, however, are temporary.

One common side effect of chemotherapy is the reduction of the bone marrow's ability to produce the normal amount of blood cells. This may put your child at greater risk for anemia (if significantly fewer red blood cells are being produced), bleeding (if production of platelets is down), or infection (if the white cell count, particularly that of the neutrophils, is low). No medications or special diets are known to reverse chemotherapy's effect on the bone marrow and the resulting

---

* *See chapter entitled, **Chemotherapy and You**. Consult CONTENTS for page location.*

lowering of blood counts. Your physician will let you know if the blood counts are so low that special precautions must be taken. In general, you should be particularly alert to any signs of infection, bruising, or bleeding and notify your physician if they occur. Anticancer drugs, their routes of administration, physical descriptions, and side effects are listed in the foldout drug chart starting on page 69.

Many side effects from anticancer drugs are possible, and the following points are good to keep in mind:

1. Most side effects can be lessened by taking appropriate measures before, during, and after chemotherapy. (See the following section for how to control side effects.)

2. Side effects vary in severity and type from person to person and treatment to treatment. Your child will not necessarily have the same reactions as another child, but it is important for you to be aware of those problems that occur commonly so you can recognize their occurrence early.

3. Most side effects are reversible and will improve after the drug is stopped. Some, such as hair loss and bone marrow depression, may lessen or disappear even without discontinuing chemotherapy.

4. Slightly decreasing the drug dosage because of serious, persistent, and unreasonable side effects usually will not decrease a drug's ability to be effective. Consequently, even if your child's dose is reduced in an effort to lessen or eliminate these side effects, the chance of recovery will not be changed.

5. Side effects of chemotherapy may be classified as common or uncommon and as acute (immediate) or delayed (days to weeks after chemotherapy):

Common acute side effects:

- Nausea and vomiting
- Pain and burning at injection site

Less common acute side effects:

- Allergic reactions (hives; rash; swelling of eyelids, hands, and feet; shortness of breath)
- Drug extravasation (leaking of drug out of vein into skin)

Common delayed side effects:

- Hair loss
- Mouth soreness and ulcers
- Constipation (especially with the drug vincristine)
- Bone marrow depression (low blood counts)

Uncommon delayed side effects:

- Jaundice (yellow tint to skin and eyes due to liver problems)
- Hemorrhagic cystitis (bloody urine due to bladder irritation – especially with the drug cyclophosphamide)
- Mental or nervous system changes (lethargy, tiredness, lack of coordination)

Each drug has the potential of producing its own side effects. Your doctor can tell you which ones your child is most likely to experience.

6. Daunorubicin or its chemical cousin adriamycin may cause heart damage if the cumulative dose over time exceeds certain levels. Your physician should keep a careful record of the cumulative dose and should warn you if your child passes the usual limits.

7. Recent research has raised the possibility of long-term effects of treatment on such areas as reproductive and intellectual abilities. Your physician can tell you more about these in relation to your child's specific care and treatment.

Controlling the Side Effects of Chemotherapy

Certain side effects, although not dangerous, are bothersome, and you can try to avoid or control some of these through specific measures:

1. Constipation from vincristine: Encourage increased consumption of fluids and roughage (juices, fruits, vegetables, bran cereals) starting the day before injection and continuing for a week. If the child does not have a bowel movement for a considerably longer period of time than is usual, contact your physician. If constipation is a common problem, the regular use of a stool softener may be necessary while the child is on vincristine.

2. Pain: Aspirin should not be used for pain or fever because it can affect blood clotting and upset the stomach. Acetaminophen (aspirin-free pain reliever) is usually used instead. If pain is severe or persistent, contact your physician. If the child has a fever as well as pain, contact your physician before giving any medication for pain.

3. Tissue burns from vincristine, daunomycin, or adriamycin leaking at the site of injection: Any swelling, redness, or pain occurring during an injection or up to a few days afterward should immediately be brought to the attention of the doctor or nurse. Prompt treatment may be necessary to prevent a severe burn and ulceration of the skin.

4. Heartburn and stomach-ache from prednisone and dexamethasone: To prevent this, give ½ glass of milk or 1 or 2 tablespoons of an antacid with each dose.

5. Hair loss from vincristine, adriamycin, methotrexate, cyclophosphamide, etc: This will occur in varying degrees in each child, depending on which drugs and which schedule of drugs is received. There is no way to prevent hair loss, short of discontinuing medication. Experimental attempts to prevent hair loss, such as wearing a special headband or ice cap during drug administration, are being undertaken, but their results are inconclusive. The hair will grow back, but adequate regrowth takes months. In the interim, emotional stress exists, especially in teenagers. If marked hair loss appears to be occurring, your child may want to consider wearing a wig. Caps or scarves may also be worn. The wearing of a wig will *not* hamper hair regrowth.

6. Mild to severe mouth soreness is caused occasionally by several drugs (e.g., methotrexate, adriamycin). Good oral hygiene is important during this period. Many people use special mouth-rinses to ease the discomfort. (See the discussion of mouth care in "Common Health Issues" for more information.) No particular regimens are known to prevent mouth soreness from occurring.

7. Nausea and vomiting, also caused by several drugs, can often be relieved and sometimes prevented by certain medications. Unfortunately, no perfect drug exists to prevent nausea and vomiting. Those that are effective are most helpful if given before chemotherapy. If these symptoms are marked, ask your physician about prescribing medication to counteract them. Hypnosis and relaxation exercises are used in some treatment centers to alleviate these symptoms.

8. Hemorrhagic cystitis (irritation and bleeding from the bladder) from cyclophosphamide: The likelihood of this occasional side effect may be reduced by seeing that the drug does not rest in the bladder for a long time. This is best done by giving the drug early in the day and seeing that urination is increased by encouraging your child to drink plenty of fluids throughout the day (thirst cannot be relied on). This will assure elimination of the drug from the bladder. The amount of liquids to be given depends on the child's size, so discuss this with your physician. This complication may occur shortly after the drug is given or show up weeks or months after the patient receives cyclophosphamide, so pink or bloody urine occurring at any time after therapy should be immediately reported to the doctor.

9. Some drugs increase sensitivity to the sun, so a complete sun-blocking lotion containing PABA (check the product's list of ingredients) should be used to prevent burning.

Finally, it is helpful to discuss with your physician any of the listed side effects and any other changes that you observe in your child.

Radiation Therapy*

Radiation therapy is treatment by high-energy X-rays. The basic principles of radiation therapy are simple: X-rays, radium, and other sources of ionizing radiation are used to destroy cancer cells. The interaction between the radiation rays and the cellular tissue damages the DNA within cells (the genetic code that directs development), causing the cells to die as they are about to divide. The doses used kill the cancer cells but have a minimal effect on the surrounding normal tissues. The result is a reduction of the tumor's size.

Radiation may be used alone, in combination with surgery or chemotherapy, or both. There is no pain or discomfort during the treatment. It is much like having an ordinary X-ray taken, except that the child needs to hold still for a few minutes longer. In some cases, young children need to be sedated in order to hold still for the radiation treatment. You will not be allowed in the room during treatment, because this would expose you to needless X-rays. Younger children may find it frightening to be left alone in the room during radiation therapy. If you accompany your child to treatment, it may be reassuring to explain

---

* See chapter entitled, **Radiation Therapy and You.** Consult CONTENTS for page location.

that you are just outside the room. In some hospitals, closed-circuit television or viewing windows allow you to watch your child receive treatment, and in these cases, the child may feel easier knowing that you can see him or her all during the treatment. Most radiation departments are willing to give you and your child a tour of the treatment area before the first treatment. During this time, the technologist will explain the machines. A trip to the radiation therapy room ahead of time may also help quiet fears about the equipment, especially its large size.

Before therapy is started, a physician specializing in radiation therapy will talk with you and explain the details of the treatment. The physician will also use dye to mark the area to be irradiated. Once in place, this dye should not be washed off for the duration of the treatments, because it will be used as a guide for aiming the radiation. While radiation therapy is being received, soap or lotion should not be used on these lines or within the radiation field, where the skin will become tender. The area should also be kept dry.

Areas of the body not being treated are often protected from radiation by special shields made of lead.

Side Effects of Radiation Therapy and Controlling Them

Your child will not be radioactive after or during radiation therapy. Neither you nor anyone else need fear contact with the child. Among the real side effects of treatment, which vary according to the site receiving the radiation, are:

1. *Skin Damage.* The skin in the treated area may be somewhat sensitive and therefore should be protected against exposure to sunlight and irritation. During treatment, it should not be exposed to sunlight. After treatment is completed, the skin will still be sensitive, and a sun-blocking lotion containing PABA should be used to prevent burning. If the head is affected, soft hats and scarves are comfortable and fashionable. Your physician may also prescribe baby powder or cornstarch, an antibiotic ointment, or steroid cream to relieve itching and pain and to speed healing. Nothing, however, should be applied to the treatment area without the recommendation of the person in charge of the treatment.

2. *Sore mouth* (if the head and neck are within the irradiated area). Your physician may prescribe a mouthrinse, and the hints on mouth care provided in "Common Health Issues" will also help.

3. *Hair loss.* Hair is frequently lost from the area receiving the radiation therapy. This loss is usually temporary, with hair growth beginning about 3 months after the completion of treatment. Initial adjustment to even temporary hair loss can be difficult, but after a time, children are able to play, work, and go to school without undue embarrassment. Some will want to wear a wig, cap, or scarf.

4. *Nausea, vomiting, and headaches.* A few children have these symptoms following radiation therapy

661

to specific sites, such as the head or abdomen. These problems may last for about 4 or 5 hours and can be relieved by medicines prescribed by your doctor. In terms of diet, small, frequent meals are recommended. You may want to see that your child eats 3 to 4 hours before treatment.

5. *Diarrhea, after radiation to the abdomen* (or pelvic area). This condition usually responds to simple measures such as nonprescription drugs or medications prescribed by your doctor. A low-residue diet avoiding fresh fruits, vegetables, and fried foods may also help. Occasionally, treatment will have to be suspended until the symptoms subside.

6. *Late effects.* Following irradiation to the brain and/or central nervous system, some children seem to be drowsy and need more sleep. This symptom may begin at various times, even as late as 5 to 7 weeks after therapy has been completed. It usually lasts about 5 to 10 days. Several days before the drowsiness occurs, the child may lose his appetite, have fever or headache, have nausea and vomiting, and be irritable in general. This is a temporary condition; nevertheless, *it is important to report such symptoms to your physician*. Other posttherapy symptoms your doctor will want to evaluate are dizziness, sight disturbances, increased appetite, and stiff neck. None of these may occur, but if they do, you should contact the physician.

7. *Long-term effects.* Recent research suggests that radiation therapy to the head may affect intelligence and/or coordination, depending on several factors, including the age of the child at the time of exposure. Research also points to the increased possibility of developing a second tumor in an area treated with radiation. A second tumor usually develops several years after the exposure. Your child's physician or radiation therapist can tell you more about these long-term effects in relation to your child and the treatment.

New Treatments

The search for new and more effective drugs to treat cancer is a continuing one. Each year, thousands of drugs are tested in experimental animals for activity against cancer. The most promising of these are further studied to determine whether they might be safe and effective for human use and to establish the proper dosage.

Newspaper and magazine reports of such research can be unintentionally misleading. A so-called new drug "cure" may refer to an agent that is effective against animal leukemia and has not yet been tested in patients. Or it may be a drug with limited usefulness in one particular type of cancer or in cancer at one particular stage. If you have any questions, discuss such reports with your child's physician, who is in the best position to evaluate them.

Some parents are concerned that if a cure for cancer is found in one hospital, it will not be known in another. Actually, the medical world is relatively small, and in this age of rapid communications, the discovery of a successful new treatment method will become generally known almost immediately.

Unproven Treatments

Unusual remedies and approaches to cancer treatment often achieve public notoriety. As the parent of a child with cancer, inevitably you will hear of these yourself or have them brought to your attention by others. Patients, particularly older ones, may also hear of such treatments.

These treatments may involve unusual forms of therapy or strict dietary regimens that are reported to cure cancer. As a group, these treatment techniques are often called "unproven" methods, because they have not been tested in the same strict method as have treatments employed by your physician. Reports of cures seldom provide enough information to compare their effectiveness with that of more conventional therapies.

The guarantee of cure these treatments offer may seem attractive when judged against the difficult treatment course of conventional therapies and the fact that your physician cannot absolutely predict the results of that treatment. If you develop an interest in an unconventional treatment or have any questions, discuss it with your physician, who should be able to provide or direct you to relevant information. The treatment team's primary concern is that your child receive the most effective treatment possible. If some magical, easy cure for cancer existed, caregivers would be the first to make it available.

Because many people have heard of unproven methods of cancer treatment, you, or occasionally the older patient, may find yourself in the position of defending your decision to follow conventional treatment methods. This can be a frustrating situation and place a burden on you during an already stressful time. It is important to remember that suggestions are usually well intentioned and that they come from those who are not well informed about treatment advances. The best way to deal with this may be to provide these people with more information and make it clear that you appreciate their interest but that you feel your child is already receiving the best treatment available.

Common Health Issues

A number of routine health-related matters are common to all young people with cancer. Some of these are discussed below and should provide you with general information on issues of concern to you. You may want to check with your physician or others in the treatment center to see how these general statements apply to your child's specific situation.

Infections

Because of lowered white blood cell counts from chemotherapy, infections can be particularly serious in a child with cancer who is receiving chemotherapy. Your child may handle most infections as well as other children. Still, there is the potential for the development of serious and unusual infections, and any sign of infection, such as fever, should be reported to your child's physician as soon as possible.

To determine the cause of the infection, the physician may ask that cultures be taken of any sores as well as of the blood, urine, throat, and stool. If it is a bacterial infection, antibiotics will be given to control it. These may be given either orally or intravenously. Depending on the severity of the infection and your physician's policy, your child may be hospitalized. The cultures taken earlier will usually be repeated to check the course of the infection and the effectiveness of the antibiotic treatment.

Antibiotics will not be used if the infection is caused by a virus, because antibiotics are ineffective in treating viral infections. In these cases, chemotherapy may be stopped for a time and medication given to ease the symptoms while your child's blood counts and general condition are closely monitored.

Some viral infections, such as chickenpox, can be particularly dangerous to a child receiving chemotherapy, because complications from the infection may arise. Notify your child's physician immediately if your child has been exposed, because certain measures can be taken, such as decreasing drug doses or using a special gamma globulin. If your child attends school, teachers should know to inform you at once if a schoolmate develops chickenpox.

Most children who have had chickenpox are immune for life and will not contract it, even if exposed while in relapse or on chemotherapy. However, some children on chemotherapy who have already had chickenpox may, when exposed to it again, develop shingles. This is a blistery-like skin rash that resembles chickenpox but, instead of appearing all over the body, is confined to one area. Although complications from shingles are less likely than from chickenpox, notify your physician if you suspect your child has shingles.

Regular or red measles (also known as Rubeola or hard 9-day measles) may also be more serious for a child on chemotherapy. If the child is exposed to this type of measles, your physi-

cian should be notified. Regular gamma globulin may be given in an attempt to prevent or control the infection.

There is no evidence that infections play any role in activating the cancer or causing a relapse. As stated earlier, your child will tolerate most infections as well as if he or she did not have cancer. Chemotherapy may be stopped during the period of infection, depending on the severity of the infection and the child's white cell count. Your physician will be the best judge of whether this should be done.

Your child may miss some oral medications because of a gastrointestinal infection. Contact the physician or treatment center if this occurs. Brief interruptions of medicine for such reasons do not seem to jeopardize the welfare of the child.

Activities

Cancer and its management may seem to consume an overwhelming amount of your time. For the child, however, the best antidote to this unwelcome (and at times painful) attention is to encourage your child to live as normal and active a life as possible. Check with your physician to see if any special precautions should be taken.

If your child feels well, there is no need to insist on extra rest. However, there may be days, especially after chemotherapy or radiation therapy, when your child may seem lethargic or appear to need more rest. This is a normal result of the treatment. Other days normal levels of energy will return, and you should encourage your child to get regular rest and pursue normal activities.

In complete remission, there are usually no restrictions on activity.

Diet

Good nutrition is an important part of your child's treatment. In general, your child's normal diet should be continued during cancer treatment unless your physician gives you a special one. A few diet hints are listed below:

1. Build meals around your child's favorite foods. Variety is not as important as intake.

2. Small, frequent meals and snacks are attractive to most children. You can freeze portions of a favorite dish and serve them when desired.

3. Smaller bites and frequent sips of water, milk, or other unsweetened drinks will make chewing and swallowing easier.

4. Avoid empty calorie foods. Such items, e.g., soft drinks, chips, candy, reduce your child's appetite without providing nutrients. By contrast, milkshakes (with eggs or yogurt in them), yogurt, fruit, juices, or instant breakfasts provide extra calories and protein.

5. Some types of chemotherapy may temporarily alter your child's sense of taste. Well-seasoned foods such as spaghetti, tacos, and pizza may seem especially good at times. Sometimes adding extra salt or sugar, or using less, may make foods taste better. However, because of fluid retention, patients on cortisone drugs should limit salt in their diets.

6. A decrease in appetite is common to some types of chemotherapy. (See the drug chart for examples.) But this must be countered with an *increase* in fluid intake beginning a few days before the chemotherapy and continuing for a few days after it.

7. If appetite is poor, the addition of a single multivitamin (one without *folic acid*, if your child is taking methotrexate) per day may be advisable. Be sure to ask your doctor before beginning vitamin supplements.

8. If your child is taking oral medication at home, the time of day that medication is given may be critical. Some are best given in the morning, some at midday, some on a full stomach, etc. Be sure to ask your doctor when and how medications should be administered.

Immunizations

Live virus vaccines (regular measles, German measles or rubella, mumps, polio) should not be given. They may be dangerous to a young person who is under medication that suppresses the normal response to these vaccines. Diphtheria, whooping cough, and tetanus immunizations (DPT or DT shots) are not "live" and are considered by some to be safe for those being treated for cancer. Ask your physician before allowing any immunizations to be given. If your child has never received the regular measles vaccine, report this to the physician.

Other Medications

A young person under treatment should not take any other medications without the physician's approval. It is important to note that some medications ordinarily used to treat common conditions should be avoided. For instance, when the child's platelet count is low, avoid aspirin and glyceryl guaiacolate (present in certain cough syrups). If your child is on prednisone or dexamethasone, avoid aspirin, because it may stimulate bleeding. If fever, pain, or aches are present, acetaminophen (aspirin-free pain reliever) may be used, but the presence of the condition (fever, pain, etc.) should be reported to the physician.

Mouth Care

It is especially important to keep the young person's teeth, mouth, and gums clean to protect from tooth decay and infection. Also, a child with a poor appetite who receives mouth care before meals may feel better about eating.

Teeth should be brushed after each meal, using a soft toothbrush. After each use, the brush should be rinsed well with cold water, shaken thoroughly, and hung to dry on the toothbrush rack. Disposable paper cups should be used for rinsing out the mouth. Dental floss may be used, if care is taken not to cut the gums.

To prevent the severe tooth decay that can result when saliva flow is reduced from radiation to the head and neck, older children should use a fluoride mouthrinse as often as recom-

mended by the physician or dentist. Fluoride gels may be prescribed for home use.

Children whose treatment has not included radiation to the head and neck should also use a mouthrinse frequently during the day. One suggested mouthrinse is a mixture of salt and baking soda (¼ teaspoon of each in a cup of water).

Infants and toddlers can be given mouth care by wrapping a soft cloth around your finger and gently wiping the teeth and gums with a solution of mouthrinse.

When the young person has low blood counts, mouth care should be especially gentle. *Very soft* bristle toothbrushes should be used. If you prefer a Toothette (a spongy swab), discard it after use. Water jet devices or dental floss should *not* be used when blood counts are low and your child is prone to infection. Watch for sore areas or red and white patches. Alert the physician to any red or white patches, mouth sores, or irritated areas that develop in the mouth.

When mouth sores, bleeding areas, or irritated areas are present, only the mouthrinse described above or one prescribed by your doctor is appropriate. Moreover, they should be used at least every 2 to 3 hours. Your child should rinse the mouth out well after every meal and before bedtimes. Also, Q-tips or glycerin swabs can help remove food particles.

If mouth sores become painful, a local anesthetic ordered by your physician may help and can be applied as often as recommended. When your child has mouth sores, it may be easier to eat if you apply an anesthetic directly to sore gums or to other *small* areas in the mouth immediately before meals.

If used as a rinse or applied to the back of the throat, however, give it to your child at least 1 hour before meals. Otherwise, the normal gag-reflex may be suppressed, and there could be a danger of choking.

If your child has dry lips, petroleum jelly or a lip pomade can prevent cracking.

Dental Care

Ideally, your child should have a thorough oral examination and any necessary dental work before cancer treatment begins. This is not always possible. Although dental work may have to be delayed because of the cancer and side effects of treatment, it should not be neglected.

When blood counts are normal, dental work is an important part of overall health care, but you should check with the physician before scheduling dental work. Even checkups should be avoided when the blood count is low.

Bleeding

A low platelet count may predispose your child to bleeding. In that case, special precautions should be taken to curtail "contact" activities. For the older child, it is wise to limit activities such as football, soccer, skateboarding, or rollerskating. To control episodes of sustained bleeding, remember the following:

● Apply pressure until the bleeding stops – a clean towel, handkerchief, or cloth *firmly* applied to the wound will slow or stop the bleeding.

● For nosebleeds, have the child sit up. Don't let your child lie down. Pinch the bridge of the nose over the bone for 10 minutes. The pressure must be tight on both sides to be effective.

● Notify the doctor promptly if bleeding continues.

Transfusions

If necessary, transfusions of whole blood or specific components of blood can be given to cancer patients. Blood transfusions may be given to control the anemia that may result from a low red blood cell count. The blood may be given as whole blood, which includes the plasma or liquid portion of the blood, or as "packed cells," a transfusion of blood from which the liquid portion has been removed.

Platelet transfusions may be given if your child has a low platelet count because of the disease or its treatment and is at increased risk for bleeding. Platelet transfusions are most commonly given if the patient is bleeding or is in a situation that will predispose to bleeding, such as preparing for surgery.

Because each individual has a characteristic blood type, tests are run to be sure the donor's blood is compatible with the recipient's. This process is called blood typing and cross-matching.

In transfusions of white blood cells, the need for compatible tissue type between donor and recipient is greater, and siblings and parents of the patient often serve as donors. In the process of collecting white cells for transfusion to the patient, the other components of the blood are returned to the donor. White cell transfusions may be given to a patient with a low white count and a serious infection that is not responding to treatment.

Tips for Clinic Visits and Medical Procedures

Listed below are some ideas for making treatment and medical procedures easier. These are based on the experience of other parents and are offered only as suggestions.

1. Bring a favorite toy or book to the clinic to comfort your child during the wait and the discomfort of treatment. Since waits are sometimes long and space is limited, reading, crafts, or quiet games can help pass the time. Teenagers may want to bring crafts, electronic games, playing cards, books, or magazines.

2. Keep a daily log of your child's temperature, activity level, feelings, sleep patterns, amount of drugs given, and any reaction, among other information. Also, record the treatments and clinic visits. You and an older child may want to work together on keeping this log. Be sure to bring this log with you on your clinic visits. It will be helpful to your child's doctors.

3. Prepare your child for medical tests. You need to become informed about a test before explaining it to your child. Ask the doctor or other health care team members for information and how best to explain the test to your child. Your child may react with anger or fear, but knowing this information in advance helps build a child's trust in adults. Using language that takes into account the child's age and understanding, you can tell what will be done and why. You may still want to use dolls and puppets or other playthings. Be honest about the amount and type of pain the treatment will bring. Above all, listen to your child's questions and encourage your child to express feelings about what was just heard.

4. Plan to stay with your child during a test or treatment. Your presence can do much to reassure and comfort your child and can make discussion afterward easier for you. Encourage your child to take part and make choices wherever possible. for example, your child may want to hold a gauze pad or watch for a signal. This helps children feel as if they have some control.

5. Become involved in the health care of your child. Begin by informing yourself about your child's diagnosis and treatment. Your child's doctor or other members of the health care team can provide you with current information from books or pamphlets. Next, participate in decisions about your child's treatment. Remember, you and your child and the health professionals are partners in your child's health care. You may want to

set up a meeting with the health care team, which may include nurses, doctors, social workers, nutritionists, and others, to discuss your concerns. Before that meeting, make a list of questions.

6. Be discreet when talking with other parents or with patients in the waiting room. Don't discuss aspects of your child's illness that you haven't discussed with your child.

When To Call Your Doctor

Ask when your physician should be called. Call when you have questions or if you are unsure whether something should be reported.

In general, you should let a physician or other team member know if your child has any of the following:

1. A fever or other sign of infection or just doesn't "look well" when the white cell count is low. When the white cell count is adequate, you should report a fever or any other signs of infection that persist or become worse.

2. Exposure to a contagious infection, especially chickenpox or measles, unless your child is known to be immune from prior exposure or develops a contagious infection.

3. Persistent headaches, pain, or discomfort anywhere in the body.

4. Difficulty in walking or bending.

5. Pain during urination or bowel movements.

6. Reddened or swollen areas.

7. Vomiting, unless you have been told that your child might vomit after chemotherapy or radiation.

8. Problems with eyesight, such as blurred or double vision.

9. Bleeding. In addition to obvious bleeding such as nosebleeds, signs of bleeding can be seen in the stools (red or black), in the urine (pink, red, or brown), in vomit (red or brown, like coffee grounds), or the presence of multiple bruises.

10. Other troublesome side effects of treatment, such as mouth sores, constipation (beyond 2 days), diarrhea, and easy bruising.

11. Marked depression or a sudden change in behavior.

You should also check with your physician when your child is due to receive any kind of vaccination or any form of dental care.

Common Medical Procedures

Evaluation and treatment of a young person with cancer involve a variety of diagnostic procedures. Many of these are repeated at intervals over the course of treatment to monitor progress and response to therapy. These procedures should be carefully explained to you and your child before they are carried out. If you have any questions, do not hesitate to ask your physician or another member of the treatment team.

Angiograms

Angiograms reveal blocking, deviation, or abnormal development of blood vessels, which may indicate the presence of a growing tumor. The blood vessels are injected with dye and then X-rayed. A similar type of study, *lymphangiography*, can be used when cancer involving the lymphatic system is suspected.

Biopsy

Biopsy is a surgical procedure used to determine whether tumor tissue is benign or cancerous. For this test, a small piece of tissue is removed from the tumor and then examined under a microscope to check for the presence of cancer cells. The tissue is examined by a pathologist, a physician who is an expert at identifying the changes in body tissue caused by disease. This microscopic study of the tissue confirms or rules out a diagnosis of cancer.

Blood Studies

Blood studies evaluate the young person's blood and the components of the blood using a variety of tests. The blood studied in these tests is obtained by drawing blood from a vein with a syringe or by a "fingerstick," in which a small prick is made in a fingertip and a few drops drawn off.

Different tests that may be performed to study the blood include:

White Blood Cell Count (WBC)

Blood cells ("blood smear") are stained on a slide and examined under a microscope. The white blood cells, those components of the blood that fight infection, are counted, and the number of those cells per cubic millimeter of blood is established. Young people receiving chemotherapy generally have a lower white cell count than normal. This test is also used to detect the presence of leukemic blasts.

Hemoglobin

Measurements are taken of the amount of hemoglobin, the substance in the red blood cell that caries oxygen and is responsible for the blood's red color. Lower amounts than normal of this substance in the red blood cells indicate anemia. If the patient shows a low hemoglobin, physicians may do other tests to find out why and give medication (iron supplements in some cases) to correct it. A sudden appearance of anemia may suggest a relapse or be a side effect of chemotherapy.

Hematocrit

This is a measure of the amount of red blood cells and is expressed as

670

the percentage of the whole blood that is made up of red cells. A low count may indicate anemia.

Platelet

The number of platelets (the component of the blood that helps stop bleeding in case of injury) per cubic millimeter of blood is counted. A platelet count below normal range may be due to relapse, side effects of medication, or infection. If platelet counts are low, more tests may be necessary to find out the reason.

Bone Marrow Aspiration

Bone marrow aspiration evaluates the stem cells that mature into normal blood cells. The procedure is used to diagnose leukemia and to check the response to treatment. In young people with other cancers, it determines whether the disease has spread to the bone marrow.

Bone marrow aspirations in young people are usually done in the pelvis (hip bone). The patient lies on the stomach with a pillow under the pelvis, and the area is cleaned with an iodine solution to kill skin bacteria. Then the skin is numbed with a local anesthetic, and the bone marrow needle is put through the skin and into the spongy part of the bone. A sensation of pressure is felt; some patients also complain of pain. Once the needle is in place, marrow is quickly drawn into a syringe. This is the most painful phase, but lasts only a second or two.

The entire procedure usually takes less than 5 minutes and is not dangerous, but it may be stressful to the patient. Attempts to reduce a patient's anxiety and get him or her to relax may reduce the pain of this procedure and certainly the stress. Usually

there is only temporary tenderness at the site, and the young person can get up and go immediately afterward.

Computerized Axial Tomography

Computerized axial tomography (CAT scan) is an X-ray technique for detecting masses in the body. While the young person lies still, a narrow X-ray beam directed by a computer revolves around him or her. In a matter of seconds the machine registers thousands of bits of information, which are translated into a cross-sectional picture on a viewing screen. The physician can also refer to a printout for more detailed analysis.

Lumbar Puncture

Lumbar puncture (L.P. or spinal tap) is used to determine whether cancer cells or infection is present in the cerebrospinal fluid (CSF) that surrounds the brain and spinal cord. It is also used to deliver anticancer drugs directly to the brain and spinal cord.

An L.P. is done while the patient is lying on one side or sitting. In either instance, it is very important that the patient be in a tight ball so the lower back is rounded and the backbone projects backward. After the young person is in position, a local anesthetic is applied to the lower back. The patient is held in a tight ball and the needle is inserted between the vertebrae into the fluid space around the spinal cord. A sample of CSF is collected and examined for blood and cancer cells and levels of sugar and protein and can be cultured to check for infection. After the fluid is collected, medicines may be given through the puncture. As with bone marrows, this can be painful and produce anxiety in

671

the patient. Some of this may be alleviated if the patient can learn to relax during the procedure.

Usually there are no after effects, but sometimes the young person may get a headache when sitting or standing. Sometimes the headache can be prevented by lying flat for about an hour after the procedure and by increasing fluid intake for 24 hours afterward. Fortunately, headaches are uncommon, and usually the young person can return to normal activity. When anticancer drugs are given into the spinal fluid, nausea and vomiting may occur. Antinausea medicines may be prescribed by your physician.

Scans and Radioisotope Studies

Scans or radioisotope studies are used to discover abnormalities in the liver, brain, bones, kidneys, and other organs. In these tests, chemicals that collect in particular organs can be sound waves above the range of human hearing can be bounced off tissue and then changed electronically into images. Ultrasound is particularly effective in diagnosis because it can "recognize" masses that are not cancerous. "labeled" with a harmless radioactive material. The young person swallows the material or is injected with it. After a short waiting period, electronic devices are used to track the radioactive material as it collects within the body. Looking at how the material distributes itself in the body, the physician can then "see" whether an organ is functioning correctly or if it contains an abnormal mass or masses. Your child will *not* be radioactive after or during these tests.

Ultrasound Studies

Ultrasound studies determine the presence of tumors in the young person's body. Because tumors generate different "echoes" than normal tissue.

Coping With Cancer

Dealing With the Diagnosis

Even though many parents suspect what the outcome of their child's diagnostic tests will be, the diagnosis confirming these fears comes as a shock. Initial explanations of the disease and treatment may be lost as parents try to come to grips with the reality that their child has cancer. This initial confusion is common, and repeated explanations of the diagnosis, treatment, and possible outcome of the disease may be necessary. Because this is a time when many important decisions must be made, as a parent, you should not be hesistant or embarassed about asking and reasking questions about your child's disease and its treatment. Treatment centers often provide printed materials that give further explanations about cancer and its treatment that allow parents to absorb details at their own pace. A selected list of such materials, is available free of charge from the National Cancer Institute.

Parents' Initial Reaction

Parents may experience many feelings upon hearing that their child has cancer. Common reactions are denial, anger, guilt, grief, fear, and confusion. These reactions are natural and may be a way of helping you cope with the necessity of accepting a situation that you want to change but cannot. It is important to remember, however, that this is a time when your child needs your support and is particularly sensitive to your moods and feelings. Expressing these feelings too strongly may create problems for the child. A child, particularly an older child, who senses that parents do not want to acknowlege the disease, may try to protect them by not discussing his or her own feelings and fears. This feeling isolates the child from an important source of support and may only increase concerns, because the child may imagine the situation to be far worse than it actually is.

Although the diagnosis is usually definite once the test results have been examined, parents occasionally ask for a second opinion from another physician. Your physician or treatment center can recommend someone to you, or you may wish to get a recommendation from another source. Second opinions may be useful for confirming the diagnosis and reassuring parents about its accuracy and for confirming recommended treatment or exploration of another approach to treatment. However, once the diagnosis and treatment have been agreed upon by two physicians, seeking a third opinion may in fact reflect a parent's need to find another, more acceptable diagnosis. This puts an unfair burden on the sick child and delays treatment.

Accepting the Diagnosis

Gradually parents realize that their child has cancer and nothing can change it. At this point they begin to cope with the diagnosis and their feelings about it. Some parents become angry. Targets for this anger may vary and can include God, themselves, the physician, or even the sick child for becoming ill. Because it is difficult to express anger toward the sick child, spouses and healthy children can become the scapegoats for unresolved feelings. Parents sometimes lose their tempers. Letting the anger out may occasionally be helpful. It is important to remember, however, that other members of the family experience similar feelings. Realizing that some reactions stem from this anger and talking things through with family members, treatment staff, or others who can give support may help in dealing with these feelings.

Feelings of guilt may stem from thinking that the child's illness is retribution for the parents' past mistakes. Parents may worry about how they treated the child or whether the child should or should not have received a certain vaccine. It may be difficult to accept that, despite all their efforts to understand the cause of their child's cancer, it will largely remain unexplained. One thing parents should remember is that, as far as scientists can determine, *nothing they did or didn't do caused their child's illness.*

Parents frequently blame themselves and their physicians for delays in diagnosis. All parents want to know when the cancer began, but there is no definite answer. The onset can be rapid or gradual. Because the early symptoms of cancer are often the same as those for common childhood illnesses, early diagnosis is sometimes very difficult – even for physicians. Furthermore, medical evidence suggests that in most cases of childhood cancer, the success of therapy depends more on the type of tumor and appropriate treatment than the time of diagnosis.

Telling Your Child

One of the most difficult decisions facing parents after diagnosis is what to tell their child. In the past, there were strong cultural tendencies to shelter children from painful realities.

Today, there is general agreement that the patient should be told as much about the illness as the child's age allows him or her to understand. In fact, recent studies have shown that, even when children are not told about their disease, they learn its name and its implications within the first few months of treatment. It is virtually impossible to keep from children the knowledge that they are seriously ill, because their environment has already told them they are: they take special medicines, and their parents are likely to show extra concern about their health. At home and at school, they have opportunities to overhear discussions about their condition. In the hospital, they may see and talk to other children with the same disease.

The question, then, is not whether to talk about the diagnosis, but rather how to let your child know that concerns are shared and understood and that you are willing to talk about these things with your child. The single most important and basic approach is gentle, honest communication. Failure to answer a child's question in an honest fashion undermines the parent-child relationship at a time when the child desperately needs to communicate with the parents.

As a parent, you are the best judge of your child's moods. But you may want to keep in mind that, just because your child does not talk about the illness and the fears related to it (including death), you cannot assume he or she does not have these fears. The child who knows the illness is more serious than the usual childhood illness is undoubtedly afraid, and secrecy tends to isolate and increase fears.

Exactly when and what to tell will depend on your child's age and maturity and your attitudes. You may prefer to tell the child yourself, with or without the physician present, or you may want the doctor to do it. Use the method that makes you feel most comfortable.

Age-Related Concerns of Children

Your physician or other members of the treatment team may be able to help you determine what and how to tell the child. Some of this will depend on the child's age. In general, toddlers need only be told that they are sick, that they have to take medicine to get better, and that needles hurt, but only for a minute. Separation, abandonment, and loneliness are especially frightening to children under 5. They need to be reassured that, even if you have to leave for a while, you will be back. Children between the ages of 6 and 10 and perhaps as young as 5 have fears relating to physicial injury and bodily harm. They understand that theirs is no ordinary illness; it is very serious and very threatening. Thus, they need to know that they have cancer, a serious but treatable disease. They may also be told that the cause of cancer is unknown, that they will require a lot of medicine, and that it may take some time before they really feel well again. Much can be said with honesty and hope.

Older children and adolescents are old enough to understand their diagnosis and treatment, and also its implications. They may equate cancer with dying, and they need to know not only about their diagnosis and treatment, but also that cancer can often be successfully treated and about treatment advances and increased survival rates. To these young people, the impact cancer and its treatment will have on their normal activities, appearance, and relationships with peers may also be especially important.

Reassuring Your Child

Whatever you tell your child about the illness, he or she may bring up the issue of death and the fears it creates. Be prepared to cope with questions about death, even if they are painful. Refusing to discuss death may deny your child an outlet for some strong and possibly frightening feelings, and it will deny you the opportunity to offer comfort or reassurance. In addition to discussing the child's feelings and fears, it is important to stress to all young people with cancer the fact that cancer can be treated, that research for better methods is ongoing, and that new treatments are becoming available all the time.

Finally, young people of all ages tend to feel guilt and anger at the time of a severe illness. Guilt feelings may stem from the often subconscious feeling that disease is a punishment for being bad. Your child, therefore, needs *frequent* reassurances that he or she has done nothing wrong and is loved. The child may direct anger inward or at you for letting the illness happen. It is important for you to remember that even when your child is angry with you, your child loves you.

Many parents fear they will say something wrong that will upset their child or cause undue distress. In honest discussions this rarely happens. Even if initially upset or angry, the child will eventually benefit from the sharing of concerns with loved ones.

By handling the situation as openly as possible, the parent and child are free to resume as normal a life as possible. Shared awareness among the young person, parents, and medical personnel frequently has a soothing effect. The child seems happier knowing about the disease than fearing the unknown. Medical care is more successful because the child can actively participate. Parents do not carry the extra burden of concealing the truth. Despite the uncertainties and the heartaches, everyone becomes more comfortable with the disease and with the future.

In addition to talking with their parents and caregivers, young people with cancer may want to read about cancer and hospitalization.

Telling the Brothers and Sisters

The diagnosis of cancer affects the entire family. For the siblings, the initial period can be a time of confusion and fear. Children, even young ones, are sensitive to what is happening. They are aware of a brother's or sister's hospitalization and of trips to the doctor and clinic. They notice their parents crying and trying to comfort one another. They may overhear parts of conversations that are difficult to understand. Children often conspire to figure out what is going on. Pieces of information are gathered, pooled, and analyzed. Because of this, it is important to take time early in the diagnosis and treatment process to have an honest discussion of the situation with the siblings. Encourage them to ask questions and answer these as honestly as possible. Explain the facts about cancer, keeping in mind the age and maturity of each child, and update the information periodically as the siblings and patient

get older and are able to understand more. If the siblings are very young, it may be enough to say that their brother or sister is sick, will have to stay in the hospital for a while, and will need to take medicine for a long time. Older children will require more detailed information about cancer and its implications. Siblings should be prepared for physical changes in the patient, such as hair loss or amputation. If you wish, the doctors or nurses who care for the patient may be called upon to explain the diagnosis, prognosis, and treatment to the siblings or to discuss it with the entire family.

All of the children need to know that cancer is not contagious and that they will not become sick from contact with the patient. They need to be reassured that they are healthy themselves and that the possibility of cancer running in the family is highly unlikely.

Siblings also need to be told emphatically that they are in no way responsible for the illness. Angry outbursts, such as "Drop dead!" or "I hate you," which are said by all normal children at one time or another, frequently haunt a child after learning about a sibling's illness. Feelings of guilt or wrongdoing need to be dealt with immediately. Failure to do so may result in problems later on.

Continuing Life

One of the challenges facing the family of a child with cancer is maintaining a normal life. This is not always an easy task, particularly during moments of high stress such as at the time of diagnosis and during the hospitalizations and relapses. Even when treatment is going successfully, the lives of the patient and family members are influenced by the disease and its treatment and side effects. Schedules are rearranged to accommodate hospitalization or clinic visits, family members may be separated, siblings may feel neglected. Everyone may be worried or tense.

Despite all this, the continued development of family members demands that life continue as normally as possible under the circumstances. To see that this happens, the sick child should be treated as normally as possible, the needs and feelings of the patient's siblings attended to, and prediagnosis sources of support kept open for both the parents and the child. In addition, new sources of support, such as other parents of children with cancer and treatment team members, can help parents cope.

The Parents

To cope with the child's illness and the changes this brings in your own life, you may want to consider the following suggestions:

1. Make a special effort to find private times to communicate with your spouse, or if you are a single parent, with others close to you. Don't allow all your discussions to revolve around the sick child. Make time to do things you enjoyed doing together before your child became sick.

2. Find ways to reduce the frustration you may feel when clinic visits require waiting for procedures, test results, or consultations with physicians. When your child is hospitalized, try to make it as easy on yourself as possible. Bring something to read or do while the child is sleeping or doesn't need your individual attention.

3. If work schedules permit and the distance between hospital and home is close enough, you and your spouse may alternate staying with the hospitalized child. Weekends may be a good time for a switch: the parent who has been at home or work can stay at the hospital, and the other parent can spend time at home with the other children and rest. This also allows both parents to become familiar with the child's life in the hospital and various aspects of treatment. It reduces the gap that may grow between parents when one becomes much more actively involved in the treatment than is the other. If you are a single parent, other family members or friends who are close to the child may be able to stay at the hospital occasionally so you can rest.

4. Don't hesitate to turn to treatment staff for support. Most treatment centers have psychologists, psychiatrists, social workers, nurse clinicians, or chaplains available to talk over special concerns.

5. You may want to look for other sources of support. Talk to other parents of children with cancer informally in the hospital or clinic. Your treatment center may have a parents' group supervised by a staff member for more formal discussions. In addition, organizations outside the center may also exist. Such groups may provide support and information on how others have dealt or are dealing with situations you are facing. One national group, the Candlelighters (see "Sources of Information, Support, and Assistance" for a full description), has local chapters. Treatment center staff may be able to help you locate such a group.

When your child is in remission, it may be tempting to put all thoughts of the cancer out of your mind. And, indeed, this is a good time to get a rest from it and focus your attention on other segments of your life. However, this is also a good time to clear up any misconceptions about the cancer that the patient, siblings, or other family members and friends may have.

This is particularly true for the patient and siblings when treatment has been a lengthy process. You may need to initiate discussions to update information if you feel that this has not happened naturally during the course of treatment and that the child is concerned but reluctant to raise questions.

The Patient

Although the diagnosis of cancer will change your child's life for a time, the child still has the same needs as other young people – for friends, school, and the activities enjoyed before the illness. You can help by encouraging your child to continue a "normal" life as much as possible.

Friendships may be maintained during hospitalization or when your child is sick at home through letters or telephone calls.

The School

For the school-age child, continuing with school is vital. School is the major activity of children the same age, and continuing to attend school will reinforce the child's sense of well-being. Furthermore, it prevents the child from falling behind others the same age in learning and in the emotional development that comes from participating in school and school activities. When your child is hospitalized, a special hospital school program may be available. If your child is receiving frequent treatments or is too ill to attend school while at home, a home tutor may be available through the school system (the treatment center may be able to help you arrange for this). But home tutoring should be undertaken with the understanding that it is directed toward easing the eventual return to school.

When the young person returns to school, the teachers, counselor, school nurse, and principal may need information about the cancer and its treatment, any absences necessary for treatment, and any restrictions on activity. Teachers should be encouraged to give normal, equal attention instead of granting special favors that the child's condition does not warrant. *Students with Cancer: A Resource for the Educator*, a publication for school personnel designed to ease your child's return to school, is available from the National Cancer Institute (see listing in "Additional Reading Materials").

Both you and your child may be anxious about the return to school. Your child may be uneasy about how classmates will react to any change in appearance, such as hair or weight loss, weight gain, or loss of a limb through amputation. You may find yourself reluctant to allow the return because you are afraid your child will become ill or you find separation difficult. Both reactions are common, but your child should return to school. Accept the child's fear of rejection and try to help dealing with it. Most young people and parents find that their fears are unwarranted. Usually, classmates accept the patient and condition, and the child gains a sense of self-confidence by resuming the former role as a student. Because classmates may have questions about the child's cancer and any changes in appearance, you may want to help your child anticipate these questions and answers to them.

Discipline

Discipline is important to the normal development of all children. This is no less true when they have cancer. However, the special circumstances of these children's lives may make maintaining discipline more difficult. Having seen their child ill and in pain, parents may attempt to make up for this by giving extra presents or allowing behavior they would not tolerate in another child. They may find it difficult to discipline the child with cancer because of the uncertainty of the future. Although it is true that for many of these young people the future is uncertain, and some will die, discipline is an important part of seeing that the quality of life is maintained.

It may also be tempting to overprotect your child, to keep the child with you and away from situations you cannot control. This may deny your child the opportunity to participate in normal activities necessary for growth and development.

Some parents say that discipline and the setting of boundaries for behavior and activity are all the more difficult because they do not know what they can reasonably expect of their child. Ask your physician or other members of the treatment staff whether therapy may be making your child behave differently and whether any limits should be set on activities. If "contact" sports should be avoided because the child's platelet count is low, you will want to see that he avoids them. But if there is no reason not to go skateboarding or participate in sports, denying this may be overprotection on your part at a time when your child should be enjoying normal activities. Some medications may cause tiredness. In these cases, the child may not have the energy to participate in some functions. Some children, however, may occasionally complain of being tired to avoid chores they do not enjoy or activities they are reluctant to try. When you know what to expect, you will be able to treat your sick child as you would any other child.

Adolescents

Many teenage patients complain that their parents are overprotective. Although this is a common cry of adolescents, it may be especially true with teenage cancer patients who are at a stage in their lives when they are naturally striving for independence, but have a disease that forces them to be dependent on you and caregivers. Adolescents' attempts to achieve independence and make some of their own decisions should be encouraged within the limits set out by medical personnel.

With adolescents, certain special questions may arise. Those with driver's permits may want to go to the clinic alone or with a friend. Frustration over the disease-related dependence may increase their need to rebel against authority figures, which in this case could include physicians and other hospital personnel as well as you and other family members.

As with many teenagers, the questions of sexuality and drug use (including alcohol) may arise. In general, these are neither more nor less complex than when these issues are faced by adolescents who do not have cancer. In terms of drug use, however, the issue of marijuana may take on extra importance if the patient is on chemotherapy and has heard that marijuana helps prevent vomiting after chemotherapy. There is some evidence that THC, the active ingredient in marijuana, may be effective in controlling chemotherapy-induced nausea and vomiting. Researchers at various treatment centers are studying the effectiveness and side effects of oral THC capsules.

Siblings

Siblings of cancer patients may have many different feelings about the patient, the illness, and the attention the patient receives. While sympathizing with their brother or sister who is ill, they may still feel some resentment and believe that they are being neglected. In many cases, this is true. During times of hospitalization or when the patient is not feeling well, attention may focus on the sick child. As parents, you may not be able to pay as much attention to the siblings as you did before. You may have to miss school functions or ball games in which the siblings are participating. You may have little emotional reserve left after dealing with your sick child to talk with siblings about their concerns, to play with them, or help with their homework.

When you do have the energy, try to make special time for the siblings. Encourage them to become involved in outside activities and make a point of recognizing their achievements.

When you can, make plans to spend time alone with them and do things that interest them.

Others may focus special attention on the sick child. It is not unnatural, then, for siblings to resent the "privileged status" of the sick child in the family, neighborhood, and school, and the lack of attention to their own needs. Talking with siblings about the special attention paid to the sick child, letting them know that feelings of resentment are natural, and enabling them to share in the family crisis will encourage healthy growth and maturity. Efforts should be made to give equal attention, or explanations when this is not possible.

One way to help them to understand their brother's or sister's illness is by involving them in the treatment. Older children in particular welcome the opportunity to be taken into their parents' confidence and will often respond in helpful ways. Finding things for them to do for their sick brother or sister, or their worried parents, gives many young people a sense of belonging and usefulness that might otherwise be lacking in the family's focus on cancer.

Siblings may accompany you to the clinic when the patient gets treatment or, if possible, visit when the patient is hospitalized. This will allow them to see for themselves what the hospital, clinic, and treatment are like. If this is not possible because of distance, try to describe the setting and situation. Siblings may need such concrete experiences or explanations to prevent the construction of fantasies about the hospital and the hospital experience. Fantasies may range from fearing that the patient is being tortured to believing that the patient is having a good time; siblings may be terrified or jealous.

Remember, the patient's brothers and sisters may be asked questions about the illness by schoolmates or others in the community. They should have enough information to answer these questions. In fact, you might want to help them anticipate questions or comments and discuss possible answers.

Behavior Changes in Siblings

Behavior changes among siblings of young people with cancer are common and can indicate that they are having trouble dealing with the situation. They may become depressed, have headaches, or begin to have problems in school. If necessary, counseling can help them cope with their feelings, and treatment center staff can help with this. If their teachers are aware that a brother or sister has cancer and that this might affect the student, teachers can alert you if problems arise at school.

Remember that siblings, like all children, don't care about tomorrow and want equal treatment and attention today. It helps to appreciate them as individuals and to make a special effort to keep in touch with their needs.

Family and Friends

A diagnosis of cancer affects not only the patient's parents and siblings, but also the grandparents, other relatives, and family friends. Ideally, these people can provide support and assistance. They can babysit and spend time with the siblings, stay with the sick child to relieve you, or assist in the many practical problems that arise

when a household must continue to function under stress.

Unfortunately, they are not always able to do this. Grandparents may feel particularly lost and helpless, because they are concerned about their grandchild and at the same time cannot stop the suffering of their own child. If grandparents do not understand and accept the situation, you may find yourself in the difficult position of dealing with your own emotional difficulties while attempting to support the grandparents. Treatment team members can help, for instance, by offering to explain the child's condition to the grandparents. Being allowed to participate in meetings of parents' groups may also help grandparents deal with their feelings about the child's illness.

Each family has its own way of relating to relatives, friends, and neighbors. Above all, initial honesty is of real value in the long-term handling of any problems. People want and need to help, but they may need assistance from you to do so. They will need information about the disease and its treatment. Some may have to be told such basics as the fact that cancer is not contagious.

In general, you and your sick child must take the lead in showing others how you want to be treated.

You may need to point out to family and friends that too much attention or indulgence does not help the patient. For yourself, you may need to show others that you want to be treated as you were before, and although your time may be limited, you would like to be included in activities you previously enjoyed together.

Your employers may also need to

be told about your child's sickness so they can understand the reason for requests for time off from work. If you feel it is necessary, the child's doctor may write your employer and explain the situation.

Finally, in their efforts to help, people will give all sorts of advice. If their comments are confusing or upsetting, make a point of discussing them with medical personnel.

Finances

The cost of your child's treatment may cause additional pressure in an already tense situation. The desire to have the best in care may be offset by fear about the costs and how they will be met. As soon as financial questions arise, ask your doctor or the social worker for help.

Because health and life insurance questions can influence major health decisions, you'll need a clear understanding of the coverage your policies offer. Caregivers, particularly medical social workers, can clarify individual policies and help you fill out forms.

You should also keep complete records; store your bills and insurance forms together for easy reference at tax time. Keeping track of bills, your payments, and insurance payments by date and type of charge will simplify this further. Current records of bills and payments can be kept by listing them on a single sheet using the following format suggested in Nina Cottrell's *Coping at Home with Cancer* (listed in the section on additional reading materials):

Treatment center staff may also be able to help you with other costs associated with cancer treatment. Check with them to see if you are eligible for special rates for parking or food at the hospital. If your child is hospitalized or needs daily treatment away from home, lodging costs for parents may be substantially reduced if a Ronald McDonald House (described in "Sources of Information, Support, and Assistance") is available or other special arrangements have been made. Medical social workers may be familiar with other programs, such as those of voluntary cancer-related organizations (including those listed in "Sources of Information, Support, and Assistance") or state or local programs, that may be able to assist you.

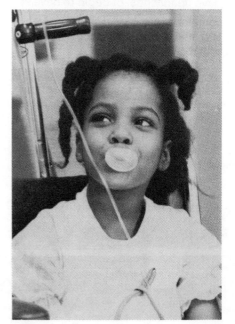

Date	Paid	Bill From	Total Charge	Ins. Paid	We Paid
7/1/78	Ch. 213	XYZ Surgery	$408.00	$365.42	$42.28

Sources of Information, Support, and Assistance

Candlelighters

Candlelighters is a national organization of parents whose children have or have had cancer. Now numbering over 100 chapters and affiliates in 40 states, the organization formed almost simultaneously in Washington, D.C., Florida, and California, in 1970. The name is taken from the saying that "It is better to light one candle than to curse the darkness."

Not all groups are called Candlelighters; the Wisconsin organization, for example, is LODAT (Living One Day At a Time).

The Candlelighters Foundation was created in 1976. Headquartered in Washington, D.C., it maintains communications between parents and professionals through quarterly newsletters and between groups through bimonthly newsletters. It publishes a teens newsletter and an annual cumulative bibliography for parents, operates a parent information service, offers information and assistance in forming new groups, and makes available a variety of handbooks to such groups.

Family support groups under the aegis of Candlelighters have many functions, including:

● exchanging practical information and ways of dealing with common problems;

● providing an outlet for the frustrations of those under stress through self-help sessions;

● offering a social outlet for parents and siblings, reducing the sense of isolation often imposed by cancer;

● disseminating information through meetings featuring medical speakers, psychologists, or insurers; and

● directing families to professional counseling.

Some of the local chapters have such services as a toll-free hotline and a program that provides visits to the oncology areas of hospitals for the parents of newly diagnosed patients.

For more information on Candlelighters chapters and programs, contact:

Candlelighters Foundation
2025 Eye St., N.W., Suite 1011
Washington, DC 20006
(202) 659-5136

American Cancer Society

The American Cancer Society (ACS) is a national voluntary organization offering programs of cancer research, education, and patient service and rehabilitation.

Local ACS units conduct service programs for cancer patients and their families, including:

● information, counseling, and guidance concerning ACS services, community health services, and other resources;

● equipment loans for care of the homebound patient;

● surgical dressings; and

● transportation to and from treatment.

Depending on the facilities and resources of the units, these programs may be expanded to include home

683

health care, blood programs, social work assistance, medications, and a complete rehabilitation program.

For further information, consult local telephone directories for the closest ACS office or contact:

American Cancer Society
National Headquarters
90 Park Avenue
New York, NY 10016
(212) 599-3600

Leukemia Society of America, Inc.

Financial assistance and consultation services for referrals to other means of local support are offered by chapters of the Leukemia Society of America to cancer patients with leukemia and allied disorders. Financial coverage is reserved for outpatients and pays up to $600 per patient per year of costs not covered by other sources. The program includes payment for drugs used in the care, treatment, and/or control of leukemia and allied diseases; laboratory costs associated with blood transfusion; transportation; and up to $300 of costs for X-ray therapy for early Hodgkin's disease and up to $300 of costs for cranial radiation for children with acute lymphocytic leukemia.

For more information about the program and its local chapters, contact:

Leukemia Society of America, Inc.
733 Third Avenue
New York, NY 10017
(212) 573-8484

Cancer Information Service

The Cancer Information Service is a toll-free telephone inquiry system that supplies information about cancer and cancer-related resources to the general public, cancer patients and their families, and health professionals. CIS is administered by the National Cancer Institute. Most CIS offices are associated with Comprehensive Cancer Centers, which are special research and treatment centers recognized by the National Cancer Institute.

CIS offices do not diagnose cancer or recommend treatment for individual cases. They do provide support, understanding, and rapid access to the latest information on cancer and local resources. Telephone information may be supplemented by printed materials. All calls are kept confidential, and you do not need to give your name.

PDQ Database

The National Cancer Institute has developed PDQ (Physician Data Query), a computerized database designed to give doctors quick and easy access to:

● the latest treatment information for most types of cancer;

● descriptions of clinical trials that are open for patient entry; and

● Names of organizations and physicians involved in cancer care.

To get access to PDQ, a doctor can use an office computer with a telephone hookup and a PDQ access code or the services of a medical library with online searching capability. Most Cancer Information Service offices (1-800-4-CANCER) provide a physician with one free PDQ search and can tell doctors how to get regular access to the database. Patients may ask their doctor to use PDQ or may call 1-800-4-CANCER themselves. Information specialists at this toll-free number use a variety of sources, including PDQ, to answer questions about cancer prevention, diagnosis, and treatment.

Ronald McDonald Houses

The first Ronald McDonald House opened in 1974 as a place where out-of-town families can stay while their children are being treated at the Children's Hospital of Philadelphia. Since that time, other houses have opened in other major cities. In general, a Ronald McDonald House is available for families of seriously ill children and provides lodging at economical rates.

For further information about the Ronald McDonald House program, contact:

Mr. A. L. (Bud) Jones
Ronald McDonald House Coordinator
c/o Golin Communications, Inc.
500 North Michigan Avenue
Chicago, IL 60614
(312) 836-7100

Home Care for the Dying Child

Although treatment efforts are successful for many children with cancer, this is not always the case. When treatment is not successful and the child's disease becomes terminal, some parents may wish to have their child die at home rather than in the hospital. The patient may also prefer it. Parents who have taken their child home have shown that it is possible to provide quality care for their dying child when assisted by nurses, doctors, and other health professionals.

A home care program for children may exist in your area, but if one doesn't, you and the treatment center or a home health agency may have to work out the arrangements necessary for you to care for your child successfully. Coordination between parents and health care personnel is essential to success in caring for dying children. A home care nurse can help parents care for their child, help acquire any necessary equipment such as hospital beds or wheelchairs, and provide emotional support for parents. Basic information growing out of a research project on home care is available and may help parents who are interested in such a program. The two texts, *Home Care for Dying Children: A Manual for Parents,* and a nurses' manual, *Home Care: a Manual for Implementation of Home Care for Children Dying of Cancer*, may be purchased from:

Research Center
School of Nursing
University of Minnesota
3313 Powell Hall
500 Essex Street, S.E.
Minneapolis, MN 55455

Chapter 35

Diet and Nutrition for Young People With Cancer

Nutrition Advice and Special Diets

Introduction

This information is about diet and nutrition for children with cancer. It was written for the parents of these children in recognition of the fact that parents are both willing and able to make an important contribution to their child's care and recovery. At the same time, many parents who want to be involved in their child's care are uncertain about what to do. The purpose of this information is to assist you, the parent, in meeting your child's nutritional needs at a time when good nutrition is especially important.

Diet and nutrition are not quite the same thing. Diet is all the food and liquid you swallow. Some of this is used by the body and some goes to waste. Food is used to build the body, keep it in working order, and provide energy.

Nutrition is the process by which the body takes in and uses food. Good nutrition (that is, the intake and assimilation of required amounts of food and drink) is required for the normal growth and development of all children. When a child has cancer, good nutrition becomes even more important. Not only is the child's body growing, but it is also coping with the effects of the disease and possibly the side effects of cancer treatment as well.

Cancer may also stop the body from using as well as it should the food that is taken in. Altogether these effects cause malnutrition, which means that the body is getting too little nourishment or the wrong kind. When this happens, the child may lose weight, become weak, and lack energy.

Preventing or limiting nutritional problems is one of the large tasks facing you as the parent of a child with cancer. Among the problems you are likely to encounter are the child's reluctance to eat and the body's tendency to reject some foods because of the cancer and its treatment. This book contains information and suggestions which may be helpful in dealing with these problems.

Some of the advice in this book applies to wise eating by anybody — young or old, sick or well — and much of it would apply to any cancer patient. But there are special concerns with children. One is that they are more likely to be affected by loss of appetite than adults. Children are finicky eaters at the best of times. Another concern is that children are growing and need good nutrition to develop normally. Cancer is a long illness, and if the body falls behind in its development, it may never quite catch up.

The book also contains information on special diets which are sometimes prescribed for children with cancer. If your child is placed on such a diet, one of the diet sheets in this booklet may be a handy reference for planning meals.

Some advice before we begin. Your child's doctor or dietitian will know what foods your child should eat and what must be avoided. Ask for instructions and feel free to discuss changes in your child's diet with the doctor. You can do a lot to help in finding the proper diet for your child. Watch closely how your child reacts to different foods, and tell the doctor about these and other things you notice about your child's eating habits.

And finally a word of caution. Every situation is different, and it may be a long time before you find the best answers to your child's eating problems. Some of the ideas in this book will be helpful; others may not. What works for one child may not work for another. And what works one day may not the next. Be patient — with yourself and with your child. As a concerned and loving parent you have much to offer in planning and providing the best possible care for your child.

The Importance of Nutrition

We have already pointed out that good nutrition is vital to the normal growth and development of children and even more important to the child with cancer. One reason is that good nutrition helps maintain the body's natural defense system. These defenses can help the body resist infections. A well-nourished child may also tolerate the side effects of cancer treatment much better than a poorly nourished one.

Nutritional needs of children depend on their age, sex, body size, activity, heredity, and general state of health. Your child's needs are also influenced by the type of cancer, stage of the disease, and type of treatment.

The amount of food a young child needs is frequently less than some parents think. A general guide to how much your child should eat is that for each year of age a child normally will eat about one tablespoon of each food included in a meal. For example, a 2-year-old's dinner might include 2 tablespoons each of meat, one or two vegetables, a fruit, plus milk or juice and perhaps a slice of bread.

What foods your child eats is just as important as how much. Small amounts of some foods are very nutritious. This chapter is designed to help you select nutritious foods by understanding the role that different foods play in your child's health.

Nutrients, Their Functions and Sources

Nutrients are substances that support the body's life-sustaining processes. They are proteins, carbohydrates, fats, vitamins, minerals, and water. These nutrients are found in foods, but most foods do not contain all of them. In fact, some foods may contain almost none of them.

Nutrition refers to the whole process of food intake (eating and drinking), release of nutrients from the food, and the absorption and use of nutrients by the body. This process is basic to life. Good nutrition means that the body is receiving enough of the nutrients it needs and is using them properly.

Diet is a general term for foods eaten. A normal, well-balanced diet includes a broad variety of foods which provide the nutrients needed for good health. In disease, special diets may be necessary to meet specific nutritional requirements pro-duced by the illness. These diets may include or exclude certain foods, increase or decrease specific nutrients, limit the amount of food intake, change the texture or the energy value of foods eaten. Such diets should be prescribed by a physician, dietitian, or nutritionist.

Calories are a measure of food energy and are present, in varying amounts, in carbohydrates, fats, and protein. They are required to maintain normal body function (although they are not nutrients). Each of us requires enough energy in the form of calories to keep the body alive and to perform physical activity. A child also needs energy for growth and development. In addition, fever and other disease-related stresses increase the body's demand for energy. The sick child's caloric (energy) intake must be enough to meet normal growth demands and the requirements created by the disease.

The following chart is adapted from the 1974 Recommended Daily Dietary Allowances of the National Academy of Sciences. It can guide you in determining your child's normal energy (or caloric) needs. Bear in mind, however, that energy needs vary somewhat with each child and depend on the same factors influencing general nutritional requirements. Also remember

691

that these energy recommendations are for healthy children.
Children with cancer or other
chronic diseases often have
greater energy requirements.

	Weight		Height		Energy
	kilograms	*pounds*	*centimeters*	*inches*	*in calories*
Infants					
0-6 months	6	14	60	24	702
6 months-1 year	9	20	71	28	972
Children					
1-3 years	13	28	86	34	1,300
4-6 years	20	44	110	44	1,800
7-10 years	30	66	135	54	2,400
Boys					
11-14 years	44	97	158	63	2,800
15-18 years	61	134	172	69	3,000
Girls					
11-14 years	44	97	155	62	2,400
15-18 years	54	119	162	65	2,100

Protein is the basic substance of every cell in the body and is made up of small units called amino acids. When eaten, protein in food is broken down (digested) into its amino acid components. These are used by the body to build and maintain tissues; to form enzymes, antibodies, and some hormones; to regulate body processes, and to provide some energy if necessary.

The major function of protein is to build new body tissue and repair existing tissue. This continues throughout life. In a normal, healthy person the amount of protein needed in relation to body weight is greatest during the childhood years of rapid growth. When the diet does not contain enough fats and carbohydrates to meet the body's energy demands, protein may be used for energy instead of body building. To avoid this, enough energy must be provided in the form of carbohydrates and fats.

Carbohydrates are starches and sugars. They provide the most easily used source of body energy. When eaten, some carbohydrate—in the form of glucose—is used for immediate energy needs. Some is stored in the liver and muscles, and the rest is converted to fat. Since carbohydrates are a good source of energy, one of their most important functions is to "spare" protein from being used to provide body energy so that it is available to build and repair body tissue.

Fats are important dietary elements. They supply compounds known as fatty acids which are essential to many body functions, and they are carriers for certain fat-soluble vitamins. Fats are also the most concentrated source of energy, providing about twice the number of calories in an equal weight of protein or carbohydrates.

Vitamins play a vital role in maintaining body health. They are present in many foods, and adequate amounts are usually contained in a well-balanced diet. Vitamins are called fat-soluble (A, D, E, and K) or water-soluble (the B vitamins and vitamin C). Fat-soluble vitamins can be stored by the body for later use, but unused water-soluble vitamins are excreted in the urine. Foods containing the water-soluble vitamins must be eaten often in order to provide the body with a constant supply.

When a child's appetite is poor, both fat-soluble and water-soluble vitamins may be added to food or given separately. However, you must remember that too much vitamin can be as dangerous as too little. High doses of vitamins or minerals should not be given without first consulting your doctor.

Vitamin A is needed for normal vision and to keep the skin and inner linings of the body healthy and resistant to infection. It is obtained from foods of animal origin such as whole milk, butter, egg yolk, whole-milk cheese, and liver. Carotene, a substance found in dark green and deep yellow vegetables and fruits, can be converted to Vitamin A by the body.

Vitamin D is important in building strong bones and teeth. It must be present for the body to use calcium from food and to release calcium stored in the bones. Some Vitamin D can be produced by the body through the action of direct sunlight on the skin.

If a person is not exposed to enough sunlight, a dietary source of Vitamin D is necessary. The best source is fish liver oils; however, these are not included in ordinary diets and are often refused by children. Another excellent source is milk fortified with Vitamin D. A quart provides the recommended daily amount. Milk is also rich in calcium and phosphorus, which require the presence of Vitamin D for their use by the body. Other foods fortified with this vitamin are margarine and some breakfast cereals and dairy products.

Vitamin E prevents destruction of certain other nutrients in the body and aids in the proper use of energy supplied by glucose and fatty acids. It is also necessary for healthy red blood cells. This vitamin is found primarily in foods of plant origin such as vegetable oils, wheat germ, nuts, whole grain breads and cereals, and dark green, leafy vegetables.

Vitamin K is essential for blood to clot properly. Dietary requirements for this vitamin are normally quite small because it is formed in the intestine. It is found in a variety of vegetables such as cabbage, cauliflower and spinach.

The Vitamin B complex is a group of eight water-soluble vitamins: thiamine, niacin, riboflavin, B_6 (pyridoxine), B_{12} (cyanocobalamin), folic acid, pantothenic acid and biotin. Some of the B vitamins are necessary for the release and use of energy from foods. Others are important for the formation of red blood cells and the promotion of healthy skin and good digestion.

Specifically, thiamine is needed for energy release from carbohydrates and for healthy nerves, heart, and blood vessels. Both niacin and riboflavin contribute to healthy skin; riboflavin is also essential for growth. Vitamins B_6 and B_{12} are both important for a healthy nervous system. B_{12} and folic acid are particularly important for the proper development of red blood cells. Pantothenic acid is needed for the production of certain hormones and aids in energy release. Biotin aids the body in using carbohydrates, fats, and proteins.

Organ meats such as liver are excellent sources of all the B vitamins; pork is a rich source of thiamine; and milk is one of the best sources of riboflavin. Other sources of the B complex include enriched and whole-grain cereal products, meat, and green leafy vegetables.

Minerals, like vitamins, are essential for health but are not needed in large amounts. A balanced diet usually supplies enough. Different minerals are needed by the body for growth and maintenance of good health. Calcium, phosphorus, sodium, potassium, iron, chlorine, magnesium, and sulphur account for most of the minerals in the body. Other minerals used by the body, such as iodine, manganese, copper, zinc, cobalt, and fluorine are called trace minerals because they are present only in very small amounts.

Calcium is the mineral found in the largest amount in the body. It is essential for the formation of strong bones and teeth. It also aids in blood clotting, transmis-sion of nerve impulses, and the regulation of muscle contraction.

Phosphorus also adds to the mineral content of bones and teeth by combining with cal-cium to form a compound that gives strength and rigidity to these structures. Milk and milk products are the best source of calcium and phosphorus; phosphorus can also be ob-tained from other high-protein foods.

Sodium is important in main-taining fluid balance in body tissues. Most of this mineral is found in the blood and in fluids outside the cells. Children nor-mally take in enough sodium; however, a lot can be lost dur-ing long periods of diarrhea and vomiting. The major source of sodium is in salt added to foods at the table or in cooking. Bread, pastry, milk, and cheese are other sources.

Potassium has a number of important roles in the body, including the transmission of nerve impulses. Like sodium, it is involved in fluid balance, and the body's supply of potas-sium may be too low following prolonged diarrhea or vomiting. Most plant and animal foods contain potassium. Good sources are fruits (especially bananas), milk, meat, and potatoes.

Iron is needed to make hemoglobin, the substance in red blood cells that carries oxygen to the tissues. Liver and other organ meats are especially rich in iron. Egg yolks, green leafy vegetables, dried fruits such as prunes, raisins, and apricots, and enriched breads and cereals are also good sources.

Other minerals are just as important for various body functions. However, so little is needed by the body that a normal diet will usually provide enough.

Water is essential for life. In fact, the body's need for water is much more urgent than its need for food. One can survive only a few days without water. Water helps regulate body temperature, aids in digestion and elimination of body wastes, and is essential to the survival of all cells. It is present in all foods—particularly soups, juices, milk, fruits, and vegetables.

The requirement for water obtained from all sources varies with the age and size of a child. For example, a six-month-old infant will need approximately one quart of water per day, most of which will be obtained from milk or formula. A child 6 years old will need about 2 quarts per day, obtained from drinking water, milk, juice, and other water-containing foods.

Fiber contributes bulk or roughage to the diet. A diet high in fiber helps promote regular bowel movements. Fiber intake can be increased by eating more whole grain products, raw and dried fruits, raw vegetables and nuts. A low-fiber diet is sometimes recommended in cases of severe diarrhea or certain intestinal problems.

Digestion, Absorbtion, Metabolism

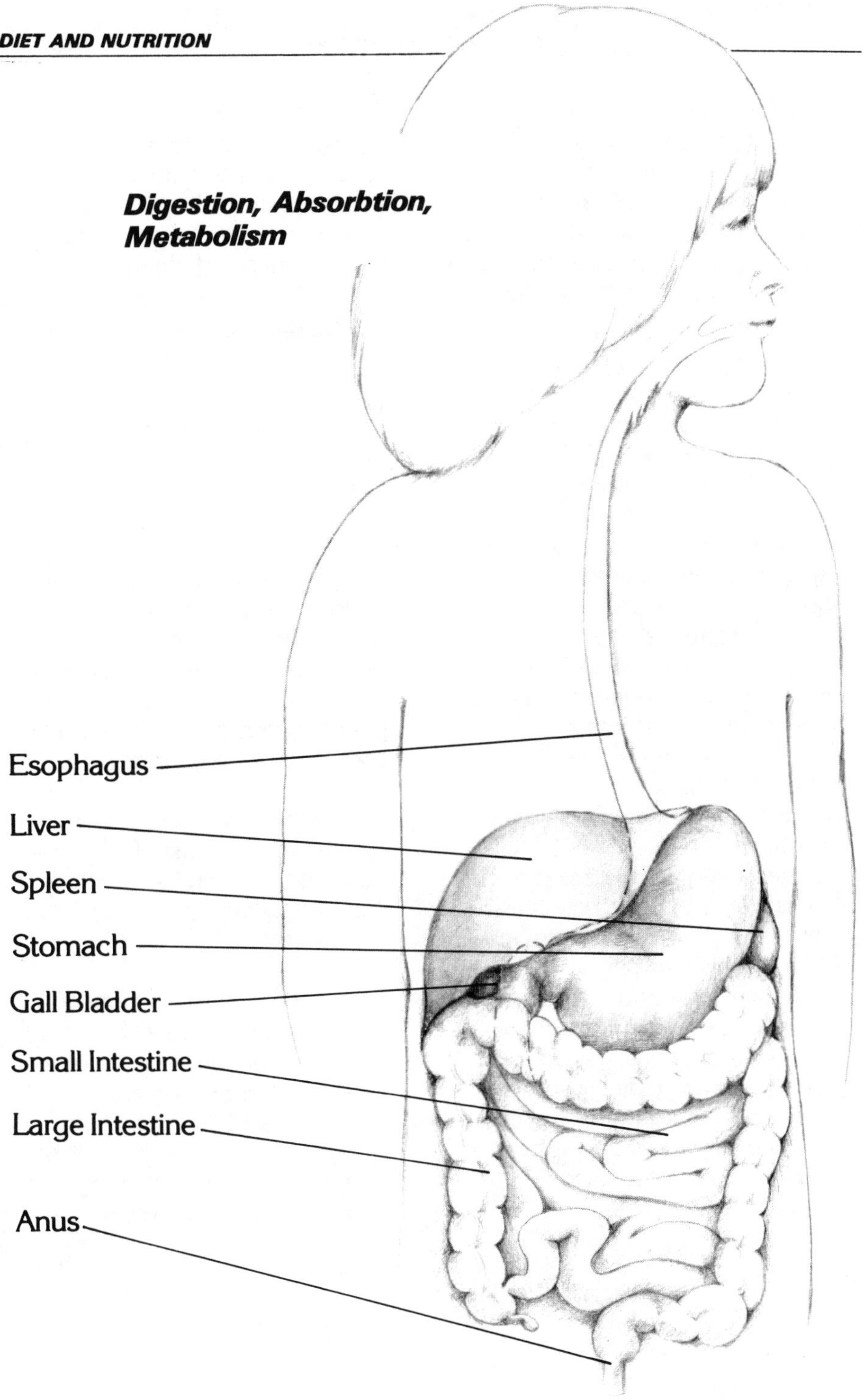

Esophagus

Liver

Spleen

Stomach

Gall Bladder

Small Intestine

Large Intestine

Anus

Before food can be used by the body it must be in a form that can enter the blood and be carried to all the cells and tissues. The process by which the body breaks down food into these simpler forms is called digestion.

Digestion takes place in the gastrointestinal (GI) tract, which is much like a long tube running through the body. Digestion begins in the mouth, where chewing and moistening with saliva prepare the food to pass easily down the esophagus to the stomach. In the stomach muscle contractions churn the food, breaking it up further and mixing it with gastric juices. The gastric juices contain chemicals which begin the process of changing fat, carbohydrate, and protein into simpler substances.

The food mixture passes from the stomach to the small intestine where it mixes with bile from the liver and with more chemicals which further change its form. The products of these chemical reactions—simple sugars, amino acids, glycerol, and fatty acids—are then ready for use by the body through absorption and metabolism. Undigested material such as fiber passes from the small intestine into the large intestine, where absorption of nutrients is completed. Body wastes are added to the remaining unusable material, and the material is concentrated by removal of some water. It is eliminated as stool (feces) through the anus.

Absorption is the movement of the nutrients from the GI tract into the blood and lymph systems. Most absorption takes place in the small intestine. The long tube of intestine has an interior surface which resembles velvet in texture, because it is covered with billions of tiny projections, each of which contains vessels of the blood and lymphatic systems. The products of carbohydrate and protein digestion enter the blood vessels; the products of fat digestion enter the lymph vessels. Most of the products are then transported to the liver for further chemical processing.

Metabolism refers to all of the chemical changes that take place after absorption. Absorbed products of digestion are used to build, maintain, and repair tissues, or to provide energy. The body must constantly metabolize nutrients to support life.

Side Effects of Cancer and Cancer Treatment

A healthy child's body is able to store nutrients, conserve energy, and regulate metabolism. During short periods of illness when a child may eat too little food, nutrients are redistributed to maintain the body's most important tissues and organs.

When a child is ill with a chronic, long-term disease like cancer it becomes more difficult for the body to make up for lack of enough food being eaten, digested, or absorbed. The child's appetite may be affected and the body's ability to store and use nutrients reduced. Side effects associated with cancer and cancer treatments may also interfere with normal nutritional processes.

This chapter contains brief discussions of the three major forms of cancer treatment (radiotherapy, chemotherapy, and surgery) and identifies some of the side effects associated with each one which may affect nutrition. It also contains suggestions for coping with some of the most common side effects resulting from cancer or cancer treatment.

Anorexia, or loss of appetite, is one of the most common problems associated with cancer and its treatment. Causes are not altogether understood but include biochemical, psychological, and emotional factors, as well as the side effects of treatment. A child suffering from nausea, vomiting, mouth ulcers, or other side effects will understandably find food less appealing.

Cachexia (severe weight loss and wasting of body tissues) may result from loss of appetite, other effects of the disease or from treatment. If the child cannot eat properly, weight loss and possibly muscle tissue wasting will result. Additional energy requirements during the course of disease place even more stress on the young patient's body. It is difficult to halt and reverse this condition once it appears. That is why it is so important to see that the young cancer patient gets enough calories and protein to prevent this weight loss and wasting process from the beginning.

15

Radiotherapy
(Radiation Treatment)

Radiation is frequently used to destroy cancer cells. It can be administered from outside the body, or radioactive material can be inserted in body cavities or implanted in diseased tissue. In all forms of radiotherapy, care is taken to protect normal healthy cells as much as possible while exposing the cancer cells to the radiation.

Some young patients experience no immediate side effects from radiation treatment. Side effects are common, however, and may affect a child's nutrition. The site treated is one important factor in this. Radiation treatment to the abdominal area, for example, sometimes causes nausea, vomiting, and diarrhea, and may interfere with the absorption of nutrients. Treatment of the head, neck, or chest areas may affect mucous membranes in the mouth, throat, or esophagus. If these areas become sore and dry, swallowing may be painful and taste may be altered.

Radiation treatment of the head and neck area also contributes to increased tooth decay and other dental problems. Careful attention to oral hygiene is therefore important both during and after treatment.

It is easy to see why a child suffering from these side effects of radiotherapy may lose interest in food. Yet the child's nutritional requirements actually increase at this time because of the stress of treatment. It is therefore important to encourage eating and to find ways of making foods more appealing and acceptable.

Sometimes appetite may be poor at normal mealtimes and much better at other times. Radiation treatment generally lasts less than 2 months. During this period, flexibility in mealtimes can help maintain normal nutrition.

Radiation therapists are interested in helping their patients maintain good nutrition, and they should be consulted when nutritional problems arise. These physicians may recommend a special diet to lessen the side effects, or they may prescribe drugs, including those for nausea or diarrhea.

Chemotherapy
(Drug Treatment)

Chemotherapy is the treatment of cancer with drugs, which may be administered by mouth, by injection into a muscle or infusion into a vein. Children respond differently to drug treatment. Some children experience side effects while others are able to take the drugs with little problem. Drug therapy often continues for several years. A child who has no side effects initially may develop problems with time. The side effects result from the action of the drugs on some normal tissues, as well as on cancer cells.

Among the normal tissues of the body most susceptible to the effects of anticancer drugs are the linings of the intestine and other parts of the GI tract. Irritation of the GI tract may result in mouth sores, bleeding gums, or other problems that can interfere with your child's ability to eat.

Nausea and vomiting are the most common side effects affecting nutrition. When nausea and vomiting are severe, loss of body fluid, general weakness, and weight loss become major nutritional concerns. In some cases drug treatment can be scheduled so that nausea and vomiting will not occur at mealtimes. However, when a child is undergoing intensive chemotherapy this is often not possible. In these cases, good nutritional status before and in between treatments is especially important. Maintaining liquid intake during treatment will help to prevent dehydration.

Certain drugs, such as prednisone, will cause a child to gain weight. The extra weight is in the form of water which the drug stops the body from eliminating in the normal ways. When

this occurs, the doctor may restrict the amount of salt the child eats, since salt also causes the body to retain water.

Some drugs cause diarrhea or constipation and consequently may affect the intestinal absorption of nutrients. Prolonged diarrhea results in dehydration, mineral deficiencies and malnutrition. Severe malnutrition may increase the risk of infection and may also affect a child's normal growth and development.

Some hints for coping with side effects such as nausea, vomiting, and diarrhea are discussed later in this chapter.

Surgery

Surgical removal of a malignant tumor is an important treatment method for many types of cancer. Children tend to tolerate surgery better and recover more rapidly than adults. However, a child's nutritional status will influence both the speed and ease of the recovery process. Good nutritional status helps prevent complications, improves wound healing, and shortens recovery time.

Stress associated with surgery—loss of blood, tissue breakdown, vomiting, and fever—increases the need for nutrients. Confinement to bed and restriction of food intake after an operation does not allow the nutritional deficiency created by surgery to be corrected immediately.

If appetite and nutritional status are poor before surgery, an additional strain is placed upon the patient. If this is the case with your child, the doctor may recommend a special diet before performing surgery. For example, if there is severe weight loss, a high protein-high calorie diet for 1 to 4 weeks before the operation may be helpful. In this way the child's body is better prepared to meet the need for increased energy and tissue repair following surgery.

Nutrition after surgery is planned to meet individual needs. The most immediate concern is replacement of body fluids to prevent dehydration. Intravenous (IV) fluid replacement is a standard procedure following surgery. The IV fluid provides water, some calories, and perhaps medications and important minerals, especially sodium and potassium.

Food is often not given by mouth right after the operation since the digestive system requires some time to begin functioning normally again. Frequently surgical patients are first given a clear liquid diet and then gradually progressed to a normal diet. Diet after surgery should provide enough calories and protein to allow rapid repair of damaged tissue, resumption of normal body functions and return of muscle strength. Vitamin intake after surgery is also important since

vitamins are necessary for the proper use of protein. We have already mentioned two minerals—sodium and potassium—which are of special concern following surgery. Iron, used in the formation of red blood cells, is another mineral which is especially important at this time.

While a child is in the hospital, the dietary planning is the responsibility of the doctor and the dietitian. They will make certain that needed nutrients are included in the meals and medications your child receives. As a parent you can help by encouraging your child to eat and, if the child's appetite is poor, discussing with the doctor, nurse, or dietitian your child's food preferences.

In some cases, perhaps when a child has difficulty in swallowing, food may be given through a tube inserted in the nose and extending into the stomach. Less frequently, the tube may be inserted directly into the stomach through a surgically created opening in the abdominal wall.

Recently some doctors have begun using intravenous techniques for providing complete nutritional support to certain patients. This new form of IV treatment, called total parenteral nutrition (TPN) or hyperalimentation, provides protein, calories, and other essential nutrients. While these feeding methods may seem strange and frightening to you and your child, they may be necessary to prevent malnutrition and speed up recovery from major surgery.

Coping with Side Effects of Cancer and Cancer Treatment

As we have already seen, side effects of cancer and cancer treatment often affect the patient's desire or ability to eat. Cancer or its treatment can also affect the way the body uses food which is eaten. These side effects vary, and it is impossible to predict just how a child will react to either the disease or its treatment. Your child may or may not experience the side effects described here, or may have a response that is more or less severe than that of other children with the same form of cancer or undergoing the same treatment.

Ways for successfully treating side effects vary as much as the side effects themselves. What works for one child may not work for another. Sometimes the approach you used yesterday with great success will prove less helpful today. Suggestions offered on the following pages are ones that have proved effective in a number of cases. While this in no way guarantees that they will work for you and your child, they do provide a starting point for trying to control side effects related to nutrition.

Nausea is a common side effect of drugs or radiation and may also be caused by the disease itself. Nausea may also be caused by other conditions unrelated to your child's cancer or therapy. Control of nausea is important to enable your child to eat adequate amounts of food and help prevent vomiting. If your child experiences nausea, some of these suggestions may be helpful:

● Encourage the child to eat small amounts frequently and slowly.

● Avoid feeding the child in a stuffy, too-warm room or one filled with cooking odors or other smells that might be disagreeable.

● Don't serve liquids with the child's meals, since the liquids can cause a full feeling.

● Encourage drinking or sipping liquids frequently throughout the day, *except* at mealtimes. Using a straw may help.

● Serve beverages cool or chilled. Try freezing favorite beverages in ice cubes.

● Serve foods at room temperature or cooler; hot foods may contribute to nausea.

● Don't force the child to eat favorite foods when nauseated; it may cause a permanent dislike of the food.

● Encourage rest periods after meals. (Activity can slow digestion.)

703

• Many cancer patients, children and adults, feel at their best in the morning. If this is true of your child, use breakfast as the opportunity for a high protein-high calorie meal.

• If nausea should be a problem for your child in the morning. eating dry toast or crackers before getting up may help.

• If your child tends to be nauseated and vomits during radiation or chemotherapy, food should be avoided for several hours before treatment.

• Ask your child's doctor about an antinausea drug if the problem is a continuing one.

• Try these foods: low-fat foods, such as vegetables, fruits, skinned chicken (baked or broiled, not fried), sherbet, pretzels, angel food cake; dry foods (like toast and crackers); salty foods (pretzels are salty as well as low-fat); cold foods.

• Avoid these foods: fat, greasy, or fried foods; overly sweet foods; spicy, hot foods, and others with strong odors.

• Observe if there is a pattern or regularity to when your child becomes nauseated or what causes it (specific foods, events, surroundings). If possible, make appropriate changes in the child's diet or schedule.

• Share your observations with your child's doctor.

Vomiting often accompanies nausea and may be brought on by food odors, gas in the stomach or intestine, motion, or therapy. In very sensitive individuals, certain surroundings (such as the hospital) may produce vomiting. If nausea can be controlled, vomiting is usually prevented. At times, however, your best efforts may be unable to prevent either nausea or vomiting. If vomiting occurs, try these hints for making your child comfortable and preventing further vomiting.

• Help your child find a restful, comfortable position with head slightly elevated. Positioning on one side often works.

• Loosen any tight, restricting clothing.

• Change clothing and bed linen as needed to remove all reminders of vomiting.

• Be sure the room is well ventilated, with no unpleasant sounds or smells.

• Gently wipe the child's face with a cool, damp cloth.

• Rinse the child's mouth with cool water or mouthwash to remove the bad taste. (The water or mouthwash should not be swallowed.) If rinsing is not possible, use mouthswabs or a cool, damp cloth to gently wipe the inside of the child's mouth and tongue.

• Withhold all liquids and food until vomiting is well under control.

• Once vomiting is controlled, small amounts of clear liquids should be tried. Begin with a teaspoonful every 10 minutes, gradually increase the amount to a tablespoon every twenty minutes, and finally, 2 tablespoons every 30 minutes.

• When clear liquids are well tolerated, a full liquid diet may be tried and the child gradually progressed to his or her normal diet. Continue the "small amounts frequently" approach. (See the section on Special Diets for descriptions of the clear liquid and full liquid diets.)

Weight Gain has already
been mentioned as a possible side effect of treatment with certain anticancer drugs. This weight gain is actually water retention, and does not necessarily mean the child is eating too much. If you think your child is gaining weight, bring this to the attention of the doctor. He or she may recommend that your child's intake of salt be limited, since salt holds water. Medication may also be prescribed to help eliminate excess water. The best solution to this problem will depend on what the doctor determines to be the cause.

Diarrhea is a side effect
that may be caused by chemical or bacterial toxins, infections, drugs, radiation to the abdomen, food sensitivity, malabsorption, or even emotional or psychological factors. Some cancer therapy causes an intolerance of lactose, a substance in milk. Lactose intolerance may result in diarrhea when milk and milk products are eaten. If diarrhea is severe or prolonged, loss of fluid and minerals—especially potassium—may occur. Long-term, chronic diarrhea can result in other nutritional deficiencies since the rapid passage of food through the intestine prevents adequate absorption of nutrients. Here are some suggestions for coping with diarrhea.

• Bed rest will help reduce intestinal contractions (called *peristalsis)* which move food and waste products through the intestine.

• Use the "small amounts frequently" approach to giving your child both liquids and solid food.

• Try a clear liquid diet during the first 12 to 14 hours following acute (sudden, short-term) diarrhea. This allows the bowel to rest while replacing essential body fluids lost as a result of diarrhea.

• Gradually advance the child's diet to full liquids, then soft foods low in roughage and bulk, as bowel movements return to normal.

- Serve liquids at room temperature.

- Don't serve liquids with your child's meals, but encourage liberal fluid intake during the rest of the day. Children can quickly become dehydrated as a result of diarrhea unless care is taken to replace fluid loss.

- Since diarrhea causes loss of sodium and potassium as well as fluids, these minerals need to be replaced. Most people in the United States use enough table salt to provide sufficient sodium when eating a normal diet. Foods high in potassium which also don't cause diarrhea include bananas, peach and apricot nectar, boiled or mashed potatoes.

- Be cautious in giving your child milk and milk products, since the diarrhea may be a result of lactose intolerance.

- Try foods low in fiber, such as fish, chicken, tender or ground beef, eggs, pureed vegetables, canned or cooked fruit without skins, ripe bananas, cooked cereal, smooth peanut butter, bread made with refined flour.

- Avoid greasy, fatty, or fried foods; citrus juices; carbonated beverages; raw vegetables and fruits; cooked vegetables high in fiber, such as broccoli, corn, cauliflower.

- Contact your child's physician if the diarrhea is extremely severe or lasts for more than 2 days.

Constipation may be caused by some anticancer drugs, and may also occur if the diet lacks adequate fluid or bulk. Certain other medications, lack of exercise, obstructions, or intestinal spasms due to irritants or emotional stress may also cause constipation. The following suggestions are useful in both preventing and treating constipation.

- Encourage your child to take plenty of liquids.

- A hot beverage in the morning or evening when bowel movements normally occur may stimulate a bowel movement.

- Be sure your child gets some exercise every day. A bedridden child should receive assistance and encouragement to perform arm, leg, and neck exercises to retain muscle tone as well as help regulate bowel movements.

- Try high fiber foods such as raw fruits and vegetables, whole grain breads and cereals, nuts, dried fruit, corn chips, oatmeal cookies.

- Add bran to foods such as casseroles, homemade breads.

- If none of these efforts work, ask your child's doctor about medication to eliminate constipation. Do not give the child a laxative unless recommended by the doctor.

Some laxatives may actually make the constipation worse, especially if the constipation is the result of other medications.

706

Dehydration, an excessive

loss of body fluid, may be due to diarrhea, severe vomiting, or excessive sweating brought on by fever. When the body loses too much water, serious and even life-threatening conditions can result. Minerals, especially sodium and potassium, may also be lost. Dehydration can occur quickly in a child and it is important to replace lost fluids as rapidly as possible.

The discussions here of nausea, vomiting, and diarrhea offer a number of suggestions for coping with the fluid loss that accompanies those conditions and can lead to dehydration. Most of these suggestions call for encouraging your child to take fluids, and to do so in a way that will reduce the risk of their being lost again through a new attack of diarrhea or vomiting. When either of these conditions continues for more than a day or two, or if they are particularly severe, your child's doctor should be notified.

Mouth Sores, tender gums and

inflammation of the throat and esophagus are often caused by infection, drugs, or radiation. Certain foods will irritate a tender mouth and swallowing may be difficult. These conditions can understandably make a child less interested in eating. While some foods increase the discomfort

caused by these problems, careful selection of foods and good care of the mouth area can make your child feel better and more like eating.

- Be sure your child sees the dentist, who can advise you on mouth care and identify problems that need special attention.

- If your child's gums and teeth are sore, clean them with a cotton swab and a mixture of hydrogen peroxide and water. Your child's dentist may recommend a special product for this purpose.

- Encourage your child to rinse his mouth frequently to remove food and bacteria and promote healing. For older children, a mixture of hydrogen peroxide and warm water is good for this purpose. **It Should Not Be Swallowed.**

- Soft foods (like mashed potatoes, custards, scrambled eggs) are easier to chew and swallow.

- Use a blender to puree your child's food if the problem is severe.

- Have your child use a straw to drink beverages and liquids.

- Cut foods into small pieces.

- Butter, thin gravies, and sauces can make foods easier to swallow.

- Cook foods until soft and tender.

- Cold foods, or those at room temperature, may be better tolerated than hot foods, which can irritate tender tissues in the mouth and throat.

- If swallowing is difficult, encourage your child to tilt his head back or move it forward.

• Try these foods: ice cream, milk shakes, bananas, peach, pear and apricot nectars, watermelon, cottage cheese.

• Avoid these foods: tomatoes, citrus fruit and fruit juices (oranges, grapefruit, tangerines) which are acidic and can burn or sting sensitive tissues; hot spices or highly salty foods; rough, coarse, or dry foods such as raw vegetables, granola, toast.

Mouth Blindness or taste
blindness is a term used to describe a changed sense of taste which can occur with chemotherapy or radiation of the head and neck area. Cancer itself may also produce this condition. Foods may be harder to taste or develop a bitter, unpleasant taste. If your child says a food does not taste good, this may well be a symptom of mouth blindness. Finding ways to deal with this problem requires experimenting and observing how your child responds to different foods. Which suggestions here will work for your child will depend on how his or her taste has been affected.

• Select and prepare foods that look and smell appetizing.

• Drinking fluids with meals may help take away a bad taste in the mouth.

• If red meat (like beef) tastes strange to your child, substitute chicken, turkey, eggs, dairy products, or fish that doesn't have a strong smell.

• Tart foods like oranges or lemonade may have more taste. Try them if your child is not also suffering from tender mouth and gums. A tart lemon custard might taste good and will also provide needed protein and calories.

• Foods may taste better cold or at room temperature, rather than hot.

• Enhance the flavor of meat, chicken, or fish by marinating in sweet fruit juices, sweet wine, Italian dressing, or sweet and sour sauce.

• Try using strong seasonings such as basil, oregano, rosemary, or lemon juice.

• Onions, bacon, or ham add flavor to vegetables.

• Tell your child's doctor and dentist about this problem.

Dry Mouth is another side effect
that can affect the way foods taste to your child. It may be caused by drugs or radiation decreasing the flow of saliva. When this happens foods also become more difficult to chew and swallow. Some of the suggestions below may be helpful in dealing with this problem. Also try some of the suggestions for coping with mouth and throat sores, since these are designed to make foods easier to swallow.

• Very sweet or tart foods like lemonade may stimulate the production of saliva in the mouth. **Don't Try This If Your Child is Also Suffering From a Tender Mouth or Sore Throat.**

• Sucking on hard candy or pop-sicles, or chewing sugar-free gum, can also stimulate production of saliva.

• Soft and pureed foods may be easier to swallow.

• Gravies, sauces, and salad dress-ings make foods easier to swallow.

• Ask your child's doctor or dentist about an "artificial saliva" prepara-tion if this problem is severe.

• A humidifier in the child's bed-room may help.

Tooth Decay can become a greater problem when a child has cancer. Not only may treatment have a bad effect on teeth and gums, but altered eating habits may also add to the problem. If your child is eating frequently or prefers sweets, more frequent brushing is needed to keep teeth healthy. In addition to frequent brushing — after every meal or snack if possible — here are some other suggestions for preventing dental problems.

• Have your child see the dentist regularly.

• Select a soft toothbrush for your child or — if gums are extremely sensitive — clean the child's teeth with Q-tips or mouthswabs de-signed especially for this purpose.

• Rinse the child's mouth with a mixture of hydrogen peroxide and warm water when mouth and gums are sore. **This Mouthwash Should Not Be Swallowed.**

• If your child is not having a problem with loss of appetite or weight loss, limit the amount of sugar in his or her diet.

• Avoid giving your child foods that tend to stick to the teeth, such as caramels or chewy candy bars.

• Have your child use a good flouride toothpaste and mouthwash.

• Remember that good nutrition promotes healthy teeth and gums.

Encouraging Your Child to Eat

When a child loses interest in food, or when eating becomes an unpleasant experience because of side effects, special efforts have to be made to encourage eating. The point cannot be overemphasized that the young patient must obtain enough nutrients—in food or supplemental form—not only for normal growth, but also to cope with the stress of the disease and its treatment. Many of the suggestions offered here have been made by parents of children with cancer who have firsthand experience in motivating finicky eaters. They are included in the hope that other parents will find them helpful in coming up with workable solutions of their own. While all these suggestions are intended to improve the nutritional status of children with cancer, some of them may not apply to your child. Before making any major changes in your child's diet consult the doctor.

Emotional Influences on Your Child's Appetite

Most cancer patients experience lack of appetite at some stage of treatment. It can have medical or emotional roots. You, the parent, play an important role in creating a reassuring, relaxed environment for your child and in reducing the anxieties of the young patient.

Children get depressed and anxious just as adults do when confronted with a major illness. Most children with cancer seem to sense the seriousness of their illness, even when parents try to protect them from this knowledge. In fact, the child may try to protect the other family members from his or her own understanding of the illness, and may experience feelings of guilt for imposing a burden on the family. This can result in the child feeling isolated, cut off from family and friends.

Brothers and sisters, while worried, may also be resentful of the changes in the family routine and the demands on parents' time made by the sick child. Parents may have resentful feelings, generally followed by guilt and always accompanied by worry about the child, the rest of the family, and other responsibilities. These are normal feelings shared by all parents facing a crisis in the life of one of their children. Finding ways to cope with the stress and strain of the child's illness is a difficult task for all family members, but is also an important part of the child's therapy.

The first step in helping to lessen the child's anxieties is open, honest communications. According to the child's age and level of understanding, explain as much as you can about the treatment. Be optimistic

710

but honest in your answers to questions, and be just as positive and honest in your dealings with your other children and the rest of the family.

Try to minimize your child's fears of being different and isolated from family and friends. Involve him or her in as many of your normal family and neighborhood activities as practical. You may have to juggle schedules or other priorities to do this, but keep those problems behind the scenes. Try not to make the child feel a burden or an inconvenience to others.

Maintaining a calm, positive attitude in both yourself and your child is especially important at mealtimes. Try not to discuss disturbing and upsetting topics at mealtimes. Your child may feel happier and less isolated if included in the normal family mealtimes. If not, don't press the issue.

Try changing time, place, and surroundings of meals. If your child has favorite TV shows, he or she may be happier and more willing to eat while watching them. Try small, positive rewards, such as a favorite dessert or reading a new story, when your child eats well. And don't forget words of praise and encouragement.

Never argue or nag about eating. Forcing foods on a child who feels sick will often result in negative feelings about foods eaten at such times. A favorite food may then be distasteful even when the child's appetite is somewhat improved.

Never punish lack of eating by withholding affection or activities the child enjoys. We all remember being told as children to "sit there until you finish what's on your plate." For a child who is ill and already under stress, this strategy will only magnify the problem.

Making Foods More Nutritious and Appealing

Dietary changes can often offset side effects of cancer treatment that spoil a child's appetite and tolerance for food. Modifying a child's diet may help to ease physical distress and discomfort, promote better nutrition and encourage the return of normal appetite. And remember that it is often the child who knows best which foods he or she can tolerate.

The child's favorite foods may not always be the most nutritious, but there are ways to increase their nutritional quality, and the most important thing is to have the child eat something. Serving nutritionally complete meals may be less important for a while than providing enough food to meet energy and protein requirements. Choose foods that are high enough in calories and protein to prevent tissue wasting. If necessary, essential vitamins and minerals can be given in tablet, capsule, or other form as recommended by the physician.

Small portions of food served at frequent intervals instead of three large meals may avoid overwhelming the child with the quantity of food to be eaten. Small meals also help reduce nausea and vomiting.

Nutritious snacks can actually become small meals in themselves. Have milk shakes ready in the refrigerator to drink whenever the child feels like it during the day. Snacks may help to stimulate the appetite as well as increase food intake.

Explain to your child that eating slowly will lessen feelings of nausea. Praise or a reward when food is eaten will encourage the child to try to eat more. If eating problems are an after-effect of treatment and last no more than a few hours, timing of meals should be arranged to avoid the period of nausea, vomiting, or lost appetite. When these effects are more prolonged, different approaches to feeding the child must be found.

One approach is to prepare the child for upcoming treatment by encouraging eating while appetite is good. Building up the body's energy stores at this time will lessen demands on body protein as a source of energy during periods of poor appetite. Including the child in food

selection and preparation often helps. Old favorites as well as new foods, or a "theme" or ethnic meal, may be helpful depending on the age level and interest of the child. In addition, a change in location, style, and table setting may make meal-time more fun.

Foods prepared with flavorings favored by children such as chocolate syrup or vanilla may help if taste is impaired. All foods should be attractively prepared and presented so that they have eye appeal in terms of color, texture, and arrangement. High calorie garnishes such as deviled eggs or cheese cubes often make a plate of food more interesting, and add to the nutritional quality of the meal.

The following pages contain suggestions for:

- *increasing protein and calories*
- *increasing calories*
- *nutritious snacks*

Most of the items are foods many people normally keep on hand or include in weekly shopping lists. Many of the foods are dairy products which are high in protein and also high in calories because of the fat content. Dairy products are often readily accepted by cancer patients. One exception is patients with "lactose intolerance". Patients with this disorder have difficulty digesting milk and milk products.

This is a good point at which to re-emphasize the importance of protein and calories. Protein is necessary for growth and the maintenance and repair of body tissues. Calories must be supplied in sufficient amounts to prevent protein from being used as energy instead of for tissue building. While a high-fat diet is not generally recommended, fat is a good source of calories. For this reason, a number of the suggestions included here call for foods with a high fat content, such as butter and cream. Their use should be guided by your doctor's recommendations and whether your child seems to have a problem in obtaining enough calories to meet his or her energy needs.

Many of the foods listed are also excellent sources of particular vitamins and minerals.

Increasing Proteins and Calories

Cheese	Melt on sandwiches, hamburgers, hot dogs, other meats or fish, vegetables, eggs, desserts like stewed fruit or pies; grate and add to sauces, casseroles, vegetable dishes, mashed potatoes, rice, noodles, meatloaf, breads, muffins.
Cottage Cheese	Mix with or use to stuff fruits or vegetables; add to casseroles or egg dishes like quiche, scrambled eggs, souffles; add to spaghetti or noodles; use in gelatin, pudding type desserts, or cheese cake; add to pancake batter; stuff crepes and pasta like shells or manicotti.
Cream Cheese	Spread on sandwiches, fruit slices, and crackers; add to egg or vegetables; roll into balls and coat with chopped nuts, wheat germ, granola.
Milk or Cream	Add to water used in cooking, or use in place of water in preparing foods such as hot cereal, soups. Serve cream sauces with vegetables and other appropriate dishes.
High Protein Milk	Blend whole milk with dry skim milk powder using 1 cup dry powder for each quart of milk; substitute for regular milk in beverages and in cooking whenever possible; substitute for water in soups, cocoa, and pudding mixes; use on cereals, jello, and stewed fruits.
Powdered Milk	Add to regular milk and milk drinks such as eggnog and milk shakes; use in casseroles; add to meatloaf, breads, muffins, sauces, cream soups, pudding and custards, and milk based gelatin salads or desserts.
Egg	Add chopped, hardcooked eggs to salads and dressings, vegetables, casseroles, creamed meats; beat eggs into mashed potatoes or vegetable purees; add an extra egg to French toast and pancake batter, or milk shakes.
Egg Yolks	Beat into sauces; add extra yolks to quiche, scrambled eggs, custards, puddings, pancake and French toast batter; a rich boiled custard made with egg yolks, high protein milk and sugar is a good source of calories and protein. Add extra hardcooked yolk to deviled egg filling and sandwich spreads.

Ice Cream	Use in beverages such as sodas, milk shakes, or other milk drinks; add to cereals, fruits, gelatin desserts, and pies; blend or whip with bananas and soft or cooked fruits; sandwich between enriched cake slices, cookies, or graham crackers.
Peanut Butter	Spread on sandwiches, toast, muffins, crackers, waffles, pancakes, fruit slices; use as a dip for raw vegetables like carrots, cauliflower, celery; add to meatloaf, appropriately flavored soups and sauces, cookies, breads, muffins; blend with milk drinks and beverages; swirl through soft ice cream and yogurt; top cookies and cakes.
Wheat Germ	Add to casserole, meat, bread, muffin, and pancake or waffle recipes; sprinkle on fruit, cereal, ice cream, or yogurt; sprinkle on top of vegetables and toast to add a crunchy topping; use in place of breadcrumbs.
Nuts	Serve as snacks; add chopped or ground nuts to ice cream, yogurt, puddings, breads, muffins, pancakes, waffles, cookies, meatloaf and hamburgers, vegetable dishes, salads, sandwiches; blend with parsley or spinach, herbs and cream for a noodle, pasta or vegetable sauce; roll banana in chopped nuts.
Meat or Fish	Add small pieces of any cooked meat or fish to vegetables, salads, casseroles, soups and biscuit ingredients; use in omelets, souffles, quiches, sandwich fillings, chicken and turkey stuffings; wrap in pie crust or biscuit dough as turnovers; add to stuffed baked potatoes. Liver is an especially good source of protein and other nutrients if accepted.
Textured Vegetable Protein	Add to hamburgers, meatloaf, meatballs, spaghetti sauce, and ground or chopped meat dishes, casseroles, sandwich fillings.
Legumes	Dry peas, beans, and bean curd (tofu) can be cooked and made into soup or added to casseroles, pastas, and grain dishes which also contain cheese or meat. Mash with cheese and milk.
Plain or Sweet Yogurt	Add to fruits and desserts; use to top cereal, pancakes, waffles, fill crepes; add to milk-based beverages and gelatin dishes.

Increasing Calories

Butter and Margarine	Add to soup, mashed and baked potatoes, hot cereal, grits, rice, noodles, and cooked vegetables; stir into sauces and gravies; combine with herbs and seasonings and spread on cooked meats, hamburgers and fish; use melted butter as a dip for raw vegetables, seafoods such as shrimp, scallops, crab, lobster.
Whipped Cream	Use unsweetened on soups and sweetened on cocoa, desserts, gelatin, pudding, fruits, pancakes, waffles; fold unsweetened into mashed potatoes or vegetable purees.
Table Cream	Use in soups, sauces, egg dishes, batters, puddings, and custards; put on cereal; mix with pasta and rice; add to mashed potatoes; pour on chicken and fish while baking; use as binder in hamburgers, meatloaf, and croquettes; substitute for milk in recipes. Make cocoa with cream, add marshmallows.
Sour Cream	Add to soups, baked potatoes, vegetables, sauces, salad dressings, stews, baked meat and fish dishes, gelatin desserts, bread and muffin batter.
Mayonnaise	Add to salad dressing; spread on sandwiches and crackers; combine with meat, fish, or vegetable salads; use as binder in croquettes; use in sauces and gelatin dishes.
Honey	Add to cereal, milk drinks; fruit deserts; glaze for meats such as chicken; add to yogurt as dessert.
Granola	Use in cookie, muffin, bread batters; sprinkle on vegetables, yogurt, ice cream, pudding, custard, fruit; layer with fruits and bake; mix with dry fruits and nuts for a snack; substitute for bread or rice in pudding recipes.
Dried Fruits	Cook and serve for breakfast or as dessert; add to muffins, cookies, breads, cakes, rice and grain dishes, cereals and puddings, stuffings; bake in pies and turnovers; combine with cooked vegetables such as carrots, sweet potatoes, yams, acorn and butternut squash, combine with nuts or granola for a finger snack.

Nutritious Snacks

Cream cheese and other
  soft cheeses
Sandwiches
Peanut butter
Gelatin salads, desserts
Cheese cake
Bread products including
  muffins, crackers
Cake and cookies
  made with whole grains, fruits,
  nuts, wheat germ, granola
Cereal

Creamed soups
Baby foods
Buttered popcorn
Pizza
Dips made with cheese,
  beans, or sour cream
Nuts
Juices
Raw vegetables
Fresh and canned fruits
Dried fruits such as raisins,
  prunes, or apricots

Hard boiled and deviled eggs
Puddings and custards
Yogurt
Ice cream
Whole milk and milk shakes
Chocblate milk
High protein milk
All hard and
  semisoft cheeses
Cottage cheese
Applesauce

Special Dietary Modifications

When a child's ability to eat properly is severely impaired, the doctor may prescribe a special diet or a commercially prepared nutritional supplement to prevent malnutrition. Occasionally it may be necessary to feed a child intravenously (through the veins) or by a tube inserted into the stomach. These are usually temporary measures, and as soon as the child is able to eat properly a regular diet is resumed.

Special Diets

The use of special diets to correct nutritional problems is common in the treatment of many diseases, including cancer. Usually these diets are used only for a few days. Often they do not provide adequate nutrients for use over a long period of time. A special diet should be given only at the doctor's direction.

Some of the diets commonly prescribed during cancer treatment are included in this handbook. Each diet sheet can be removed and displayed in the kitchen for handy reference. The illustrations are intended to make the idea of a special diet more interesting and appealing to a child.

It is important that the need for such a diet not be interpreted by the child as another sign of being different. Encourage positive feelings about the diet and its role in recovering good health. This will make the limitations and restrictions on food more acceptable.

Clear Liquid Diet

Clear liquid diets are used when there is a severe intolerance for food, such as after surgery, during an infection, or when a child is experiencing severe nausea and vomiting. This diet is usually used for 1 to 2 days, or until the child is able to consume a more liberal liquid diet.

Broth, clear soups, carbonated beverages, tea with lemon and sugar, and fruit-flavored drinks are the usual liquids tolerated. In addition, strained fruit juices, fruit ices, and plain gelatin are often included. This diet is intended to prevent dehydration and to minimize the amount of undigested material in the digestive tract. It is not nutritionally adequate for an extended period of time.

Clear Liquid
Diet
Suggested Meal Pattern For Children Five to Nine Years of Age

Breakfast	½ C. juice ½ C. clear broth, if desired	Hot tea Sugar
Lunch	½ C. juice ½ C. clear broth	Popsicle
Dinner	½ C. juice ½ C. clear broth	½ C. flavored gelatin Dessert

Clear Liquid Diet

Food Group	Allowed Foods	Excluded Foods
Beverages	Carbonated beverages, cereal beverages, decaffeinated coffee, fruit-flavored drinks, strained lemonade, limeade, and fruit punches, tea, water.	Milk, milk drinks, all others
Breads Cereals Flours	None	All
Cheeses	None	All
Desserts	Plain gelatin desserts, fruit ices without milk or pieces of fruit.	All others
Eggs	None	All
Fats	None	All

Fruits Fruit Juices	Apple, cranberry, grape juice, strained citrus juices if tolerated.	All others
Meat Poultry Fish Legumes	None	All
Milk Products	None	All
Potatoes Rice or Pasta	None	All
Soups	Bouillon, clear fat-free broths, consomme.	All others
Sweets	Honey, jelly, syrups, plain sugar candy in small amounts.	All others
Vegetables	Tomato juice, strained vegetable broth.	All others
Miscellaneous	Salt	All others

NOTE: No limitation on amounts allowed per day.

721

Full Liquid Diet

A full liquid diet is suggested when a child has had surgery, is acutely ill or unable to chew and swallow solid food. It includes all foods that are liquid at room or body temperatures. When properly planned for nutritional content, this diet can be used for relatively long periods of time. Iron and vitamins, however, need to be supplemented.

The protein content of the diet can be increased by adding non-fat dry milk to beverages and soup. Strained meats like those in baby food may be added to broths.

The caloric value of the diet may be increased by:
- Adding butter to cereal gruels and soups.
- Substituting cream for part of the milk allowances.
- Including sugar or syrup (glucose) in beverages.
- Using smooth ice cream in desserts or in beverages.
- Using prepared breakfast mixes in milk or milkshakes.

Full Liquid Diet

Suggested Meal Pattern For Children Five to Nine Years of Age

Breakfast	½ C. juice	Hot tea
	½ C. cereal	Sugar and cream
	1 C. milk	Salt
Lunch	½ C. juice	1 C. milk
	½ C. strained soup	Salt
	1 serving allowed dessert	
Dinner	½ C. juice	1 C. milk
	½ C. strained soup	Salt
	1 serving allowed dessert	
Snack	½ C. juice	1 C. milk

Full Liquid Diet

Food Group	Allowed Foods	Excluded Foods
Beverages	Cereal beverages, decaffeinated coffee, fruit drinks, strained lemonade, limeade, or fruit punches, coffee, tea, water.	None
Breads Cereals Flours	Refined or strained cooked cereal for gruels.	Breads and cereals in solid form
Cheeses	Cheese Soup	Others
Desserts	Plain gelatin desserts, Junket, soft or baked custard, sherbets, plain cornstarch pudding, fresh or frozen yogurt, ice milk, smooth ice cream.	All others, particularly those with fruits or seeds
Eggs	Pasteurized eggnog.	Fried, scrambled, hard boiled eggs
Fats	Butter, cream; oils; margaine.	All others
Fruits Fruit Juices	Citrus fruit juices, strained fruit juices, thin fruit purees, all juices and nectars.	All others

Meat **Poultry** **Fish**	Small amounts of strained meat in broth or gelatin.	All others
Milk **Milk Products**	Chocolate, buttermilk, skim and whole milk, ice milk, milk shakes, plain yogurt.	All others, yogurt with pieces of fruit
Potatoes **Rice or Pasta**	Potatoes pureed in soup.	All others
Soups	Bouillon, broth, clear soups, cream soups. Any strained or blenderfied soup.	All others
Sweets	Honey, jelly, syrups in small amounts.	All others
Vegetables	Vegetable puree for cream soups, tomato juice, vegetable juice.	All others
Miscellaneous	Flavoring extracts, salt.	All others

Soft Diet

This diet is usually a transitional diet between a liquid diet and a regular diet. The foods included are lightly seasoned, easy to chew, and modified in consistency. Fried or "greasy" foods are avoided.

Foods may be made soft by cooking, mashing, pureeing, or homogenizing the foods used in normal diets.

Soft Diet

Suggested Meal Pattern For
Children Five to Nine Years of Age

Breakfast	½ C. fruit or juice	1 tsp. butter or margarine
	1 serving cereal	Jelly
	1 egg	1 C. milk
	2 strips bacon	Sugar and cream
	1 slice toast	Salt and pepper
Lunch	½ C. juice and/or soup	1 tsp. butter or margarine
	2 oz. meat or substitute	1 serving fruit or dessert
	½ C. vegetable and/or allowed salad	1 C. milk
		Salt and pepper
	2 slices bread	
Dinner	3 oz. meat or substitute	1 tsp. butter or margarine
	½ C. potato or substitute	1 serving fruit or dessert
	½ C. vegetable and/or allowed salad	1 C. milk
		Salt and pepper
	1 slice bread or roll	
Snack	½ C. juice	

Soft Diet

Food Group	Allowed Foods	Excluded Foods
Beverages	All	None
Breads	French, Vienna, Italian; seedless rye, white, refined whole wheat, cornbread, or any except whole-grain. If tolerated, muffins, French toast, crackers, biscuits, rolls, pancakes, waffles.	Brown, cracked wheat, pumpernickel, raisin, rye with seeds, buckwheat, whole-grain crackers, rolls with coconut, raisins, nuts, or whole grains, tortillas
Cereals	Refined, cooked or ready-to-eat.	Whole-grain or bran
Flours	All except whole-grain, bran, wheat.	Whole-grain, bran or wheat
Cheeses	All, except those excluded.	Sharp or strongly flavored cheeses, or those containing whole seeds and spices
Desserts	Ice milk, ice cream, sherbet, ices, custards, gelatins, or others with allowed fruits.	Desserts made with prohibited fruits, nuts, coconut
Eggs	All, except fried.	Raw, fried
Fats	Butter, cream, cream substitutes, vegetable shortenings and oils, margarine, mayonnaise, sour cream, commercial French dressing.	Other salad dressings, salt pork. Fried foods
Fruits Fruit Juices	All juices and nectars. Avocado, banana. Canned or cooked apples, apricots, cherries, grapefruit and orange sections without membrane, peaches, pears, seedless grapes.	All raw fruit except avocado and banana. All dried fruit, berries, crabapples, coconut, figs, grapes, melons, pineapples, plums, rhubarb.
Meat	Tender beef, lamb, veal or liver that is baked, broiled, creamed, roasted or stewed. Roasted or stewed pork.	Fried, salted and smoked meats. Chitterlings, corned beef, pork, sausage, cold cuts

	Allowed	Avoid
Poultry	Chicken, cornish game hen, duck, turkey, chicken livers.	Game birds, goose
Fish	Cooked, fresh or frozen fish without bones. Tuna, salmon.	Fried fish, shellfish, anchovies, caviar, herring, sardines, snails, skate
Legumes Nuts	Creamy peanut butter, refined soy products.	All other legumes; nuts and seed kernels
Milk Products	All.	None
Potatoes Rice Pasta	Baked, boiled, creamed, scalloped, mashed, au gratin, mashed sweet potatoes. Dumplings, noodles, brown or white rice, spaghetti.	French fries, hashbrowns, potato salad, whole sweet potatoes or yams. Bread stuffing, fritters, chow mein noodles, wild rice, barley.
Soups	Bouillon, broths, consomme, strained cream and vegetable.	Bean, split pea, onion. Bisques, gumbos, unstrained chowders
Sweets	Apple butter, butterscotch, candy, caramels, chocolate, fondant, plain fudge, lollipops, marshmallows, mints. Honey, jelly, syrups, sugars in small amounts.	Candied fruits, nut brittle, chewing gums, jams, preserves, marmalade, marzipan, fruit sauces with prohibited fruits
Vegetables	Canned or cooked asparagus, beans, carrots, beets, eggplant, mushrooms, parsley, pumpkin, spinach, squash, tomatoes. Tomato juice, vegetable juice cocktail. Raw lettuce if tolerated.	All raw vegetables except lettuce. All canned or cooked vegetables not specifically allowed.
Miscellaneous	Aspic, catsup, chocolate, gelatin, gravy, pretzels, soy sauce, vinegar. Brown, cheese, cream, tomato and white sauces. All finely chopped or ground leaf herbs and spices.	Garlic, horseradish, olives, pickles, popcorn, potato chips, relishes. Chili, A-la-king, creole, barbecue, coktail, sweet-sour, Newburg, Worcestershire sauces; whole and seed herbs and spices.

Low Residue Diet

This diet is sometimes recommended following intestinal radiotherapy. It is used to decrease the amount of fiber which passes through the intestinal tract. Fiber or roughage may cause irritation leading to diarrhea and/or cramping. Other foods, especially milk and milk products, may also be difficult to digest.

Fiber and milk products can be gradually increased in the diet according to the child's tolerance. It is best to consult your dietitian concerning the gradual addition of foods.

Low Residue Diet

Suggested Meal Pattern For Children Five to Nine Years of Age

Breakfast	½ C. fruit juice	1 tsp. butter or margarine
	1 serving allowed cereal	Jelly
	1 egg	1 C. milk
	2 strips bacon	Sugar and cream
	1 slice toast	Salt
Lunch	½ C. juice and/or soup	1 tsp. butter or margarine
	2 oz. meat or substitute	1 serving allowed fruit
	½ C. allowed vegetable	or dessert
	2 slices bread or roll	Salt
Dinner	3 oz. meat or substitute	1 tsp. butter or margarine
	½ C. potato	1 serving allowed fruit
	1 slice bread or roll	or dessert
		1 C. milk
		Salt
Snack	½ C. juice	

Low Residue Diet

Food Group	Allowed Foods	Excluded Foods
Beverages	Fruit flavored drinks, milk drinks, carbonated beverages, coffee, decaffeinated coffee, tea. *2 cups milk or milk products allowed per day. All others: no limitation*	None
Breads	French, Vienna, Italian, refined whole wheat, white and rye breads without seeds. Crackers, biscuits, French toast. Plain hard, rusk and zweiback rolls.	Breads, crackers, rolls or cereals containing whole grain or graham flour, bran seeds, nuts or raisins, corn bread
Cereals	All refined, cooked or dry cereals, oatmeal.	All cereals made from prohibited flours or other foods
Flours	All except bran, graham, whole wheat or whole grain flours.	Bran, graham, whole wheat or whole grain flours
Cheeses	Cottage, cream, American, Swiss, muenster, or other mild cheeses. *1 oz. may be substituted for 1 cup milk.*	All others
Desserts	Custards, gelatin puddings, plain cookies and cakes, sherbets. Pastry without nuts.	All desserts containing seeds, nuts, coconut or raisins. Tough skinned fruits
Eggs	All except fried.	Fried eggs
Fats	Crisp bacon, butter, oils, cream, dry cream substitutes, margarine, mayonnaise, shortenings, smooth salad dressings, sour cream.	Salad dressings made with prohibited ingredients, tartar sauce
Fruits Fruit Juices	All juices and nectars. Canned, or cooked fruit, peeled fruit without seeds. Apples, apricots, avocados, bananas, cherries, grapefruit, oranges, tangerines, fruit cocktail, grapes, melons, cantaloupe, honeydew, peaches, pears, pineapple, plums. *2 servings allowed per day.*	All other fresh fruits, dried fruits, berries, figs, grapes with seeds

	Allowed	Prohibited
Meat Poultry	Tender beef, ham, lamb, liver, poultry, or veal that is baked, broiled or stewed.	Fried meats and poultry, other smoked or cured meats, cold cuts, corned beef, frankfurters, pastrami, sausage
Fish	Fresh or frozen fish without bones, canned tuna or salmon, cooked shellfish.	All fried or smoked fish, sardines, herring
Legumes Nuts	None	All dried legumes, lima beans, peas, nuts
Milk Milk Products	Buttermilk, chocolate, skim and whole milk, yogurt. *2 cups including that used in cooking allowed per day.*	Yogurt containing prohibited fruit
Potatoes Rice Pasta	Broiled, creamed, mashed, scalloped. Baked and sweet potatoes without skin, macaroni, noodles, white rice, spaghetti. *1 serving potato allowed per day. All others: No limitation.*	Potato cakes, French fries, hash browns, potato salad, fibrous sweet potato, brown and wild rice, barley, hominy
Soups	Cream and broth based soups made with allowed foods.	All others
Sweets	Honey, jelly, syrup. candy.	Jams, preserves and candies with fruits, coconut, raisins, or nuts, candied fruits
Vegetables	Canned or cooked asparagus, beans, beets, carrots, mushrooms, peas, pumpkin, squash, spinach, tomatoes, turnip greens. Tomato juice, raw lettuce if tolerated. *No limitation on juices. 1 serving whole vegetables allowed per day.*	All raw vegetables except lettuce. Canned or cooked vegetables not specifically allowed.
Miscellaneous	Ground or finely chopped herbs and spices, salt, flavoring extracts, catsup, chocolate, mild gravy, white sauce, soy sauce, vinegar.	All other spices and condiments, olives, pickles, potato chips, popcorn

Lactose-Restricted Diet

Lactose or milk sugar is found in all milk products. A lactose-restricted diet may be recommended following intestinal radiotherapy which often produces a temporary lactose intolerance. Fermented milk products are often tolerated by individuals who cannot tolerate whole milk. Lactose is frequently used as a filler in many products such as instant coffee and some medicines. Labels should be read carefully.

Lactose intolerance may vary from child to child. Consult the physician or dietitian for more flexibility in the choice of allowed foods.

Lactose-Restricted
Diet *Suggested Meal Pattern For Children Five to Nine Years of Age*

Breakfast	½ C. fruit juice 1 serving cereal 1 egg 2 strips bacon 1 slice toast 1 tsp. butter or margarine	Jelly 1 C. acidophilus milk Sugar Salt and pepper
Lunch	½ C. juice and/or broth-based soup 2 oz. meat or substitute ½ C. vegetable and/or salad 2 slices bread or roll	1 tsp. butter or margarine 1 serving fruit or dessert 1 C. acidophilus milk Salt and pepper
Dinner	3 oz. meat or substitute ½ C. potato or substitute ½ C. vegetable and/or salad 1 slice bread or roll	1 tsp. butter or margarine 1 serving fruit or dessert 1 C. acidophilus milk Salt and pepper
Snack	½ C. juice	

Lactose-Restricted Diet

Food Group	Allowed Foods	Excluded Foods
Beverages	Lactose-free carbonated beverages, fruit-flavored drinks, fruit punches, lemonade, limeade, decaffeinated coffee, tea, coffee, nondairy product drinks.	Artificial fruit drinks containing lactose. All beverages made with milk and milk products with the exception of buttermilk or yogurt
Bread	All	None
Cereals	Any cooked or dry cereal not containing lactose.	Instant hot cereals, high protein cereals. All cereals with added milk or lactose
Flours	All	None
Cheeses	Fermented cheeses (cheddar and any cheese aged with bacteria).	Others
Desserts	Fruit ices, gelatins, angel food cake, desserts made with nondairy products, buttermilk or sour cream.	Ice cream, puddings and other desserts containing milk or milk products
Eggs	All except eggs prepared with milk or milk products.	Creamed, scrambled, omelets or other eggs prepared with milk
Fats	Margarine not containing milk solids, vegetable oils, mayonnaise, shortening.	All others: cream, half-and-half, table and whipping cream
Fruits Fruit Juices	All fresh, canned or frozen fruits that are not processed with lactose.	Any canned or frozen fruits and fruit juices that are processed with lactose

Meat **Poultry** **Fish** **Legumes** **Nuts**	Any except those specifically excluded.	Creamed or breaded fish, poultry, meat. Cold cuts, hot dogs, liver, sausage or other processed meats containing milk or lactose. Gravies made with milk.
Milk **Milk Products**	Protein hydrolysate formulas. Fermented milk products as acidophilus milk, buttermilk, yogurt and sour cream.	All milk, milk products except fermented milk products
Potatoes **Rice** **Pasta**	White or sweet potatoes, macaroni, noodles, spaghetti or other pasta, rice.	Any prepared with milk as creamed or scalloped; commercial potato products containing dried milk
Soups	Broth based soups.	Cream soups, chowders, commercially prepared soups that contain milk or milk products
Sweets	Honey, jams, preserves, syrups, molasses.	Candy containing lactose, milk or cocoa. Butterscotch candies, caramels, chocolates. **Read all labels carefully**
Vegetables	All vegetables, except those prepared with milk.	Any prepared with milk as creamed or scalloped. Any processed vegetables containing lactose
Miscellaneous	Catsup, chili sauce, horseradish, olives, pickles, vinegar, gravies prepared without milk, mustard, all herbs and spices, peanut butter, unbuttered popcorn.	Chocolate, cocoa, milk gravies, cream sauces, chewing gum, instant coffee, powdered soft drinks, artificial juices containing milk or lactose

NOTE: No limitation on amounts of allowed foods.

Gluten-Restricted Diet

This diet is sometimes recommended following intestinal radiotherapy. It may also help to control or stop cramping and diarrhea which may occur after abdominal radiotherapy.

The protein gluten is found in most breads and flours. It is eliminated from the diet by omitting wheat, rye, barley, oats, buckwheat, and foods prepared with these grains. Rice, corn and products made from these may be substituted for the grains omitted. Products made from soy flour, tapioca flour, cornstarch, potato flour, arrowroot, wheat starch and gluten-free flour may also be included.

Gluten-Restricted
Diet *Suggested Meal Pattern For Children Five to Nine Years of Age*

Breakfast	½ C. fruit or juice	1 tsp. butter or margarine
	1 serving rice cereal	Jelly
	1 egg	1 C. milk
	2 strips bacon or 1 oz. meat	Sugar and cream
	1 cornmeal muffin or substitute	Salt and pepper
Lunch	½ C. juice and/or clear soup	1 tsp. butter or margarine
	2 oz. meat or substitute	1 serving fruit or dessert
	½ C. vegetable and/or salad	Salt and pepper
	2 slices gluten-free bread or substitute	
Dinner	3 oz. meat or substitute	1 tsp. butter or margarine
	½ C. potato or substitute	1 serving fruit or dessert
	½ C. vegetable and/or salad	1 C. milk
	1 rice muffin or substitute	Salt and pepper
Snack	½ C. juice	

Gluten-Restricted Diet

Food Groups	Allowed Foods	Excluded Foods
Beverages	Decaffeinated coffee, fruit juices, lemonade, limeade, tea, coffee, cocoa, carbonated beverages.	Cereal beverages (Postum, Ovaltine), malted drinks. Alcoholic: ale, beer
Breads	Breads, cakes, muffins, rolls made from allowed flours.	Breads, crackers, doughnuts, muffins, pancakes, pretzels, rolls, waffles. Bread crumbs containing barley, oats, rye, or wheat. Any product made from prohibited flours
Cereals	Cereals made from corn or rice, hominy grits, cream of rice, granulated rice.	Bran or cereal made from bran, cream of wheat, farina, oatmeal, wheatena. Any other cereals derived from barley, buckwheat, oats, rye, wheat germ
Flours	Flours made from arrowroot, cornmeal, cornstarch, potatoes, rice, soya, tapioca, wheat starch, flours that are gluten-free.	Buckwheat, graham, rye, white or whole wheat flours
Cheeses	All except processed cheese spreads.	Processed cheese spreads
Dessert	Desserts made with allowed flours. Milk, cream and fruit desserts made with eggs, gelatin, rice, cornstarch, tapioca or wheat starch.	Fruit desserts, cakes and cookies prepared with prohibited flours, starches or milk products
Eggs	All except those prepared with wheat flour or other prohibited foods.	Creamed egg dishes and souffles prepared with wheat flour
Fats	All fats.	Commercial salad dressings containing prohibited flours

Category	Foods Allowed	Foods Prohibited
Fruit Juices		
Meat Poultry Fish Legumes Nuts	All meat, fish and poultry that is not breaded, creamed or served with thickened gravy or bread dressings. Meat analogs that do not contain wheat, rye, barley or oats. All legumes and nuts.	Commercial products containing prohibited cereals. The following foods frequently contain gluten: bologna, canned meat mixtures, frankfurters, liverwurst, luncheon meats, meat analogs, meat loaf made with bread-crumbs, sausage, scrapple, gravy or cream sauces thickened with prohibited flours
Milk Milk Products	Buttermilk, canned milk, dry milk, skim and whole milk, yogurt, cocoa made with milk, cocoa powder.	Milk drinks made with cereal additives, chocolate milk, or malted milk
Potatoes Rice Pasta	White and sweet potatoes, potato chips, rice.	Creamed potatoes made with flour, potato salad made with commercial salad dressing, commercial potato products containing prohibited flours. Barley, bread stuffing, dumplings, fritters, macaroni, noodles, spaghetti, Yorkshire pudding
Soups	Homemade meat or chicken broth, chowders, cream soups thickened with egg yolks or allowed flours and starches.	Soups made with wheat, rye, oats or barley. Commercial soup and soup mixes
Sweets	Honey, jams, preserves, hard candy, molasses in small amounts.	Commercial candies containing cereal products. **Read labels**
Vegetables	All, except those with prohibited flours.	Vegetables containing prohibited flours
Miscellaneous	Catsup, pure chocolate, cocoa, garlic, gelatin, mustard, olives, pickles, popcorn, soy sauce, vinegar, Worcestershire sauce. All herbs, spices and extracts.	Cream sauces and gravies prepared with prohibited flours. **Read labels**

High Fiber Diet

This is essentially a normal diet but includes an additional two or three daily servings of food high in bulk and roughage. A high fiber diet contains nondigestible material such as that found in fruits, vegetables and whole grain cereals, which produce bulk in the intestinal tract to stimulate bowel movements. This diet may be useful when constipation occurs from medications or inactivity.

The emphasis in this diet is on increasing the amount of cereal, fruit, and vegetable bulk. Whole grain and bran breads and cereals should be increased in the diet and the consumption of refined breads, cereals, sugars and sweets should be reduced. Raw, canned or dried fruits and vegetables should also be increased in the diet.

High Fiber
Diet *Suggested Meal Pattern For Children Five to Nine Years of Age*

Breakfast	½ C. stewed fruit or citrus fruit ½ C. whole grain cereal 1 egg 2 strips bacon 1 slice whole grain toast	1 tsp. butter or margarine Jelly or jam 1 C. milk Sugar and cream Salt and pepper
Lunch	½ C. juice and/or soup 2 oz. meat or substitute Raw vegetable and/or salad 2 slices whole grain bread	1 tsp. butter or margarine Fruit 1 C. milk Salt and pepper
Dinner	3 oz. meat or substitute ½ C. potato or substitute Raw vegetable and/or salad 1 slice whole grain bread	1 tsp. butter or margarine Fruit or dessert 1 C. milk Salt and pepper
Snack	Raw fruits and vegetables	½ C. juice

High Fiber Diet

Some
General
Guidelines

1 Use whole-grain cereals such as bran, bran flakes, shredded wheat. Use whole-grain bread products such as cracked wheat and rye.

2 Use potatoes, brown or wild rice, whole-wheat pasta and other cooked whole cereal grains rather than refined products.

3 Include two salads daily, emphasizing raw fruits and vegetables.

4 Eat whole fruits including skins.

5 Include stewed or dried fruits and juices such as stewed prunes, prune juice, apricots, figs, raisins and nuts.

Commercial Food Supplements and Liquid Diets

Commercially prepared diets and dietary supplements are designed for persons with special nutritional requirements. These are sometimes called *medical foods, chemically defined diets,* or *defined formula diets*. They provide different amounts of calories, protein, fat, carbohydrate, vitamins, and minerals.

These products are also designed for use in particular ways and are by no means interchangeable. Many were developed exclusively for use in the hospital. Some are for use only in tube feeding and may be bitter-tasting. Others, to be taken by mouth, are flavored like milk shakes.

Still others may have little or no taste and can be added to other foods to increase their nutritional value without altering their flavor.

These food supplements must never be used without the doctor's approval. However, if you are worried about your child's nutrition and are looking for ways to increase the intake of calories or protein, ask the doctor or dietitian about food supplements. They will be able to tell you if such supplements would be appropriate for your child, recommend specific brands, and suggest ways of using them effectively.

Parenteral and Enteral Nutrition

Total Parenteral Nutrition

(TPN), or hyperalimentation, is a form of intravenous feeding now in use by some doctors as a preventative measure when nutritional problems are expected.

The TPN solution is administered through a large vein, usually one near the neck. In this way nutrients are introduced directly into the blood stream, bypassing the stomach and intestine entirely. TPN is not recommended for all cancer patients, and its role in cancer therapy is still being investigated.

We should mention that most intravenous fluids received by hospital patients are not TPN, but simply sterile solutions of glucose, electrolytes, and medications. They provide fluid as well as a route for administering drugs, but do not include large amounts of calories, protein, or other nutrients.

Enteral nutrition refers to eating, digesting, and absorbing food through the gastrointestinal (GI) tract. Thus, normal eating of foods by mouth is a form of enteral nutrition. However, in the therapeutic sense enteral nutrition usually refers to various methods of tube feeding. Such methods may be necessary

when a patient with a normally functioning digestive tract refuses to eat or cannot eat enough. Nutrient solutions are given via a tube inserted through the mouth, nose, or an opening in the esophagus, stomach, or small intestine. If all nutrients are supplied in this manner, it is referred to as total enteral nutrition (TEN).

The most common form of tube feeding is the nasogastric, in which a small flexible tube is passed through a nostril of the nose into the esophagus and then to the stomach. At regular intervals, or continuously, a prescribed amount of a liquid diet is poured into the tube. Under certain circumstances, as when severe irritation of the esophagus exists or when tube feeding is to be used for an extended period of time, the feeding tube is inserted into the stomach through an abdominal incision. In this way the child is relieved of the discomfort from a tube inserted through the nose or mouth.

None of these special feeding techniques is as desirable as the normal methods of eating and drinking. When necessary, however, their use is as important to your child's care and recovery as other forms of treatment.

Glossary

Absorption-The process by which the products of digestion are transferred from the intestinal tract into the blood and lymph circulation.

Acute-Occurring suddenly or over a short period of time.

Alimentary Canal-The tubular passage that extends from mouth to anus and functions in digestion and absorption of food and elimination of waste. It is also called the gastrointestinal tract.

Alkylating Agents-A group of highly reactive chemical compounds that combine with nucleic acids in the cell to affect the cell's production of protein, thus slowing or stopping tumor cell growth.

Alopecia-The loss of hair.

Ambulatory-Being able to walk; not confined to bed.

Amino Acids-Organic compounds of carbon, hydrogen, oxygen and nitrogen; the building blocks of protein molecules.

Anemia-A condition in which blood is deficient in red blood cells, hemoglobin, or total volume.

Anorexia-Loss of appetite for food.

Antibiotic-Class of drugs derived from microorganisms; specific antibiotics are toxic to specific organisms; some antibiotics inhibit growth of tumor cells.

Antibody-One of the many substances produced by the body which help to defend the body against infections.

Antigens-Substances the body recognizes as foreign and which can cause production of antibodies.

Antimetabolite-Anticancer agents that closely resemble substances needed by cells for normal growth. The tumor cell uses the drug instead, and "starves" for lack of proper substance.

Basal Metabolic Rate (BMR)-The minimum energy needed to carry on the body processes vital to life.

Benign-Referring to a non-malignant condition.

Biopsy-A process that involves the removal of tissue, cells, or fluid from the body for pathological examination.

Bone Marrow-The material which fills the cavities of the bones and is the substance from which the circulating blood cells are formed.

Burkitt's Lymphoma-A type of cancer of the lymphatic system.

Cachexia-A condition characterized by malnutrition and wasting of body tissues which may occur during the course of an illness.

Calorie-A unit of heat measurement.

Cancer-Malignant disease marked by abnormal growth of cells. Normal tissues can be invaded by abnormal cells; the abnormal cells can also leave the original site and form new colonies elsewhere in the body. (See metastasis.)

Carbohydrate-A class of substances which includes sugars, starches, and cellulose.

Carcinogen-A chemical or other agent that causes cancer.

Carcinoma-Cancer of the tissues which cover or line the body surface and internal organs.

Cat Scan-Diagnostic X-ray procedure in which a computer is used to generate a 3-dimensional image.

Catheter-A tube used to permit injection or withdrawal of fluid; a catheter can be rubber, plastic, glass or metal.

CBC (complete blood count)-A series of tests to examine components of the blood. The tests are useful in diagnosing certain health problems and in following the results of treatment.

Cell-The smallest unit of living material that can function independently.

Chemotherapy-The use of chemical agents in treatment of disease.

Chronic-A term that is used to describe a disease of long duration or one that is progressing slowly.

CNS-Central nervous system; refers to the brain and spinal cord.

Cobalt Treatment-Radiation that uses gamma rays generated by cobalt-60, a radioactive isotope of the element cobalt.

Colostomy-A temporary or permanent opening in the colon and the abdominal wall to permit elimination of wastes.

Congenital-A condition existing at, or dating from birth.

Culture-A laboratory procedure in which samples of blood, secretions or other body fluids are cultivated in special nutrients; used to determine the presence and type of infectious agents.

Cyst-A fluid-filled sac which can be malignant or benign.

Cystitis-Inflammation of the urinary bladder. It is accompanied by pain and frequent urination.

Dehydration-A condition resulting from loss of water; often results from severe diarrhea or from prolonged nausea and vomiting.

Diet-A general term for all foods eaten, including both liquid and solid forms.

Digestive Tract-The organs involved in the digestive process including the esophagus, stomach, intestine, colon, liver, gall bladder and pancreas. Also referred to as alimentary canal or gastrointestinal tract.

Diuretics-Drugs that increase the elimination of water and salt from the body.

Dumping Syndrome-Reaction in which food is "dumped" from the stomach into the intestine too quickly after being swallowed. This condition, which can result in severe diarrhea, often occurs after partial or total surgical removal of the stomach, and is due to the fact that the remaining stomach or esophagus can hold only a small amount of food.

Dyspepsia/Indigestion-Upset stomach.

Dysphagia-Difficulty in swallowing.

Edema-The accumulation of excess fluid within the tissues.

Electrolytes-A general term for the minerals necessary to provide the proper environment for body cells and proper fluid balance.

Emaciation-Wasting of the body; excessive leanness.

Enteral Nutrition-Refers to feeding by way of the digestive tract.

Enzymes-Complex organic compounds (proteins) produced within an organism and which control the rate of chemical reactions in the body.

Essential Fatty Acids-Specific components of dietary fats which are vital to normal metabolism; they cannot be produced by the body and must be obtained from the diet.

Etiology-The study of causes of diseases.

Excision-Surgical removal of tissue.

Flatulence-Bloating of the stomach or intestines by air or gas; act of passing or eliminating gas.

Food Aversion-A dislike for food in general or a specific type of food.

Fortified Refers to the addition of nutrients to foods.

Gamma Globulin A class of protein components of the blood; most antibodies are gamma globulins.

Gastrectomy Surgical removal of all or part of the stomach.

Gastrointestinal Tract-The mouth, esophagus, stomach, and intestines — commonly abbreviated to GI tract.

Glucose-A simple sugar occuring in some fruits and honey; the sugar found in blood.

Gluten-A protein in wheat and other cereals that gives an elastic quality to the dough.

Gram-A metric unit of weight; there are approximately 28 grams in an ounce. Abbreviated g. or gm.

Hematologist-A physician specializing in the study of blood diseases.

Hematology-The study of blood and blood-forming organs.

Hemoglobin-The iron-protein component in the red blood cells which carries oxygen to the tissues.

Hemorrhage-Refers to a loss of blood due to injury to the blood vessels.

Hodgkin's Disease-A form of cancer that arises in a single lymph node and which may spread to nearby and then distant lymph nodes. It may reach other tissues, most commonly including the spleen, liver, and bone marrow.

Hormone-A chemical substance produced by the endocrine glands and carried in body fluids to other organs or parts of the body. Hormones help to regulate various bodily functions.

Hyperalimentation-Intravenous administration of nutrients, bypassing the gastrointestinal tract. It is also called Total Parenteral Nutrition (TPN).

Immune Reaction-A reaction of normal tissues to "foreign" substances such as bacteria or viruses.

Immunity-The body's ability to resist and overcome infection.

Immunology-Study of the body's natural defense mechanisms against disease.

Immunotherapy-A method of cancer therapy which involves stimulating the body's immune defenses.

Infection-Refers to the invasion of the body by disease-producing organisms.

Informed Consent-Refers to the permissions given by a person before surgery or treatment. The patient, or a parent or guardian, must understand the potential risks and benefits of the treatment or surgery and legally agree to accept those risks.

Infusion-Continuous slow introduction of a substance into a vein or artery.

Injections-The administration of medications through a needle into a muscle, vein, or tissue under the skin.

Intramuscular (IM)-Refers to the injection of a drug into muscle tissue where it is absorbed into the blood stream.

Intravenous (IV)-The administration of a drug or fluid directly into a vein.

Isotopic Scan-A diagnostic procedure for examining organs, the brain, or bones. In this procedure, a radioactive substance is introduced intravenously and is then studied by X-ray or fluoroscope.

Kilogram-A metric unit of weight equal to 1,000 grams or 2.2 pounds. Abbreviated kg.

Lactose -The form of carbohydrate in milk; milk sugar.

Laparotomy-Surgical procedure that involves cutting through the abdominal wall.

Lethargy-Inactivity, drowsiness, forgetfulness.

Leukemia-An acute or chronic disease characterized by abnormal numbers of immature white blood cells (leukocytes) in the tissue or bloodstream.

Leukocyte-White blood cell or corpuscle.

Lipid-A term for fats and fat-like substances including neutral fats, oils, fatty acids and cholesterol.

Lumbar Puncture-A diagnostic procedure which involves taking and examining a sample of spinal fluid.

Lymph-A transparent, almost colorless fluid found in the lymphatic vessels of the body. It consists chiefly of tissue fluid and proteins, and bathes body cells.

Lymphatic System-Refers to the lymphoid organs and the circulatory network of vessels that carry lymph fluid. It is involved in the body's immune responses.

Lymphoid Tissue-Tissues such as tonsils and lymph nodes that are important in defense against disease.

Lymphoma-A tumor of the lymphatic system.

Malignant-Tending to become progressively worse; in the case of cancer, it implies ability to invade, disseminate, and actively destroy surrounding tissue.

Malnutrition-Condition in which the body is receiving too little nourishment or the wrong kind.

Melanoma-A cancer of the pigment cells of the skin, often arising in a pre-existing pigmented area as a mole.

Metabolism-Refers to the process by which the cells of the body use absorbed nutrients to maintain the body and its activities.

Metastasis-The spread of cancer cells through the blood and lym-phatic vessels and establishment of new groups of those cells at locations distant from the primary tumor.

Microorganisms-Very small organisms such as bacteria, viruses, yeasts, and molds.

Modality-A general term for a type or method of treatment. The basic modalities of cancer treatment include surgery, radiotherapy, chemotherapy, and experimental immunotherapy. Multimodality treatment refers to the use of more than one type of treatment.

Mucous Membrane-Type of tissue lining body passages such as the gastrointestinal tract.

Neoplasm-New or abnormal uncontrolled growth, such as a tumor.

Neuroblastoma-A solid tumor derived from tissues of the symphathetic nervous sytem. Frequently found in the abdomen.

Non-Hodgkin's Lymphoma-A tumor which can develop in any lymphatic tissue in the body.

Nucleic Acid-Class of substances found in cells which carry the biochemical codes for heredity and day-to-day function of cells.

Nutrient-A substance that is necessary for growth, normal functioning, tissue repair, and maintaining life. Essential nutrients are proteins, minerals, fats, carbo-hydrates, and vitamins.

Nutrition-The process of food intake (eating and drinking), release of nutrients from the food, and the absorption and use of nutrients by the body.

Oncologist-A physician or surgeon who specializes in cancer.

Oncology-The study of physical, chemical, and biological properties and features of cancer.

Organ-Several tissues grouped together to perform one or more functions in the body.

Osteoporosis-A loss in body substances producing brittleness and softness of bones.

Osteosarcoma-A tumor of the bone.

Ostomy-A suffix which refers to a surgically created passage connecting an internal organ with the skin of other internal organs.

Pathologist-One who studies and interprets disease-caused changes in tissues.

Pathology-The branch of medicine involved with examining and classifying disease-caused and normal characteristics of tissue.

Peptic Ulcer-An ulcer of the stomach, duodenum or lower end of the esophagus.

Pharmacology-The study of drugs including their absorption, distribu-tion throughout the body, and excretion.

Plasma-The liquid portion of the blood which contains numerous proteins and minerals and is necessary for normal body functioning.

Platelets-Particles in the blood which play a role in blood clotting.

Proctitis-Inflammation of the anus and rectum.

Prognosis-An estimate of the outcome of a disease; a prediction.

Radiation-The release of energy through waves (such as ultraviolet rays or X-rays) or energetic particles (such as electrons or neutrons).

Radical Surgery-An operation to remove a tumor, plus adjacent tissues and lymph nodes.

Radioresistant-Describes a cancer that does not readily respond to radiation.

Radiosensitive-Describes a cancer that responds readily to radiation.

Radiotherapy-A treatment which is based on the capacity of atomic particles and rays to destroy living cells.

RDA (Recommended Daily Allowances)-quantities of specified vitamins, minerals, and other nutrients needed daily for good nutrition.

Relapse-The reappearance of a disease after a period when symptoms had lessened or ceased.

Remission-Refers to the period when the symptoms of a disease have lessened or ceased.

Renal-A term which refers to the kidneys.

Resection -The surgical removal of tissue.

Retinoblastoma-A malignant tumor which occurs in the retina of the eye in children.

Rhabdomyosarcoma-A tumor of the soft tissues of the body, generally muscle.

Sarcoma A cancer of connective tissue, bone, cartilage, fat, muscle, nerve sheath, blood vessels, lymph system or glands.

Secretion-A discharge of a substance by a cell or gland.

Septicemia-Widespread infection involving the bloodstream.

Stomatitits -The inflammation of the mucous membranes in the mouth.

Syndrome-A set of symptoms occurring together.

Systemic-Pertaining to the body as a whole.

Therapeutic-Refers to a treatment or therapy for the cure or control of a condition or disease.

Thoracic-Pertaining to the thorax: the chest, the rib cage and the organs within the rib cage.

Tissue-A collection of cells similar in structure and function.

Tolerance -The ability to endure or withstand a particular drug or treatment without ill effects.

Toxicity -The quality of a substance which causes ill effects.

TPN-Total Parenteral Nutrition; procedure in which nutrients are supplied directly to the bloodstream.

Tumor-A mass or swelling; the word "tumor" carries no connotation of being either benign or malignant.

Ulcer-An erosion of normal tissue resulting from acids, infection, impaired circulation, or cancerous involvement.

Vitamin-Any one of a group of chemical substances vital for the maintenance and growth of the body.

Wilms' Tumor-A malignant tumor of the kidney usually occurring in children under 6 years of age.

WBC (white blood count)-A test that determines the number of leukocytes in the peripheral blood; the term WBC may also refer to white blood cells.

Chapter 36

Students With Cancer

A Resource for the Educator

Introduction

At some point in your career as an educator, you may have a
young person with cancer in your classroom or school. You
may be concerned about the effects of this disease on the young
person and the ways you can help. Depending on your prior
experiences with cancer, you may be apprehensive about your own
ability to handle your student's illness. You may, understandably,
know little about cancer in the young and wonder what to do
or say.

This has been prepared to answer some of your questions and to indicate other sources of information and support. It
will help you contact others who are close to your student to facili-
tate the young person's continued education.

What follows are explanations of the disease, its treatment and
effects; suggested approaches for dealing with the young person,
classmates, and parents; guidelines for school reentry; and referral
to additional materials and organizations.

Much of this material is purposefully general. Medical explanations, for instance, are not detailed because there are many types
of cancer in the young, and wide variations in response to treatment for each individual. Approaches to your student will also
depend on the facilities and philosophy of the school, different
teaching styles, and preferences of the parents and student.

In any case, you will undoubtedly need more specific information on the student's situation. With parental permission, school
personnel can establish contact with caregivers who can further
explain the young person's medical condition and answer other
questions as they arise. Members of the health care team may
be available on a continuing basis to assist you with any other
concerns. Parents and, in some cases, the student can keep
you informed. Another important resource is the school nurse,
who can also act as a liaison.

Outlook

Today the young person with cancer stands a good chance of surviving the disease. Long-term survival rates for several childhood cancers are well in excess of 50 percent. Advances in all types of treatment, including surgery, radiation therapy (cobalt or X-ray) and chemotherapy (anticancer drug therapy), have produced dramatic increases in survival rates.

Despite the outcome of the disease, it is important to pay attention to the quality of the young person's life. Despite a serious illness, your student is still growing and developing and has the same educational and social needs as his peers.

Cancer in the Young and Its Treatment

Cancer is actually a group of diseases, each with its own name, its own treatment, and its own chances for control or cure. It occurs when abnormal cells begin to multiply and grow uncontrollably, crowding out the normal cells.

Leukemias (cancers of the blood-producing tissues), lymphomas (cancers of the lymphatic system, the network carrying fluid that bathes body cells and is important in the body's defense against disease), and brain tumors account for a large proportion of all cancers in young people. Solid tumors (e.g., bone) affecting other parts of the body such as arms or legs constitute most of the remainder of cancers occurring in young persons.

Early diagnosis is often difficult because many cancer symptoms mimic those of other illnesses. If cancer is suspected, many pediatricians or general practitioners refer the young person to a medical center which has teams of cancer specialists who confirm the diagnosis and design a specific treatment plan. If the family lives some distance from the center, the local physician often administers medicines and participates in care. Periodically the young person returns to the cancer center for reevaluation.

The goal of treatment is to remove or destroy the abnormal cells by surgery, radiation, or chemotherapy (anticancer drug therapy), or some combination of these methods. Initial treatment may be intense and then may become more moderate depending upon the young person's response. It may be necessary to continue some form of treatment for many years.

Remission and relapse (or recurrence) are terms used to describe different phases of the disease. A patient is in remission when no evidence of cancer is detectable. Relapse refers to the return of the disease after apparent improvement or a period of remission. Following relapse, the young person again undergoes treatment in an attempt to bring about remission. Although increasing numbers of young people are maintaining their initial remissions, others go through several cycles of remission and relapse. Some respond to treatment but do not attain a state of complete remission. Failure to control a relapse often results in progression of the disease and eventual death. However, if a complete remission continues for a number of years, the patient's doctor may begin to think of the young person as "cured."

Effects of the Disease and Treatment

Both the disease and treatment can produce physical changes in the patient such as nausea, vomiting, and fatigue, which decrease energy levels and the ability to participate in school activities. Other possible changes, which are usually temporary, include weight gain or loss, mood swings, facial fullness and distortion, problems with coordination, difficulties with fine and gross motor control, body marks resembling tattoos which identify sites of radiation therapy, and muscle weakness. Patients with solid tumors may have surgical changes, such as amputation or scars.

Hair loss occurs in many patients undergoing chemotherapy and is, perhaps, to them the most disturbing aspect of their treatment. The hair may fall out suddenly or over a period of weeks or months. It may grow back while the patient is still receiving therapy, but doesn't usually return to normal until after chemotherapy is completed. The young person will often wear a wig, hat, or scarf to hide the loss.

Any of these physical changes can result in teasing and rejection by peers and can create a reluctance to resume friendships and return to school.

Young people with cancer also must face emotional challenges. They fear relapse and the subsequent repetition of treatments. Emotional energy usually spent mastering basic developmental skills now is used to cope with the illness. For example, teenagers have difficulty attaining the independence so important to their development when the disease forces them to be dependent on parents and caregivers. In addition, the young person must learn to deal with others who treat them differently because of their disease; they may subsequently seem to withdraw, regress, or become belligerent.

School Reentry

Young people with cancer can benefit from attending school throughout their illness. They feel better if they are productive in the role of learner, gaining the satisfaction that academic achievement brings.

Frequent absences for medical reasons, overprotection and/or overindulgence by parents, limitations on physical activity, and social isolation tend to be common obstacles to regular school attendance. But these obstacles are not insurmountable. Successful reentry is possible given strong family reinforcement and positive support from educators and caregivers.

The Teacher

Planning for the student's return to class may cause you to address your feelings about life-threatening illness. You might find it helpful to share your concerns with a physician, social worker, or nurse from the student's treatment center. In your own school, assistance can be provided by the school nurse, counselor, or an educator who has taught young people with cancer or other chronic illnesses. These professionals may also be able to suggest classes to attend and helpful literature.

Still, no matter how prepared you are, having a student with cancer in the classroom can be emotionally demanding and time-consuming. There may be times when you feel unequal to the task or depressed about your student's situation. At these times, it may help to know that health professionals who work with young patients also are subject to these same emotions and rely on each other and outside sources for support.

Just as caregivers do, you should remind yourself that you're part of a team which includes parents, treatment center personnel, and other school staff members. Whether you are working through your own feelings, looking for advice, or sharing loss, support and guidance should be available from others on your team.

What to Find Out

When planning for the student's return, it is important to gather information about the young person's situation. You should contact parents and treatment center staff (if available) to find out:

☐ Specific type of cancer and how it is being treated;
☐ When treatment is administered, what potential side effects are, and effects on appearance and behavior;
☐ Approximate schedule of upcoming treatment, procedures, or tests that may result in the student's absence from the classroom;
☐ Limitations, if any, on the student's activities (Periodic updates from parents are also helpful.);
☐ What the student knows about the illness (Although current policy is to be honest with young people who have cancer, there are exceptions.);
☐ For younger students, what the family would like classmates and school staff members to know;
☐ For adolescents, whether the student wishes to talk directly with teachers about any of the above points.

Dealing With Parents

When talking with parents, usually a sympathetic but direct approach is best. Most parents want teachers to ask about their child and the disease and are willing to supply information. Also, remember that if they are angry or sad (even to the point of tears), these feelings are not necessarily caused by or directed to you.

If parents are depressed, hostile, or overly anxious, a united approach by school and health professionals can be reassuring. Treatment center psychologists and outreach professionals can suggest additional strategies appropriate to the situation.

What To Do

Once the information about the situation has been obtained, planning can proceed. If the treatment center is close, doctors, nurses, or social workers, along with school personnel and parents, can meet to prepare a joint plan. Even if including caregivers is not possible, a *consistent* plan or approach should be developed at a meeting of school personnel including:

☐ Designating one teacher, counselor, administrator, or school nurse as the liaison between the school, the student's family, and the treatment center. Whatever the choice, the liaison person should have the time and be willing to assume the responsibility for keeping *all* the young person's teachers and teachers of siblings informed.

This is especially important for junior and senior high school students, who come in daily contact with several teachers, all of whom should have accurate information on the student's condition. Another means of ensuring information dissemination is to arrange a meeting at the beginning of each semester between a member of the medical staff and all teachers of the junior or senior high school student. The family and student, of course, should give consent for the meeting and ideally can also be involved.

☐ Asking the principal and counselor to assist with special needs, such as transportation. Young people with cancer also may need places to rest, have snacks, or be by themselves for a while.

762

Students with cancer should be accepted as young people with a chronic disease who require periodic treatment. If the cancer is ignored, a major part of the young person's life is overlooked. On the other hand, if the cancer is an overwhelming concern, other important aspects of the young person's life may be neglected. Although some concessions may be necessary, a balance must be struck between what students can reasonably do and what they *must* do to maintain their self-image.

Like their peers, young people with cancer need love, support, and understanding. But they should not be overprotected; the same limits on behavior apply to students with cancer as to their classmates. Teachers should discipline and hold reasonable academic expectations for young patients. Doing less will rob them of pride in learning and accomplishment and will prevent camaraderie with their peers. Obvious special treatment will create resentment among classmates and can be devastating to the student with cancer. For example, assignment deadlines may need to be correlated with a student's treatment schedule. However, the completed work should be evaluated by the same criteria used for the rest of the class.

Teachers should also be alert to any new learning or behavioral problems (peer fighting, hostility, irritability), which should be brought to the attention of the person acting as liaison between the school, family, and treatment center.

It is also important for students with cancer to feel a part of their class, even if absences for medical reasons preclude full-time attendance. You should consider sending assignments to the young person at home or to the hospital; many medical centers have programs for students to continue schoolwork. Other approaches can be used, depending on the school and the situation, including attending school for part of the day or being tutored.

The Student in the Classroom

The parents of the young person with cancer and the student should be consulted before you discuss the illness with class members. Some school districts also require prior written permission from the parents of each class member. The content and manner of conducting discussions will vary according to students' ages, preferences of the parents and the student with cancer, and your wishes.

The following suggestions from educators who have taught

students with cancer may be useful:

☐ Begin by asking students in the class how they want to be treated when they are ill or how they feel when they are around someone (of any age) who is sick. Use answers to these questions as bases for discussing how classmates might treat their friend with cancer.

☐ Explain to classmates the type of cancer their friend has, the kind of treatment received, and the ways the disease and treatment may affect the student's appearance and/or behavior. This is particularly useful in dealing with embarrassing side effects such as temporary weight gain or hair loss. Classmates who know that these changes come about because of the lifesaving therapy their friend is receiving are less likely to tease and may even defend the student against the ill-considered remarks of outsiders. Also, reassure classmates that they can't "catch" cancer and emphasize that no one knows what causes it.

☐ Prepare a health or science unit for the study of cancer. Assign groups of class members to develop research reports on a specific type of cancer treatment and side effects, making sure that source material is up-to-date. When completed reports are shared with the class, students will have basic knowledge about cancer as well as their classmate's disease.

☐ Invite personnel from the treatment center or another organization (one teacher involved the social worker from the local American Cancer Society office) to make a presentation to the class. This approach should be a supplement, rather than substitute, for class discussion led by the teacher.

Classmates

Classmates are sure to have questions and be concerned about their friend at other times during the illness. Most young people with cancer prefer answering questions directly rather than having to deal with mute stares or turning away.

If teasing occurs, find out if classmates feel the student with cancer gets unfair attention, pampering, or special consideration beyond what is really necessary. Are they frightened and putting distance between themselves and the student as a defense? Are they normally aggressive? Through stories, discussion, and role playing, you can help teasers understand their own motives and discover more desirable ways of coping with the situation and the feelings which give rise to teasing.

Keeping in Touch

Prolonged, unexplained absences of the young person with cancer may be anxiety-provoking for other students. Encourage classmates to write to their friend and, if it is convenient for the parents and the student with cancer, a few classmates might plan a visit. Whatever the arrangements, it is vital for the young person with cancer to feel part of the class. In the words of one teacher:

> My student was present in my classroom only 36 days of the school year due to cancer and subsequent breakages of his leg. However, he was a class member *every* day. My students wrote him every other week. We sent Halloween candy, Christmas cards, Valentines, birthday cards and get-well cards. We visited him at home (as a class) which his parents wanted. It made his later return to school much easier. I encouraged telephone calls by students and refused to let the children forget him.

Other Medical Concerns

You may have other health-related concerns about the student with cancer. The most common are:

Activities. In general, young people with cancer should be encouraged to undertake all activities suited to their age. Most set a pace that is comfortable for them and do not have to be cautioned against overexertion. Do not assume what the patient can or cannot do. Through the school liaison, maintain contact with the parents and treatment center concerning special limitations.

Infections. No special precautions are necessary with the following three exceptions: shingles (herpes zoster), chickenpox, and regular measles. Actual or suspected exposures *must* be reported immediately to the parents and treatment center, because young people on chemotherapy are especially vulnerable to these diseases. It may be possible to take measures that will prevent serious complications if the exposure is reported immediately. Sibling exposure to these diseases *must* also be reported to the parents *without delay.*

Medical Crises. It is unusual for the young person with cancer to have a medical crisis in the classroom. Ask the parents or school or hospital liaison if there are any potential medical problems.

Treat minor medical problems (e.g., nausea, headaches) as you would for any other student. However, if these problems persist, they should receive medical attention.

Health Screening. The student with cancer is subject to the same health concerns and maladies of any other young person and requires routine health screening. For example, vision and hearing tests are necessary on a routine basis just as they are for other young people.

Communicability of Cancer. Cancer is not contagious. In this respect, consider your student as someone recovering from a broken bone rather than having a cold or the flu.

Special Concerns of Junior and Senior High School Students

In some ways, the experiences and needs of adolescents with cancer differ from those of younger students. These differences reflect the developmental issues facing adolescents (i.e., independence, peer acceptance, body image, and self-worth), as well as the mechanics of secondary as opposed to elementary schools.

Cancer often interferes with the adolescent's attempts to achieve independence from parents and other adults. The illness and treatment many involve limitation of activites and temporarily place the adolescent in the position of being cared for like a younger child. Since the parents fear losing the young person to cancer, they may tighten their control even more, leading to inevitable conflict. If you notice or suspect this situation with your student, counseling from the medical center or school can help open lines of communication. Once the dynamics of the situation are understood by parents, counselors can assist all concerned to allow the student more freedom of choice in school and home life.

At a time when peer pressure assumes vital importance, the adolescent with cancer is quickly classified as "different," both by the fact of the illness and by any visible manifestations of treatment, such as hair loss or weight gain. Also, certain types of cancer are more common among adolescents than young children, and treatment results in obvious body changes. For example, adolescents are more likely to develop a bone tumor requiring amputation and a lengthy rehabilitation process. Physical limitations can interfere with participation in sports and other school activities, creating a sense of isolation. Teasing or rejection by peers can result in varying degrees of withdrawal from extracurricular activities, or even from school. You can help by encouraging the young person's participation wherever possible in social activities that foster peer acceptance. If you are aware of problems with other students, you can intercede to try to resolve the conflict. Simple solutions will not always be readily apparent or even workable. If, for example, the student was a "loner" before diagnosis, encouraging acceptance by classmates becomes very difficult.

The size and complexity of junior and senior high schools also influence the student's ability to reenter school successfully. Secondary students must deal with many teachers, some of whom are new each quarter or semester and may have no information about the illness and treatment.

Teachers cannot easily inform all students in the school of the young person's illness. Although immediate classmates may be understanding and supportive, ridicule can come from students in other classes or grade levels.

Policies necessary to the operation of a large school can create problems for the young person if communication is poor and special arrangements are not made. For instance, rules against wearing hats in class may create embarassment for the student without hair, when a teacher who is unaware of the illness demands that the hat be removed. Schedule changes, necessary for medical care, can sometimes be difficult to arrange. Although physical education requirements may be waived completely, it is often difficult for faculty members to allow the student limited participation or alternatives to active involvement.

The larger classes and greater number of teachers may make it more difficult for the young person to maintain contact with the school during periods of extended absence. This can lead to a reluctance on the student's part to return to school when well again for fear of social awkwardness and difficulty in "catching up."

For students with motor problems (weakness, impaired coordination, or leg amputation), the size and structure of the school building may pose problems in arriving at classes on time.

Part of the solution to many of these problems is communication. As previously mentioned, one person in the school should be made responsible for contact with the student's medical staff and for disseminating information to all teachers involved with the student.

Ongoing contact between medical staff, faculty representative, and other faculty members is essential throughout the year, especially at the beginning of semesters and when the student's medical condition changes, e.g., when complications from treatment, relapse, or secondary illness occurs.

A single individual who has rapport with the young person should meet frequently with the student to discuss academic progress and social interaction. Other teachers should become aware that this individual is the "trouble shooter" to whom problems concerning the young person should be referred.

Terminal Illness

Despite improvements in survival rates, cancer in some patients cannot be controlled and is ultimately fatal. This raises the questions of how to manage the terminally ill student in the classroom during the later stages of the illness and how to respond to parents and classmates after death. Even in the final phase of illness, school can remain a rewarding experience for the young person. Often simple measures can help the student get the most from life remaining. For example, those who become too fatigued to attend school for a full day can often benefit from half-days or even an hour's attendance each day. As energy ebbs, assigned work should be adjusted accordingly. The young person who has lost a great deal of weight may be uncomfortable sitting in a wooden desk-chair, but may do quite well if allowed a pillow or two to sit on.

When a student dies, classmates may express their grief in a bewildering variety of ways. Some are quite open, while others may appear almost indifferent to the loss of their classmate. Such responses are a normal variation in the gamut of young people's grief reactions. They may assimilate the information about a death gradually, as they become able to deal with the event and its implications. Feelings of loss for the young person with cancer should be acknowledged, but no attempt should be made to force classmates to talk about the death or to deal with grief before they are ready. Most young people do so in their own way and at their own pace, if they are allowed but not forced or hurried.

Attending the memorial service or funeral of the student is another way of helping classmates understand the meaning of the death. For very young children, especially if they have not seen their sick friend for a long time, the service may help them realize that death is irreversible. In addition, it provides an opportunity for saying a last goodbye and for expressing sorrow for the loss of a friend. This is not to say that every friend or classmate should attend the service. The decision to do so rests with each individual and with each student's parents. No young person should be forced to go to the service.

As in the period of the student's illness, classmates are likely to have many questions after death. Again, most are best able to cope with this distressing event if they are given honest, simple, straightforward answers to their questions. Classmates may also want to create a memorial to their friend, such as a tree to be planted on the school grounds or some piece of equipment to be donated to the school. Organizing such a project and raising funds for it can be a valuable experience for classmates as well as provide the parents, brothers, and sisters of the young person with tangible and usually greatly appreciated evidence of the extent to which others share their feelings of loss.

Conclusion

Educators who have worked closely with young patients have found the experience rewarding and enriching. Working with the family and health care team, educators can maintain and improve the quality of life for the student. In turn, young people with cancer have much to teach those around them. Their sharpened sense of values and purpose is thought-provoking for peers and educators alike. The courage and strength they display while coping with the illness affirm the richness of life and learning.

Additional Information

Progress and developments in cancer in the young have been so rapid and information printed before the mid-1970's is often outdated and generally more pessimistic than current information. Local chapters of the American Cancer Society and the Leukemia Society of America have materials on pediatric cancers that are available free of charge. Additional sources of information include:

CANDLELIGHTERS FOUNDATION
2025 Eye Street, N.W., Suite 1011
Washington, D.C. 20006

A mutual support and self-help group of parents of children with cancer dedicated to improved communications, information, and treatment. Bibliographies of materials on death and dying are available free of charge for children and teachers of young people with cancer.

Cancer Information Service

The National Cancer Institute sponsors a toll-free Cancer Information Service (CSI), open 7 days a week to help you. by dialing

1-800-4-CANCER

(1-800-422-6237), you will be connected to a CIS office, where a trained staff member can answer your questions and listen to your concerns.

In Alaska, call 1-800-638-6070; in Hawaii, on Oahu call 524-1234 (on neighboring islands, call collect).

Spanish-speaking staff members are available to callers from the following areas (daytime hours only): California, Florida, Georgia, Illinois, northern New Jersey, New York, and Texas.

Selected Bibliography for Educators

Bernstein, Joanne E. *Books to Help Children Cope with Separation and Loss.* 2nd edition. New York: R.R. Bowker, 1983.

Chessler, Mark A. and Oscar A. Barbarin. "Parents' Perspectives on the School Experiences of Children with Cancer." *Topics in Early Childhood Special Education.* Vol. 54 (4), Winter 1986, pp. 36-48.

Greenlee, Karen M. *An Annotated Bibliography of Identifying and Meeting the Needs of the Student with Chronic Health Problems.* Arlington, VA: ERIC Document Retrieval Service, 1983.

Moffit, Karen. *Childhood Cancer: A Medical, Psychosocial and Educational Approach.* (Paper presented at the Council for Exceptional Children/Division for Early Childhood, National Early Childhood Conference on Children with Special Needs, Denver, CO, October 6-8, 1985). Arlington, VA: ERIC Document Retrieval Service, 1985.

Ott, Jeanne S., et al. "Childhood Cancer and Vulnerability for Significant Academic Underachievement." *Journal of Learning Disabilities.* Vol. 15 (6), June-July 1982, pp. 363-364.

Ross, Judith W. and Susan A. Scarvalone. "Facilitating the Pediatric Cancer Patient's Return to School." *Social Work*. Vol. 27 (3), May 1982, pp. 256-261.

Ross, Judith W. "Resolving Nonmedical Obstacles to Successful School Reentry for Children with Cancer." *Journal of School Health*. Vol. 54 (2), February 1984, pp. 84-86.

Schowalter, John E., et al. (editors). *"The Child and Death."* New York: Columbia University Press, 1983.

Wass, Hannelore and Charles Core (editors). *Helping Children Cope with Death: Guidelines and Resources*. 2nd edition. Washington, DC: Hemisphere, 1984.

Zwartjes, Georgia M., et al. "Students with Cancer." *Today's Education*. Vol. 70 (4), November-December 1981, pp. 18-23.

Selected Bibliography for Young People

The titles listed below include true-life as well as fictional stories and books. They are listed here because the are representative of available materials of potential interest to children with cancer. Your local library or bookstore should be able to get these books for you.

Books for Children

Fine, Judylaine. *Afraid to Ask: A Book about Cancer*. New York: Lothrop, Lee and Shepard, 1986. (Ages 10+).

Gravelle, Karen and Bertram A. John. *Teenagers Face to Face with Cancer*. New York: Julian Messner, 1986. (Ages 12+).

Howe, James. *The Hospital Book*. New York: Crown, 1981. (Ages 6 – 12).

Hyde, Margaret O. and Lawrence E. Hyde. *Cancer in the Young: A Sense of Hope*. Philadelphia: Westminster, 1985. (Ages 10 – 16).

Lancaster, Matthew. *Hang tough!*. New York: Paulist Press, 1983. (Ages 8 – 12).

Silverstein, Alvin and Virginia Silverstein. *Cancer*. New York: Harper and Row, 1977. (Ages 8+).

Simonides, Carol. *I'll Never Walk Alone*. New York: Continuum, 1983. (Ages 14+).

Swenson, Judy H. and Roxanne B. Kunz. *Cancer: The Whispered Word*. Minneapolis: Dillon, 1985. (Ages 7+).

Books for Friends

Beckman, Gunnell. *Admission to the Feast*. New York: Dell, 1973. (Ages 12+).

Bunting, Eve. *The Empty Window*. New York: Warne, 1980. (Ages 8 – 12).

Carter, Alden R. *Sheila's Dying*. New York: Putnam, 1987. (Ages 13+).

Strasser, Todd. *Friends Till the End*. New York: Delacorte, 1981. (Ages 12 – 16).

Slote, Alfred. *Hang Tough, Paul Mather*. New York: J. B. Lippincott, 1973. (Ages 12 – 14).

Stretton, Barbara. *You Never Lose*. New York: Knopf, 1982. (Ages 12 – 16).

On the Death of a Friend or Sibling

Bernstein, Joanne E. *Loss: And How to Cope with It*. New York: Clarion, 1981. (Ages 10+).

Clardy, Andrea. *Dusty Was My Friend: Coming to Terms with Loss*. New York: Human Sciences Press, 1984. (Ages 8 – 12).

Levy, Erin Linn. *Children Are Not Paper Dolls: A Visit with Bereaved Siblings*. Greeley, CO: Counseling Consultants, 1982. (Ages 8+).

Lawry, Lois. *A Summer to Die*. Boston: Houghton-Mifflin, 1977. (Ages 8 – 13).

Vogel, Ilse-Margaret. *My Twin Sister Erika*. New York: Harper and Row, 1976. (Ages 5+).

Acknowledgement

Special credit must go
to Linda Bartlett
who contributed her creative
talents.

Chapter 37

Advanced Cancer

Living Each Day

Introduction

Advanced cancer affects everyone whose life it touches—the patient, family, and friends. Dealing with the changes and the problems caused by a terminal disease and facing the future are difficult challenges.

This aims to help make living with advanced disease easier by providing practical information and by addressing questions that are often asked. It does not attempt to minimize the seriousness of having advanced cancer or deny its difficulty.

"Living Each Day" is based on the most current written information, and on interviews with advanced cancer patients and those close to them. Throughout the booklet, several messages and suggestions are stressed:

- Try to live each day as fully and normally as possible.

- Many of your concerns can be eased with medical skill, emotional support, knowledge, faith, and love.

- A decision to make the most of the time available can help you help yourself live with advanced cancer.

It is possible to live with a sense of purpose and the hope that good relationships will continue, that family, friends, and caregivers will be available to provide the support you need, and that each day will offer its measure of happiness.

Not everyone will want all the information in this chapter, nor will all find it suited to their needs. Perhaps parts of it will spark a new thought, relieve anxiety, or help solve certain problems for you. Even at this difficult time, there are many things that can be done to help you and your loved ones.

Living With Advanced Cancer

Few people like to think about dying. We all know that death will come, but most of us spend little time thinking about it. Many of us think of dying as something that happens to other people, believing that we will live on and on.

While this belief may be comforting, it is no longer useful when you have weeks or months—not years—to live. Approaching death often requires changing how we look at life and what we value. You will need time to think about death and adapt to its approach.

One patient with advanced cancer expressed his philosophy about dying this way:

The death rate for any generation is 100 percent. We all die. However, I know what will probably kill me, while most people don't. We have no guarantee of how long we will live. But I believe it is truly the quality of life, not the quantity, that is most important.

There are no right or wrong ways to face the end of life. You need to do what is right for you. Many people with a terminal illness have been able to find peace of mind by coming to terms with their emotions and beliefs about their lives, and about dying. You may be able to do this too, in your own way and at your own pace.

How Others Have Coped With Advanced Cancer

There are probably as many ways to cope with advanced cancer as there are people trying to do so. Each of us is unique, and we each find our own way to live and to die. Still, we have many feelings in common and may approach the knowledge that our time is limited in similar ways.

Many people find it easier to concentrate on the present, and do not focus on the distant future. They think of the future as the end of each day, and live one day at a time. As one patient explained,

Before this happened I had a 5 year plan, a 10 year plan, even a 20 year plan. No more . . . what I realized was that I could only die in the future, but I was alive right now and I would always be alive in the here and now.

Others find it more helpful to plan ahead—within limits—days, a month, 6 months, possibly a year. They find that it reaffirms, to themselves and to others, that there are still things they want to do. Their plans may be general, such as enjoying family and social relationships and talking about their thoughts and feelings, or specific, such as reading a certain book, or finishing some needlepoint.

Some view having cancer as a challenge to be met or a battle to be fought. They think of each day they survive as a victory. One woman expressed her outlook this way:

> *I get satisfaction by being engaged in the fight. It's me and my doctors against cancer, and we know we might not win in the end; but by God, we're going to give it a run for its money.*

Others cope by rethinking what is important in their life and what is not. "Disease rearranges your values, and you cast off things. You reduce the trivia to a minimum, you simplify life. . . ."

Still others may not be able to accept the seriousness of the situation. They may deny the fact that they are dying until their final moments.

Many people are emotionally overwhelmed when they first learn their diagnosis. With time, their reactions may change to acceptance and a desire to do as much as possible in the time that remains.

Others, instead of accepting, lose their ability to cope and their will to live. This does not have to happen. You can choose the way you wish to face each day. Even if you are very ill, you may still have physical and emotional reserves. Deciding to call on these reserves can help revive your spirits and your will to live.

We are all born with the will to live. Exactly what influence this force has in curing disease—especially cancer—has long been debated, but there is little argument that a strong desire to live can enhance the quality of life. Those who are determined to live fight harder and sometimes seem to do better.

There are many people with advanced cancer who have lived far longer than expected. A positive attitude about the value of life, along with a combination of hope, endurance, willpower, and courage, are common characteristics of such people. When asked to explain how they have managed, these people often give answers such as "I'm needed too much at work" or "I can't die until my grandchild is born" or "I need to help my daughter." They do not seem to want to give up or retreat from living. A keen interest in daily events appears to keep them from giving up.

Others have approached illness and dying from a different point of view. They believe that life is so precious, under any conditions, that they simply will not let it go. This intense need to go on may be present with or without the help of family, friends, concerned caregivers, or effective treatment. It may even exist without any apparent sources of encouragement. These people seem to generate their own hope and keep going through sheer willpower.

This does not mean that a positive mental attitude will necessarily lengthen your life. Neither does it mean that you are inadequate if you are sick and not getting better. But trying to emphasize the positive aspects of your life can add meaning, purpose, and comfort to the time remaining.

What You Can Do

Accepting responsibility is one way to help yourself. By actively participating in daily activities with your family and friends and in your care, you say "I care about myself."

Set goals for yourself that are realistic so you do not become discouraged. Find out what caregivers, friends, and family are doing for you and what you can do to help yourself. Let them know what you need; this may include their presence, concern, and honesty.

You can also accept responsibility for your frame of mind. Set the tone for those around you. As one patient said, "You have to do this because no one knows how you want to be treated, and they may be waiting for a cue. No one else will talk about it unless you do. . . ."

Your caregivers may recommend a regular exercise program (even if you are in bed most of the time), medications to be taken at certain times, and nutritious food. These measures or others prescribed for you may, at times, seem unimportant in the face of declining health, but they will help you to keep your strength and your independence for as long as possible. Working with your caregivers and family can help you maintain a sense of control, purpose, and hope. Encouraging honest and open communication will help you to live the way you want to, and it will let others know how you want to be treated.

Living with serious illness can be very discouraging. You will have good times and bad times too, and your ability to deal with these changes may vary. In the morning you may feel down, but by the afternoon you may feel much better. On one day you may have little energy, but on another your mood and spirit may rebound. During a bad time, try to remember the good moments and remind yourself that there can be more good times ahead.

Sharing Your Thoughts

Many people with cancer have found it easier to live with their problems by sharing them with someone. The weight of your problems may be lightened just by talking them over with family members or a close friend. They may even think of a way of dealing with a problem that has not occurred to you.

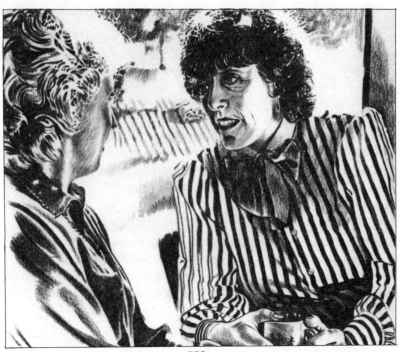

779

You may find this kind of sharing difficult, and sometimes it may also be hard for family members or friends. If this is the case, you might want to talk to a member of your medical team or with someone who is professionally trained in counseling, such as a nurse, social worker, psychologist, a member of the clergy, or other community and hospital caregivers. Many people have found support by attending self-help groups where people meet to share common concerns. They say sharing and learning from each other gives them strength and reassurance.

Sometimes people prefer to work through their feelings alone, but it often helps to share. The emotions and thoughts that go along with advanced cancer are understandable and expected, and it is not necessary to hide them. Letting your feelings out can be a great release.

If You're Alone

It may be very hard to keep up your spirits and be positive if you live alone. Loneliness is not easy to deal with at any time and may be especially difficult during illness. Many people have found this time less lonely with the help of an adopted family, friends, a volunteer, or a member of the clergy.

If you need to rely on yourself for encouragement, try to cheer yourself on. It may be very hard to do, but it's far from impossible. There are people who have learned to cope by thinking positively, helping others, and remaining as active as possible. Focusing on small pleasures—a delicious meal, a good book, a beautiful sunrise—has helped many people.

Intimacy

Advanced cancer affects all aspects of life including sexuality. You may find yourself unable or unwilling to express yourself sexually as you did before because of physical changes and emotional concerns. This does not mean, however, you must deny sexual needs and desires. There are many ways to show love and to find satisfaction.

Open, honest communication is the key. Being willing to reexamine your attitudes about intimacy will help you and your partner maintain the closeness, warmth, and sense of belonging generated in a loving relationship. Physical satisfaction can be sought in a variety of ways and may or may not include intercourse. Touching, kissing, stroking, and holding can also bring great comfort and pleasure.

Sexual problems may stem from feelings about your medical condition or treatment, rather than the condition or treatment itself. With patience and communication between partners, many of these problems can be solved. An understanding that intimacy may not be the same as it was before can prevent unrealistic expectations and relieve some of the self-consciousness you or your partner may be feeling.

Don't be afraid to seek help or advice. Ask—you are entitled to all the information you need or want. You may wish to seek counseling, and your doctor, nurse, social worker, or patient representative in the hospital may be able to guide you to a professional in this area. The library has many books on sexuality and you may find some of them helpful.

Living Each Day

Choose small goals and constructive ways to use your time, instead of dwelling on your illness. Sometimes, asking yourself "What do I cherish?" or "What is important to me right now?" can help you focus on meaningful goals. Try thinking of the needs of your family and others close to you. You may enjoy looking through and arranging family albums, scrapbooks, or hobby collections. Pets still need to be cared for and plants watered.

Some people keep a daily journal of their feelings and experiences. You may want to try this, to share with someone close to you now, or to leave them as a remembrance. Try directing your energy into living each day as it comes, and make each day count for what you can put into it.

The will to live is a part of each one of us. Some people think of it as a small flame that we carry within ourselves. For many, it is a source of strength that can make it possible to look forward with hope to each day.

Common Concerns

Some say it is not death we fear, but the days, weeks, or months that precede it. Many of us are afraid there will be pain during this time, and we wonder if we will become a burden. We may think about the unknown, about isolation and abandonment, and that life will be over before we are ready.

Family and friends can help you to work out concerns and control fear—by listening when you want to talk and by being honest and sensitive to your feelings. But they may have fears, too. They need to know about your disease, what they can and cannot do for you, and what to expect.

Knowledge and understanding may help you gain perspective on these concerns. If there is something you want to know from a member of your health care team, ask. Let your doctors, nurses, and others know what information you want and need. It is your right to receive answers, even to the most direct questions about your prognosis.

It may be a good idea to include those close to you in talks with your doctor. Talking directly to your caregivers may ease your family's and friends' concerns, give them a clearer understanding of how they can help you, and help them feel less helpless in a difficult situation. The value of honest communications for all those involved cannot be stressed too much.

Facing the Unknown

Many people with advanced cancer wonder what experiences they will miss in life, what the moment of death will be like, and what their fate will be after death. They wonder, too, what will become of their family and friends, and how these people and others will react to their death.

It may help you to talk about these thoughts with a person you feel comfortable with. While some questions can be answered—immediately or in time—others have no answer. A definite answer to practical, spiritual, and religious issues may not be possible, but discussing them—with a friend, partner, member of the clergy, or caregiver—may help you to explore these questions and feel less alone with them.

Dealing With Loneliness and Isolation

As cancer progresses, it disrupts the activities that have made up your daily routine. This can lead to feelings of loneliness and isolation. Sometimes this happens even if you are surrounded by family and friends because they can't share your experience.

One way to minimize these feelings is to try to live as normally as possible. Keep close at hand the things you have always enjoyed—photos, art, magazines, music. Surround yourself with familiar things. Even in the hospital you can wear your own clothes, have your own blanket and pillows, and keep mementos and pictures nearby. You may want to keep up with local or national news, or watch a favorite television program with a friend.

Don't be afraid to call and ask friends and relatives to visit. They may not have contacted you because they don't know what to say or how to act, or are not sure you want visitors. If you do, let them know. At first, you may wish to suggest specific activities—reading aloud, playing cards, watching television—until you and your visitor feel comfortable with each other again.

Despite all your efforts, you may still feel lonely and isolated or feel that your family and friends cannot understand your problems. Some days you may just want to be left alone, and that is okay too. On other days, talking to others with cancer might provide the understanding and companionship you need. You may wish to join a support group for cancer patients. Some of these are listed in the resource section at the back of this booklet. The American Cancer Society, a local hospice, your doctor, a social worker, a visiting nurse, or a member of the clergy may also be able to put you in touch with another person or group that would be right for you.

Maintaining Self-Respect

It can be very hard for you to accept that your body is no longer as strong and reliable as it once was. As cancer progresses, your appearance may change and you may not be as independent as you once were. This may affect your self-respect. If this happens, remember that the qualities that make you a good friend, a loving parent, or a caring mate are still there. One woman with advanced cancer had this to say:

*It shouldn't take a fatal diagnosis to . . . find self-aware-
ness, self-concern and self-love. . . . But I'm afraid for
most of us it does. I think I've straightened myself out in
these areas. In fact, I've discovered . . . that I'm a stronger
person than I might have anticipated. I am just a bit gut-
sier than I thought and I'm delighted to know that.*

Even if you are bedridden, you can exercise a degree of independence and initiative. You can maintain control in little
ways—setting up a schedule for getting up, shaving, bathing,
and resting. (If you can't do these things for yourself, you can
let others know when you would like to have help.) Decide for
yourself which television programs to watch, which books to
read or have read to you, and how long to exercise.

Whether at home or in the hospital, let those caring for you
know which foods you prefer, whether you are comfortable, and
if there is something you need.

Many people with advanced cancer are not bedridden. You
may be able to do things you used to, but in a more limited way.
Conserve your strength for those activities you really want to
pursue.

Ultimately you will have to let others care for you. Dependence on others is natural when you are not as strong as you
once were.

The Grieving Process

Sadness and grief come with the unavoidable losses that occur
with advanced cancer and are not unusual reactions. Fortunately, the losses are usually gradual. You may be able to accept the losses and your feelings about them a little more each
day.

Dealing with a particular source of sorrow and working
through the emotions surrounding it may help you set it aside.
Grief about the people and things you must eventually give up
does not have to be denied or hidden, but try to balance it with
activities and relationships that have meaning for you and bring
you happiness.

Managing Pain

Many people with advanced cancer are afraid they will experience physical pain. However, some cancer patients, even those
with advanced cancer, do not have any pain at all, or very little.

If pain reaches the point where it disturbs you, it needs to be treated. It can almost always be minimized and often managed so that it does not recur.

The combination of appropriate pain relief methods, the opportunity to make personal and spiritual peace, and someone willing to listen and offer comfort and advice are probably the most potent pain relievers known.

There are many medicines that can be used alone or in combination to relieve your discomfort. Physical therapy and biofeedback, relaxation techniques, and self-hypnosis may also help. Caregivers may be able to help you with these therapies, and you may want to see what the local library has to offer. The librarian can help you or a family member locate books and records on these topics. The level of pain, your willingness to help manage your pain, and the cooperation of caregivers and family will determine which method is best for you.

Your doctor may prescribe narcotics (pain-relieving drugs) for you. When used under proper medical supervision, the chance of addiction to narcotics is small. Most people can stop taking these drugs or decrease the amount of medication taken if their pain can be controlled by other means. If narcotics are the only way to relieve pain, your comfort is more important than the possibility of addiction. If you and your doctor decide narcotics are a proper choice for you, use them as directed.

A booklet on handling pain, *Questions and Answers About Pain Control*, is available from the American Cancer Society. Contact your local ACS office listed in the telephone directory to obtain a copy.

Emotions and Pain

People with advanced cancer may be sad, depressed, angry, scared, or all of these. These are normal reactions when you are very ill and realize you probably won't live as long as you had expected. When your emotions become overwhelming they can make your pain seem more intense. Talking about your feelings may help give you, family, and caregivers guidance about what you need. It can also help to relieve sadness and depression, and may reduce pain. Writing about your emotions in a diary may help too. Occasionally you may feel like kicking or punching a pillow, or screaming and crying. Go ahead and do it.

Personal and spiritual problems may be troubling you as well. These can contribute to pain. You may want to bring up unresolved conflicts that have developed over the years between you and a friend or family member. Approached with kindness and openness, old hurts can possibly be put to rest. At the least, some level of understanding can be established between the two of you along with happier, more peaceful feelings.

Your family or caregivers can arrange for a priest, rabbi, minister, hospital chaplain, or other appropriate person to visit with you. Many people find comfort in expressing and trying to resolve personal spiritual issues.

A Theory About Dying

Each of us must face death and accept it in our own way, answering questions as best we can about the meaning of life, love, suffering, and struggle. We can hope to find some measure of peace, and acceptance of the coming of death. Unfortunately, the journey toward these goals is not easy or steady. And sometimes, it is not possible for us to reach all our goals.

The emotions that many people with advanced disease experience have been examined by trained professionals. One whose theories have become well-known to the public is Dr. Elisabeth Kübler-Ross. You may have heard about the feelings she believes dying people experience. Her work has provided guidance and comfort for many patients and their families, but it is important to remember that her theory is only one perspective on dying.

You may not experience all of the emotions that are discussed here. They are presented to reassure you and those close to you that your reactions are not unusual, but a part of the way we try to make peace with ourselves.

When patients are first told or realize they are dying, they often react with disbelief. It is a common way to cope with an overwhelming situation and can be helpful at first. Eventually, however, you must face reality, and in time many do. One patient explained it this way:

The reality of death does not go away by denying it. When you do this you can miss the comfort you get from sharing fears and concerns and missing the sense of well-being you get knowing you have taken care of your loved ones.

This feeling of "No, not me!" often changes to "Why me?" You may feel angry, resentful, even enraged. These strong emotions need to be expressed if they are to be relieved. This can be a very difficult time for you and those around you. It will help everyone to understand that your anger is not meant for those close to you but for the situation.

People may make all kinds of promises to God or to themselves with the hope of a longer life: "If I can live one more year, I'll go to church every day" or "If I can just live to see my son married, I won't ask for more." It is not unusual at all to do this.

At times you may feel depressed, because you have lost your independence, or because your savings were spent on medical care. You can help yourself at this time by valuing what you have, rather than dwelling on what you cannot change.

As you move closer to death, depression over losses that have already occurred may give way to grief over the friends, family, and life you are going to lose. This grieving should not be discouraged—it must be worked through in order to say a peaceful goodbye.

During this time it will help not to be alone, though you may find yourself gradually needing fewer people around you—perhaps just those you feel especially close to. It may help your family and friends to understand that this type of withdrawal often occurs toward the end of life and it is not due to something they have done or should feel badly about. Conversation may not be necessary, just the reassurance that someone is there for you who cares. Reassurance can be communicated by the presence of another, by holding someone's hand, by a gentle touch.

Not all people facing death are able to find peace and acceptance. However, with time and help you may be able to come to the feeling that you have accepted what must be. At this time you need reassurance, more than ever, that you will not be left alone and all that can be done for your peace and comfort will continue to be done.

The People in Your Life

Family and close friends are a primary source of emotional support for people with advanced cancer. One young woman says, "My husband and friends who love me are like a circle . . . they form a protective shield around me. I don't know what I'd do without them."

Those who are close to you need understanding and consideration as much as you do. Your expectations about what they can and should do for you should be tempered with knowledge about their feelings, abilities, and limitations. They may need time, just as you do, to adjust to your illness, and any feelings of confusion, shock, or anger they may have. Letting them know that you want them close and that you need their support will help them with their own emotions.

How Children React

Children who have a parent with advanced cancer are almost always aware of a great change in their daily lives. Even preschool children sense when something is wrong. They may be frightened by this change or become angry at you for being ill. Others, especially younger children, worry that they might have caused your illness.

Because of these possible reactions it is best to be honest and encourage communication. Try to let your children know that they are allowed to ask questions, and that you will answer them as honestly and thoroughly as you can. Tell your children as much as you think they can understand. Keep in mind that many people tend to underestimate how much children do understand.

You may want to try telling them a little at a time. A partner or relative may be able to help—together you can watch for clues that the children have absorbed as much information as they can at that time.

Children need to know that they are still loved and important, and that they will continue to be cared for. A favorite relative or friend can help by devoting time and attention to a child who needs comforting, affection, and guidance. Perhaps this person can offer to help with homework or attend important school events if you cannot.

Taking the time to listen to a child's triumphs, problems, and fears is important. This holds true for adolescents as well as for younger children. Teenagers are sometimes expected to assume responsibilities that are beyond their maturity. If you can avoid imposing too much responsibility on them, while maintaining a sense that they are important family members and still entitled to their independence, you may be able to keep their problems to a minimum.

If this kind of support is not enough, professional counseling may be necessary. Your doctor, social workers, other community and hospital caregivers, and state or community mental health departments can guide you to a counselor who is right for you and your children.

Partners

Communication is a two-way street between you and your partner. Being honest about the emotions both of you are feeling can help you draw support from each other. Endearments, hugs, and kisses can also bring a sense of comfort and togetherness.

Be realistic about demands on your partner who is, undoubtedly, having a hard time too, and may be feeling guilty about your illness and any time spent away from you. Communication is especially important if you and your partner have been separated by hospitalization for prolonged periods of time. Sometimes in the absence of their partners, patients begin to draw more support and relate more personally to members of their health care team. This pattern of relating may be difficult for partners to adjust to if they no longer feel needed.

Partners need time to meet their own needs, along with those of other family members. If these needs are neglected, your partner will have less energy, cheer, and support to give. Another family member or friend can sit with you for short periods of time while your partner attends to other details of daily life—a shower, a walk, phone calls to friends, or business matters.

The time away will replenish both of you, and give you the opportunity to visit with others. Remember, you didn't spend 24 hours a day with your spouse before your illness. You still have many of the same emotional and personal needs that you did before your illness and may need some time apart. It is better to try to maintain your relationship as it was before, as much as possible. If you are in the hospital, your doctor and nurses can provide support during the time your partner may be away.

Your partner may not be your only or primary source of emotional support. Sometimes it is a mother or father, brother or sister, or best friend. It may be one of your adult children.

These people have feelings, too, and other responsibilities. Keep demands as realistic as possible and try to keep communication flowing. Express your emotions and let them express theirs if they wish. Well-deserved praise, a hug, kiss, or hand squeeze are not out of place and can provide warmth, good feeling, and renewed energy.

Options for Care

Hospitals and machines that sustain life have become such an accepted part of illness that we sometimes forget there are other places and ways to live with advanced disease and approaching death. Many patients are most comfortable in the hospital, where they feel assured of the care and comfort they need. Others want to remain, or return home, and this kind of care can be arranged with the cooperation of the patient, family, and professional caregivers. Still others may have a hospice organization in their area and may wish to avail themselves of this kind of care. You may want to think about the choices available, and what would be best for you.

The Hospice Concept of Care

Hospices provide specialized care for dying patients and their families. In hospices the primary concern is quality of life, not prolonging life. They stress controlling pain and other symptoms so the patient can remain as alert and as comfortable as possible. Emotional, social, and spiritual health and followup care for the family are important too.

Hospices offer both inpatient and home care. There are freestanding hospices, hospices within a hospital or skilled nursing facility, or at-home care arrangements.

In 1978, the National Hospice Organization (NHO) was established to promote and maintain quality hospice care and to encourage support for patients and family members. For information about NHO or about hospice concepts and practices, contact the National Hospice Organization, 1901 North Fort Meyer Drive, Arlington, VA 22209, (703) 243-5900.

Making Treatment Decisions

Family, friends, and caregivers may find it hard to accept, but the time may come when continuing to live is no longer a patient's top priority. A patient may opt for experimental drugs and methods, or decide to end treatment. This point may be reached when standard therapy is no longer effective, when the quality of life is no longer acceptable to that person, or at some other time.

Refusing Treatment

It is your right to refuse further treatment. If you make this decision, treatment will be given only to relieve pain and other symptoms and to keep you as comfortable as possible. If your condition stabilizes, therapy can always be started again. Your doctors will, almost certainly, have recommendations, information, and advice to give you about this course of action, but they cannot act against your wishes.

Many religious groups have issued statements about the decision to end treatment. Most do not oppose such a decision. If you want to know more, ask your priest, rabbi, minister, or other counselor.

Patient's Rights

You have other rights, too. You are entitled to be given complete information about your illness and your prognosis and to withhold that information from others if you wish. You should also be informed about any procedures and treatments that are planned, and how much they will cost.

The American Hospital Association has prepared "A Patient's Bill of Rights." You can get this document from a library, hospital, or directly from the American Hospital Association, 840 North Lakeshore Drive, Chicago, IL 60611, (312) 280-6000.

The Living Will

A Living Will is a legal document that states you do not wish to be kept alive by artificial means or heroic measures. It is a recognized statement of your right to forego treatment and has been upheld in court.

If you sign a Living Will, tell everyone close to you and give them copies. Your health care team and lawyer should also be informed and given copies. This is to ensure that your wishes will be carried out.

You can obtain a copy of the Living Will, in the form preferred by your state, from Concern For Dying (CFD), 250 West 57th Street, New York, NY 10017, (212) 246-6962. Signing a Living Will will not, according to CFD, adversely affect any life insurance policy and will not be interpreted as suicide.

CFD recommends appointing someone who can make binding decisions for you about medical care in the event you can no longer do so (power of attorney). Name a person who knows your views about specific treatments and any religious considerations that need to be taken into account.

Practical Concerns

Careful planning can help to minimize the financial, legal, and emotional difficulties your family and friends may face after your death. However difficult it may be, discussing practical matters now can eliminate many problems. Advice from professional counselors and advisors—lawyers, members of the clergy, funeral directors, insurance company representatives—can help you make decisions that fulfill your requests and help those close to you.

You can help your family and loved ones by gathering copies of records, documents, and instructions they will need. A large envelope can be used to store copies of your important papers. Only photocopies should be placed in the envelope. Originals should be stored in a fireproof place such as a safety deposit box. Be sure to tell one or more people where you keep the envelope. If you cannot gather all these items, list where they can be found. You can use the following form as a guide for collecting your personal records.

Personal Inventory

Name_____ Date_____

Address_____

Date of Birth_____ Place of Birth_____

Social Security Number_____

Next of Kin: Name_____

                Address_____

Employer

Address_____

Company Benefits_____

Personal Papers

Item: (Veterans' discharge papers, birth certificate, Living Will) Location:

_____

_____

_____

Insurance

Life: Company (Name and Address)

_____Policy Number _____

Health and Accident: Company

_____Policy Number _____

Automobile: Company

_____Policy Number _____

Other: Company

_____Policy Number _____

Banking Papers

Kind of Account	Bank Name/Address	Account Number
_____	_____	_____
_____	_____	_____
_____	_____	_____

Other Accounts

Type	Where	Account Number
Safety Deposit Box	_____	_____
_____	_____	_____

Automobiles (Make, Model, Year)

_____

_____

Real Estate Papers

_____

_____

Personal Items of Value

_____

_____

_____

_____

Counselors Who Can Help With My Affairs

Attorney _____

Banker _____

Insurance Agent _____

Doctor _____

Clergy _____

Other (Broker, Business Associate, Accountant) _____

_____

Funeral Arrangements

_____

_____

_____

_____

Special Requests

_____

_____

Resources

American Cancer Society
90 Park Avenue
New York, NY 10017
(212) 736-3030

A voluntary organization offering a variety of patient services, also involved in cancer education and research. The ACS sponsors:

I Can Cope—addresses the educational and psychological needs of people with cancer.

CanSurmount— "team approach" composed of patient, family member, trained volunteer (also a cancer patient), and health professional. On physician referral, a trained CanSurmount volunteer meets with the patient and family in the hospital and home.

Cancer Care, Inc. and the National Cancer Care Foundation, Inc.
1180 Avenue of the Americas
New York, NY 10036
(212) 221-3300

A voluntary social service agency providing professional counseling and planning to advanced cancer patients and their families.

Leukemia Society of America, Inc.
733 Third Avenue
New York, NY 10017
(212) 573-8484

Supplemental financial assistance and consultation services are offered to cancer patients with leukemia and related disorders.

Make Today Count
P.O. Box 222
Osage Beach, MO 65065
(314) 348-1619

The goal of this organization is to help patients with incurable diseases and their families cope with illness and improve their quality of life.

The Candlelighters Childhood Cancer Foundation
Suite 1011
2025 I Street, N.W.
Washington, DC 20006
(202) 659-5136

A voluntary organization that provides practical information and psychological support for parents of children with cancer.

General References

Kelly, Orville. *Make Today Count,* and *Until Tomorrow Comes,* available from Make Today Count, P.O. Box 222, Osage Beach, MO 65065. These books relate how Orville Kelly reacted to his diagnosis of cancer and his goal to "live each day as fully and completely as possible." His philosophy is to promote honest and open communication between patients, family, and caregivers.

Morra, Marion, and Potts, Eve. *Choices. Realistic Alternatives in Cancer Treatment,* New York, NY; Avon Books; 1987. A comprehensive guide for cancer patients and their families. Sections on different kinds of cancer treatment options including experimental and unproven treatments, coping with pain, questions to ask caregivers, and where to get help.

Rosenbaum, Ernest, M.D. *Living With Cancer,* St. Louis, MO; C.V. Mosby Co.; 1982. Focuses on individual cancer patients and how they have coped with their illnesses. Many first-person accounts of their emotions and thoughts.

Rosenbaum, Ernest, M.D., et al. *A Comprehensive Guide for Cancer Patients and Their Families,* Palo Alto, CA; Bull Publishing Co.; 1980. A thorough discussion of the questions and problems faced by cancer patients and their families.

Nutrition Information

American Cancer Society. *Nutrition for Patients Receiving Chemotherapy and Radiation Treatment,* available from local units. Describes the importance of maintaining nutritional intake while receiving chemotherapy and radiation and how these treatments affect caloric needs.

Office of Cancer Communications. *Eating Hints—Recipes and Tips for Better Nutrition During Cancer Treatment,* National Cancer Institute, Building 31, Room 10A24, Bethesda, MD 20892. Includes recipes designed to help you increase protein and caloric intake and suggested ways to stimulate your appetite.

Rosenbaum, Ernest H., M.D., et al. *Nutrition for the Cancer Patient,* Palo Alto, CA; Bull Publishing Co.; 1980. Practical advice about how to maintain weight, and why it's so important for the person with cancer.

Children and Death

Grollman, Earl. *Explaining Death to Children,* Boston; Beacon Press; 1965. No matter how young, children sense the impact of serious illness. This book offers a practical approach for explaining death and dying to them.

Le Shan, Eda. *Learning to Say Goodbye, When a Parent Dies,* New York; Macmillan Publishing Co., Inc.; 1976. Designed to help children through a difficult time.

Moving Toward Death

Duda, Deborah. *A Guide to Dying at Home,* Santa Fe, NM; John Muir Publications; 1982. Practical considerations for seriously ill patients who want to remain at or return home.

Kubler-Ross, Elisabeth. *On Death and Dying.* New York, NY; Macmillan Publishing Co., Inc.; 1969. Discusses the emotions that many dying people experience.

Hospice

Hamilton, Michael, and Reid, Helen, editors. *A Hospice Handbook*, Grand Rapids, MI; Eerdmans Publishing Co.; 1980. A guide designed to help the patient and family evaluate if hospice care is an option for them.

Stoddard, Sandol. *The Hospice Movement—A Better Way of Caring for the Dying*, New York, NY; Random House; 1978. Discusses the history and philosophy of the hospice movement and the kind of care the hospice has to offer.

PART IV—
A STATISTICAL OVERVIEW

Chapter 38

Cancer Rates and Cancer Risks

U.S. and International Statistics by Types of Cancer

Cancer Rates

Cancer Death Rates in 20 Countries

All Sites

Cancer occurs throughout the world; no country, no population is free of it. Cancer does not, however, occur with the same frequency in all countries; there are wide variations in total cancer death rates from country to country. There are also wide variations among different countries in the death rates for specific cancers. The bar graphs that follow show some of these variations.

The cancer death rates that are displayed in these 10 graphs were derived from the number of cancer deaths per 100,000 population in each country for the years 1971-1977. The 20 countries were chosen because all have major populations with good, nationwide reporting systems, and each of the countries reports to the World Health Organization. To make meaningful comparisons between countries, the rates were all age-adjusted to a standard age distribution. Cancer deaths occur most often in older age groups, but not all countries have the same age proportions. Age-adjusting corrects for these differences.

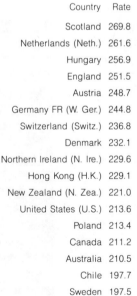
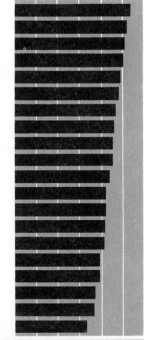

Country	Rate
Scotland	269.8
Netherlands (Neth.)	261.6
Hungary	256.9
England	251.5
Austria	248.7
Germany FR (W. Ger.)	244.8
Switzerland (Switz.)	236.8
Denmark	232.1
Northern Ireland (N. Ire.)	229.6
Hong Kong (H.K.)	229.1
New Zealand (N. Zea.)	221.0
United States (U.S.)	213.6
Poland	213.4
Canada	211.2
Australia	210.5
Chile	197.7
Sweden	197.5
Norway	188.0
Japan	186.7
Israel	170.5

Male

0 50 100 150 200 250 300

Death rates per 100,000 population for all cancers in 20 countries, 1976–77, age-adjusted to U.S. standard 1970 population.
From: World Health Statistics Annual 1979–80 as adapted by American Cancer Society 1983.

Cancer death rates indicate only the number of persons who die from cancer in a given year; they do not necessarily coincide with the incidence of new cases of cancer in that year. But tumor registries are needed to monitor cancer incidence, and not all countries have them. Most countries do have systems for reporting vital statistics. Cancer death rates thus provide a way to make international comparisons. (The U.S. cancer death rates in these charts are for all races.) The first graph shows death rates for all cancers, by sex, among the 20 countries. The nine graphs following show death rates for specific cancers.

Country	Rate	Female
Denmark	170.9	
Scotland	165.8	
Hungary	163.6	
England	156.0	
Austria	155.3	
W. Ger.	154.8	
Chile	153.8	
N. Zea.	150.7	
N. Ire.	150.4	
Neth.	142.6	
Israel	141.3	
Sweden	140.9	
U.S.	136.3	
Canada	135.3	
Switz.	134.2	
Norway	131.2	
Australia	129.2	
Poland	126.4	
H.K.	125.3	
Japan	108.7	

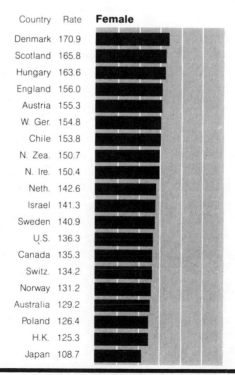

0   50 100 150 200 250 300

Cancer Death Rates in 20 Countries
Breast

Female breast cancer is rare in much of Asia, but it has been the most common cause of cancer death in North America and most of Europe. In the United States, lung cancer is overtaking breast cancer as the most common cause of cancer death among women. Breast cancer is very rare in men.

The highest breast cancer death rates have been found among Caucasian women in Hawaii and in British Columbia, both with death rates greater than 80 per 100,000 population. Among the countries listed below, the highest death rate is seen in Denmark, followed by Great Britain. The lowest are seen in Hong Kong and Japan. Low death rates also prevail in Africa. The breast cancer death rates for Chinese and Japanese women in the United States are three times higher than in Singapore or Japan, but not so high as the death rates among whites in the United States. The breast cancer death rate among U.S. black women is lower than among white women, but is increasing.

Death rates per 100,000 population for female breast cancer in 20 countries, 1976–77, age-adjusted to U.S. standard 1970 population.
From: World Health Statistics Annual 1979–80 as adapted by American Cancer Society 1983.

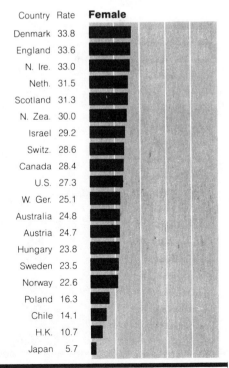

Country	Rate	Female
Denmark	33.8	
England	33.6	
N. Ire.	33.0	
Neth.	31.5	
Scotland	31.3	
N. Zea.	30.0	
Israel	29.2	
Switz.	28.6	
Canada	28.4	
U.S.	27.3	
W. Ger.	25.1	
Australia	24.8	
Austria	24.7	
Hungary	23.8	
Sweden	23.5	
Norway	22.6	
Poland	16.3	
Chile	14.1	
H.K.	10.7	
Japan	5.7	

0   20   40   60   80   100

Cancer Death Rates in 20 Countries
Colon and Rectum

Risk factors, incidence, and death rates vary for cancers of the colon and the rectum, but the two are often considered together, as colorectal cancers. They are considered diseases of economically developed countries: death rates are highest in western Europe, North America, and New Zealand, and lowest in Asia, Africa, and most Latin American countries. In this country, deaths from colorectal cancers rank second only to lung cancers in the total number of deaths, but death rates vary widely by geographic area in this country. Death rates are highest, for example, in Northeast urban areas and lowest in the South and Southwest.

Death rates per 100,000 population for colorectal cancer in 20 countries, 1976–77, age-adjusted to U.S. standard 1970 population.
From: World Health Statistics Annual 1979–80 as adapted by American Cancer Society 1983.

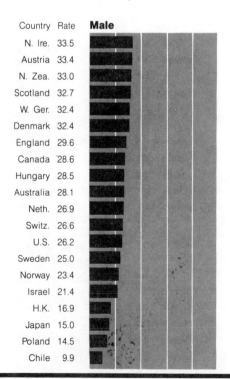

Country	Rate	Male
N. Ire.	33.5	
Austria	33.4	
N. Zea.	33.0	
Scotland	32.7	
W. Ger.	32.4	
Denmark	32.4	
England	29.6	
Canada	28.6	
Hungary	28.5	
Australia	28.1	
Neth.	26.9	
Switz.	26.6	
U.S.	26.2	
Sweden	25.0	
Norway	23.4	
Israel	21.4	
H.K.	16.9	
Japan	15.0	
Poland	14.5	
Chile	9.9	

0   20   40   60   80   100

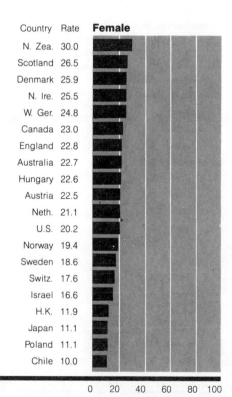

Country	Rate	Female
N. Zea.	30.0	
Scotland	26.5	
Denmark	25.9	
N. Ire.	25.5	
W. Ger.	24.8	
Canada	23.0	
England	22.8	
Australia	22.7	
Hungary	22.6	
Austria	22.5	
Neth.	21.1	
U.S.	20.2	
Norway	19.4	
Sweden	18.6	
Switz.	17.6	
Israel	16.6	
H.K.	11.9	
Japan	11.1	
Poland	11.1	
Chile	10.0	

0   20   40   60   80   100

Cancer Death Rates
in 20 Countries
Esophagus

Cancer of the esophagus is characterized by wider variations in incidence and death rates than any other cancer. There are geographical "pockets" of very high death rates in parts of the Soviet Union, Iran, China, and France. In some of these pockets the male-female ratios are very high. Among the countries listed below, male death rates are highest in Hong Kong and Chile, and lowest in Israel. Relatively high death rates from esophageal cancer are also seen among women in Hong Kong and Chile. In the United States, the male death rate from esophageal cancer is 1.6 times higher than for women. A pocket has been found in this country among black men in Washington, D.C., who have a death rate of 28.6 per 100,000.

Death rates per 100,000 population for esophageal cancer in 20 countries, 1976–77, age-adjusted to U.S. standard 1970 population.
From: World Health Statistics Annual 1979–80 as adapted by American Cancer Society 1983.

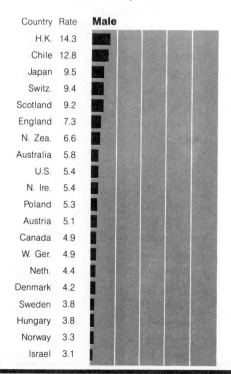

Country	Rate	Male
H.K.	14.3	
Chile	12.8	
Japan	9.5	
Switz.	9.4	
Scotland	9.2	
England	7.3	
N. Zea.	6.6	
Australia	5.8	
U.S.	5.4	
N. Ire.	5.4	
Poland	5.3	
Austria	5.1	
Canada	4.9	
W. Ger.	4.9	
Neth.	4.4	
Denmark	4.2	
Sweden	3.8	
Hungary	3.8	
Norway	3.3	
Israel	3.1	

0 20 40 60 80 100

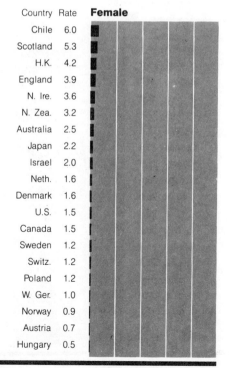

Country	Rate	Female
Chile	6.0	
Scotland	5.3	
H.K.	4.2	
England	3.9	
N. Ire.	3.6	
N. Zea.	3.2	
Australia	2.5	
Japan	2.2	
Israel	2.0	
Neth.	1.6	
Denmark	1.6	
U.S.	1.5	
Canada	1.5	
Sweden	1.2	
Switz.	1.2	
Poland	1.2	
W. Ger.	1.0	
Norway	0.9	
Austria	0.7	
Hungary	0.5	

0 20 40 60 80 100

Cancer Death Rates in 20 Countries

Larynx

Death rates from cancer of the larynx, or "voicebox," vary widely throughout the world. The highest death rates in the world are found among men in Sao Paulo, Brazil (14.1) and in parts of Spain (13.6). In the United States, the highest laryngeal cancer death rate is now

found among black men in the San Francisco Bay area. Historically, laryngeal cancer has been a male disease. In the table below, for example, the highest male death rate, among Hungarian men, is 10 times greater than the highest female death rate, and the lowest male death rate, in Sweden, is 2 times greater. There are indications, though, that death rates from laryngeal cancer are now rising in women.

Death rates per 100,000 population for cancer of the larynx in 20 countries, 1976–77, age-adjusted to U.S. standard 1970 population.
From: *World Health Statistics Annual 1979–80* as adapted by American Cancer Society 1983.

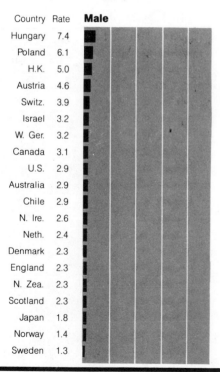

Country	Rate	Male
Hungary	7.4	
Poland	6.1	
H.K.	5.0	
Austria	4.6	
Switz.	3.9	
Israel	3.2	
W. Ger.	3.2	
Canada	3.1	
U.S.	2.9	
Australia	2.9	
Chile	2.9	
N. Ire.	2.6	
Neth.	2.4	
Denmark	2.3	
England	2.3	
N. Zea.	2.3	
Scotland	2.3	
Japan	1.8	
Norway	1.4	
Sweden	1.3	

0 20 40 60 80 100

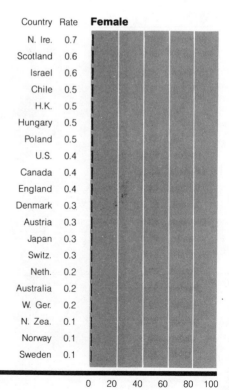

Country	Rate	Female
N. Ire.	0.7	
Scotland	0.6	
Israel	0.6	
Chile	0.5	
H.K.	0.5	
Hungary	0.5	
Poland	0.5	
U.S.	0.4	
Canada	0.4	
England	0.4	
Denmark	0.3	
Austria	0.3	
Japan	0.3	
Switz.	0.3	
Neth.	0.2	
Australia	0.2	
W. Ger.	0.2	
N. Zea.	0.1	
Norway	0.1	
Sweden	0.1	

0 20 40 60 80 100

Cancer Death Rates in 20 Countries

Lung

Lung cancer is a major cause of death in most Western countries, particularly, as this graph shows, among men. (Cancers of the lung, bronchus, and trachea are grouped together in the World Health Organization reporting system.) In the United States, lung cancer is the leading cause of cancer death among men and is expected, in 1984 or 198, to outstrip breast cancer as the leading cause of cancer death among women (Horm and Asire, 1982). Lung cancer is one of the three most common cancers in men throughout the world, and probably outranks stomach cancer as the most common cancer in men (Fraumeni and Blot, 1982). Men in Scotland have the highest lung cancer death rate in the world, followed by men in the Netherlands, England, Wales and Northern Ireland. The lung cancer death rates are relatively low in Chile and in other Latin American countries. They are also low in China, India, and most African countries.

Death rates per 100,000 population for lung cancer in 20 countries, 1976–77, age-adjusted to U.S. standard 1970 population.

From: World Health Statistics Annual 1979–80 as adapted by American Cancer Society 1983.

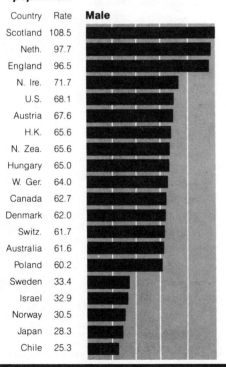

Country	Rate	**Male**
Scotland	108.5	
Neth.	97.7	
England	96.5	
N. Ire.	71.7	
U.S.	68.1	
Austria	67.6	
H.K.	65.6	
N. Zea.	65.6	
Hungary	65.0	
W. Ger.	64.0	
Canada	62.7	
Denmark	62.0	
Switz.	61.7	
Australia	61.6	
Poland	60.2	
Sweden	33.4	
Israel	32.9	
Norway	30.5	
Japan	28.3	
Chile	25.3	

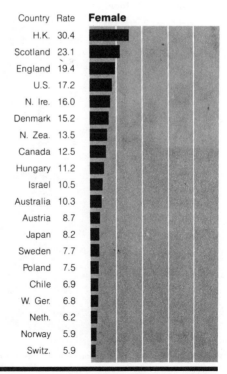

Country	Rate	**Female**
H.K.	30.4	
Scotland	23.1	
England	19.4	
U.S.	17.2	
N. Ire.	16.0	
Denmark	15.2	
N. Zea.	13.5	
Canada	12.5	
Hungary	11.2	
Israel	10.5	
Australia	10.3	
Austria	8.7	
Japan	8.2	
Sweden	7.7	
Poland	7.5	
Chile	6.9	
W. Ger.	6.8	
Neth.	6.2	
Norway	5.9	
Switz.	5.9	

0   20   40   60   80   100   0   20   40   60   80   100

Cancer Death Rates in 20 Countries
Oral Cavity

Cancers of the oral cavity generally refer to cancers located in the mouth and throat. The highest death rates in the world–three times higher than death rates found anywhere else–are found among both men and women in Hong Kong. In all other countries, the death rate among men is three or more times higher than for women. The high death rates from oral cancers in Hong Kong are chiefly due to cancers of the nasopharynx, a cancer that is rare among North Americans and Europeans. High death rates from nasopharyngeal cancers have also been found in parts of China. Death rates from oral cancers are lowest in Japan and in the Netherlands.

Death rates per 100,000 population for oral cancer in 20 countries, 1976–77, age-adjusted to U.S. standard 1970 population.
From: World Health Statistics Annual 1979–80 as adapted by American Cancer Society 1983.

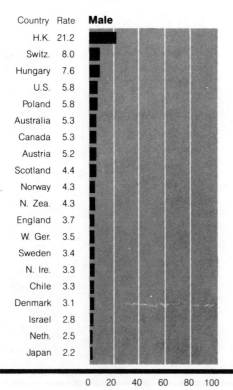

Country	Rate	Male
H.K.	21.2	
Switz.	8.0	
Hungary	7.6	
U.S.	5.8	
Poland	5.8	
Australia	5.3	
Canada	5.3	
Austria	5.2	
Scotland	4.4	
Norway	4.3	
N. Zea.	4.3	
England	3.7	
W. Ger.	3.5	
Sweden	3.4	
N. Ire.	3.3	
Chile	3.3	
Denmark	3.1	
Israel	2.8	
Neth.	2.5	
Japan	2.2	

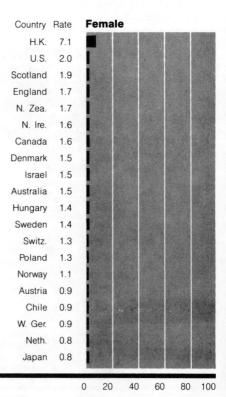

Country	Rate	Female
H.K.	7.1	
U.S.	2.0	
Scotland	1.9	
England	1.7	
N. Zea.	1.7	
N. Ire.	1.6	
Canada	1.6	
Denmark	1.5	
Israel	1.5	
Australia	1.5	
Hungary	1.4	
Sweden	1.4	
Switz.	1.3	
Poland	1.3	
Norway	1.1	
Austria	0.9	
Chile	0.9	
W. Ger.	0.9	
Neth.	0.8	
Japan	0.8	

0   20   40   60   80   100   0   20   40   60   80   100

Cancer Death Rates in 20 Countries

Prostate

Cancer of the prostate is one of the most common cancers among men. Of the 20 countries listed below, the highest death rates from this cancer are seen among northwest European men: Swedes, Norwegians, Swiss, East Germans, Hungarians, and Dutch in the Netherlands. In the United States, cancer of the prostate is the second most common cause of cancer death among men. This cancer is rare in east Asia: the death rate among Japanese men is 3.6 per 100,000 a year, and the death rate of 2.9 in Hong Kong is the lowest in the world.

Death rates per 100,000 population for cancer of the prostate in 20 countries, 1976–77, age-adjusted to U.S. standard 1970 population.
From: World Health Statistics Annual 1979–80 as adapted by American Cancer Society 1983.

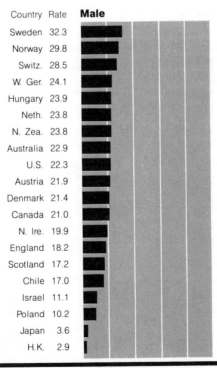

Country	Rate	**Male**
Sweden	32.3	
Norway	29.8	
Switz.	28.5	
W. Ger.	24.1	
Hungary	23.9	
Neth.	23.8	
N. Zea.	23.8	
Australia	22.9	
U.S.	22.3	
Austria	21.9	
Denmark	21.4	
Canada	21.0	
N. Ire.	19.9	
England	18.2	
Scotland	17.2	
Chile	17.0	
Israel	11.1	
Poland	10.2	
Japan	3.6	
H.K.	2.9	

0   20   40   60   80   100

Cancer Death Rates in 20 Countries

Stomach

The Japanese have the highest death rates in the world for stomach cancer: 70.2 deaths per 100,000 population for men and 34.9 for women. Stomach cancer causes more deaths among the Japanese than all other types of cancer combined. Americans, in contrast, have stomach cancer death rates among the lowest in the world. The death rates for this cancer are relatively high for both men and women in Chile, Hungary, Austria, Germany, and Poland. They are significantly lower, for both sexes, in Israel, Canada, and Australia. The U.S. death rates from stomach cancer were high until the 1930s; they have since been declining steadily.

Death rates per 100,000 population for stomach cancer in 20 countries, 1976–77, age-adjusted to U.S. standard 1970 population.
From: World Health Statistics Annual 1979–80 as adapted by American Cancer Society 1983.

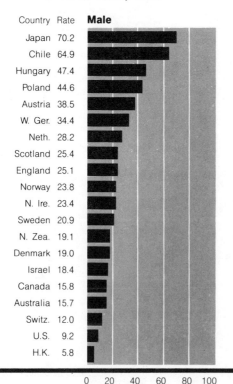

Country	Rate	**Male**
Japan	70.2	
Chile	64.9	
Hungary	47.4	
Poland	44.6	
Austria	38.5	
W. Ger.	34.4	
Neth.	28.2	
Scotland	25.4	
England	25.1	
Norway	23.8	
N. Ire.	23.4	
Sweden	20.9	
N. Zea.	19.1	
Denmark	19.0	
Israel	18.4	
Canada	15.8	
Australia	15.7	
Switz.	12.0	
U.S.	9.2	
H.K.	5.8	

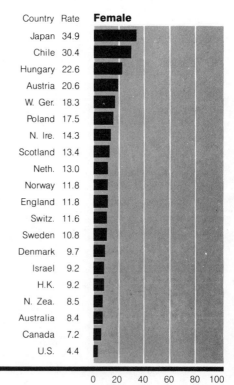

Country	Rate	**Female**
Japan	34.9	
Chile	30.4	
Hungary	22.6	
Austria	20.6	
W. Ger.	18.3	
Poland	17.5	
N. Ire.	14.3	
Scotland	13.4	
Neth.	13.0	
Norway	11.8	
England	11.8	
Switz.	11.6	
Sweden	10.8	
Denmark	9.7	
Israel	9.2	
H.K.	9.2	
N. Zea.	8.5	
Australia	8.4	
Canada	7.2	
U.S.	4.4	

Cancer Death Rates in 20 Countries

Uterus

Cancers of the uterine cervix and of the uterine corpus, or endometrium, differ in type, cause, and risk factors. Some countries, however, do not distinguish between the two in their reporting, thus limiting the usefulness of international comparisons. Both types are included in the chart above. Among the countries represented, Chilean women have the highest death rate for the two cancers combined, and Israeli women the lowest. Death rates for these two cancers are relatively low in the United States. Both the incidence and death rate for cervical cancer have been decreasing in the past several decades in the United States and in some other Western countries, but rising in others.

Death rates per 100,000 population for cancer of the uterus in 20 countries, 1976–77, age-adjusted to U.S. standard 1970 population.
From: World Health Statistics Annual 1979–80 as adapted by American Cancer Society 1983.

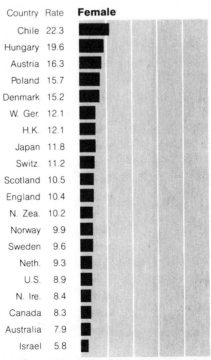

Country	Rate	Female
Chile	22.3	
Hungary	19.6	
Austria	16.3	
Poland	15.7	
Denmark	15.2	
W. Ger.	12.1	
H.K.	12.1	
Japan	11.8	
Switz.	11.2	
Scotland	10.5	
England	10.4	
N. Zea.	10.2	
Norway	9.9	
Sweden	9.6	
Neth.	9.3	
U.S.	8.9	
N. Ire.	8.4	
Canada	8.3	
Australia	7.9	
Israel	5.8	

0   20   40   60   80   100

Cancer Incidence

International Range of Cancer Incidence

Although cancer occurs in every country in the world, there are wide geographic variations in incidence. Among men, for example, lip cancer occurs at a rate of 22.8 cases per 100,000 population in Newfoundland and 0.1 cases per 100,000 in Osaka, for a high-low ratio of 228.

The incidence of cancer of the prostate is highest among black men living in Alameda County, California, and lowest among men in Shanghai. The high-low ratio is 125.3. Stomach cancer occurs at a rate of 100.2 cases per 100,000 among Japanese men in Nagasaki and 5.7 cases per 100,000 among U.S. white men in Atlanta, for a high-low ratio of 17.6.

Both the world's highest and lowest incidence rates of lung cancer in men are found in the United States: the highest incidence rate- 107.2 cases per 100,000 is found among black men in New Orleans and the lowest--8.1 per 100,000--is found among American Indians living in New Mexico. This latter group has the world's highest incidence rate of gallbladder cancer.7 cases per 100,000 compared with 0.5 cases per 100,000 among men in Bombay.

Among women, the greatest worldwide variation in incidence is found for cancer of the nasopharynx. It occurs at a rate of 0.1 cases per 100,000 population in Trent, England, and at a rate 144 times greater, 14.4 cases per 100,000, among women in Hong Kong. The highest incidence rate of breast cancer in the world, 87.5 cases per 100,000, is found among Hawaiian women and the lowest rate, 8.9 cases per 100,000, is found among Japanese women in Osaka. The high-low ratio is 9.8.

Cancer of the uterine corpus, or endometrium, occurs at a rate of 38.5 cases per 100,000 among white women in Alameda County, California, and at a rate of 1.0 cases per 100,000 among rural Japanese women in Fukuoka, a 38.5-fold difference.

The world's highest incidence of melanoma is found in New South Wales, Australia. It occurs there at a rate of 19.1 cases per 100,000 among women and 17.2 cases per 100,000 among men. The lowest incidence of this cancer is found among Japanese men and women in Osaka.

By comparing the worldwide incidence of cancer among men and women, it can be seen that cancer is generally less common among women. The table also shows that the United States has the highest incidence rates in the world of a number of cancers: breast and bladder cancers among women, prostate and kidney cancers among men, and cancers of the colon, pancreas, and gallbladder and myeloid leukemias in both sexes. The U.S. incidence rates for stomach cancer among men, lung cancer among American Indian men, and cancer of the esophagus among women are the lowest in the world.

The charts on the following two pages are based on data obtained by the International Agency for Research on Cancer (IARC), a part of the World Health Organization. IARC was formed in 1965 to collect and evaluate international data on cancer and to identify potential risk factors through epidemiologic and laboratory studies.

International range of incidence for selected sites of cancer around 1976 by sex.

Males

Site	High Population	Rate	Low Population	Rate	Ratio H/L
Lip	Canada, Newfoundland	22.8	Japan, Osaka	0.1	228.0
Tongue	India, Bombay	10.2	Romania, County Cluj	0.5	20.4
Mouth	France, Bas Rhin, Urban	13.0	Japan, Miyagi	0.5	26.0
Oropharynx	France, Bas Rhin, Urban	13.4	Norway	0.3	44.7
Nasopharynx	Hong Kong	32.9	Japan, Miyagi	0.3	109.7
Hypopharynx	France, Bas Rhin, Rural	11.0	Israel, All Jews	0.2	55.0
Esophagus	Shanghai	24.7	Hungary, Szabolcs, Rural	1.1	22.5
Stomach	Japan, Nagasaki	100.2	U.S., Atlanta, White	5.7	17.6
Colon	U.S., Connecticut	32.3	India, Poona	3.1	10.4
Rectum	Canada, N.W. Territory & Yukon	22.6	Israel, Non-Jews	3.1	7.3
Liver	Hong Kong	34.4	Australia, New South Wales, Rural	0.6	57.3
Gallbladder	U.S., New Mexico, Amerindian	7.7	India, Bombay	0.5	15.4
Pancreas	U.S., Bay Area, Black	18.3	India, Bombay	2.0	9.2
Larynx	Italy, Varese	16.0	U.K., North Scotland	1.8	8.9
Lung & Bronchus	U.S., New Orleans, Black	107.2	U.S., New Mexico, Amerindian	8.1	13.2
Melanoma	Australia, New South Wales, Urban	17.2	Japan, Osaka	0.2	86.0
Prostate	U.S., Alameda, Black	100.2	Shanghai	0.8	125.3
Testis	Switzerland, Vaud, Rural	10.5	Cuba	0.3	35.0
Penis	Jamaica, Kingston	5.7	U.S., Los Angeles, White	0.2	28.5
Bladder	Switzerland, Geneva	30.2	India, Poona	2.4	12.6
Kidney, etc.	U.S., Hawaii, White	11.2	India, Bombay	1.3	8.6
Brain	Australia, South	8.2	Japan, Miyagi	0.9	9.1
Thyroid gland	U.S., Hawaii, Chinese	7.8	India, Poona	0.4	19.5
Lymphosarcoma	Switzerland, Geneva	8.5	Poland, Warsaw, Rural	1.2	7.1
Hodgkin's disease	Switzerland, Vaud, Urban	4.9	Japan, Miyagi	0.5	9.8
Multiple myeloma	U.S., Bay Area, Black	8.4	India, Poona	0.6	14.0
Lymphatic leukemia	Switzerland, Neuchatel	7.9	Japan, Fukuoka, Urban	0.5	15.8
Myeloid leukemia	U.S., Hawaii, Hawaiian	8.7	Romania, County Cluj	0.7	12.4

*Age-standardized to the Standard World Population (Waterhouse et al, 1982).

International range of incidence for selected sites of cancer around 1976 by sex.

	High		**Low**		**Ratio**
			Females		
Site	**Population**	**Rate**	**Population**	**Rate**	**H/L**
Lip	Romania, County Cluj	2.3	U.K., Birmingham	0.1	23.0
Tongue	India, Bombay	4.1	Czechoslovakia, W. Slovakia	0.2	20.5
Mouth	India, Bombay	5.8	Yugoslavia, Slovenia	0.2	29.0
Oropharynx	U.S., Hawaii, White	2.7	Japan, Osaka	0.1	27.0
Nasopharynx	Hong Kong	14.4	Trent, U.K.	0.1	144.0
Hypopharynx	India, Bombay	2.2	Canada, British Columbia	0.1	22.0
Esophagus	India, Bombay	10.7	U.S., Utah	0.4	26.8
Stomach	Japan, Nagasaki	51.0	Israel, Non-Jews	2.4	21.3
Colon	U.S., Bay Area, Japanese	27.4	India, Poona	2.8	9.8
Rectum	Switzerland, Neuchatel	13.4	Israel, Non-Jews	1.5	8.9
Liver	Shanghai	9.1	Norway, Rural	0.4	22.8
Gallbladder	U.S., New Mexico, Amerindian	22.2	India, Bombay	0.7	31.7
Pancreas	U.S., New Mexico, Amerindian	10.4	India, Bombay	0.9	11.6
Larynx	India, Bombay	2.6	Norway	0.2	13.0
Lung & Bronchus	New Zealand, Maori	48.8	Spain, Navarra	2.6	18.8
Melanoma	Australia, New South Wales, Rural	19.1	Japan, Osaka	0.2	95.5
Breast	U.S., Hawaii, Hawaiian	87.5	Japan, Osaka, Rural	8.9	9.8
Cervix uteri	Colombia, Cali	52.9	Israel, Non-Jews	2.1	25.2
Corpus uteri	U.S., Alameda, White	38.5	Japan, Fukuoka, Rural	1.0	38.5
Ovary	Israel, Jews born in Europe & America	17.2	Japan, Osaka, Rural	2.1	8.2
Bladder	U.S., New Orleans, White	6.5	Hungary, Szabolcs, Rural	0.5	13.0
Kidney, etc.	Canada, N.W. Territory & Yukon	15.3	India, Poona	0.6	25.5
Brain	Poland, Warsaw City U.S., Hawaii	6.6	Japan, Miyagi, Rural	0.6	11.0
Thyroid gland	Hawaiian	17.6	Poland, Warsaw, Rural	0.7	25.1
Lymphosarcoma	U.S., Hawaii, Hawaiian	6.3	Poland, Katowice	0.5	12.6
Hodgkin's disease	Switzerland, Vaud, Rural	4.3	Japan, Osaka	0.3	14.3
Multiple myeloma	U.S., Hawaii, Hawaiian	5.9	Poland, Katowice	0.4	14.8
Lymphatic leukemia	U.S., New Mexico, Other White	3.3	Japan, Fukuoka	0.4	8.3
Myeloid leukemia	New Zealand, Maori	5.4	Hungary, Szabolcs	0.8	6.8

*Age-standardized to the Standard World Population (Waterhouse et al, 1982).

U.S. Cancer Incidence
Age-Specific, All Sites, by Age and Race

Cancer is chiefly a disease of middle and old age, rare in children and young adults. More than half of all cases of cancer are diagnosed after age 65. Up to age 50, the incidence of cancer is higher in women. After age 60, there is a dramatic increase in cancer incidence among men.

Average annual age-specific cancer incidence per 100,000 U.S. population, all sites combined, by race and sex, 1973–77.
From: SEER.

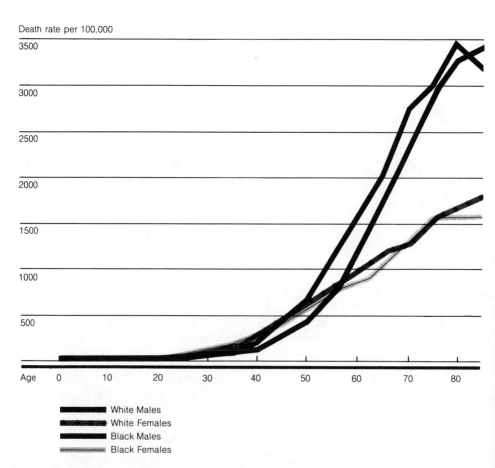

Death rate per 100,000

Age 0 10 20 30 40 50 60 70 80

White Males
White Females
Black Males
Black Females

U.S. Cancer Incidence

By Age Group for All Races and Both Sexes

Data in this chart are set up on a logarithmic scale to display percentage changes in cancer incidence in five different age groups; the log scale yields a truer picture of time changes than do arithmetic scales. The greatest changes in incidence in the years covered were among adults aged 65 to 74. Lesser increases are seen in adults aged 45 to 64, while incidence has remained stable for ages 15 to 44. Incidence has decreased for children under age 14 (the 1975 dip for this age group may be due to changes in the population surveyed by SEER).

Incidence of cancer per 100,000 U.S. population, all sites combined, all races and both sexes, by age group, 1973–79.
From: SEER.

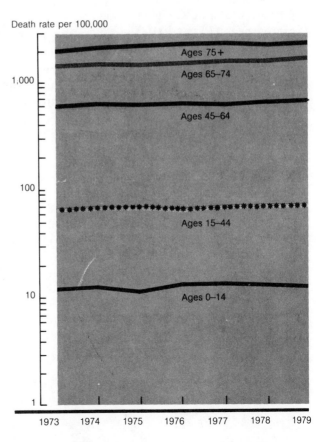

819

U.S. Cancer Incidence
10 Most Common Cancers by Sex Among Whites, Blacks, and Hispanics, 1973-77

Cancer of the lung is the most common type of cancer among black and white men with an incidence of 110 cases per 100,000 population among blacks and 76 per 100,000 among whites. Hispanic men are at less risk for this cancer.

Cancer of the prostate is the most common cancer among Hispanic men with an incidence approaching 59 cases per 100,000. Among black men, the incidence of cancer of the prostate is almost as high as lung cancer, near 110 per 100,000. Colorectal cancers are the third most common cancers among both black and white men, and the fourth among Hispanic men.

Stomach cancer is the third most common cancer among Hispanic men, the fourth among black men, and the seventh among white men. White men are at far greater risk for bladder cancer than either black or Hispanic men.

Breast cancer is the most common cancer among women of all three groups. It occurs most frequently among white women, with an incidence of 85 per 100,000 population, compared with 75 per 100,000 in black women and 48 per 100,000 in Hispanic women. Colorectal cancers are the second most common among all three groups of women.

Cancer of the uterine corpus is the third most frequent cancer among white women; cervical cancer is third among black and Hispanic women. Lung cancer is fourth among all three groups of women.

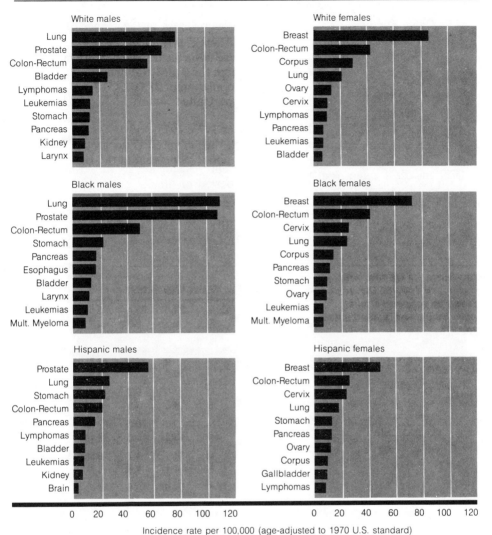

Incidence rate per 100,000 (age-adjusted to 1970 U.S. standard)

Incidence per 100,000 U.S. population of 10 most common cancers among whites, blacks, and Hispanics, by sex, 1973–77, age-adjusted to 1970.
From: SEER.

U.S. Cancer Incidence

Changing Patterns by Site Among Whites and Blacks, Men and Women

The incidence of cancers by site for men and women, white and black, for five different time periods appear in these two charts. The data for 1969 and 1971 came from the Third National Cancer Survey, covering a population of 21,003,451 from nine

major areas in the United States.

The data for 1973, 1975, and 1977 came from SEER, which then covered Il geographic areas representing about 10 percent of the U.S. population. The populations are not strictly comparable, but they can be used to give an idea of changes in cancer incidence, by site, over a period of time.

Incidence for whites, both sexes, per 100,000 U.S. population by year and site, all ages combined, age-adjusted to 1970.
Data for 1969 and 1971 from TNCS. Data for 1973–1977 from SEER.

Cancer Site	Sex	Incidence per 100,000				
		1969	1971	1973	1975	1977
Bladder	M	23.8	23.4	25.5	25.8	26.3
	F	6.3	6.3	6.1	6.9	7.2
Breast	F	73.9	75.1	81.0	86.2	82.7
Colon	M	34.5	32.4	34.2	35.5	38.5
	F	30.6	28.6	29.7	30.6	32.1
Kidney	M	9.0	8.2	9.4	9.0	9.4
	F	4.3	3.8	4.4	4.0	4.6
Lung	M	70.6	70.0	72.3	76.4	79.4
	F	13.3	15.5	17.7	21.8	24.5
Melanoma	M	4.4	4.7	5.8	6.4	7.6
	F	4.1	4.8	5.1	6.0	6.7
Ovary	F	14.9	13.6	14.2	14.2	13.7
Pancreas	M	12.1	12.3	12.7	12.5	11.6
	F	7.5	7.0	7.5	7.2	7.5
Prostate	M	59.0	56.7	61.0	64.8	70.4
Rectum	M	17.5	18.1	18.8	18.3	19.1
	F	11.1	10.6	11.3	12.0	11.2
Stomach	M	15.4	13.4	13.8	12.7	11.6
	F	7.1	6.3	6.1	5.4	5.2
Total Leukemia	M	13.2	12.2	13.2	12.5	11.7
	F	8.0	7.2	7.8	7.3	7.6
Uterine Cervix	F	16.0	14.3	12.6	10.7	9.5
Uterine Corpus	F	22.6	24.6	29.0	32.4	28.5

- Melanoma incidence has almost doubled for white men and women.

- Breast cancer incidence has increased sharply among women of both races but is more frequent among white women.

- The incidence of cancer of the uterine cervix has decreased markedly among black and white women but its incidence remains more than two times higher in black women.

- Cancer of the uterine corpus, or endometrial cancer, has increased in incidence among women of both races. Its incidence is markedly higher among white women.

Incidence for blacks, both sexes, per 100,000 U.S. population by year and site, all ages combined, age-adjusted to 1970.
Data for 1969 and 1971 from TNCS. Data for 1973–1977 from SEER.

| Cancer Site | Sex | Incidence per 100,000 | | | | |
		1969	1971	1973	1975	1977
Bladder	M	13.2	9.9	10.6	13.0	16.4
	F	4.2	5.0	3.8	5.2	5.5
Breast	F	62.1	54.9	66.9	75.9	71.5
Colon	M	29.0	26.0	31.9	31.8	42.9
	F	28.1	29.0	29.5	32.4	29.8
Kidney	M	7.4	7.2	8.7	8.1	9.4
	F	3.8	4.0	4.4	4.0	4.5
Lung	M	78.6	102.8	108.4	107.4	112.7
	F	13.5	15.0	21.7	21.7	28.4
Melanoma	M	0.5	0.8	0.4	0.8	0.3
	F	0.8	0.8	0.7	0.7	0.6
Ovary	F	9.5	10.9	9.9	10.1	8.6
Pancreas	M	15.1	16.8	15.8	15.3	17.7
	F	8.4	11.1	11.9	12.0	12.1
Prostate	M	99.9	94.1	107.6	111.9	115.8
Rectum	M	14.4	14.4	11.2	13.5	14.1
	F	9.7	8.7	11.9	11.2	10.7
Stomach	M	22.1	24.2	27.2	21.7	19.8
	F	8.0	10.8	9.7	10.4	9.6
Total Leukemia	M	11.6	9.8	12.5	11.4	10.0
	F	6.2	5.5	8.3	6.4	5.6
Uterine Cervix	F	35.2	32.8	30.3	27.2	22.2
Uterine Corpus	F	11.3	14.5	14.7	17.2	16.8

- Ovarian cancer incidence has dropped slightly among black and white women.

- Incidence of cancer of the prostate has increased among men of both races but most markedly among black men.

- Bladder cancer incidence has increased for all four groups. It is higher among whites than among blacks.

- Leukemia incidence has decreased for all four groups.

- The incidence of kidney cancer has increased slightly among all four groups.

- Stomach cancer incidence has declined among black and white men and among white women. It has increased among black women.

- Colon cancer incidence has increased sharply among black men since 1969. It has increased gradually among white men. Colon cancer incidence has increased slightly among white and black women.

- The incidence of cancer of the rectum has increased among white men and women and black women; it has decreased slightly for black men.

- Pancreatic cancer incidence has decreased slightly among white men and remained constant among white women. It has increased significantly among black men and women.

- Lung cancer has more than doubled among black women in the 8 years covered by these data, and has almost doubled among white women. Marked increases are also seen for black and white men.

Changing Cancer Patterns by Age Group for All Races and Both Sexes, All Sites Combined

Data reflected in this chart are displayed on a logarithmic scale to show percentage changes in cancer death rates in five different age groups.

The death rates for children and younger adults have both declined markedly since 1964, and appear to be leveling off.

There have been slight declines in death rates among persons aged 45 to 64 in the past several years, while death rates for persons aged 65 to 74 have remained almost constant since 1964.

Death rates for persons 75 and over have risen slightly since 1970.

Cancer death rates, by age group, per 100,000 U.S. population for all races and both sexes, all sites combined, 1965–1979.
From: NCHS, USBC.

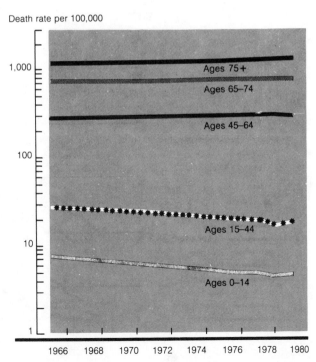

Death rate per 100,000

825

Changing Patterns for Eight Major Cancers in All U.S. Men

The lung cancer death rate for all U.S. men has climbed fourteenfold in the past 50 years, from 5 deaths per 100,000 population in 1930 to almost 70 deaths per 100,000 in the late 1970s.

Stomach cancer was the leading cause of cancer deaths among men from 1930 until 1947. Deaths from this cancer, however, have decreased markedly since 1930, from 37 deaths to 9 deaths per 100,000 population.

Deaths from colorectal cancers and cancers of the prostate both peaked in the late 1940s, then dropped and leveled off.

Deaths from cancer of the pancreas and from leukemia rose slightly from the 1930s into the 1960s and then leveled off.

Esophageal and bladder cancer deaths have remained almost constant since 1930.

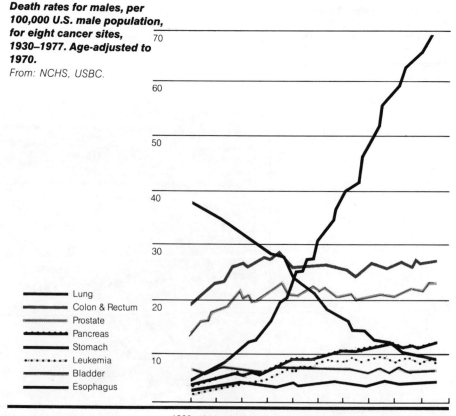

Death rates for males, per 100,000 U.S. male population, for eight cancer sites, 1930–1977. Age-adjusted to 1970.
From: NCHS, USBC.

Lung
Colon & Rectum
Prostate
Pancreas
Stomach
Leukemia
Bladder
Esophagus

1930 1935 1940 1945 1950 1955 1960 1965 1970 1975 1980

U.S. Cancer Death Rates
Changing Patterns for Eight Major Cancers in All U.S. Women

Until about 1945, cancer of the uterus was the major cause of cancer death among all U.S. women, but deaths from this cancer have been declining steadily since 1930.

Breast cancer deaths have risen only slightly since 1930, but breast cancer has been the major cause of cancer deaths among all U.S. women since about 1945.

Lung cancer deaths, meanwhile, have been climbing sharply since the early 1960s, and are expected to overtake breast cancer deaths sometime in 1984 or 1985.

Stomach cancer deaths have been declining steadily since 1930, from 28 to less than 5 deaths per 100,000 population. Cancer of the uterus, once the major cause of cancer deaths among U.S. women, now accounts for less than 10 deaths per 100,000.

The death rates from leukemia and ovarian cancer both rose slightly from 1930 to 1955 but have since leveled off.

Pancreatic cancer deaths rose slightly over the period and are still rising slightly. The death rate for this cancer is still less than 8 per 100,000 each year.

Deaths from colorectal cancers rose in the 1930s and 1940s but have been declining since 1945.

Death rates for females, per 100,000 U.S. female population, for 8 cancer sites, 1930–1977. Age-adjusted to 1970.
From: NCHS, USBC.

Legend:
- Breast
- Colon & Rectum
- Lung
- Uterus
- Ovary
- Pancreas
- Leukemia
- Stomach

1930 1935 1940 1945 1950 1955 1960 1965 1970 1975 1980

U.S. Five-year Survival Rates
Changes for 19 Sites Among Whites

The overall, 5-year relative survival rate for cancer patients in the United States is now 48 percent or greater. These data show the changes in survival rates for all whites in this country for 19 major cancers. There have been some gains in survival rates for almost all cancers in the 20 years spanned by these data.

The most notable gains have been seen for endometrial, cervical and breast cancers among women, testicular and prostatic cancers among men, and for Hodgkin's disease, melanoma skin cancer, and bladder cancer among both men and women.

Survival for colorectal cancer patients has improved over the 20-year period but is still less than 50 percent. Survival rates for cancers of the lung, stomach, pancreas, and esophagus remain low.

Five-year relative survival rates for selected sites for white cancer patients.

	1960–63*	1970–73*	1973–79*
Bladder	53	61	71
Brain	18	20	20
Breast (females)	63	68	72
Cervix	58	64	66
Colon	43	49	48
Endometrium (corpus)	73	81	87
Esophagus	4	4	4
Hodgkin's disease	40	67	68
Kidney	37	46	48
Leukemia	14	22	28
Lung	8	10	11
Melanoma of the skin	60	68	76
Non-Hodgkin's lymphoma	31	41	43
Ovary	32	36	34
Pancreas	1	2	2
Prostate	50	63	64
Rectum	38	45	46
Stomach	11	13	13
Testicular cancer	63	72	80

*Data for 1960–63 and 1970–73 are from three hospital registries and one State registry, and appear in Cancer Patient Survival Experience, 1980. Data for 1973–79 are from SEER, and represent 10 percent of the U.S. population. Thus, the earlier data and the SEER data are not strictly comparable, but each set represents the best available data for the time period covered.

U.S. Five-year Survival Rates

Changes for 19 Sites Among Blacks

Substantial gains in 5-year survival rates can be seen for endometrial, cervical and breast cancers among women and for cancer of the prostate among men.

Some gains in survival are also apparent for bladder cancer, kidney cancer and colorectal cancers in both sexes. The outlook for stomach cancer and for cancers of the lung, pancreas, ovary and esophagus remains poor.

Although white patients survive longer than black patients for more than half of these sites, the survival rates are almost equal for cancers of the stomach, lung and esophagus, and for Hodgkin's disease and non-Hodgkin's lymphoma. Black patients with cancers of the pancreas, ovary, kidney, and brain survive slightly longer than whites.

The differences in survival rates is a subject of concern and is under intense study at the National Cancer Institute.

Five-year relative survival rates for selected sites for black cancer patients.

	1960–63*	1970–73*	1973–79*
Bladder	24	36	43
Brain	19	19	21
Breast (females)	46	51	60
Cervix	47	61	61
Colon	34	37	44
Endometrium (corpus)	31	44	54
Esophagus	1	4	3
Hodgkin's disease	**	**	66
Kidney	38	44	49
Leukemia	**	**	24
Lung	5	7	9
Melanoma of the skin	**	**	**
Non-Hodgkin's lymphoma	**	**	43
Ovary	32	32	35
Pancreas	1	2	4
Prostate	35	55	54
Rectum	27	30	35
Stomach	8	13	14
Testicular cancer	**	**	62

*Data for 1960–63 and 1970–73 are from two hospital registries and appear in Cancer Patient Survival Experience, 1980. The later data are from SEER, and represent 10 percent of the U.S. population. Thus, the earlier data and the SEER data are not strictly comparable, but each set represents the best available data for the time periods covered.

**Rates could not be calculated because the number of cases was too small.

U.S. Five-year Survival Rates
Changes for White Children Under Age 15

Dramatic improvements in 5-year survival rates have been achieved in the past 20 years for white children under age 15. (Black children were omitted from this analysis because of the small numbers of patients.)

Major gains in survival are seen for acute lymphocytic leukemia, or ALL, the most common leukemia among children. The outlook for acute granulocytic leukemia remains grave.

The outlook for children with cancers of the brain and central nervous system, Wilms' tumor, neuroblastoma, bone cancers, and Hodgkin's disease has improved over 1960.

Survival rates for children with non-Hodgkin's lymphomas have improved but are still only 38 percent.

Five-year relative survival rates for cancer in white children under age 15.

	1960–63*	1970–73*	1973–79*
Acute lymphocytic leukemia	4	34	56
Acute granulocytic leukemia	3	5	19
Bone	20	30	45
Brain and central nervous system	35	45	51
Hodgkin's disease	52	90	83**
Neuroblastoma	25	40	46
Non-Hodgkin's lymphoma	18	26	38
Wilms' tumor	57	69	72

*Data for 1960–63 and 1970–73 are from three hospital registries and one State registry, and appear in Cancer Patient Survival Experience, 1980. Data for 1973–79 are from SEER, which represent 10 percent of the U.S. population. The earlier data and the SEER data are not strictly comparable, but each set represents the best available data for the time periods covered.

**An apparent decrease in 5-year relative survival for children with Hodgkin's disease appears because of the change in data bases. The latest data can be applied to the U.S. population. The 1970–73 data reflect the inclusion of results from an outstanding research center, one of the four registries used for the earlier data.

U.S. Costs of Cancer
Major Medical Expenditures, 1980

Americans spent about $219.4 billion on health care in 1980. This figure includes costs for diagnosis, hospitalization, physicians, drugs, long-term care, and rehabilitation.

Costs for the four major causes of death in this country-heart disease, cancer, strokes and injuries-together accounted for about a quarter of the total health care bill.

Accidents and injuries, the leading cause of death among children and the fourth leading cause of death among adults, cost Americans $19.2 billion, or 9 percent of the total bill.

Heart disease, the leading cause of death among adults, cost $14.5 billion or 7 percent, and cancer, the second leading cause of death among adults, cost $13.1 billion, or 6 percent.

These costs are derived from the records of health insurance companies, hospitals, physicians, and state and federal health care plans. The data were compiled by the National Center for Health Statistics of the U.S. Public Health Service.

Medical care expenditures for cancer, heart disease, stroke, and injuries, 1980 (in billions).
From: NCHS.

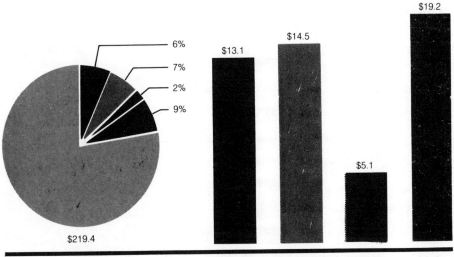

U.S. Costs of Cancer
By Cancer Sites and Age Group

This chart shows, by cancer type, the $13.1 billion spent on cancer in 1980. Costs for each cancer type are also figured for by sex and age-- under 65 and over 65.

To some extent, these costs reflect the incidence of specific cancers. Breast cancer, for example. is the major cause of cancer among women, and accounts for a major portion of the health care dollar spent on cancer.

Costs of care for benign tumors include diagnosis and treatment of non-cancerous skin tumors in both men and women, and of *in situ* carcinonia of the cervix. The cost figure also includes biopsies for benign breast disease.

Medical care expenditures (in billions) for cancers and benign tumors, 1980; total $13.1 billion, excluding nursing home care.
From: NCHS.

Care for colorectal cancer, the second most frequent cancer among women and the third among men, is included in the figure for cancers of the digestive organs and peritoneum.

Care for lung cancer, a major cancer in both men and women, accounts for most of the care costs for cancers of the lung, bronchus and trachea.

The figure for female genital organs includes care for cancers of the uterine corpus, or endometrium, and ovarian cancer. That for other genitourinary organs includes cancers of the bladder and kidney in both men and women, and for cancer of the prostate and testicular cancer among men.

The lymph and blood systems category includes leukemia and lymphomas.

*Medical care for benign tumors includes care for non-malignant skin and brain tumors and *in situ* carcinoma of the cervix, and biopsies for benign breast disease.

	■ Male <65
	■ Male ≥65
	⚊ Female <65
	— Female ≥65

	Percent		
	<65	**≥65**	
Digestive organs	48%	52%	$1.1
	26%	74%	$0.9
Lung, bronchus, and trachea	55%	45%	$1.0
	74%	26%	$0.6
Skin, bone, and connective tissue	61%	39%	$0.4
	66%	34%	$0.5
Breast	66%	34%	$1.2
Female genital organs	72%	28%	$0.9
Other genitourinary orgrans	32%	68%	$0.9
	40%	60%	$0.2
Lymph and blood systems	61%	39%	$0.5
	61%	39%	$0.5
Other and unspecified sites	69%	31%	$0.8
	69%	31%	$0.7
Benign tumors*	72%	28%	$0.6
	87%	13%	$2.2

<u>U.S. Costs of Cancer</u>
Earnings Lost Due to Cancer in 1977

The value of lost earnings due to cancer and benign tumors was estimated to be $26.4 billion in 1977. "Lost earnings" are those lost because of premature death from cancer. They are computed by multiplying the number of cancer deaths at various age levels by adjusted projections of lifetime earnings.

Even though 60 percent of 1977 cancer deaths occurred in persons 65 and older, that age group accounted for only 11 percent of lost earnings. Those aged 45 to 64 accounted for 34 percent of deaths and for 62 percent of lost earnings. Persons under age 45 at time of death were responsible for 6 percent of cancer deaths and for 27 percent of lost earnings.

Lung cancer deaths accounted for the largest single portion of lost earnings: almost $6 billion. Cancers of the digestive organs include colorectal cancer and cancers of the stomach, esophagus, and pancreas.

Earnings lost (in billions) due to cancers and benign tumors, 1977; total: $26.4 billion.
From: NCHS.

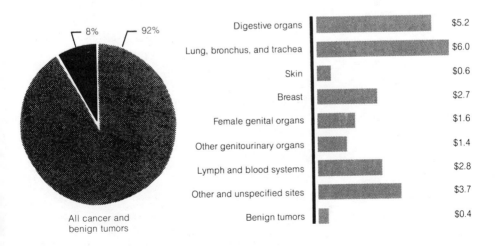

Digestive organs	$5.2
Lung, bronchus, and trachea	$6.0
Skin	$0.6
Breast	$2.7
Female genital organs	$1.6
Other genitourinary organs	$1.4
Lymph and blood systems	$2.8
Other and unspecified sites	$3.7
Benign tumors	$0.4

8% 92%

All cancer and benign tumors

■ **Morbidity**　　■ **Mortality**

Cancer Risk Factors

Air and Water

As a nation we have learned that the air around us may become contaminated with industrial and automotive emissions, and that this may happen to our seas, lakes, rivers, and groundwater supplies as well. Americans are becoming increasingly concerned with this issue, but there is still very little conclusive information about the effects of such pollution on the incidence of cancer.

Each of us, at various times, may be exposed to potential carcinogens in the air we breathe and the water we drink. Though the number of such substances is large, the levels are generally small—much smaller, for example, than the levels found in some workplaces. On the other hand, carcinogens in air and water may be harder to avoid than those found in specific workplace locations. It has been estimated that pollution accounts for at most 1 to 5 percent of all cancer deaths (Doll and Peto, 1981).

Air Pollution

There is little evidence to date that ambient air—the circulating air around poses serious cancer risks. The ambient air in specific areas may contain industrial plant emissions, automobile exhaust, and other pollutants linked to cancer, but in most places, the air we breathe does not contain high levels of carcinogens. In fact, the strongest link between air pollution and cancer is found among smokers, who inhale particulates in their tobacco smoke.

Much of what we know about the health effects of large amounts of pollutants in the air comes from workplace studies of coal gas, tar, pitch, and coke oven emissions. Certain workers may be at some risk but workplace exposures are often 10 to 1000 times the levels found in ambient air.

Asbestos is a known carcinogen found in the air around some workplaces. Levels vary, but are highest near asbestos mines, mills, waste dumps, and manufacturing plants. Asbestos is the only known cause of mesothelioma, a form of cancer that affects the membrane lining of the chest and abdominal cavities. It is rare in the general population, but found frequently among workers exposed to high levels of airborne asbestos. Asbestos can also cause lung cancer Studies of shipbuilders in coastal areas of Georgia, Florida, and Virginia, many of whom were exposed to asbestos insulation, showed an increased risk of lung cancer in all areas, and of mesothelioma in Virginia, particularly among employees who worked during World War II (Blot and Fraumeni, 1981). There may also be risks of exposure during demolition of buildings that contain asbestos used for fireproofing in walls and ceilings. There has been concern, for example, about children's exposure to asbestos in older school buildings. It is sometimes safer to cover interior asbestos than to try to remove it.

Benzo(a)pyrene, or B(a)P, is a combustion product. B(a)P levels in ambient air in this country have decreased since the 1930s and 1910s when oil and natural gas—which burn more cleanly—placed coal for home heating (Shy and Struba, 1982). A study of roofers exposed to high levels of B(a)P in hot pitch showed a higher incidence of lung cancer among them than in the general population (Hammond et al, 1976).

Lung cancer incidence is higher in cities than in the country, but this is not necessarily due to urban air pollution. Workplace exposures and other lifestyle factors of city dwellers, like cigarette smoking, may be more important (Buell, 1967; Cederlof, 1975). The "urban factor" is much weaker than cigarette smoking on lung cancer incidence.

Increased death rates from chronic, non-malignant lung diseases like bronchitis, particularly among the elderly, have been linked with "brown-outs," smogs, and other episodes of serious air pollution. Sulfur dioxide from older power plants and smelters is the main component of acid rain. It can also aggravate chronic lung disease. Few cancer studies have looked at any link with acid rain, but it produces other effects like damage to trees and to aquatic life in lakes and rivers.

Exposure to radioactive emissions from radon in uranium mines has been shown to be responsible for the increased risk of lung cancer in miners. Recent concern has focused on radon exposures in homes, particularly those that have been made airtight by efficient insulation. The radon can enter the home from soil, water or building materials. Some researchers estimate that as many as 10,000 cancers a year may result in this country from indoor radon pollution. Cigarette smoke is another form of indoor pollution that has been linked to increased lung cancer, but the extent of the hazards from both radon and passive smoking is not now clear.

Water Pollution

Drinking water contains complex mixtures of known and suspected carcinogens including asbestos, metals, radioactive substances, and industrial chemicals. Even the process of treating water may create small quantities of chemicals linked to cancer, but the levels are so small that there is probably a low risk, if any, associated with most drinking water supplies.

Trihalomethanes, or THMs, can be formed when chlorine used to purify drinking water reacts with organic compounds in water. At levels normally found in chlorinated city water supplies, there is some suspicion that THMs may increase the risk of gastrointestinal and urinary tract cancers (Crump and Guess, 1982). THMs are also used as indicators of more hazardous compounds that are difficult to measure directly. To reduce the levels of THMs, water is often filtered so that less chlorine is needed to purify it.

A few other chemicals that have been found in drinking water from a small number of supplies are known to cause cancer in humans (Harris et al, 1977). Vinyl chloride, for example, may be introduced into drinking water from industrial plants, or, in very small amounts, by seepage from polyvinyl chloride piping used in some water distribution systems. Benzene and bis(2-chloroethyl)ether are other carcinogens that are occasionally found in drinking water (Kraybill et al, 1980).

Nitrates are seldom removed during the water treatment process. Nitrates themselves do not cause cancer, but they can be transformed in the body into nitrosamines, which are powerful carcinogens. Although some studies have found a link between high levels of nitrates in drinking water and gastric cancer (Cuello et al, 1976; Geleprin et al, 1976), there is no indication that the low levels sometimes found in drinking water pose a risk of cancer.

Asbestos fibers are widely distributed in water supplies in this country, with higher levels often found near cities and industrial centers. But studies have not shown consistently that asbestos in drinking water affects cancer risk (Shy and Struba, 1982).

The trace metals arsenic, chromium, and nickel are found in drinking water in varying amounts. They may come from industrial plants, mines, seepage from soil or piping, by mineralization from rocks, or from water treatment processes. High levels of arsenic in drinking water in some other countries have been linked with skin cancer (Tseng et al, 1968; Tseng, 1976) but the much lower concentrations in U.S. drinking water have not been linked with cancer in humans.

Radioactive substances may be found in water depending on local rock type and on the use and disposal of radioactive compounds by nearby industries, hospitals, and nuclear power plants. Radioactive strontium and radium, sometimes found in some water supplies, can accumulate in bone tissue but even the cumulative dose from radium would result in so few fatal bone cancers that they would probably not be detected in epidemiologic studies. Naturally occurring radon gas is found dissolved in water in some parts of the United States. Ingestion of radon in water does not pose much of a hazard, because of its low concentration. Radon can be released, though, from water into household air via showers and washing machines. Studies are trying now to evaluate the risk of such exposures.

Water that percolates down below the earth's surface, known as groundwater, is often the source of spring and well water. Aquifers—rock formations that hold water in underground "lakes—may also be sources for springs and wells. Contamination of these water sources with pesticides, industrial solvents, and other industrial chemicals such as polychlorinated biphenyls, or PCBs, can become a serious problem. Disposing of such wastes in lagoons or landfills can contribute to groundwater contamination.

Burying hazardous wastes on land is the most common method of disposal in this country because it is inexpensive. Disposal sites can leak, however, contaminating groundwater with toxic substances. Contamination of groundwater could become more widespread as older disposal sites begin to leak, but cleanups and better disposal methods can prevent contamination. Environmental Protection Agency regulations now require that hazardous waste disposal be completed in safer ways than in the past.

The major United States water supplies are continually monitored for carcinogens under Environmental Protection Agency guidelines. National Cancer Institute scientists have been studying the possible link between cancer and drinking water quality (Cantor et al, 1978). Except for some drinking water supplies that contain unusually high levels of carcinogens, the evidence to date suggests that our drinking water now poses little cancer risk to us.

Risk Factors
Alcohol

Consumption of alcoholic beverages increases the risk of cancer, particularly of the mouth, pharynx, larynx, and esophagus (Tuyns, 1982). Ethanol, by itself, does not cause cancer in animals, but very few people drink pure ethanol. They consume drinks flavored with congeners—chemical compounds or contaminants produced during fermentation—and many people who drink also smoke. It has therefore been difficult to evaluate the role of drinking alone, but there is no doubt that drinking and smoking together have a synergistic, or combined, effect, and do contribute to the high incidence of some cancers.

This combined effect of drinking and smoking was shown clearly in a case-control study (Rothman and Keller, 1972) of patients with cancers of the mouth and pharynx. Their risk increased with the amount of alcohol consumed and number of cigarettes smoked. Even among the nonsmokers in this study, though, an effect of alcohol could be seen.

Risk for developing cancer of the larynx also increases with alcohol consumption (Wynder et al, 1976), although tobacco is a more powerful determinant.

Esophageal cancer has been closely linked to drinking in a number of studies. Studies of black men in Washington, D.C. (Pottern, Ziegler et al, 1981), where esophageal cancer rates are the highest in the United States, showed that heavy drinking was chiefly responsible for the increased risk of esophageal cancer. In parts of China and Africa, where esophageal cancer incidence is also high, there is some link with "home brews"—"samshu," a Chinese rice wine combined with grain alcohol (De Jong et al, 1974), and in the Sudan, "aragi," a distillate made from dates (Malik et al, 1976). In Puerto Rico, a case-control study (Martinez, 1970) showed that alcohol and tobacco were the major factors associated with esophageal cancer, with alcohol having the greatest effect. And studies in France (Tuyns et al, 1977 and 1979) showed synergistic effects of alcohol and cigarette smoking in increasing the risk of esophageal cancer, with local wines and ciders particularly implicated.

Other cancers are also linked to alcohol consumption, although the evidence is not always clear cut. An increased incidence of liver cancer, for example, has been seen among patients with alcoholic cirrhosis. And a study done in Denmark (Jensen, 1979) reported a relative risk of 1.5 for primary liver cancer among more than 14,000 brewery workers who were entitled to drink a beer "ration" each working day. But another study of brewery workers in Dublin (Dean et al, 1979) who consumed above-average amounts of stout failed to show a link with increased risk of liver cancer. About a fifth of the workers, who worked in the brewhouse, did have higher risks of cancer of the rectum.

It is not now clear if one type of alcohol is riskier than another, chiefly because most of the populations studied have drunk one type of alcohol only—wine, applejack, beer, grain alcohol. The Washington, D.C., study (Pottern et al, op cit) did show that men who drank equivalent amounts (in terms of ethanol content) of hard liquor, or of hard liquor and beer, had a greater risk of esophageal cancer than did those who drank only wine and beer.

Since ethanol does not cause cancer in lab animals, it is suspected that alcohol acts as a cocarcinogen, enhancing the effects of other cancercausing agents like tobacco. It is also hypothesized that poor nutrition may contribute to the effects of alcohol by failing to provide protective nutrients.

Risk Factors
Diet

It has become clear that what we eat—or don't eat—for breakfast, lunch, and dinner may have profound effects on our chances of developing cancer. One estimate (Doll and Peto,

1981) is that the death rate from all cancers in this country might be reduced more than a third by practical changes in our diet. These are some of the diet components that are believed to affect the cancer process:

Carotenoids and Vitamin A

Carotenoids are found in carrots, sweet potatoes, peaches, cantaloupes, and other yellow-orange fruits and vegetables, and in some dark green vegetables like broccoli, kale, and spinach. Beta-carotene and some of the other carotenoids are provitamins, or precursors, of vitamin A. When ingested, some of them are converted to vitamin A in the body.

Preformed vitamin A, or retinol, occurs only in foods of animal origin—chiefly whole milk, cheese, butter, egg yolks, and liver. Preformed vitamin A, in the form of retinyl acetate or retinyl palmitate, is also present in many multiple—vitamin pills and in some fortified foods.

In many cultures, carotenoids from fruits and vegetables are the source of most of the vitamin A, and particular plant foods often account for most of them. Dark green, leafy vegetables are the main source of beta-carotene among some Chinese, for example, as are carrots in this country, a red palm oil used for cooking in West Africa, and

yellowgreen vegetables in Japan (Peto and Doll, 1981).

Inverse associations have been found, in a number of studies, between dietary vitamin A or carotenoids and the incidence of a number of cancers—those of the oral cavity and pharynx, the larynx, and lung (Doll and Peto, 1981; Shekelle et al, 1981). These findings suggest that either or both of these substances may protect against cancer A study of esophageal cancer has suggested that deficiencies of a number of micronutrients may increase risk for that cancer (Ziegler et al, 1981).

To examine the effects of adding beta-carotene to the diet, the National Cancer Institute (NCI) began a study in 1982 of physicians enrolled in a National Heart, Lung, and Blood Institute (NHLBI) study. The NHLBI portion of the study is looking to see if regular aspirin use protects against stroke and heart attack; the NCI portion is looking at how beta-carotene affects cancer development. Other case-control studies are looking to see if fruits and vegetables, beta-carotene, or other factors are most strongly associated with decreased cancer risk, and to examine which cancers are or are not influenced by diet factors.

Vitamin C

Some studies show an inverse association between fresh fruit and vegetable consumption and some cancers, including stomach cancer (Kolonel et al, 1981), though no studies have implicated vitamin C deficiency in the etiology of this cancer. Animal studies show that ascorbic acid—vitamin C—can inhibit the formation of carcinogenic N-nitroso compounds from ingested nitrates.

Fats

Surveys of various populations in this country and in others have suggested a link between dietary fat intake and some cancers, particularly those of the breast, colon, endometrium, and prostate gland. Animal studies tend to confirm these associations. A link between per capita fat intake and breast cancer risk is also supported by a number of international studies, although case-control studies do not, in general, support this link.

Animal studies have shown that high levels of fat in the diet enhance the development of both spontaneous and chemically induced mammary cancers in mice. This was true even if the fat was fed after tumor initiation, lending support to the hypothesis that dietary fat acts as a cancer promoter.

Correlations of international incidence and death rates with diet components indicate that colon cancer and, to a lesser extent, rectal cancer, are associated with total dietary fat intake. Some case control studies have also suggested a

relationship between dietary fat intake and risk of colon and rectal cancers (Palmer and Bakshi, 1983), but the evidence is not clear-cut.

Varying levels of fiber intake may help to explain some of the conflicting data on fat intake and colon and rectal cancers, because fiber is thought to protect against these cancers. Thus, fat intake—particularly milk fat—was found in one study to be about the same for individuals in rural Finland and in Copenhagen, Denmark, but the Finns, who eat large amounts of high-fiber, unrefined rye bread, had a much lower incidence of colon cancer (MacLennan et al, 1978).

An association between the incidence of prostate cancer and high dietary fat intake in humans has been seen chiefly in international surveys. Both prostate cancer incidence and fat intake are higher among Japanese living in Hawaii than among Japanese living in Japan (Waterhouse et al, 1976). And prostate cancer incidence has been linked with the consumption of animal fat and protein among several ethnic groups in Hawaii (Kolonel et al, 1981).

Most population studies of dietary fat intake and cancer incidence have not been able to differentiate the effects of saturated and unsaturated fats, but consumption of the two often go hand in hand. Total fat intake accounts for about 40 percent of total calories in the U.S. diet, compared with only 20 percent in the Japanese diet. Meat, eggs, dairy foods, and oils used in cooking and in salads are the chief sources of fat in the American diet.

Fiber

Dietary fiber appears to protect against some forms of cancer, particularly colon cancer. Which types of fiber, and how they may work, are not clear.

Fiber is found in fruits, vegetables, nuts, legumes (peas and beans), brown rice, and wholegrain breads and cereals. Some studies have shown an inverse association between the consumption of vegetables and the occurrence of colon cancers (Graham, 1972; 1978). But it has been difficult to single out the role of fiber in many of the studies that measure total fruit and vegetable intake. Individuals who eat diets high in fruits, vegetables, legumes, and whole grains usually eat less fat and protein and tend not to be overweight. And a diet high in fruits and vegetables is likely to be high in carotenoids and vitamin C.

If some fiber component does protect against colorectal cancer, it may do so by speeding the transit time of fecal matter through the bowel, thus decreasing the time that food carcinogens stay in contact with bowel walls; by increasing the bulk of the stool and thus decreasing the concentration of carcinogens; or by changing the different bacterial species in the bowel, some of which

may destroy carcinogen metabolites (Doll and Peto, 1981). It has also been postulated that dietary fiber intake decreases the production of mutagens in the stool (Ehrich, 1979).

Cured, Pickled, and Smoked Foods; Molds and Fungi

Studies in different parts of the world show an apparent link between frequent consumption of pickled, cured, and smoked foods and an increased risk of stomach cancer. This association could be due either to the curing agents or to molds and fungi toxins that may form in these foods if they are not refrigerated. The decrease in stomach cancer incidence in the United States since the 1930s has been attributed to the wide use of refrigeration, although there is no proof.

Vitamin E and Selenium

Both vitamin E and an enzyme that depends on selenium for its activity act as antioxidants, able to block damage to cellular DNA from some carcinogens. These substances can also keep cultured cells treated with chemicals from becoming cancerous. There is no evidence that "megadoses" of either of these substances help to protect humans against cancer. Selenium is known to be toxic in high doses, and vitamin E, which is fat-soluble, is potentially toxic.

Obesity

Obesity has been associated with increased cancer death rates in animals in a number of studies over the past 45 years (Doll and Peto, 1981). It is also suspected that obesity is associated with increased death rates for some cancers in humans, particularly those of the prostate, pancreas, breast, and ovary. One large study, of three-quarters of a million men and women observed over a 13-year period (Lew and Garfinkel, 1979), has lent some support to these suspicions.

Risk Factors

Drugs

The development of "miracle" drugs that effectively treat a variety of illnesses has been one of medicine's major achievements. Unfortunately, when chemically altering or arresting the course of one disease, these drugs can contribute to the development of other diseases, including cancer. Estrogenic hormones, immunosuppressive agents, and, ironically, anticancer drugs designed to kill tumor cells are the classes of drugs most often linked to human cancer.

Drugs are believed to account for fewer than 2 percent of all cancers. When deciding to use drugs, the informed patient and physician must carefully weigh the benefits of a medication against its possible risks.

Hormones

Estrogens are hormones, produced mainly by the ovaries, that help regulate menstruation and pregnancy. They are also responsible for the development of feminine body features. The ovaries produce several different estrogens—estradiol, estriol, and estrone—but because they have similar functions and chemical structures, they are collectively referred to as estrogens.

Many middle-aged and older women take synthetic "replacement" estrogens to relieve symptoms of menopause that may develop when their ovaries decrease production of these hormones. Such use has been linked to cancers of the endometrium, the lining of the uterus. One study reported that women who take replacement estrogens for more than 7 years increase their risk of endometrial cancer 14 times (Zeil and Finkle, 1975). It appears, though, that women who stop taking replacement estrogens decrease their risk of this cancer to the level of a nonuser after 2 years (Stolley and Hibberd, 1982).

It is not clear if replacement estrogens increase the risk of breast cancer in menopausal women. Several studies have shown a slightly increased risk (Hoover et al, 1976; Brinton, 1981; Ross, 1980; Thomas, 1982; Hoover, 1981; Jick and Walker, 1980; Hulka and Chambless, 1982) especially in long-term users. The groups these studies looked at differed, and other investigators have failed to show an association (Kelsey et al, 1981). Thus, results are not conclusive.

Synthetic estrogens are the chief ingredient of birth control pills. The most effective and most widely used birth control pills are "combination" pills that contain both estrogen and a second ovarian hormone, progestin. Pills that contain only progestin, called "minipills," are also available.

Combination pills may actually decrease a woman's risk of developing some cancers. Women who take these pills are only half as likely as nonusers to develop cancer of the ovary or endometrium; their use is estimated to prevent 1,700 cases of ovarian cancer and 2,000 cases of endometrial cancer each year (CDC, 1983).

A different form of birth control pills, known as "sequential" pills, were available at one time. They were taken off the market by the U.S. Food and Drug Administration in the late 1970s because studies linked them to an increased risk of endometrial cancer. Sequential pills provided separate estrogen and progestin in sequence: during the first weeks of her menstrual period, a woman took the estrogen pills, and in the last week took the progestin.

One study showed a sevenfold increase in risk of endometrial cancer among women who took one brand of sequential pills, but failed to find an increased risk among users of other brand (Weiss and

Sayvetz, 1980). The risk was associated with the brand that contained the most potent form of estrogen and the weakest progestin.

The link between birth control pills and breast cancer is less clean. Most of the evidence suggests that women who use oral contraceptives do not have an increased risk of breast cancer despite duration of pill use and other variables. In some studies, though, specific groups of women who use these pills have been adversely affected: those with a family history of breast cancer or those with benign breast disease. A recent study suggested a foulfold increase in breast cancer incidence among women under age 36 who were long-term users of combination pills containing a "high" dose of progestin (Pike et al, 1983). Other recent studies have linked oral contraceptives with an elevated risk of cervical cancer, even after sexual activity and other risk factors for this cancer were taken into account.

DES (diethylstilbestrol), an estrogen-like compound, has been widely publicized as a cancer-causing drug. During the 1940s and 1950s, doctors prescribed DES to pregnant women because they believed the drug helped prevent miscarriages. Although studies in the 1930s had shown that DES caused cancer in laboratory animals, the problem received little attention until the 1970s, when a rare vaginal and cervical cancer was found in a number of young women living in areas where DES had been widely prescribed. Histories showed that the patients had been exposed to DES *in utero* when their mothers took the drug (Herbst et al, 1971). It is now thought that between four and six million Americans—mothers, daughters, and sons—may have had pregnancy-related exposure to DES. The DES findings also provided the first evidence that a carcinogen could travel across the placental barrier from the mother to the fetus.

There have been few studies of the effects of DES on women who took it, and those studies produced conflicting results. One study showed some increased risk of cancer of the breast and reproductive organs in these women (Bibbo et al, 1978); another showed no such link (Brian et al, 1980).

DES has not been associated with cancers of the reproductive tract in sons of women who took it, but anatomic abnormalities of the sperm and reproductive tract have been reported in these men. Studies to see if these abnormalities affect their fertility have been delayed because, as a group, these DES sons seem to have postponed starting families (DES Task Force, 1978).

Androgens, a class of male hormones, are structurally related to estrogens. Synthetic androgens are used to treat various cancers, some genetic diseases, and some blood and endocrine disorders. Some athletes use androgens to increase body mass and athletic performance.

Studies have shown an increased incidence of liver cancer among children who received androgens for the treatment of some types of anemias (Johnson et al, 1972). It is not known, though, if the liver cancer these children developed resulted from the androgens or the disease.

Anticancer Drugs

In the last decade, anticancer drugs have prolonged the lives of many thousands of cancer patients. A number of these patients have developed second cancers.

Alkylating agents are a class of drugs used to treat a variety of cancers. They work by inserting foreign molecules into the genetic material of dividing cancer cells. These foreign molecules act like wrenches thrown into the machinery of the cell, preventing growth and division.

Alkylating agents may also cause mutations in the cell's genetic material, similar to the mutations caused by ionizing radiation, and lead to cancer. Several studies have shown that Hodgkin's disease patients treated with alkylating agents have an increased incidence of acute myelocytic leukemia (AML).

Not a single case of AML was found in more than 3,000 Hodgkin's disease patients studied before 1962 (Moertel and Hagedorn, 1957 and Berg, 1967). But a study done between 1961 and 1973 showed that Hodgkin's disease patients were developing AML at a rate of 156 cases per 100,000 population (Weiden et al, 1973). The greatest incidence of AML in this 12-year study occurred from 1970 to 1973, a few years after the MOPP regimen (nitrogen mustard, vincristine [Oncovin], prednisone, and procarbazine) was introduced in 1967. Both nitrogen mustard and procarbazine are alkylatin agents. The risk of leukemias after treatment of Hodgkin's disease has continued to increase, especially among patients who receive both MOPP and radiation therapy.

Alkylating drugs used to treat other cancers have also been linked to cancer. Epidemiologic studies showed a hundredfold increase in AML among multiple myeloma patients after the drug melphalan was introduced (Adamson and Sieber, 1977). A recent survey of women treated for ovarian cancer showed that melphalan and chlorambucil increase the leukemia risk in steps that correlate with dose (Greene et al, 1982).

The risk of acute leukemia has also been shown to rise after use of alkylating agents to treat lung cancer (Stott et al, 1977), the blood disorder known as polycythemia vera (Berk et al, 1981), and non-Hodgkin's lymphoma (Greene et al, 1983).

The alkylating agent methyl-CCNU (semustine), used to treat cancers of the stomach, colon, and rectum, was recently shown to increase a patient's risk of developing leukemia by sixteenfold (Boice et al, 1983). Most surveys of chemotherapy-related cancers have focused on leukemia because it develops within 4 to 5 years after exposure. The risk of other cancers has not been evaluated in a systematic way because most exposed patients have not lived long enough to develop other cancers.

Immunosuppressive Drugs

Drugs that suppress the immune system are given to organ transplant patients to help them accept a foreign organ. Azathioprine and adrenal corticosteroid hormones were widely used in the past for kidney transplant patients, and cyclosporin A has been used recently. Non-Hodgkin's lymphoma, the most common type of cancer in these patients, occurs 32 times more often among them than in the general population (Hoover and Fraumeni, 1973). The lymphoma often arises rapidly-within a year or two-after the transplant operation, and often develops in the brain, an unusual site for this type of cancer (Hoover, 1977). Some other cancers—skin cancers, Kaposi's sarcoma, and lung cancer—also occur at a high rate in transplant recipients.

Other Drugs

Radioactive drugs contain a molecule "tagged" with a radioactive isotope so

Other Drugs

Radioactive drugs contain a molecule "tagged" with a radioactive isotope so the isotope can be counted or imaged in diagnostic tests. Radioactive drugs can concentrate in body tissues and, depending on their strength and half-life, may injure those tissues. Radioactive drugs are also used to treat bone tuberculosis, thyroid cancer, and the blood disorder polycythemia vera. Some of these radioactive drugs have been shown to cause various cancers, including osteogenic sarcoma, a type of bone cancer; leukemias; and a rare form of liver cancer (Hoover and Fraumeni, 1981).

In 1964, chlornaphazine, a drug used to treat polycythemia vera and Hodgkin's lymphoma, was withdrawn from the market because it was found to cause bladder cancer. Chlornaphazine is chemically related to beta-naphthylamine, a chemical earlier associated with bladder cancer among workers in the dye industry.

Other drugs have also been found to increase the rate of human cancers. Pain-killing drugs that contain phenacetin have been linked to kidney cancers, and methoxypsoralens, used with ultraviolet-A radiation in the PUVA regimen for psoriasis, have been linked with skin cancer.

Risk Factors
Familial Factors

Most cancers are caused by a variable mix of hereditary and environmental factors. Some rare cancers are inherited, and usually appear at an early age. A number of rare hereditary disorders may predispose a person to cancer but the added action of one or more environmental factors is often needed for the cancer to develop. Other individuals seem to be resistant to some cancers. Subgroups of some of the common cancers have a genetic component but may also require an environmental trigger. Some nonhereditary cancers seem to run in families, but this may reflect chance or a common environmental exposure. How a person reacts to his environment is also a part of the equation.

As an example of the interactions of genetic and environmental factors, consider the Australian woman who develops nonmelanoma skin cancer She inherited her fair skin; that is the genetic component. She lives near the equator, where sunlight is intense and prolonged; that is an environmental factor. She fails to avoid the sun at noontime or to protect her skin with clothing and sun screens, and that is yet another factor: how the individual interacts with her environment. This mix of factors can apply to the origins of many cancers, and suggests various possible preventive measures.

Retinoblastoma, an eye cancer, is one of the very rare inherited cancers. About 40 percent of all

Predispositions for certain rare cancers also are inherited but seem to require an additional environmental event (Miller, in press). These include the hereditary form of Wilms' tumor, a childhood kidney cancer; xeroderma pigmentosum, which makes individuals extremely sensitive to sunlight and to nonmelanoma skin cancer; dysplastic nevus syndrome, a precursor of melanoma; and ataxiatelangiectasia, an inherited immune deficiency syndrome that predisposes individuals to lymphoma, leukemia, and stomach cancers.

Certain "cancer families" have also been identified and followed. The pattern of their cancer occurrences indicates that the cancers were inherited, though the family members may develop different forms of cancer (Li and Fraumeni, 1982).

Subgroups of breast cancer, colon cancer, and brain cancer also appear to be heritable. And with some of the other common cancers, such as stomach cancer and lung cancer, a familial component is strongly suspected, though it could reflect exposure to a common cause. Thus, the risks of developing breast cancer or colon cancer may be twenty- to thirtyfold greater than normal in persons with familial risks. In one family with kidney cancer, followed for four generations, the youngest members are being closely watched because their chances of developing it are so great.

Some ethnic groups seem to possess traits that protect them against some cancers. Thus, chronic lymphocytic leukemia is extremely rare among Orientals, and Ewing's sarcoma is very rare among blacks.

Genetic "markers" help to identify family members who are at high risk of developing certain heritable cancers so that they can be watched for signs of early disease. A "marker" for retinoblastoma, for example, is a missing chromosome segment. In instances where a predisposition is inherited, care can be taken to prevent exposure to the environmental event or "insult" that causes cancer. Removal of precursor moles for melanoma, or of polyps for colon cancer, are ways to prevent development of disease, even though the predisposition for it has been inherited.

Meanwhile, on another front, basic researchers are trying to learn exactly what happens at the level of the gene. Recent oncogene research has led to the hypothesis that normally "quiet" genes found in all vertebrate cells may be triggered—by viral infection, by environmental events or by some other mechanisms—at some step in the cancer process.

Risk Factors
Ionizing Radiation

Ionizing radiation is a known cause of cancer, and of other adverse effects as well. It is one of the most extensively studied human carcinogens and may account for about 3 percent of all cancers. Ionizing radiation is able to remove electrons from atoms and to change the molecular structures of cells. It is these cellular changes that may cause cancer to develop. The genetic DNA in the cell nucleus is thought to be the critical target for radiation-induced damage.

Some radiation comes from natural sources, like that from cosmic rays and from radioactive substances in the earth's crust. Each of us is exposed to this "background" radiation at a rate of about 0.1 to 0.2 rad per year. (The rad is a unit of measurement for the amount of radiation energy absorbed by body tissues.)

Very high doses of radiation (hundreds of rads) received all at once may be fatal, but if spread out over a period of time, a high dose of radiation may be less damaging to healthy tissues. A single, 500-rad dose of whole-body irradiation, for example, would cause about half the people exposed to it to die within 30 days. But patients who receive daily radiation therapy treatments of 200 rads a day directed to a small area of the body can be exposed to thousands of rads over a period of weeks. It is difficult to measure the effects of low-level radiation—of less than 25 rads, say—from common sources like medical X-rays.

Some of what we now know about the effects of radiation exposure was learned by studying patients who received medical treatments with radiation in the past. Some of the first quantitative evidence that radiation causes cancer came from studies of patients who received radiation therapy before 1954 for a spinal disorder (Court Brown and Doll, 1965; Smith and Doll, 1982). Researchers noticed that these patients had more leukemia and cancers of the stomach, pancreas, lung, and other highly irradiated organs than would be expected in a healthy population.

Between 1935 and 1954, fluoroscopy, an X-ray procedure, was used to monitor treatment of patients with tuberculosis; the women who were thus treated could receive an average dose of 150 rads to the breast. Ten to 15 years later these women had a high incidence of breast cancer (Boice and Monson, 1977).

There is a high risk of thyroid cancer many years after childhood exposure to radiation for therapy of noncancerous conditions of the head and neck. Exposure during childhood can be particularly damaging because rapidly growing cells may be more sensitive than slower growing cells irradiated later in life. Before 1950, individuals with enlarged thymus glands were treated with intense radiation. An elevated risk of thyroid cancer and leukemia has since been found in this population. Females were at greater risk than males, and the risk among Jews was especially high (Hempelmann et al, 1975).

Those who think they may have received radiation treatments for thymus conditions or other childhood problems, such as scalp ringworm or enlarged tonsils, should tell their physicians.

The radiologists who first used X-rays extensively before 1920, when the potential dangers of radiation were not recognized, had high rates of leukemia, a blood cancer. Today, precautions are taken to reduce the exposure to patients, radiologists, and X-ray technicians.

A classic study of women who painted radium dials before 1930 showed high rates of bone sarcomas and head cancers. They had swallowed large quantities of radioactive radium by licking their paint brushes to make fine tips; it has been estimated that the average dose reaching their bone tissues was 1700 rads (BEIR, 1972).

Most of our information about the effects of radiation comes from studies of atomic bomb survivors in Japan, among whom have been found increased rates of acute leukemia and cancers of the breast, thyroid, lung, stomach, and other organs (Boice and Land, 1982). Female survivors who received a single dose of radiation from the blast were found to be at the same risk for breast cancer as the women with tuberculosis who had repeated fluoroscopy exposures over a 3- to 5-year period (Boice et al, 1979). This suggests that in the case of breast cancer—but not necessarily other cancers—repeated small doses over the years may be as hazardous as a single, large dose.

Today, many women at risk of developing breast cancer are periodically examined with mammography, or low-dose breast X-rays. But for high-risk women, particularly over age 50, the benefits of detecting cancer early outweigh the small risk of developing cancer from repeated mammograms.

Exposure to low levels of radiation before birth is associated with the development of cancer during childhood, especially leukemia (Bithell and Stewart, 1975), but not all researchers are convinced that prenatal irradiation is the cause of childhood cancer. Individuals exposed prenatally during the atomic bomb blasts in Japan do not have higher cancer rates. Now, though, ultrasound is used during pregnancy instead of X-rays when possible.

There are other environmental and occupational exposures to radiation. Radioactive fallout, for example, is produced during nuclear weapons tests when airborne radioactive particles settle to the ground. One study showed that persons accidentally exposed to very high levels of fallout had an increased risk of thyroid cancer, and that females were especially susceptible (Boice and Land, 1982).

Uranium miners inhale radioactive radon gas produced underground by the natural decay of uranium, and have high rates of respiratory cancer (Archer et al, 1976). There may also be an interaction between inhaled radioactive gas and smoking that increases the risk (Wittenmore and McMillan, 1983). Radon is becoming a public health concern in some locations because of its presence in ground water and building materials.

In general, the breast, thyroid, and bone marrow are most sensitive to the effects of ionizing radiation. There may be a minimum lag time after exposure of about 2 years before leukemia develops, and 10 to 15 years before other cancers develop.

Reducing exposure to unnecessary medical X-rays is one of the best ways to reduce exposure to ionizing radiation. In many instances, though, the benefits outweigh the risks, as in mammography for some women, as a tool for diagnosis of various diseases or injuries, and as a way to treat some cancers.

Risk Factors
Occupation

In 1775, London surgeon Percivall Pott published a report on a rare cancer of the scrotum that he found was common among chimney sweeps, a disease known at the time as "soot-wart" (Shimkin, 1977). A century later, two other scientists noted similar cancers among gas plant workers in Germany and oil shale workers in Scotland. Yet another 40 years later, certain constituents of

tar, soot, and oils, known as polycyclic aromatic hydrocarbons, were found to cause cancer in laboratory animals.

This brief detective story has become a model for many later investigations of workplace carcinogens: observation of unusual cancers, or a high incidence of more common cancers, among groups of workers; a search for a responsible agent; and finally, demonstration that the agent can cause cancer in laboratory animals.

A postscript to the chimney sweep story deals with the ultimate goal of workplace cancer studies: prevention. Spurred by Pott 's report, the Danish chimney sweeps guild in 1778 urged its members to take daily baths (Clemmesen, 1951). A report in the 1892 British Medical Journal, "Why Foreign Sweeps Do Not Suffer From Scrotal Cancer," noted that the sweeps of northern Europe seemed to benefit from this hygiene measure, but English sweeps, who apparently ignored such implications, continued to develop cancer.

Industrial workers are, in a sense, flagmen for our society. In this age of chemicals, metals, plastics, and fibers, we all run the risk of exposures to industrial carcinogens in our air, water, food, and homes. But the exposures of the industrial worker may be intense and prolonged. If a substance used in the workplace is a carcinogen, the cancers it can cause will most likely be seen first in workers.

Since 1971, the International Agency for Research on Cancer (IARC), an agency of the World Health Organization headquartered in Lyons, France, has been publishing critical reviews of data on the carcinogenicity of chemicals to which humans are exposed, and IARC working groups of scientists have been evaluating these data in terms of human risk. A summary of these reviews was published in 1982 (IARC, Supplement 4).

The IARC scientists assessed the data from epidemiologic studies of humans, from studies in experimental animals, and from short-term tests or assays. Based on these data, they assigned individual chemicals, chemical groups, industrial processes and occupational exposures to one of three categories of risk. (See tables on next two pages.) When there was enough evidence from epidemiologic studies to support a causal association with cancer, the chemical, chemical group, process, or exposure was assigned to Group 1. The scientists placed the chemicals, chemical groups, processes, or exposures that they considered probably carcinogenic to humans in Group 2. Those with data to support the highest carcinogenic risk to humans appear in Group 2A; those with lower risk are in Group 2B.

The carcinogenic agents included in the tables do not fall into any particular class of substances; they may be metals, solvents, dyes, organic and inorganic dusts, pesticides or herbicides. Space here is too short for a detailed discussion of each of the agents in Tables I and II, and such information can be found in the IARC series.

But to illustrate briefly how exposures occur, how risk is ascertained, and how exposures can be minimized or prevented, four types of workplace carcinogen, each from Group I, are discussed here in some detail: a mineral fiber (asbestos), a chemical (benzene), a metal (chromium), and an industrial process (furniture manufacture).

TABLE I

Group 1:

Industrial processes and occupational exposures causally associated with cancer in humans:

Auramine manufacture
Boot and shoe manufacture and repair (certain occupations)
Furniture manufacture
Isopropyl alcohol manufacture (strong-acid process)
Nickel refining
Rubber industry (certain occupations)
Underground hematite mining (with exposure to radon)

Chemicals and groups of chemicals causally associated with cancer in humans:

4-Aminobiphenyl
Arsenic and arsenic compounds
Asbestos
Benzene
Benzidine
N,N-Bis(2-chloroethyl)-2-naphthylamine(Chlornaphazine)
Bis(chloromethyl)ether and technical-grade chloromethyl
    methyl ether
Chromium and certain chromium compounds
2-Naphthylamine
Soots, tars and oils
Vinyl chloride

TABLE II

Group 2A:	Chemicals, groups of chemicals or industrial processes *probably* carcinogenic to humans with at least limited evidence of carcinogenicity to humans:

Acrylonitrile
Benzo*(a)*pyrene
Beryllium and beryllium compounds
Diethyl sulphate
Dimethyl sulphate
Manufacture of magenta
Nickel and certain nickel compounds
ortho-Toluidine

Group 2B:	Chemicals, groups of chemicals or industrial processes *probably* carcinogenic to humans with sufficient evidence in animals and inadequate data in humans:

Amitrole
Auramine (technical grade)
Benzotrichloride
Cadmium and cadmium compounds
Carbon tetrachloride
Chlorophenols
DDT
3,3'-Dichlorobenzidine
3,3'-Dimethoxybenzidine (*ortho*-Dianisidine)
Dimethylcarbamoyl chloride
1,4-Dioxane
Direct Black 38 (technical grade)
Direct Blue 6 (technical grade)
Direct Brown 95 (technical grade)
Epichlorohydrin
Ethylene dibromide
Ethylene oxide
Ethylene thiourea
Formaldehyde (gas)
Hydrazine
Phenoxyacetic acid herbicides
Polychlorinated biphenyls
Tetrachlorodibenzo-*para*-dioxin (TCDD)
2,4,6-Trichlorophenol

Asbestos

Derived from the Greek word meaning "incombustible," asbestos is the generic name for a group of minerals composed of silicate fibers that are heat-stable, non-conductive and can be woven. Asbestos occurs widely in mineral formations found throughout the world and has been used since the late 1800s. In 1976, more than 5,500 tons of asbestos were produced (IARC, Vol 14, 1977), the bulk of it by Canada and the Soviet Union. About two-thirds of the asbestos produced is used in the construction industry for cement sheets and pipes, insulating materials, and floor and ceiling tiles. It is also used for friction applications, like clutch and brake facings for cars and machinery. It is used widely in the shipbuilding industry, chiefly for insulating and fire-proofing. In the past, it was often sprayed on for insulation, fire-proofing, and decorative and acoustic uses, but its use in many of these settings is now decreasing.

The presence of asbestos in various materials does not necessarily pose a health risk. The health risk arises when the asbestos fibers are set free during mining, drilling, sawing, or spraying or when materials with asbestos in them start to decompose.

Reports linking asbestos with lung cancer and asbestosis, a lung disease, have been appearing since 1935. The earlier studies reported these diseases mostly among asbestos workers and miners, but as the uses of asbestos multiplied, particularly in shipbuilding during World War II, the numbers of workers who suffered the injurious effects of asbestos exposure continued to grow. Mesothelioma, a rare cancer that affects the lining of the chest and abdominal cavity, has been linked with asbestos exposure since the early 1960s. Inhaled asbestos fibers produce these cancers in a number of different laboratory animals.

Lung cancer and mesothelioma both have latency periods of up to 30 years or more; this means it may take that long for cancer to develop after exposure. But the duration of the exposure needed to cause cancer may be very brief. In some cases, individuals who were exposed to asbestos for only a few months have developed cancer. Men who worked in shipyards for only a few years during World War II, for instance, have been found to be at high risk of lung cancer (Blot et al, 1982). Some cases of lung cancer and mesothelioma have also been found to occur among "bystanders": the families of workers who carried asbestos fibers home on their clothing; workers who were nearby when asbestos materials were sawed, drilled, or sprayed; individuals who lived near asbestos mines or factories where asbestos was fabricated.

Cigarette smoking and asbestos exposure have a synergistic effect: smoking plus asbestos exposure creates far more risk than either one alone. Some other cancers have also including cancers of the esophagus, stomach, colon, larynx, and kidney.

Asbestos exposure is now regulated by the Occupational Safety and Health Administration (OSHA), which sets standards for the number of fibers that may be present in the workplace air. It also requires personal protective equipment for workers. The National Institute for Occupational Safety and Health (NIOSH), the research arm of OSHA, recommends that all non-essential uses of asbestos be eliminated.

Benzene

A clear, colorless liquid, benzene was first isolated by Faraday in 1825 from a liquid condensed by compressing oil gas (IARC, Vol 7, 1974). It is now produced from petroleum. Up until World War II, benzene was used chiefly in this country as a gasoline additive. Now it is also used widely as a solvent in the chemical and drug industries, and as an intermediate reactant in the synthesis of resins, adhesives, and plastics.

Case reports linking leukemia with occupational exposure to benzene have appeared in the literature since the late 1920s; such reports have come from a number of countries. The major route of absorption of benzene is through the lungs; most of the affected workers had breathed its fumes. Among those exposed who later developed leukemia were workers who made artificial leather

or made shoes using rubber cements that contained benzene. Case-control and cohort studies (IARC, Vol 7, 1974) have supported this association.

Benzene causes chromosomal abnormalities, but not mutations, in some short-term assays (IARC, 1982) and has recently been found to be carcinogenic in assays with laboratory animals (NTP, 1984).

Some two to three million workers may be exposed to benzene in petrochemical, rubber, and coke plants. Shoemakers, furniture finishers, and gas station attendants are also exposed to it. OSHA regulates workplace exposures.

Chromium and Chromium Compounds

The element chromium is the 20th most abundant element and occurs, mostly in chromite ores, throughout the world. The Republic of South Africa and the Soviet Union are now the two major producers. Chromium and its compounds are used widely in industry because of chrome's hardness, resistance to corrosion, high melting point, and wide availability. Its name is derived from the Greek word "chroma," for color, because of the reds, oranges, yellows, and blues of its salts when it is combined with other minerals.

Most chromium compounds are used in the metallurgical industry, particularly to make stainless steel and alloys. Chromium compounds are also used in the manufacture of bricks, glass, ceramics and certain iron-containing metals. The colored chromate salts of various metals, like zinc and potassium, are used in the pigment, paint, tanning and dyeing industries (IARC, Vol 23, 1980).

An increased incidence of lung cancer has been seen among workers in the chromate-producing industry. There are also indications of high risk among chromium platers and chromium alloy workers.

Furniture Manufacture

For many centuries, furniture and cabinet-making were performed by craftsmen and artisans working at home or in small shops. With the advent of the Industrial Revolution and the development of circular saws and planers, furniture and cabinet-making became an industry. Advances in mechanization were most rapid after World War I. With the development of bandsaws, routers, lathes, and sanders, furniture-making became an assembly-line process, a process that created more furniture and more hazards: high noise levels, accidents, and dust pollution. It was not until the 1960s that the cancer-causing effects of furniture dust began to be recognized.

An increased incidence of cancers of the nose and nasal cavities was first reported among furniture makers in England. Later reports came from Italy, Canada, the Netherlands, Denmark, France, Germany, Sweden, and other parts of England (IARC, Vol 25, 1981). A study in this country (Brinton et al, 1984) showed high nasal cancer risks among furniture workers, particularly in North Carolina. There have also been reports of high incidence of cancers of the larynx, lung, and gastrointestinal tract among furniture workers in the United States, England, and Germany, although these associations are not clear.

From the epidemiologic data available, IARC has concluded that nasal adenocarcinomas have been caused by employment in the furniture-making industry, and that the excess risk of these cancers occurs mainly among those workers exposed to dust from certain hardwoods.

Suction devices, particularly near saws and sanders, can markedly reduce the amount of airborne dust at the workplace (Hounam and Williams, 1974) and masks worn by workers can further reduce the amount of dust inhaled.

The remaining chemicals or processes listed in Tables I and II each fall into the four categories discussed above. Ways to reduce workplace exposure to them, including labeling, venting, and individual protective measures, are regulated by a number of Federal agencies. NCI studies are attempting to gain further understanding of workplace carcinogens, and are looking at ways to counter the cancer risks of workers who have already been exposed to workplace carcinogens. Also, some industries are testing substances in short-term cell-culture assays before introducing them to the workplace.

Risk Factors
Solar Radiation

Solar radiation is the chief cause of nonmelanoma skin cancer responsible for about 90 percent of cases. It has also been linked with skin melanoma, but that relationship is more complex.

Though nonmelanoma skin cancers are now considered to be 98 percent curable, they still accounted for as many deaths in the United States during the 1950s and 1960s as did melanomas, which are far rarer but far more lethal (Mason et al, 1975). More than 400,000 new cases of nonmelanoma skin cancer are thought to occur in the United States each year and this number is rising. Nonmelanoma skin cancer is the most common form of cancer among Caucasians

The relationship between sun exposure and nonmelanoma skin cancer has been clarified greatly in the past decade. Observers had noted in the late 1800s that sailors exposed to the sun developed "Seamanshaut," or "sailor's skin," and in the early 1900s an excess risk of skin cancer was observed among farmers. The greater risk for Caucasians exposed to sun had also been observed (Hyde, 1906).

By 1928, scientists were able to demonstrate the cancer-causing effects of ultraviolet radiation on the skin of lab animals, using both sunlight and artificial light sources (Findlay, 1928). These carcinogenic effects were produced by ultraviolet-B (UV-B) radiation in the 290 to 320 namometer range, the same range that produces burning in human skin.

Though latitude, or distance from the equator, generally determines the amount of UV-B radiation in a given location, altitude and sky cover are also determining factors. Atlanta, Georgia, and El Paso, Texas, for example, are in the same general latitude (32 to 33° N). But El Paso, which is higher and drier, has an annual UV-B count 38 percent higher than Atlanta.

Time of day and time of year also affect the amount of UV-B radiation in any location. The greatest amount, of course, occurs during the summer months, and a third of the day's total amount occurs between the hours of 11 a.m. and 1 p.m. (or 12 noon and 2 p.m. DST).

In 1973, special meters designed to measure UV-B radiation were set up in a number of U.S. cities by Temple University in collaboration with the National Cancer Institute and other government agencies. Data from these meters permitted precise correlations, for the first time, with NCI data on skin cancer incidence in four of these cities, thus affording observations on human populations (Scotto et al, 1976).

The most striking association was the inverse relationship between latitude and nonmelanoma skin cancer incidence: the lower the latitude (the equator is at zero), the higher the incidence. The data also indicated that nonmelanoma skin cancer is related to annual, cumulative UV-B exposure, while skin melanoma may be related to brief exposure to high-intensity UV radiation.

Other findings from the UV-B stations and NCI incidence data are that in some parts of the South, the incidence of skin cancer exceeds that of all other cancers combined, and in parts of the North it accounts for about 40 percent of all cancers.

Another factor that affects UV-B exposure is the amount of ozone (O_3) in the atmosphere (Scotto et al, 1982). Ozone gases absorb most of the UV light in the upper stratosphere and let only small amounts reach the earth. There has been concern in the past decade that the exhaust gases of supersonic aircraft, some fluorocarbons (particularly those used in spray propellants), nuclear weapons, and nitrogen fertilizers could deplete this ozone layer. A Federal task force warned in 1975 that if 1972 levels of fluorocarbon release were continued, the ozone concentration would be reduced by up to 7 percent within several decades. It also observed that there would be about a 2 percent

increase in UV-B radiation near the equator for each 1 percent reduction in stratospheric ozone concentration. These concerns are now being studied by a number of Federal agencies.

Solar radiation ranks high among the "lifestyle" factors associated with cancer. Most individuals have some choice in the amount of sunlight exposure they get, and too much sun is the chief cause of nonmelanoma skin cancer.

Risk Factors
Tobacco

Cigarette smoking is the single major cause of cancer mortality in the United States. Cigarette smokers have total, overall cancer death rates two times greater than nonsmokers; heavy smokers (over a pack a day) have a three- to four-times greater risk. If every smoker in this country were to stop, the overall cancer death rate in the United States would decline significantly. There is no single action an individual can take to reduce the risk of cancer more effectively than to quit smoking, particularly cigarettes (U.S. Surgeon General's Report, 1982). The American Cancer Society estimated that tobacco use contributes to more than 350,000 premature deaths each year (ACS, 1983).

Cigarette smoking increases the risk of cancer of the lung more than any other site. But cigarette smoking-as well as pipe and cigar smoking-also multiplies the risk of cancers of the lip, mouth, tongue, and pharynx, depending on the type and amount of smoking (Fraumeni, 1975). Cigarette smoking also increases the risk of cancers of the larynx and esophagus. Heavy drinking of alcoholic beverages, combined with smoking, increases the risk of cancers of the mouth and throat, larynx, and esophagus even further.

Cigarette smoking is also linked with increased incidence of cancers of the bladder pancreas, and kidney, though to a lesser degree than with cancers of the respiratory and upper digestive tracts. In addition, some epidemiologic evidence points to an association between cigarette smoking and stomach cancer and there is conflicting evidence about the role of cigarette smoking and cancer of the uterine cervix (U.S. Surgeon General's Report, 1982).

	Age 45–64	Age 65–79
Total Cancer	2.14	1.76
Lung	7.84	11.59
Mouth, pharynx	9.90	2.93
Larynx	6.09	8.99
Esophagus	4.17	1.74
Bladder	2.00	2.96
Kidney	1.42	1.57
Prostate	1.04	1.01
Pancreas	2.69	2.17

Cancer death ratios among men who smoked cigarettes compared with a risk of 1.0 for men who never smoked regularly (American Cancer Society Survey, 1966)

There are distinct dose-response relationships between cigarette smoking and cancers of the lung, mouth and throat, esophagus, bladder and larynx; the risk of developing these cancers increases with the number of cigarettes smoked each day. Those who smoke filtered, low-tar cigarettes have a lower lung cancer risk than those who smoke nonfiltered, high-tar cigarettes. The cancer risk for such smokers is still far higher than for nonsmokers, however (Wynder, 1982).

Pipe and cigar smoking, tobacco chewing, and snuff dipping also increase the risk of certain cancers. Both pipe and cigar smoking account for some lung cancer risk (though far less than cigarette smoking), and both increase risk for cancers of the mouth, esophagus, and larynx (U.S. Surgeon General's Report, 1982).

Snuff dipping, common in parts of the South and on the increase among teenagers, increases the incidence of cancers of the mouth and throat. (Snuff dipping is the practice of holding a cud of finely ground tobacco in the cheek.) The risk of cancers of the cheek and gum has been shown to be increased nearly 50-fold in long-term snuff users (Winn et al, 1981).

The number of cancers of the mouth and esophagus associated with tobacco chewing and snuff dipping is relatively small in this country. But in countries where these habits are common, such as India and Ceylon, death rates from oral cancers are extremely high (Wynder 1982).

The links between tobacco use and a number of cancers come largely from retrospective and prospective epidemiologic studies, as well as from laboratory studies and animal experiments. Analytic chemistry studies have shown that tobacco smoke consists of almost 4,000 compounds, many of which act as initiators, promoters, and cocarcinogens. The major carcinogenic activity, though, comes from the tar or particulate portion (Wynder 1982). The tar contains carcinogenic agents. Chewing tobacco and snuff may contain large parts of N-nitrosamines that may be metabolized to carcinogens.

Risk Factors
Viruses

Francis Peyton Rous of New York showed in 1911 that a virus infection could increase the incidence of cancer in chickens, and in 1972, he was awarded the Nobel Prize for this research. Other studies have shown that viruses can increase cancer incidence in a wide spectrum of animal species. Although some viruses are associated with human cancers, other factors are believed to be responsible for the development of cancer. Viruses may make cells more susceptible to the effects of radiation or chemical carcinogens, for example.

Viruses may invade the genetic material of a cell and affect the cell's protein production, causing changes that can lead to uncontrolled growth. Under this theory, a whole virus need not be present to cause a change. A single gene, the basic unit of heredity that codes for a protein, may be enough to disrupt the cell's normal function or make it more vulnerable to other carcinogens.

Epidemiologic research has focused on the possible roles of several viruses in human cancer. Among them are Epstein-Barr virus (EBV), herpes simplex type 2 (HSV2) and hepatitis B. Found throughout the world, EBV has been linked to Burkitt's lymphoma, a cancer found in African children, and to nasopharyngeal cancer which occurs mainly in adults in southern China and in parts of Southeast Asia. EBV also causes infectious mononucleosis, the benign "kissing disease" common among young adults in the United States.

A second candidate, HSV2, appears to be transmitted primarily by sexual activity and has been tentatively linked to cancer of the uterine cervix. But other factors are also important in the development of cervical cancer. The third candidate, hepatitis B virus, is linked to the high incidence of liver cancer in Africa, Taiwan, and China. A chronic infection with the virus may be necessary for most cases of liver cancer to develop (Blumberg and London, 1982).

Robert Gallo and coworkers at the National Cancer Institute have found another type of virus in certain rare forms of human leukemia and lymphoma (Poiesz, 1980) known as human T-cell leukemia-lymphoma virus, or HTLV. It infects human T-cells, white blood cells in the immune system, and is the first virus with genetic information coded as ribonucleic acid, or RNA, shown to play a role in human cancer. All other viruses linked with human cancer have genetic information coded as deoxyribonucleic acid, or DNA.

The presence of antibodies for some viruses, which often indicates earlier viral infection, is linked to the high incidence of certain cancers. In Japan and in Caribbean countries, for example, 90 to 100 percent of T-cell leukemia or lymphoma patients also have human T-cell leukemia-lymphoma antibody. And almost all Africans with Burkitt's lymphoma have large amounts of antibody to Epstein-Barr virus. African children become infected with EBV when antibodies acquired from the mother

disappear at 2 to 8 months of age (Biggar et al, 1978).

Other factors acting with viruses are probably needed for cancer to develop. The necessary "cofactor" may be another virus, a hormone, an immune system deficiency, or an environmental factor. Cofactors are thought to be necessary because only a small percentage of persons infected with these viruses ever seem to develop cancer. Thus, EBV is common in many areas that have very low incidences of the associated cancers, but the link between EBV and Burkitt's lymphoma in Africa may require a predisposing factor like malaria.

It is possible that vaccines will be developed against viruses linked to human cancers. An existing vaccine against hepatitis B virus, for example, may reduce the risk of liver cancer. One approach to preventing cancers associated with viruses may be by reducing exposure to possible cofactors as they become identified.

Cancer Risks: For Major Cancers

Biliary Tract

Biliary tract cancers are more common in other countries than in the United States where their incidence is low. In this country, American Indians and Hispanics are at greater risk than the general population.

The biliary tract consists of the gallbladder which stores bile made in the liver and the ducts, which transport the bile to the small intestine. There the bile helps to digest dietary fats. Cancers may develop in the gallbladder or in the duct cells.

Incidence increases with age; most cases of biliary tract cancer occur in persons over age 65. The epidemiology of cancers of the biliary tract closely resembles that of gallstones, but except for that association, little is known about the possible causes of these cancers.

Gallbladder Cancer

Cancer of the gallbladder is more common in women than in men, perhaps due to hormonal changes during puberty and pregnancy that affect bile production. Gallbladder cancer risk rises with the number of pregnancies.

In the United States, the incidence of gallbladder cancer is 1.8 per 100,000 for women and 1.0 for men. Among American Indians in New Mexico, the incidence is 22.3 for women and 5.9 for men. Among Hispanics in New Mexico, incidence ranges from 9.2 for women to 2.5 for men (Young et al, 1981).

Gallbladder cancer accounts for fewer than 1 percent of all cancers in the United States (Young et al, 1981), but it accounts for about 5 percent of all cancers among women in Latin American countries (Albores-Saavedra et al, 1980). Incidence is also high in Israel, central and eastern Europe, and Japan. The lowest incidence is found among Indians in Bombay (Waterhouse et al, 1982).

Gallstones are the most important known risk factor for biliary tract cancer and especially for gallbladder cancer. Only a few of the millions of persons with gallstones ever develop biliary tract cancer but about 70 percent of gallbladder cancer patients have also had gallstones (Fraumeni and Kantor, 1982). American Indians, with their very high risk for gallbladder cancer, also have a very high incidence of gallstones. Controlling the risk factors for gallstones could decrease the incidence of both gallbladder and bile duct cancers (Fraumeni and Kantor 1982).

Biliary Duct Cancers

Cancers of the bile ducts, especially in the ducts outside the liver, tend to occur more often among men than women and are less likely to be linked with gallstones. In the United States, incidence is 1.7 per 100,000 for men and 1.1 for women. But among American Indians in New Mexico, men have an incidence of 3.4 and women have an incidence of 6.1 (Young et al, 1981). In the past few decades, the incidence of biliary tract cancer in the United States has generally been decreasing among women and increasing among men (De Vesa and Silverman, 1978).

The link between gallstones and bile duct cancer is not so strong as the link between gallstones and gallbladder cancer. Only about 30 percent of patients with bile duct cancer also have gallstones (Fraumeni and Kantor 1982).

Other Biliary Tract Cancer Risks

Several risk factors have been identified for general biliary tract cancer. Typhoid carriers, for example, have been found to have a high risk of developing biliary tract cancer. In some Asian countries, infection with liver flukes appears to increase risk by causing inflammation of the biliary system, which may then lead to cancer. Patients with ulcerative colitis have about a 10 times greater risk of developing biliary tract cancer than do healthy individuals (Ritchie, 1974).

Animal studies have shown that some of the chemicals used to process rubber are linked to biliary tract cancers. A study of workers in a rubber factory also found an excess of biliary tract cancers (Mancuso and Brennan, 1970).

Risks for Major Cancers
Brain and Other Nervous System Cancers

The nervous system consists of two anatomical parts: the central nervous system, which includes the brain and the spinal cord, and the peripheral nervous system. Cancers of the nervous system are of many different types and are classified according to tumor cell type and location. Nine out of 10 nervous system cancers are brain cancers and the most common type of brain cancer accounting for more than half of all adult brain cancers, is glioma, a fast-growing cancer usually located in the upper part of the brain.

Brain cancers occur at varying rates according to sex, race and age. Overall, the incidence of brain and other nervous system cancers is 6.3 cases per 100,000 population per year among U.S. men, and 4.4 among women. The annual U.S. death rate from nervous system cancers is 4.9 per 100,000 for men and 3.2 for women (Young et al, 1981).

Except for meningiomas, a benign tumor of the membranes that surround the brain and spinal cord, men have a higher incidence than do women of all types of benign and malignant nervous system tumors. These differences in incidence suggest a possible hormonal factor in the development of nervous system tumors.

In the United States, brain cancers occur most often among whites. Among white men, they occur at a rate of 6.7 per 100,000, and among white women, 4.6. Among blacks, they occur at a rate of 4.2 per 100,000 for men and 2.7 for women (Young et al, 1981). Whites develop gliomas more often than do blacks, while blacks develop meningiomas more often.

Brain cancer is the second most common type of cancer in children after leukemia and occurs most often in children under 10. In adults, brain cancers occur most often between the ages of 55 and 79 (Young et al, 1981).

Children have a higher incidence of medulloblastoma, a cancer that affects the part of the brain connected to the spinal cord. It accounts for almost a quarter of all childhood brain cancers, but fewer than 2 percent of adult brain cancers (Schoenberg, 1982).

Little is known about the causes of brain cancers, although studies have linked them with occupational, environmental, viral and genetic factors.

Certain brain cancers appear to be more frequent among workers in particular industries. White men who worked in three oil refineries on the Texas Gulf Coast, for example, had a higher proportion of brain cancer deaths between 1943 and 1979 than did the general U.S. population (Thomas et al, 1982). Chemists (Olin and Ahlbom 1980), pharmaceutical workers (Thomas and Decoufle, 1979), embalmers (Walrath, 1983), and workers in rubber manufacturing plants who are exposed to vinyl chloride (Schoenberg, 1982) appear to have more brain cancer than the general population. Cattle and sheep ranchers, dairy farmers, and grain millers have also been found to have a greater proportion of brain cancer (Milham, 1976).

Long-term pesticide exposure of farm workers and of children raised on farms has been associated with brain cancer development (Choi et al, 1970; Gold et al, 1979). These studies link childhood brain cancer with exposure to sick pets and farm animals, thus indicating a possible viral etiology (Schoenberg, 1982).

There is some clinical evidence that lead exposure may be linked to a type of glioma in children (Schreier et al, 1977), evidence supported by laboratory studies in which rats fed high-lead diets developed gliomas. More than 30 chemical compounds have been shown in animal studies to result in a high incidence of nervous system tumors and cancers.

A few studies have shown possible genetic susceptibility for some nervous system cancers. Retinoblastoma, a rare eye cancer is known to occur more often in families than among non-related people, as do certain gliomas (Schoenberg, 1982). There is also a significant association between brain cancers in children and the presence of epilepsy in their siblings (Gold et al, 1979).

Other factors that may be related to brain cancer include high-dose X-rays; consumption of sodium nitrate, a commonly used meat preservative; head trauma; and the use of barbiturates by pregnant women and by children (Schoenberg, 1982).

Brain cancers do not usually spread outside the central nervous system, but cancers from other sites may metastasize to the central nervous system. Breast cancer for example, often spreads to the brain and spinal cord. Melanoma and cancers of the kidney and gastrointestinal tract may also metastasize to the brain (Schoenberg, 1982).

Risks for Major Cancers
Breast

Breast cancer is the most common form of cancer (after skin cancer) among American women and accounts for more deaths among them than any other type. The high incidence rates of breast cancer that prevail in the United States—85.6 per 100,000 for white women in 1973-77, and 72.0 for black women

(Young et al, 1981)—are also seen in other western and industrialized countries, including Canada, western Europe, Australia, New Zealand, and South Africa. Incidence in Asia, Latin America, and Africa is low, and intermediate in eastern and southern Europe. In the United States, breast cancer occurs more often among women who live in cities than among those who live in rural areas (Blot et al, 1977).

Though genetic factors may play some part in the variations in incidence seen in different locales, environmental factors also appear to be important. Migrant studies have shown that breast cancer incidence among women born in countries with low incidence increases when they move to the United States, where incidence is high. This has been seen among Japanese women who have moved to Hawaii and to the mainland United States (Haenszel and Kurihara, 1968), and among the daughters of European immigrants to the United States.

Epidemiologic studies have helped to identify a number of factors that carry varying degrees of risk for breast cancer. To date, no one factor or combination of factors has been found that can be used to predict the occurrence of breast cancer in any one individual. Meanwhile, these are among the major risk factors that have so far been identified:

Age: In countries where the incidence of breast cancer is high, the rate increases sharply after age

30 and continues to rise. Among population groups with low or moderate incidence, there is often a leveling off at the ages of menopause and after. For women in the United States, age is a major risk factor for breast cancer.

Family history: Risk of breast cancer is increased when close relatives have had breast cancer. A woman's risk is increased twofold if her mother or sister have had it and sixfold if both have had it.

Previous breast cancer: Women who have had cancer in one breast have a four- to fivefold risk of developing a second cancer (Kelsey, 1979).

Reproductive experience: The risk for women who have children later in life increases with their age at first birth. Women who have never had children and women who have a first child after age 30 have a risk about three times greater than women who have a first child before age 18. Breast feeding does not seem to affect breast cancer risk.

Menstrual history: Early onset of menstruation and late menopause both appear to increase breast cancer risk. Menopause induced by removal of the ovaries (usually in conjunction with hysterectomy) before age 40 reduces breast cancer risk considerably.

Benign breast disease: Women with benign fibrocystic breast disease confirmed by biopsy appear to have a three to five times greater risk of breast cancer.

Radiation: Large doses of radiation have been linked with the development of breast cancer both in studies of women exposed in Hiroshima and Nagasaki, and of women who were X-rayed many years ago for diagnosis of pulmonary tuberculosis. The much lower doses now used for chest X-rays and for mammograms, or breast X-rays, appear to carry little or no risk.

Socioeconomic status: Women with high socioeconomic status appear to be at greater risk of breast cancer but why this is so is not clear.

Estrogens and oral contraceptives: There is some evidence for an increased risk of breast cancer associated with the use of replacement estrogens, particularly in long-term users, although the data are not all consistent (Thomas DB, 1982). Generally, the use of oral contraceptives has not been linked to increased risk of breast cancer (Brinton et al, 1982), even among women who took the pill for more than 11 years (CDC, 1983). One recent study found some evidence for an increased risk of breast cancer among women under age 36 who were long-term users of combination pills containing a high dose of progestin (Pike et al, 1983).

Nutrition: There is some evidence that obesity is associated with increased breast cancer risk (de Waard, 1975), leading to speculation that high dietary fat intake contributes to increased risk. To date, most of these associations have been derived from studies of geographical groups, and evidence on an individual basis is lacking.

Overall, the evidence suggests that hormonal factors may play a part in breast cancer in addition to genetic predisposition. This hypothesis would account for the higher risk seen in women with a long menstrual history, because of the long exposure of breast tissue to hormone stimulus. Large-scale studies that would take combinations of risk factors into account have not yet been done.

Risks for Major Cancers
Childhood

The incidence of cancer among children under age 15 in this country each year is 12.4 per 100,000 among whites and 9.8 among blacks. Though low compared with the incidence of some adult cancers, cancer is second only to accidents as the leading cause of death among children (Young et al, 1978; Young and Miller 1975). More than 40 percent of childhood cancers occur in the very young—age 4 and under.

More encouraging is the fact that five-year relative survival rates for many of the childhood cancers have increased dramatically in this country from the 1960s to the 1970s (Myers and Hankey, 1980). The five-year survival rate for acute lymphocytic leukemia in children, for example,

has increased from 1 percent to almost 50 percent in some groups of patients (Young et al, 1978).

The incidence of the childhood cancers varies greatly throughout the world, depending on the type. The acute leukemias account for about 85 percent of them in this country. But in tropical Africa, Burkitt's lymphoma, a cancer of the lymph system, accounts for more than half of childhood cancers. In Ankara, Turkey, almost half are acute myelomonocytic leukemia (AMML), but AMML accounts for only 4 percent of childhood cancers in this country.

There are also varying age trends for the childhood leukemias. Among white Americans, western Europeans, and, more recently, Japanese, there is a peak in cancer incidence at ages 2 through 4 (Miller 1977). Among black children in the United States there is no such age peak.

These are the major childhood cancers in this country:

Acute Leukemias

Acute leukemias are the most frequent, and acute lymphocytic leukemia (ALL) accounts for most of these. The incidence is slightly higher among boys than among girls. About 40 percent of acute leukemia cases in children have been linked with chromosome disorders.

Ionizing radiation—energetic rays that cause molecules to gain or lose electrons—can cause leukemia. When warnings about radiation were widely publicized to the medical community in the mid-1950s, safety procedures for diagnostic X-rays were tightened and, by the 1960s, leukemia incidence had fallen among all groups under age 75. Studies of the possible effects of prenatal irradiation have not been conclusive (Li, 1982).

Some anticancer drugs and at least one industrial solvent, benzene, can cause leukemia in adults, but few drugs and chemicals have been shown to induce cancer in children (Hoover and Fraumeni, 1975).

Lymphomas

These cancers of the lymph system are the third most frequent and Hodgkin's disease accounts for about half of them (Young et al, 1978). Hodgkin's disease is rare in early childhood, peaking in frequency among young adults. Some studies have linked its occurrence to high socioeconomic status, but others have not found this link (Li, 1982). There may be an increased risk of developing Hodgkin's disease among siblings of those who get it, particularly among brothers.

The non-Hodgkin's lymphomas, or NHL, are also more common among boys and occasionally cluster in families. Like leukemias, they are linked with several rare, genetically

determined, immune system diseases. Further evidence for the link of NHL with immune system disorders comes from the observations that persons who receive kidney transplants, and have thus been deliberately immunosuppressed, have a 50-fold increased risk of NHL (Fraumeni and Hoover 1977).

Burkitt's lymphoma, the cancer common among African children, has been linked with Epstein-Barr virus, or EBV; raised levels of antibodies to the virus—indicating that an individual has been exposed to it—have been found in many children with the lymphoma. A cause-and-effect relationship has not been shown.

Central Nervous System

Cancers of the central nervous system—the brain and spinal cord—account for about a fifth of cancers in children under age 15 and tend to occur in the first 10 years of life. A number of genetic disorders seem to be linked with excess risk of developing these cancers.

Bone Cancers

These account for about 5 percent of childhood cancers. The incidence of osteosarcoma, the most common bone cancer peaks in late adolescence after a period of rapid bone growth (Glass and Fraumeni, 1970). It usually develops in the weight-bearing bones of the legs and pelvis, and particularly in the bone areas where most growth takes place. Ewing's sarcoma, another form of bone cancer accounts for about a third of bone cancers in U.S. white children, but is rare in black children anywhere.

Soft Tissue Sarcomas

Of the soft tissue sarcomas, rhabdomyosarcoma is the most common. This cancer shows two distinct age peaks—one before age 5 and the other in the teens (Li and Fraumeni, 1969(a)). Rhabdomyosarcomas of the head, neck, and genitourinary system form the first peak, and there is some suspicion that these cancers form before birth.

Genetic factors may play a role in the development of sarcomas of bone and soft tissue. There are several genetic disorders that predispose to sarcomas, and some of them also occur as components of family cancer syndromes (Li and Fraumeni, 1969(b); Blattner et al, 1979). Osteosarcoma tends to develop in some genetically caused bone lesions (Glass and Fraumeni, 1970). Because Ewings's sarcoma is seen so rarely among black children, genetic factors may play a part in its development also (Miller, 1977).

Neuroblastoma

This cancer arises in one type of immature nerve cells, and accounts for more than 5 percent of childhood cancers in both black and white children. The cancer may be present at birth, and more than half of all cases appear before age 2 (Miller et al, 1968). Neuroblastomas appear to arise during fetal life, and may be linked with inborn defects of nerve tissues (Knudson and Meadows, 1976).

Wilms' Tumor

A cancer of the kidney, Wilms' tumor is usually diagnosed between ages 1 and 3 (Young and Miller 1975). About 14 percent of Wilms' tumor patients also have congenital anomalies, among them aniridia (missing iris of the eye). Children who have aniridia and the tumor consistently lack a segment of a chromosome (number 13). But in one set of twins, both lacked an iris and both lacked the chromosome segment, yet only one of the twins developed Wilms' tumor. This finding lends support to the idea that the predisposition to the cancer is inherited, but that some second event is needed for the cancer to develop.

Retinoblastoma

About 40 percent of cases of retinoblastoma, an eye cancer are inherited. Like Wilms' tumor a small percentage of these eye cancers has been linked to a missing segment of chromosome.

Risks for Major Cancers
Colon and Rectum

The colon and rectum together make up the large bowel, or large intestine. The colon refers to the upper five or six feet of the large intestine; the rectum to the last five or six inches. Risk factors vary for the two cancers, as do their patterns of incidence, but the two are often lumped together as "colorectal cancers" to compare death rates over time and among different countries.

Colorectal cancers caused an estimated 58,000 deaths in this country in 1983 (ACS, 1983), second only to lung cancer. Five-year survival for both cancers has improved markedly over the past 20 years, but is still under 50 percent.

The incidence of colorectal cancers varies widely throughout the world, with up to twentyfold differences. In 1970, for example, the age-adjusted incidence of colon cancer among men was 30. 1 per 100,000 in the State of Connecticut, but only 1.3 in Ibadan, Nigeria (Waterhouse et al, 1976). High incidence and mortality rates are seen in the highly developed countries of North America, northern and western Europe, and New Zealand. The lowest rates are seen in Asia, Africa, and most of the Latin American countries (Logan, 1976).

In general, in areas where the incidence of colorectal cancers is high, colon cancers occur about twice as often as rectal cancers (Schottenfeld and Winawer 1982). This is true in the United States, for example. In areas where the incidence of both cancers is low, the two occur with about equal frequency.

Wide variations in death rates from colorectal cancers are found within the United States. The death rates are highest for men and women, blacks and whites, in the Northeast, particularly in New Jersey, Massachusetts, southern New York State, and urban areas around the Great Lakes; death rates are markedly lower than the U.S. average in parts of the South and Southwest (Mason et al, 1975). Studies have also shown correlations of colon cancer death rates with the degree of urbanization and socioeconomic status (Blot et al, 1976).

The incidence of colon cancer in this country has been rising slightly for white men and women and for black women over the past two decades (Young et al, 1981) and has increased sharply for black men. The incidence of rectal cancer has increased for white men, but has remained almost constant for white women and blacks of both sexes.

Among the risk factors for colorectal cancers are age, family history, ethnic background, history of inflammatory bowel disease, and degree of urbanization. In recent years, diet has come under increasing scrutiny as a major risk factor.

Age: The incidence of colon and rectal cancers increases slowly after adolescence and rises sharply after age 50. In the 55 to 59 age group, the average incidence per 100,000 for all races and sexes combined during 1973-77 (Young et al, 1981) was 60.2 for colon cancer and 32.7 for rectal cancer. By age 75 to 79, the incidence of colon cancer rose to 285.6 and that of rectal cancer to 104.7.

Family history: As with many cancers, subsets of colorectal cancer cases appear to be largely due to familial background. For example, individuals with familial polyposis—a family tendency to develop colon polyps—have an extraordinarily high risk of developing colon cancer; so high, in fact, that surgery to remove the colon is recommended as a prevention measure. There are also families in whom certain groups of cancers develop more frequently than in the general population; colorectal cancers tend to occur in some of these groups.

Ethnic background: A number of U.S. studies have pointed up disparities in colorectal cancer incidence and death rates according to ethnic background. One recent case-control study in rural Nebraska, for example, showed an increased risk of colorectal cancers among persons of Czech background (Pickle et al, 1984). It has often been difficult with these ethnic groups to separate genetic factors from environmental factors like diet.

Migrant studies may have provided more valuable clues.

A number of these migrant studies have shown that risks for colorectal cancers change as ethnic groups move from one country to another. The death rates for colorectal cancer in Japan, for example, are far lower than in the United States. But when Japanese move to this country, their risk of developing colon cancer increases markedly (Schottenfeld and Winawer 1982). Likewise, the incidence of colorectal cancers in Poland is far lower than in the United States, but in one study (Staszewski, 1972), the death rates for colorectal cancers among Polish-born immigrants to the United States were similar to the U.S. population. These and other studies indicate that migrant populations take on the colorectal cancer rates of their new country. Moreover this seems to happen quite quickly, within one generation.

This phenomenon is also being studied in "migrant" populations within the United States. When urban Northerners migrate to the South, where colorectal cancer death rates are lower the rates remain low, suggesting that the migrants assume the new, lower risk and do so in a fairly brief period of time. The National Cancer Institute is conducting a study in Florida to see what might account for this.

History of inflammatory bowel disease: Individuals who have had extensive ulcerative colitis for 10 years or more have a risk of developing colorectal cancer 10 times greater than the general population. There is also evidence that persons with Crohn's disease, a chronic inflammation of the intestine, have a heightened risk of developing colorectal cancers. Both genetic and environmental factors are believed to be responsible for these two diseases (Kirsner, 1980).

Degree of urbanization: As noted above, colorectal cancers occur more often in urban, industrialized countries than in rural countries (Japan is an exception). This differential lends more support to the importance of environmental or lifestyle factors for these cancers, but what those factors are is not clear.

Diet: In general, high dietary intake of fats—in meat, milk and milk products, salad and cooking oils, and margarine—is linked to an increased incidence of colorectal cancers, particularly colon cancer, and high intake of dietary fiber—in fruits, vegetables, legumes, and whole grain products—appears to protect against colorectal cancers, particularly colon cancer. The evidence is not always consistent, however.

International studies that correlate fat intake with colon cancer are more consistent (Armstrong and Doll, 1975; Knox, 1977) than studies of various groups within one country. A study of groups in different parts of Great Britain (Bingham et al, 1979), for example,

found no strong association between fat intake and colorectal cancer death rates. And a study of Mormons in Utah, who have less colorectal cancer than other Americans (Lyon and Sorenson, 1978), also failed to show a link; Mormons tend to eat more beef than do other Americans. Some case-control studies have shown strong links between fat intake and colon cancer and others have failed to demonstrate this link (Miller et al, 1983).

Dietary fiber intake may account for some of the conflicting data about dietary fat, if fiber has a protective effect even when fat intake is high. Intake of milk fats was found to be similar for example, for groups in rural Finland and in Copenhagen, Denmark, but colon cancer incidence was much lower among the Finns, who consume large amounts of high-fiber unrefined rye bread (MacLennan et al, 1978). If fiber protects against colorectal cancers, it may do so by speeding the transit time of fecal matter through the bowel, thus decreasing the time that carcinogens in the fecal matter are in contact with the bowel wall. Or fiber may inhibit production of fecal mutagens (Erich, 1979).

The American diet typically includes more than 40 percent of total calories in fats. In Japan, where the incidence of colorectal cancers is far lower fats make up only about 20 percent of the total calories in the diet. Some current dietary guidelines in this country are recommending that fat intake be decreased to a level of about 30 percent (Palmer and Bakshi, 1983).

Diets high in fruits and vegetables appear to protect against colorectal cancers. A cohort study in Minnesota (Bjelke, 1978) demonstrated this protective effect. It has also been shown in one study that the cruciferous vegetables—cabbage, broccoli, Brussels sprouts, cauliflower—exert a protective effect against colorectal cancers (Graham et al, 1978).

What in vegetables protects against colorectal cancers is not clear-vitamins A or C, other micronutrients, fiber or the substances found in the cabbage family. One case-control study of vitamin C consumption, for example, showed no association with colon cancer (Jain et al, 1980).

Risks for Major Cancers
Esophagus

Cancer of the esophagus is fairly rare in this country with an overall incidence—men and women, all races combined—of 3.6 cases per 100,000 population. It has remained at about this level for the past 40 years. Even with the best medical treatment, though, cancer of the esophagus is almost invariably fatal.

There is strong evidence that esophageal cancer is caused by environmental, or lifestyle, factors. The chief indication for this is the very sharp geographic variation in

incidence, with "pockets" seen in different locales (Day and Munoz, 1982). In one province in the Kazakhstan region of the USSR east of the Caspian Sea, the incidence soars to greater than 130 per 100,000 for both men and women. High rates are seen also in parts of China, northern Iran, France, and southern Africa. In most other parts of the world, the incidence ranges from 2 to 20 cases per 100,000, and occurs most often among men. In the United States, the incidence ranges from a high of 28.6 among black men in Washington, D.C., to a low of 1.9 among American Indian men in New Mexico.

If the disease is caused by lifestyle factors, it might, therefore, yield to prevention. Although the causes for all of the clusters are not known, major risk factors have been identified among some populations.

In parts of the United States, in Denmark, and in France, case-control studies have found that heavy consumption of alcohol and tobacco are major risk factors for esophageal cancer. A study conducted in the French province of Brittany (Tuyns et al, 1977) shows synergistic, or combined, effects of tobacco use and alcohol intake. In Linhsien County, People's Republic of China, a prime suspect for esophageal cancer is a pickled vegetable mix peculiar to that area (Miller 1978).

More recently, a case-control study of black men in Washington, D.C. (Pottern et al, 1981), which has a higher incidence than any other U.S. city, showed that excess alcohol consumption was the major risk factor accounting for about 80 percent of esophageal cancers. Poor nutrition was also implicated as a risk factor in this population.

In Bombay (Jussawalla, 1971), alcohol alone does not explain the risk of esophageal cancer. Smoking the local cigarette ("bidi"), coupled with drinking local brew, does seem to account for the risk in men, but not in women. In northern Iran and in northern Afghanistan, where the incidence of esophageal cancer is high for both sexes, both men and women follow the practice of eating the residue from opium pipes (Gobar 1976).

A number of other promising leads are being followed in studies of populations with esophageal cancer. Low socioeconomic status and poor nutrition—particularly diets deficient in riboflavin, vitamin C, and vitamin A—appear to be linked to increased risk of esophageal cancer in some areas. Esophageal cancer has also been linked with sideropenic dysphagia, an inflammation of the esophagus coupled with iron deficiency. Zinc deficiency has also been implicated as a risk factor in case-control studies of esophageal cancer. Most recently, vitamin A deficiency was found linked to esophageal cancer risk in a study of American men by Mettlin and Graham (1981).

Risks for Major Cancers

Hodgkin's Disease

Hodgkin's disease—a form of lymphoma, or cancer of the lymph system—is fairly rare in this country, with an incidence of 3.5 cases per 100,000 population per year among men and 2.4 among women (Young et al, 1981). It is still one of the most common cancers among young adults, however. And while extremely rare in U.S. children under age 5, it is often one of the most common cancers of childhood in less developed countries (Correa and O'Conor 1971).

Its incidence is characterized by two age peaks—one in the early 20s and another higher peak in the late 70s (Young et al, 1981). This pattern prevails throughout the world except in Japan, where only the second peak is seen. Because of this pattern of occurrence of Hodgkin's disease, there is some suspicion that there may be two, or even three, different disease processes at work (Grufferman, 1982).

Despite its rarity, Hodgkin's has received a great deal of attention from researchers. One reason is that it has yielded so well to therapy in just a decade. Overall, more than four-fifths of patients under age 35 are now living 5 years or more after treatment (Ries et al, 1983). Among patients whose disease is found early, the 5-year survival rate is even higher.

Hodgkin's disease has also interested researchers because of a persistent notion that it might be caused by an infection. These are among the etiologic leads that have been followed:

Clusters

Two apparent geographic clusters of Hodgkin's disease were identified among high school students in Albany, N.Y., and in one Long Island community (Vianna et al, 1971; 1973). The studies concluded that students and teachers at the schools were at increased risk of developing the disease because a number of cases had occurred among students. The studies implied that the schools might serve as a focal point for spread of the disease or that contact with patients can spread it.

Subsequently, though, a series of studies performed in Boston; Oxford, England; Connecticut, and Atlanta were unable to confirm the two earlier studies.

Doctors and nurses

Another study in upstate New York (Vianna et al, 1974) indicated that physicians had a greater than normal risk of developing Hodgkin's disease, presumably because of their greater exposure to patients. Later studies of British physicians (Smith et al, 1974), four groups of U.S. medical specialists (Matanoski et al, 1975), and doctors and nurses in Boston

(Grufferman et al, 1976) showed that these health-care providers were not at greater risk than the general population.

Mononucleosis.

Epstein-Barr virus (EBV), a herpes virus, has been isolated from patients with Burkitt's lymphoma, the most common cancer among African children. EBV is also linked with one type of infectious mononucleosis, known among college students as "the kissing disease." These observations led to a search for associations between mononucleosis and Hodgkin's disease.

One of the first studies (Miller and Beebe, 1973) looked at records of more than 2,000 veterans who had had infectious mononucleosis but found no convincing evidence of increased risk of Hodgkin's disease. Subsequent studies of other groups were also inconclusive, although a Danish study (Rosdahl et al, 1974) showed a twofold excess of Hodgkin's disease after mononucleosis.

Other

Possible associations between Hodgkin's disease and tonsillectomy, polio, multiple sclerosis, and some other conditions have also been explored, but without success.

Thus, no significant environmental risk factors have been identified for Hodgkin's disease, though there is an association between it and educational level: it appears to occur excessively among the well-educated. As for host factors, ataxia telangiectasia, a rare, genetic immune deficiency disease, is the only genetic condition that appears to predispose individuals to Hodgkin's disease.

Risks for Major Cancers
Leukemia

Leukemia is the term for a variety of cancers that arise in blood and bone marrow cells. The various leukemias, though, are quite different from each other in terms of cause, therapy, and outlook, depending on which cells they affect. Chronic lymphocytic leukemia, for example, seems more akin in some ways to lymphoma—cancer of the lymph system—than to other leukemias.

There are four main types: acute lymphocytic leukemia (ALL), acute myelocytic leukemia (AML), chronic myelocytic leukemia (CML), and chronic lymphocytic leukemia (CLL). Together they account for about 5 percent of the total annual cancer incidence in this country. They account for about 45 percent of cancers in children.

Geographic patterns in leukemia incidence show some marked variations that may have more to do with ethnic factors than with geography. Leukemia incidence is lower among children in Africa and Japan than in this country, and CLL is very rare in Japan and China. It is equally rare among these Asians living in other countries. And one rare type of leukemia, acute myelomonocytic (AMML), accounts for 40 percent of childhood leukemias in Ankara, Turkey, compared with only 4 percent in the United States.

In the United States, there is slightly more leukemia among whites than among blacks, and Jews have a somewhat higher incidence than other whites. The male-to-female ratio overall is about 1.7 to 1, and men have almost two times more CLL than do women (Young et al, 1981).

There are wide age variations in leukemia incidence in this country. The overall annual incidence ranges from about 2 cases per 100,000 in young adults to 30 or more per 100,000 over age 65. There is also a peak among white children of almost 7 cases per 100,000 under age 5.

The specific forms of leukemia are very different in their age patterns. Acute leukemias are common at all ages, accounting for almost all leukemias in children and young adults and for about two-fifths of those in older adults. In young children, these are usually acute lymphocytic leukemias (ALL), but after puberty most are acute myelocytic leukemias (AML). CLL is almost never seen before adulthood but is common over age 50.

The leukemias appear to be caused by a number of factors that act alone or in combination (Miller 1979). Some are host factors, such as genetic traits and immune status; others are environmental factors such as radiation, chemicals, or viruses.

A number of family "clusters" of leukemia have been investigated at various times in this country, but few, so far have shown clear evidence of a family predisposition for the disease. The near-absence of CLL among Orientals, on the other hand, argues for a genetic resistance to it among them.

Leukemias are associated in some instances with abnormal chromosome patterns, such as the Philadelphia chromosome (characterized by a translocation, or swap, of parts between two chromosomes) found in the bone marrow cells of persons with CML. Leukemia is also about 20 times more common than usual in persons with Down's syndrome. And it occurs more often in persons with rare conditions—some of them hereditary—that are characterized by increased chromosome breakage.

It has been known for some time that leukemia can be caused by ionizing radiation. This is radiation characteristic of very energetic rays—like X-rays or gamma rays—that can cause molecules to gain or lose electrons. Some of the first evidence of the leukemia-causing potential of radiation came from the effects seen on radiation

workers soon after the discovery of X-rays. For some time, U.S. radiologists had elevated rates of leukemia, but their risk has decreased with improved safety techniques. (These include better shielding, lower doses, and more concentrated fields of exposure.)

The chief sources of ionizing radiation are X-ray therapy and diagnostic X-rays. Studies of Japanese who lived through the atomic bombs (Beebe et al, 1978) at Hiroshima and Nagasaki showed that all forms of leukemia except CLL increased in incidence with a peak about 5 years later. The lag time between exposure and the development of leukemia varied according to the type of leukemia and the age at exposure.

Evidence for X-ray therapy as a cause of leukemia has come from a number of studies of persons who received such therapy some years ago. Among the earliest was a British study of men who received X-ray therapy for a rheumatic inflammation of the spine (MRC, 1956).

Evidence that diagnostic irradiation could cause leukemia came from followup studies of individuals who received the radioisotope thorium dioxide as an X-ray contrast agent during the years 1928-1955, and later showed increased rates of leukemia (da Silva Horta et al, 1974) and liver cancel

In 1956, the National Academy of Sciences-National Research Council in the United States (NAS-NRC, 1956) and the Medical Research Council in Great Britain (MRC, 1956) issued reports on the biological effects of ionizing radiation. Both cautioned against the use of routine fluoroscopy (an X-ray technique) for fitting children's shoes and against other nonessential uses of heavy radiation. There was wide publicity about these reports, and by 1960, declines in leukemia incidence and mortality for all age groups could be seen in Great Britain, the United States, and Norway.

Increased leukemia incidence has also been reported among military personnel present at nuclear tests and among populations in some areas that received fallout from such tests. A possible link with radiation is still being studied.

A number of chemicals used in the workplace are linked with increased risks of leukemia. Among them are benzene and other related solvents used in industry. Some of the anticancer drugs have also been linked in recent years with an increased risk of leukemia.

It has been thought for some time that infectious agents might play a part in human leukemia; viruses do cause leukemias in cats, chickens, mice, monkeys, and cattle. Epstein-Barr virus (EBV), which has been linked to one type of lymphoma, or cancer of the lymph system, was one of the chief suspects. Extensive studies were not able to show a link between either animal viruses or EBV virus and leukemia in humans.

Recently, though, a virus was found that appears to cause an unusual form of leukemia and lymphoma in humans (Poiesz et al, 1980). Antibodies to this virus, the human T-cell leukemia/lymphoma virus, or HTLV, have since been found among persons living in parts of Japan, the Caribbean basin, Africa, some other locales, and sporadically in the United States and Western Europe. (Finding antibodies in these individuals indicates that they have been exposed to the virus.) This finding raises the hope that the forms of leukemia or lymphoma linked with this virus may one day be prevented, and that new understanding of other human leukemias may come from these studies.

Risks for Major Cancers

Liver

Primary liver cancer is cancer that first develops in the liver and may then spread to other organs. Although it accounts for only about 0.6 percent of all diagnosed cancers in the United States, it is a leading cause of death in other parts of the world (Young et al, 1981).

There has been a steady decrease in deaths from liver cancer in the United States over the past 30 years (American Cancer Society, 1982), and primary liver cancer is now fairly uncommon in many Western countries. Incidence generally increases with age, except for a small peak during childhood. In the United States, it is highest in the elderly. Between 1973 and 1977, about 21 per 100,000 white men age 80 to 84 developed liver cancer each year. The incidence for black men age 75 to 79 was about 33 cases per 100,000 each year (Young et al, 1981). Incidence is also higher in black women than in white women.

The highest incidence in the world has been found in Mozambique, Africa. Between 1956 and 1961, there were some 110 cases of primary liver cancer per 100,000 males per year and about 29 cases per 100,000 females per year (Prates and Torres, 1965). Incidence is also very high in Hong Kong, Taiwan, and Singapore, and among some Chinese-Americans (Waterhouse, 1976; Szmuness, 1978).

The most important factor in the occurrence of liver cancer throughout the world may be hepatitis B virus. In some African populations, more than 90 percent of patients with liver cancer also have a chronic hepatitis B virus infection (Kew et al, 1979). In Taiwan, where primary liver cancer accounts for 20 percent of all cancers, persons infected with hepatitis B virus often develop cirrhosis and are at very high risk for liver cancer (Beasley, 1978; Beasley and Lin, 1981). Researchers hope that a recently developed vaccine against hepatitis B

infection will help prevent liver cancer in high-risk groups.

Men are more likely to develop primary liver cancer than women, possibly reflecting their higher exposure to risks factors. The male hormone testosterone increases the incidence of liver tumors in laboratory animals and may be a factor in humans (Falk, 1982).

Alcohol consumption is linked with cirrhosis, a liver disease, and cirrhosis is linked with liver cancer. Sixty to 90 percent of liver cancer occurs in association with cirrhosis but the relationship between the two diseases is not completely understood (Falk, 1982).

Angiosarcoma is a rare type of primary liver cancer linked to workplace exposure to vinyl chloride during the production of plastics. This type of cancer is so rare in the general population that even a few cases among exposed workers yielded evidence that vinyl chloride is carcinogenic.

Between about 1930 and 1955, Thorotrast was used as a radioactive contrast agent in diagnostic imaging. It accumulates in the liver exposing the organ to excess radiation, and causing an increased risk of angiosarcoma.

A widely distributed fungus that infests poorly stored peanuts and other foods produces aflatoxins, some of the most carcinogenic agents known. Aflatoxins cause liver cancer and other types of cancer in laboratory animals and may, in conjunction with hepatitis, be a factor in the high rates of primary liver cancer in Africa and Asia. In the United States, the Food and Drug Administration controls the amount of aflatoxin allowed in peanut butter but there have been cases of tainted animal feed and fish meal (Sinnhuber et al, 1968). Improved food handling and storage in areas where liver cancer is common could result in decreased incidence rates.

Risks for Major Cancers
Lung and Larynx

Primary lung cancer in the United States accounts for about 14 percent of all cancer cases (21 percent in males and 7 percent in females). And because of its high death rate, it accounts for 23 percent of all cancer deaths—31 percent in males and 12 percent in females (Young et al, 1981).

The incidence of lung cancer is increasing rapidly in most areas of the world, and is already the leading cause of cancer in many countries. The annual age-adjusted incidence among men exceeds 100 per 100,000 population in Great Britain, U.S. blacks, and Finland. The incidence is much lower in China, India, and a number of African and Latin American countries, where rates are less than 25 per 100,000 population. Lung cancer still ranks as one of the three most common cancers in males throughout the world, and probably now outranks stomach cancer as the most common cancer in males (Fraumeni and Blot, 1982).

The incidence is generally lower in females, whose rates are usually less than 25 per 100,000. This difference is thought to be due to differences in tobacco consumption.

In the United States, lung cancer incidence has risen more sharply in females than in males in recent years, reflecting the growing popularity of cigarette smoking among females over the past several decades. The lung cancer death rate among women in this country is expected to surpass that of breast cancer is a few years (Horm and Asire, 1982).

Cigarette smoking is the major cause of lung cancer and is estimated to cause 85 percent of lung cancer deaths. Lung cancer mortality increases with increasing doses, as determined by number of cigarettes smoked daily, smoking history, and inhalation patterns. Those who smoke two or more packs a day have death rates 15 to 25 times greater than nonsmokers. Cessation of smoking, though, reduces the risk of death from lung cancer; after 15 years, former smokers have lung cancer death rates only about two times greater than nonsmokers. Those who smoke filtered, low-tar cigarettes gain some benefit, but they still have death rates much higher than nonsmokers.

The link between cigarette smoking and lung cancer was first suspected in the 1920s and 1930s, and was supported in the 1950s by case-control studies in the United States and Great Britain. The evidence became conclusive through surveys of large cohorts of smokers. Two such studies were the 6-year American Cancer Society study of more than a million persons (Hammond, 1972) and the 20-year study of 34,000 British, male physicians (Doll and Peto, 1976). Both surveys showed an elevated relative risk of lung cancer among smokers.

Studies of occupational groups have identified several other respiratory carcinogens, although it is difficult to assess their precise impact. It has been found that tobacco smoke interacts with some of these occupational carcinogens, such as asbestos and radon.

Exposure to airborne asbestos appears to exert the largest cancer threat in the workplace, raising the risk of lung cancer and mesothelioma (a cancer that arises in the lining of the chest cavity, or mesothelium) as well as asbestosis, a lung disease (Fraumeni and Blot, 1982). Epidemiologic studies over the past 25 years have indicated that the risk of developing these three diseases is substantially higher for workers in a number of asbestos industries, including miners and millers, and textile, insulation, shipyard and cement workers. Lung cancer is the major asbestos-related disease, and accounts for death in about 20 percent of some men exposed to asbestos for long periods of their work life (Selikoff et al, 1979). Even men who worked for short periods in shipyards during World War II have a higher risk of developing lung cancer than workers never exposed to asbestos (Blot et al, 1978, 1980).

Asbestos-induced lung cancer is characterized by a lag time of 20 or more years between exposure and onset of disease. It is also evident that asbestos works synergistically with cigarette smoking; a study of lung cancer deaths among insulation workers (Hammond et al, 1979) showed that risk was increased fivefold from asbestos exposure alone, tenfold from smoking alone, and fiftyfold from combined exposure. Thus, reducing exposure to either agent could be expected to reduce risk.

An increased risk of lung cancer has been established among uranium miners in the Colorado Plateau, related to inhalation of radon daughters. (Radon daughters are decomposition products of the gaseous element radon, formed by the disintegration of radium. Radium occurs in small amounts in pitchblende and other uranium minerals.) Radon is probably responsible also for the elevated risk of lung cancer among hardrock miners in this country (Lundin et al, 1971). As with asbestos, the effects of radon seem to be potentiated by cigarette smoking.

Lung cancer is also one of the major effects of high doses of ionizing radiation. This is radiation produced by very energetic rays like X-rays or gamma rays that can cause molecules to gain or lose atoms. Besides the increased risk among uranium miners exposed to alpha radiation from radon daughters, excesses of lung cancer have been reported among some patients who received radiation therapy, and among atomic bomb survivors in Japan (Beebe et al, 1979), where both gamma rays and neutrons were released.

A number of other occupational agents contribute to the incidence of lung cancer, among them mustard gas, chloromethyl ethers, chromium, nickel, and inorganic arsenic.

Air pollution has been suspected as a cause of lung cancer, but it has been difficult to establish definite links. Major problems arise when trying to measure low-level effects of any carcinogen in a general population.

Finally, there is growing evidence of an increased incidence of lung cancer among persons with diets low in vitamin A, particularly when combined with heavy smoking (Mettlin et al, 1979). This finding agrees with laboratory studies showing that vitamin A, and its chemical cousins, as well as beta-carotene, a precursor of vitamin A, protect against the induction and progression of tumors arising in various organs (Sporn, 1977).

Cancer of the larynx, or voicebox, has an incidence pattern like cancers of the mouth and throat: it occurs more often among men than among women, and more often among blacks than among whites. The annual incidence of laryngeal cancer among U.S. white men is 8.3 cases per 100,000 population, and 1.3 among white women. Among black men, the annual incidence is 12.1 per 100,000, and 1.9 among black women (Young et al, 1981).

There is some evidence that cancer of the larynx is increasing, especially among women, in more developed countries (Austin, 1982). In the United States, the median age of onset for laryngeal cancer is 62 among whites and 58 among blacks (Young et al, 1981).

Risk factors for laryngeal cancer include tobacco, alcohol, asbestos, and nickel and mustard gas exposure (Austin, 1982). As with cancers of the lung, mouth and throat, many cases of laryngeal cancer can be attributed to cigarette smoking. Cigarette smokers have almost a tenfold greater risk for laryngeal cancer than do nonsmokers, and risk increases with increased cigarette smoking (Wynder et al, 1976). Heavy alcohol consumption is also a risk factor and tobacco and alcohol together appear to act synergistically.

Risks for Major Cancers
Melanoma

Melanoma is a cancer of melanocytes, the skin cells that produce the dark pigment melanin. Melanomas can occur almost anywhere on the body, but in light-skinned people they occur most often on the trunk in men and on the lower legs in women. The head, neck, and arms are other common sites. In dark-skinned people, melanomas occur most often on the palms of the hands and the soles of the feet.

Worldwide, whites have the highest incidence of melanoma; it is far less frequent among Africans, Polynesians, and Asians (Waterhouse et al, 1982). In this country, the annual incidence is 6.7 per 100,000 among white men and 6.0 among white women, compared with 0.6 for black men and 0.7 for black women (Young et al, 1981). In Australia, the incidence is close to 20 per 100,000 among white men and women (Waterhouse et al, 1982). And worldwide, the incidence has been rising sharply, doubling every decade over the past 30 years.

Melanoma is related to exposure to ultraviolet (UV) radiation, but not so directly as are the more common nonmelanoma skin cancers, basal and squamous cell. There is some evidence that the nonmelanoma skin cancers are related to cumulative exposure to UV radiation (Scotto et al, 1975), while melanoma is related to heavy, blistering overdoses. But other factors also seem to play a part in the development of melanoma.

One such factor is familial predisposition; a recent genetic study suggested that melanoma may occur as an autosomal dominant trait (Greene et al, 1983). Other recent studies have also identified the dysplastic nevus syndrome as a melanoma precursor among melanoma families. A nevus is a true mole, made up of a cluster of melanocytes, and is not be confused with other pigmented lesions of the skin such as seborrheic and actinic keratoses, freckles, and other "spots." (The darker color of these other lesions, as well as the tan that results from sun exposure, result from transfer of melanin from melanocytes to non-pigment-forming cells.)

Normally benign, the nevus may undergo abnormal changes, or dysplasia, which may then proceed to cancer or melanoma. The dysplastic nevus syndrome carries with it a very high risk among persons with a family history of melanoma. Suspicious moles should be surgically removed as soon as possible. The syndrome has also been found among persons without a family history of melanoma. The risk of melanoma is increased for these individuals, but is not so high as in those with a family history of melanoma. Such dysplastic moles should be watched carefully for any changes, though, and removed if changes take place.

Thus, it appears that some melanomas result from inherited traits. Large congenital nevi, present at birth, appear to carry an increased risk of melanoma compared with moles that develop later in life. Another genetic link with melanoma is xeroderma pigmentosum, a rare hereditary skin disease that predisposes a person to all forms of skin cancer. Individuals with this condition lack an enzyme that normally repairs cell DNA damaged by UV radiation.

Hormonal factors may also play a part in melanoma. In one study, women who had used oral contraceptives for 5 years or more and those who had a first child alter age 30 had a higher risk of melanoma than did a control group (Holly et al, 1983). But how these factors are related to melanoma is not clear.

Despite its potential for serious disease, melanoma is highly curable when detected and removed early. In Australia, where melanoma incidence and "melanoma consciousness" are both high, at least 90 percent of patients live 5 years.

These are some of the signs that may signal melanoma:

- Changes in the size or color of a mole, or rapid darkening.

- Ulceration or scaliness, changes in the shape or outline of a mole, or if the mole begins to flake, ooze, or bleed.

- Changes in the way a mole feels—hard, lumpy, itchy, tender.

- Changes in the skin around a mole, such as redness or swelling.

- Erosion or scabs around a mole.

- Development of a new, pigmented lesion or bulge in a normal skin area.

Risks for Major Cancers
Multiple Myeloma

Multiple myeloma is a cancer of the plasma cells found in the marrow of the long and flat bones of the ribs, skull, legs, hips and spine. These cells normally produce immunoglobulins, or antibodies, that circulate in the blood and help to ward off disease. In multiple myeloma, the plasma cells produce either too much of a single, specific immunoglobulin or produce just part of an immunoglobulin.

Symptoms of multiple myeloma include anemia, kidney failure, increased susceptibility to infection, and bone pain and fractures. The disease is also characterized by numerous bone lesions. These lesions account for the name "multiple" myeloma and for the earlier belief that this was a bone cancer.

The most common form of multiple myeloma is secretory myeloma, in which the plasma cells secrete a normal immunoglobulin at an abnormally high level. The immunoglobulins affected are IgG and IgA, and to some extent IgD and IgE. More than half of all patients with multiple myeloma have IgG secretory myeloma.

Little is known about the causes of multiple myeloma. It is known that multiple myeloma occurs more often among aged, black men than among other U.S. population groups.

The median age of onset for multiple myeloma in this country is 68 (Young et al, 1981). It is the 13th most common type of cancer among U.S. blacks, but is ranked 19th among whites (Young et al, 1981). The incidence for black men is 9.6 cases per 100,000 and for black women, 6.7. For white men it is 4.3 and for white women, 3.0 (Young et al, 1981).

Incidence varies worldwide. Blacks in the San Francisco Bay area have the highest recorded incidence; residents of Poona, India, have the lowest (Waterhouse et al, 1982). The incidence among all Asians is generally low.

One theory to explain the predominance of multiple myeloma in older individuals is that the immune system changes with age, and plasma cells are somehow altered, increasing their likelihood of becoming cancerous (Radl et al, 1975). The risk factors associated with race and gender have not been identified, and it is not known if these risks have a genetic or environmental basis. Blacks, for

example, have higher levels of immunoglobulins than whites which suggests a possible inborn susceptibility to multiple myeloma (Blattner 1981). Men also have higher levels of immunoglobulins than do women, suggesting a possible hormonal link with the disease.

Other factors reported to be associated with multiple myeloma include some occupational exposures, ionizing radiation, genetic susceptibility and immunosuppressive diseases.

Some preliminary studies link certain occupations with the development of multiple myeloma. Male compositors working for the U.S. Government Printing Office who were exposed to lead vapors had a twofold increase in rate of death from multiple myeloma (Greene et al, 1979). An increase in multiple myeloma deaths was also seen among people who live in areas near plastics manufacturing industries (Mason, 1975). Plastics and oils have been shown to produce plasma cell cancers in mice. Farmers, wood workers, leather workers, workers exposed to arsenic, asbestos or lead, and employees of rubber and petrochemical products plants have shown an increase in multiple myeloma incidence (Blattner 1982).

One of the risk factors for multiple myeloma appears to be radiation exposure. Radiologists with long-term, low-dose exposure to X-rays have shown a threefold increase in deaths from multiple myeloma

(Matanoski et al, 1975). Atomic bomb survivors also show an increased incidence of multiple myeloma (Ichimaru et al, 1982). Radiation has an immunosuppressive effect that may favor the development of multiple myeloma and possibly other immune system disorders.

Siblings of patients with multiple myeloma have an increased risk of developing the disease; this familial relationship may be due to an inherited susceptibility (McKusick, 1978).

There is also some association between multiple myeloma and other illnesses that result in overproduction of immunoglobulins. Such illnesses include systemic lupus erythematosus, a chronic connective tissue disorder; scleroderma, a disease that causes hardening and thickening of connective tissue and skin; rheumatoid arthritis; and chronic dermatitis (Blattner 1982).

Risks for Major Cancers
Non-Hodgkin's Lymphoma

Lymphomas are cancers that affect white blood cells of the immune system. They are characterized by the abnormal growth of lymphocytes, the infection-fighting cells in the lymph nodes, spleen, and thymus. The tonsils, stomach, small intestine, and skin may also be affected. Leukemias, in contrast, are cancers of circulating white blood cells that originate in the bone marrow.

Lymphomas are usually classified as Hodgkin's disease, the most common form, or non-Hodgkin's lymphoma. There are also other rare forms of the disease such as mycosis fungoides, a primary skin lymphoma. Its appearance is often preceded by a history of chronic skin rash. Burkitt's lymphoma, rare in most of the world, is the most common childhood cancer in central Africa, and is one of the fastest growing human cancers.

The non-Hodgkin's lymphomas are among the less common cancers in the United States. Incidence generally increases with age. Among white males, incidence is about 10.7 per 100,000, and 8.2 per 100,000 among white females. Incidence among black males is about 7.2, and 4.7 among black females (Young et al, 1981). Five-year survival for both white and black patients in this country is about 43 percent (Ries, 1983). Incidence, survival, and mortality statistics both here and abroad may be difficult to interpret because different systems are used to classify these diseases.

Non-Hodgkin's lymphoma may run in families but it is not known if this is due to heredity or a shared environmental factor. Some genetically determined immune system disorders can increase the risk of developing the disease (Purtilo, 1977), but most cases of familial non-Hodgkin's lymphoma cannot be attributed to these genetic disorders. Patients with primary immune system disorders may also have a high risk of developing non-Hodgkin's lymphoma and certain other types of cancer (Gatti and Good, 1971).

Kidney transplant patients, whose immune systems are suppressed with medications, develop non-Hodgkin's lymphomas 40 to 100 times more often than expected (Fraumeni and Hoover 1977; Kinlen et al, 1979). The short latent period—onset is often within one year of the organ transplant—and the fact that transplant patients are more prone to certain viruses linked with cancer suggest that some viruses may play a role in non-Hodgkin's lymphoma (Greene, 1982).

Epstein-Barr virus (EBV) and human T-cell leukemia-lymphoma virus (HTLV) have been linked with certain rare forms of lymphoma. EBV is ubiquitous—by adulthood almost everyone has been exposed to it and has developed antibodies against it. EBV has been linked to Burkitt's lymphoma in African children. HTLV is linked with certain types of adult T-cell leukemias and lymphomas that are found mostly in southern Japan, parts of the Caribbean and Africa, and the southeastern United States. Only a few of those exposed to this virus develop cancer. Researchers believe it can only be spread by prolonged intimate contact and is not highly contagious like other viral diseases.

Occupational studies have been inconclusive. Workers exposed to the herbicides phenoxyacetic acid or chlorophenol have a higher than expected incidence of lymphomas (Hardell, 1979). Chemists also appear to have a high risk, but specific exposures have not yet been identified (Li et al, 1969; Olin and Ahlbom, 1980).

Although non-Hodgkin's lymphomas account for only a small fraction of all cancers, they are regarded as models for understanding the immune response and carcinogenesis (Greene, 1982).

Risks for Major Cancers
Oral Cavity and Pharynx

Tobacco use—smoking, chewing and dipping—is the major risk factor for cancers of the mouth and throat. Depending on the amount and type of tobacco used, there is a four- to fifteenfold greater risk of developing mouth and throat cancers for tobacco users over nonusers (Mahboubi et al, 1982).

Mouth and throat cancers are primarily squamous cell carcinomas. The most common sites are the tongue, lip, floor of the mouth, soft palate, tonsils, salivary glands and back of the throat.

More than 90 percent of all oral and pharyngeal cancers occur in individuals over age 45, and risk increases with age (Mahboubi et al, 1982).

In certain parts of India, a large proportion of both men and women chew "pan," a quid of betel leaves, nuts, tobacco and lime. Indians have the highest rates of mouth and throat cancers in the world and about 75 percent of these mouth and throat cancers can be attributed to tobacco chewing habits (Jayant et al, 1977). Indian women have a death rate from mouth and throat cancers 40 times greater than do American women (Mahboubi et al, 1982).

Mouth and throat cancers occur at a rate of 16.8 cases per 100,000 population a year among U.S.white men, 6.0 among white women, 19.3 among black men, and 7.0 among black women (Young et al, 1981).

Even though men have higher rates of mouth and throat cancers, women are also susceptible to the cancer-causing effects of tobacco use. Women in the rural south who "dip snuff" by holding a pinch of finely ground tobacco between the gum and cheek have a high risk of developing cancers of the mouth and throat (Winn et al, 1981). Snuff contains N-nitroso-nornicotine, a chemical known to cause cancer in mice (Hecht et al, 1980).

Cigarette smoking, which is highly associated with lung cancer, also increases the risk for cancers of the mouth and throat. Risk increases with increasing cigarette consumption. Heavy smokers (smoking more than one pack of cigarettes a day) are one-and-a-half times more likely than light smokers to develop mouth and throat cancers, and they have a sixfold increase in risk over nonsmokers (Graham et al, 1977).

Cancers of the mouth and throat most often develop at the site directly exposed to tobacco. Snuff-dippers develop cancers of the gum and the mucosal lining of the cheek; cigarette smokers develop more throat cancers; and pipe smokers develop more lip cancers (Smith, 1979).

Alcohol drinking has been related to an increase in risk of mouth and throat cancers. Heavy drinkers often smoke, however, and the effects of the two factors cannot always be separated. It is estimated that heavy drinkers who consume more than seven drinks a week have a doubled risk of mouth and throat cancers (Graham et al, 1977). Smoking and drinking have a synergistic effect; in most studies, the risk of mouth and throat cancers is greater for the combined factors of smoking and drinking than for the simple addition of the two (Mahboubi et al, 1982). Among those who drink at least 1.5 ounces of alcohol and smoke 40 or more cigarettes a day, there is a fifteenfold increase in risk of mouth and throat cancers (Rothman et al, 1972). Poor nutrition, possibly related to a lack of vitamins A and B, has also been linked to an increase in mouth and throat cancers.

Some early studies have linked certain occupations with the

development of mouth and throat cancers. In an Australian study, bartenders, waiters and waitresses, presumed to be exposed to tobacco smoke and alcohol on their jobs, were found to have an increased risk of mouth and throat cancers (McMichael et al, 1982). Printers (Lloyd et al, 1977), leather workers (Decoufle, 1979), paper manufacturers (Blot and Fraumeni, 1977), electronics workers (Winn et al, 1982), farmers, sailors, and outdoor workers are prone to lip cancer. There has also been some suggestion that metal, textile, and steel workers, and workers exposed to asbestos and polyvinyl chloride may have an increased risk of mouth and throat cancers (Mahboubi et al, 1982).

Ill-fitting false teeth and bridges and sharp or broken teeth that can cause irritation or infection are also associated with an increased risk of mouth cancers. But the risk seems to be higher among those who also smoke and drink (Graham et al, 1977). Some slight evidence links the daily, longterm use of mouthwash among those who neither smoke or drink with mouth and throat cancers (Blot et al, 1983).

Quitting cigarettes, pipes, and snuff would drastically reduce the incidence of cancers of the mouth and throat, but tobacco use-snuff dipping and tobacco chewing among teenagers, as well as cigarette smoking among women-appears to be increasing (Economic Research Service, 1983; Horm and Asire, 1982).

Risks for Major Cancers
Ovary

In 1983, an estimated 18,000 new cases of ovarian cancer were diagnosed in this country (Silverberg and Lubera, 1983). Although ovarian cancer ranks second in incidence among gynecologic cancers, it causes more deaths—11,000 each year—than any other cancer of the female reproductive system (Young et al, 1981).

The ovaries, two almond-sized glands containing egg cells, lie in the lower abdomen, one on each side of the uterus. By 5 months after fertilization, the ovaries of a developing female fetus already contain about 7 million egg cells, her entire life's supply. The ovaries also secrete hormones that help regulate menstruation and pregnancy.

Besides egg cells, the ovaries contain several other types of cells. Although cancer can affect any of these, 80 to 90 percent of ovarian cancers arise from the layer of epithelial cells that surround the ovary.

Epithelial cancers develop in either ovary with about equal frequency, and develop in both ovaries at once about a third of the time.

The incidence of ovarian cancer in European and North American women has increased only slightly since the 1940s. White women 40 to 50 years old living in highly industrialized countries develop the disease most often. In the United States, a woman has a 1.3 percent chance of developing ovarian cancer by age 74 (Young et al, 1981).

Childbearing is the most important known factor in preventing ovarian cancer suggesting that hormones may play a role in its development. Women who have had children are half as likely to develop ovarian cancer as women who have not; several pregnancies confer even more protection. Use of birth control pills, which create a hormonal balance similar to that found during pregnancy, may reduce the risk of ovarian cancer by 10 to 50 percent (Weiss, 1982).

Breast cancer may also increase a woman's chance of developing ovarian cancer: women with breast cancer have twice the expected risk of developing ovarian cancer. Women who already have ovarian cancer are three to four times more likely to develop breast cancer (Young et al, 1982).

Studies of Japanese women in Hiroshima exposed to atomic bomb radiation during World War II revealed almost twice the expected number of ovarian cancer cases (Beebe et al, 1977). But the X-ray doses used for diagnosis are not likely to increase a woman's chances of developing the disease (Weiss, 1982).

Exposure to asbestos has been linked to ovarian cancer risk in one study of women working in asbestos-contaminated industrial areas (Newhouse et al, 1972). Particles of asbestos have been found in normal and cancerous ovaries, as have particles of talc, a mineral related to asbestos (Henderson et al, 1972). Because mineral deposits of asbestos and talc are often found near each other it is possible that talc may become slightly contaminated with asbestos during mining. Only two studies have examined ovarian cancer risk associated with talc use in women. One study found an increased incidence in talc users (Cramer et al, 1982); the other did not (Hartge et al, 1983). Talc has not been shown to cause cancer in laboratory animals (Hildick-Smith 1976).

Risks for Major Cancers
Pancreas

Cancer of the pancreas is a "silent" disease, without symptoms, until it is advanced. Very little is known about what causes it or how to prevent it.

An organ about six inches long located behind the stomach, the pancreas has two functions: it sends insulin into the bloodstream to control the amount of sugar in the blood, and sends pancreatic juice into the intestine to help digest food. Small tubes or ducts in the organ transport the pancreatic juice and if cancer develops it is usually in these duct cells.

From 1951 to 1978, the death rates for pancreatic cancer in the United States rose almost 30 percent to about 11 deaths per 100,000 men and about 7 per 100,000 women (American Cancer Society, 1982). The incidence of pancreatic cancer among U.S. blacks is about 1.5 times higher than for whites (Young et al, 1981). Hawaiians and American Indians are also at a higher risk (Young et al, 1981). Seventh-Day Adventists and Mormons have a lower-than-average death rate (Phillips et al, 1980; Lyon et al, 1981), and Jewish men have a higher-than-average death rate (Greenwald et al, 1975). Worldwide, the United States and Northern European countries, including Great Britain, have a high incidence of pancreatic cancer. Polynesians have an extremely high incidence.

The disease is usually fatal; only 4 percent of patients live more than 3 years after diagnosis (Ries et al, 1983). The very few patients whose cancers occur in the insulin-producing cells—not the duct cells—tend to live longer; about 30 percent of these patients live more than 3 years after diagnosis (Axtell et al, 1976).

After 30, the incidence of this cancer increases in both men and women in every population studied (Mack, 1982). An excess risk has been established among cigarette smokers, although the magnitude of the risk is not so great as with lung cancer. Diabetes mellitus has been linked in some studies with pancreatic cancer but it is not known if cancer causes diabetes-like changes, or if diabetes makes individuals prone to cancer. No clear association has been found between diet and pancreatic cancer. Coffee drinking has been associated with the disease in one study but that study has not been confirmed (MacMahon et al, 1981).

Research has focused on ways to diagnose pancreatic cancer before it is advanced enough to cause symptoms. Ultrasound and CAT scans are being tried, but to date only a biopsy yields a certain diagnosis. Surgery, radiation therapy, and anticancer drugs are used to treat pancreatic cancer, but so far have had little influence on outcome. In 1975, the National Cancer Institute established the National Pancreatic Cancer Project to stimulate research on the causes, diagnosis, and treatment of the disease.

Risks for Major Cancers
Prostate

Cancer of the prostate is one of the most common cancers among United States men. Its incidence increases with age and it is chiefly a disease of men over age 65.

The prostate gland, located at the base of the penis, surrounding the urethra, produces seminal fluid. Two conditions that commonly affect it are enlargement and cancer but the two do not seem to be related to each other.

Black men in the United States have the highest incidence in the world of cancer of the prostate (Greenwald, 1982). Between 1975 and 1977, the incidence among black men in Atlanta was about 133 per 100,000, compared with about 74 per 100,000 for white men in the same city (Young et al, 1981). The high incidence of this cancer among blacks has occurred only in the last few decades, suggesting that social factors, rather than genetic factors, are responsible (Ernster et al, 1978).

Cancer of the prostate is also common in northwest Europe. Incidence is lower in the Near East and in parts of Africa and South America. The lowest incidence occurs in Japan.

Studies of migrating populations have suggested that environmental factors, such as diet and lifestyle, play an important role in the risk of developing cancer of the prostate. Prostatic cancer incidence and fat intake are higher among Japanese in Hawaii than in Japan, for example (Kato et al, 1973; Waterhouse et al, 1976).

Mormons who do not use tobacco, alcohol, coffee, or tea for religious reasons, but whose fat consumption is similar to that of other white males in the United States, have about the same risk of cancer of the prostate as other white men. It is the most common type of cancer among Mormons (Enstrom, 1978).

Prostate growth and function depend on the hormone testosterone, formed in the testicles. It is possible that diet affects the production of sex hormones, and that this may then affect the risk for cancer of the prostate (Graham et al, 1983).

Cancer of the prostate, as well as cancers of the colon, rectum, and female breast, may be associated with dietary fat intake (Wynder et al, 1971; Carroll and Khor 1975; Berg, 1975). Cancer of the prostate has been linked with the consumption of animal fat and protein among several ethnic groups in Hawaii (Kolonel et al, 1981).

Workplace exposures to cadmium during welding, electroplating, and the production of alkaline batteries may increase the risk of cancer of the prostate. Dietary exposures to cadmium, from oysters for example, do not seem to increase risk (Kolonel and Winkelstein, 1977). Workers in the rubber industry may also be at increased risk (Tyroler et al, 1976).

Thus, the causes of cancer of the prostate are unclear, so there are no known methods of prevention. The possible role of diet and of workplace carcinogens are now being studied.

893

Skin Cancer (Nonmelanoma)

Nonmelanoma skin cancer is the most common cancer among whites in the United States. Since most nonmelanoma skin cancer patients are treated in doctors' offices, population-based estimates of skin cancer incidence are fairly difficult to obtain. Estimates are, though, that more than 400,000 new cases of nonmelanoma skin cancer occur in the United States each year, and that this number is rising (Fears and Scotto, 1982). Although the death rate from nonmelanoma skin cancer is about 1 percent, as many persons died from this cancer in the 1950s and 1960s, for example, as from the rarer, but more lethal, skin melanoma (Mason et al, 1975).

The incidence of nonmelanoma skin cancer varies directly with exposure to ultraviolet (UV) light from the sun and indirectly with the degree of skin pigmentation. Thus, nonmelanoma skin cancer is most common among fair-skinned whites who live in sunny locales. The highest rates in the past have been recorded among Caucasians in South Africa and Australia. Even Ireland, despite its rain and mist, has had a high incidence because of the susceptibility of persons of Celtic ancestry (Urbach, 1971).

Nonmelanoma skin cancer occurs less often in Orientals, and least often among blacks. In the United States, for example, a 1977-78 National Cancer Institute survey (Scotto et al, 1981) showed that the age-adjusted incidence was only 3.4 per 100,000 among blacks, compared with 232.6 among whites.

Most nonmelanoma skin cancers are of two types, squamous cell carcinoma and basal cell carcinoma. The basal cell type is more common, but the squamous cell type is more invasive, and may account for about three-fourths of all deaths from nonmelanoma skin cancer (Dunn et al, 1965).

Based on the 1977-78 U.S. skin cancer survey, basal cell cancer occurs about 1 to 2 times more often in white men than in white women, and squamous cell cancer occurs two to three times more often in men. Both types occur most often on the face, head and neck. Women have higher rates than men for both types of cancers on the legs, in line with their greater sun exposure, while men have more squamous cell carcinoma of the lip, in line with their risks from tobacco and outdoor work (Lindqvist, 1979).

When skin cancer incidence is plotted for U.S. cities according to annual UV-B measurements, the direct relationship is most clearly seen with squamous cell cancer and increasing radiation (Scotto and Fraumeni, 1982). Basal cell cancer incidence also reflects the increase in radiation. Melanoma incidence follows it least sharply. This is consistent with the evidence that factors other than sunlight also contribute to the development of melanoma (Greene and Fraumeni, 1979).

Thus the chief risk factor for nonmelanoma skin cancer is exposure to nonionizing UV radiation, most probably the UV-B portion of sunlight radiation, and evidence suggests that the risk increases with the annual dose (Fears and Scotto, 1983). Possible depletion of the protective ozone layer by the fluorocarbons used in aerosol propellants, refrigerators, and air conditioners is a matter of some concern.

There are other risk factors for nonmelanoma skin cancers. They were, for example, the first type of cancer related to ionizing radiation, with reports as early as 1902 among radiation workers. Other studies have shown an excess risk associated with radiotherapy for a number of diseases. Excess risks have also been noted among radiologists and uranium miners. Radiologists were at one time exposed to X-rays from their own equipment, and uranium miners were exposed to radon daughters, the radioactive products of uranium ores.

A number of chemicals induce skin cancers, particularly squamous cell carcinomas in animals, and epidemiologic studies substantiate their risk in humans. Polycyclic aromatic hydrocarbons induce cancers in animals and are found in coal tars, pitch, asphalt, soot, creosotes, and lubricating and cutting oils. Skin and other forms of cancer have been found in various worker groups exposed to these substances. A recent study has shown an excess risk of skin cancer among psoriasis patients treated with crude tar ointments (Stern, 1980).

Psoralens, which render skin more sensitive to light, have also been used in combination with ultraviolet light A (PUVA) for psoriasis patients, and an excess risk of skin cancer has been seen among these individuals also (Stern et al, 1979). This study has increased concern about the possible hazards of other photosensitizers found in tanning aids, cosmetics, and medicines.

Squamous cell skin cancer has also been found as a complication of tropical ulcers, burns, scars, and chronic infections and wounds (Malik et al, 1974). This complication has been seen chiefly among dark-skinned populations in Africa and Asia, but recent studies of black Americans have indicated that burn scars or chronic infections may predispose them to skin cancer. Actinic keratoses—brownish, hardened areas on skin exposed to excess sunlight—are considered to be precursor lesions for squamous cell skin cancer. Individuals with several rare hereditary diseases-including multiple basal cell carcinoma syndrome, xeroderma pigmentosum, and albinism—are also at heightened risk of skin cancers.

Avoiding overexposure to sunlight is the chief way to prevent nonmelanoma skin cancer. It is also important to avoid unnecessary X-rays and ultraviolet light exposure from artificial sources like sunlamps and tanning booths.

Stomach

In the 1930s, stomach cancer was the leading cause of cancer death among U.S. men, and the third leading cause among U.S. women after cancers of the uterus and breast. Since then, there has been a dramatic decrease in stomach cancer death rates in both sexes. The death rate decreased about 60 percent between 1951 and 1978, and today, U.S. death rates for stomach cancer are among the lowest in the world (American Cancer Society, 1982).

Despite the decrease, stomach cancer is still a major problem. About 25,000 new cases of stomach cancer were expected in the U.S. in 1983 (American Cancer Society, 1982), but only about 13 percent of these patients will live for 5 years after diagnosis (Ries et al, 1983). Stomach cancer has had one of the poorer 5-year survival rates of any type of cancer in the U.S. (Ries, et al, 1983). One reason is that it may not be detected until an advanced stage, when it has spread to other parts of the body.

Japan, Chile, Costa Rica, Colombia, Singapore, and Iceland are among the countries with high death rates from stomach cancer. In Japan, stomach cancer causes more deaths than all other types of cancers combined, and it is five times more common than in the U.S. When Japanese move to the United States, though, their stomach cancer rates decrease over successive generations.

Migrant studies and the marked decrease in U.S. death rates suggest that environmental factors play a dominant role. The widespread use of refrigeration since the 1930s may be partly responsible for the reduced rates. Refrigeration reduced the need for some other methods of food preservation and gave Americans access to fresh fruits and vegetables year-round. International surveys have shown an association between stomach cancer and large amounts of pickled, salted or smoked foods in the diet (Nomura, 1982). Other studies suggest that stomach cancer patients eat fewer servings of foods rich in vitamins C and A than do control subjects (Correa et al, 1982). Persons with diseases that affect the stomach lining, such as pernicious anemia and atrophic gastritis, have a higher risk of developing stomach cancer than the general population (Correa, 1982), but gastric ulcers have not been consistently associated with stomach cancer.

Nitrosamines are potent carcinogens that can form in the stomach. When nitrates, a family of chemicals found in some water supplies and in some green vegetables, cured meats, and cheeses, combine with bacteria in the mouth, different compounds known as nitrites may form. The nitrites, in turn, combine with components of some foods, drugs, and other substances to form carcinogenic nitrosamines. Vitamin C appears to be a natural defense against nitrosamines by preventing their formation in the body. Studies in several countries have shown that eating fresh fruits and vegetables containing vitamin C reduces the risk of stomach cancer (Nomura, 1982).

There may be other environmental and lifestyle factors involved. Studies in Connecticut, Hawaii, Norway, Iceland, and Japan have consistently shown that low socioeconomic status is associated with stomach cancer (Nomura, 1982). An association with cigarette smoking has also been suggested (Haenszel et al, 1972; Hammond, 1966). Evidence that radiation may increase risk comes from studies of atomic bomb survivors in Japan and of patients treated with X-rays for a spinal disorder.

Evidence for a genetic component comes from studies suggesting that blood type A, an inherited trait, may be a marker for increased risk (Nomura, 1982). Other research shows that relatives of persons who have stomach cancer have a risk two to three times higher than the general population (Nomura, 1982). Families tend to share the same environment, though, so it is difficult to distinguish between genetic and environmental influences.

Reducing the amounts of pickled, salted, or smoked foods, and of nitrates consumed, may reduce the risk of stomach cancer. A diet rich in fresh fruits and vegetables may also help reduce risk.

Risks for Major Cancers

Testes

American men have only a 0.3 percent chance of developing testicular cancer in their lifetimes (Young et al, 1981). But among young white men aged 20 to 34, testicular cancer is the most common form of cancer accounting for 22 percent of all cancers in this age group. It is the second most common cancer among men aged 35 to 39, and the third most common among young men aged 15 to 19 (Schottenfeld and Warshauer 1982).

The testes are small, oval glands that produce sperm and testosterone, the male hormone. The testes form in the abdominal cavity early in fetal development and usually descend to the scrotal sac before birth.

Almost all testicular cancers are germ cell cancers; the most common of these are a particular type called seminomas (Schottenfeld and Warshauer, 1982). The germ cells are the sperm-forming cells of the testes.

Men in rural Vaud, Switzerland, have the highest incidence of testicular cancer in the world with 10.5 cases per 100,000 (standardized to world population) a year; Cuban men have the lowest incidence, near zero (Waterhouse, 1982).

Among U.S. white men, the incidence is 3.6 cases per 100,000 a year. This is over four times the rate (0.8) for U.S. blacks (Young et al, 1981). The incidence of testicular cancer among Hispanics, native Americans and Asians lies between those of white and black men.

The death rate from testicular cancer among U.S. white men aged 20 to 29 declined about 40 percent between 1973 and 1978 even though the incidence for this high-risk group increased slightly during this time period (Li et al, 1982). The reasons for the upward trend in incidence are not clear, but the decline in deaths is due mainly to the increase in survival brought about by advances intesticular cancer treatment. The outlook for men with seminomas found early is very good.

Little is understood about the causes of testicular cancer but men aged 20 to 34 years are at the greatest risk. Possible risk factors are congenital abnormalities, hormonal drugs, and trauma.

Testicular and genital abnormalities have both been associated with testicular cancer. Cryptorchidism, failure of the testes to descend into the scrotal sac, is thought to account for one in 10 cases of testicular cancer (Shottenfeld and Warshauer, 1982). Studies have also linked inguinal hernia in children with adult onset of testicular cancer (Morrison, 1976). There is some evidence that these hernias are due to incomplete descent of the testes, so they should not be considered separately from cryptorchidism (Coldman et al, 1982). Other conditions associated with testicular cancer include some rare genetic abnormalities (like Klinefelter's syndrome, hermaphroditism and Turner's syndrome); gonadal aplasia, or failure of the gonads to develop; hypospadias, a condition in which the urethra opens on the underside of the penis; and mixed gonadal dysgenesis, a condition in which there is one developed testis plus nonfunctional female genitalia (Schottenfeld and Warshauer 1982).

Both the hormone estrogen and the synthetic estrogen diethylstilbestrol (DES) injected into pregnant mice can cause testicular abnormalities in male offspring (Henderson et al, 1979) DES exposure before birth has been linked to vaginal cancer in daughters, and to testicular abnormalities in sons of women who took it to prevent miscarriages (DES Task Force, 1978). If DES or estrogens increase the risk for testicular cancer in men is not yet clear.

Other factors that may be related to increased risk of testicular cancer are maternal bleeding during pregnancy and history of stillbirths (Swerdlow et al, 1982).

A recent study suggested that teenage participation in sports like bicycling and horseback riding may be associated with testicular cancer, but more study is needed before it can be concluded that the risk observed is a real one. The study also did not yield evidence that might explain the possible association.

Scientists have speculated from time to time that trauma might somehow increase a man's risk of testicular cancer but no studies to date have shown a definite association.

There is some contradictory evidence concerning testicular cancer and socioeconomic status. Some studies have found that those with high income and high education are two-and-a-half times more likely to develop testicular cancer than those with less income and education (Schottenfeld and Warshauer 1982). There is also some evidence that men from rural areas have higher rates of testicular cancer than city dwellers (Graham et al, 1977).

An association between exposure to viral disease like mumps orchitis and adult onset of testicular cancer has not been proved although an early case report in the 1940s suggested such a risk (Gilbert, 1944).

Risks for Major Cancers
Urinary Tract

Urinary tract cancers account for 9 percent of the new cancer cases diagnosed each year in men and 4 percent of those in women (Silverberg and Lubera, 1983). The two most common urinary tract cancers are bladder cancer and kidney cancer. The estimated 38,500 cases of bladder cancer that Americans developed in 1983 make it the 6th most common cancer in this country. Kidney cancer estimated to occur in 18,200 Americans in 1983, ranks 11th in cancer incidence.

Besides the two kidneys, the urinary tract includes the ureters that carry urine from the kidneys to the bladder, the bladder and the urethra, a tube that carries urine from the bladder. This system of organs eliminates liquid waste products and helps maintain stable chemical conditions in the fluid that surrounds body cells.

Bladder

In the United States, bladder cancer is chiefly adisease of white men over age 65. The incidence of 27 cases per 100,000 population among white men is twice the incidence among nonwhite men. There is little racial difference in incidence among women, who develop bladder cancer less than a third as often as men do (Young et al, 1981).

From the late 1940s to the early 1970s, the incidence of bladder cancer declined 21 percent for white women and 38 percent for nonwhite women. At the same time, it increased 24 percent for white men and doubled for nonwhite men (Devesa and Silverman, 1978).

Around the world, bladder cancer occurs most often in the United States and Europe and least often in Asia (Waterhouse et al, 1982).

The most important known risk factor for bladder cancer is cigarette smoking. Cigarette smokers develop bladder cancer two to three times more often than nonsmokers, and areas in the United States where cigarette sales are high also have high death rates from bladder cancer (Morrison and Cole, 1982). Smoking is estimated to be responsible for about 40 percent of the bladder cancers among men and 29 percent among women (Cole et al, 1971).

As early as 1895, workers in the dyestuffs industry showed a high risk of bladder cancer that was later associated with exposure to aromatic amines, a class of compounds used to make dyes (Rehn, 1895). Two of these chemicals, benzidine and 2-naphthylamine, are now known to be potent bladder carcinogens (Case, 1954). Workers in the rubber and leather industries also have an increased risk of developing bladder cancer. Occupations in which workers are suspected of having an elevated bladder cancer risk include painter, chemical worker, printer, metal worker, hairdresser, textile worker, machinist (Morrison and Cole, 1982) and truck driver (Silverman et al, 1983).

The possible risk of bladder cancer associated with widely used artificial sweeteners received much attention when the Food and Drug Administration removed cyclamates from the market in 1969. It was later reported that the sweetener saccharin caused bladder cancer in male laboratory rats when the animals were exposed to the chemicals before birth (Arnold et al, 1977). But recent epidemiological studies show that, overall, people who use artificial sweeteners do not appear to have a higher incidence of bladder cancer than non-users (Morrison and Buring, 1980; Hoover et a], 1980).

Although early studies showed a possible link between bladder cancer and coffee drinking, recent studies based on large numbers of individuals found little or no increase in bladder cancer incidence among coffee drinkers compared with those who do not drink coffee (Morrison et al, 1982; Hartge et al, 1983).

Other factors that may contribute to the development of bladder cancer are bladder infection with the parasitic fluke *Schistisoma haematobium*, treatment with the anticancer drugs chlornaphazine or cyclophosphamide and long-term use of pain killers containing the drug phenacetin (Morrison and Cole, 1982).

Kidney

About 85 percent of the kidney cancers diagnosed in this country are renal cell cancers. Cancer of the renal pelvis, the inner part of the kidney connected to the ureter accounts for most of the remaining 15 percent.

The incidence of renal cell cancer among white men, 9.4 cases per 100,000 population, is nearly the same as for black men, 8.7 per 100,000. Renal cell cancer occurs twice as often in men as it does in women, and develops most often in both sexes in persons over age 60 (Young et al, 1981).

Worldwide, the incidence of kidney cancer is high in North America and low in Asia (Waterhouse et al, 1982).

As with bladder cancer cigarette smoking is the most important known risk factor for kidney cancer. Smokers are twice as likely as nonsmokers to develop kidney cancer (Wynder et al, 1974; McLaughlin et al, 1984). One estimate is that 30 percent of kidney cancers in men and 24 percent in women are caused by cigarette smoking (McLaughlin et al, 1984).

Among women, obesity, or factors associated with it, appears to be a risk factor for kidney cancer (Wynder et al, 1974; McLaughlin et al, in press). Because fatty tissue can convert other hormones into estrogen, obese women may have high levels of this hormone (MacDonald and Siiteri, 1974; Schindler et al, 1972). The higher-than-expected incidence of kidney cancer among obese women could be due to excess estrogen levels. There have been few studies of occupational risk factors for kidney cancer. Workers exposed to insulation fibers such as asbestos and workers in the petroleum industry show an elevated incidence of kidney cancer (Selikoff et al, 1979; Thomas et al, 1982).

Although cancer of the renal pelvis is a fairly rare form of kidney cancer one study reported that approximately 82 percent of the cases among men and 61 percent among women could be prevented if people stopped smoking (McLaughlin et al, 1983). Other factors that may increase the risk of cancer of the renal pelvis are the long-term use of pain relievers containing phenacetin or acetaminophen (McLaughlin et al, 1983; Morrison and Cole, 1982).

Risks for Major Cancers
Uterine Cervix

Cancer of the uterine cervix, or cervical cancer has been studied extensively, but no one cause has yet been found for it. A number of factors appear to contribute to risk.

The incidence of invasive cancer of the uterine cervix and mortality from it have been declining steadily in this country for the past three decades. The incidence is still almost 2 times higher in U.S. black women than in whites, though, and the mortality is still almost three times higher in blacks, despite the declines in both groups.

901

The uterine cervix is the small cylindrical neck that leads from the uterus, or womb, into the vagina. A knob of the cervix protrudes into the vagina and can be seen during physical examination. Cell samples are taken from this part of the cervix for the Pap smear test used to detect changes in cell structure that may lead to cancer.

Researchers think that these cell changes, or dysplasias, may precede carcinoma *in situ*, or CIS, which may then develop into invasive cancer of the cervix. This has not been proved, though.

An argument for this relationship is that invasive cervical cancer occurs most often among women over age 50, and carcinoma *in situ* occurs most often among women 25 to 34 years old (Young et al, 1981). Also, the incidence of invasive cervical cancer has been decreasing while CIS incidence has risen. This might mean that Pap smears are detecting more carcinomas *in situ* and that treating these has prevented the development of invasive cervical cancer. Part of the decrease seen in cervical cancer incidence, though, might be due to the large number of hysterectomies–removal of the uterus and cervix–performed in the older age groups.

In carcinoma *in situ*, an outer layer of normal cells has been replaced by cancer cells. It is about 95 percent treatable and curable. In invasive cancer of the cervix, the cancer cells have invaded the underlying tissue of the cervix.

Whether or not CIS and invasive cervical cancer are part of a continuum representing stages, or degrees of cancer the risk factors appear to be similar.

The two major risks are multiple sex partners and early age at first intercourse. Early first intercourse is thought to be risky because the tissue of the cervix changes during puberty and may thus be more sensitive or vulnerable in young women. One study separated age at first intercourse from number of partners and found number of partners was more important (Harris et al, 1980). Frequency of intercourse with one partner does not appear to influence risk (Rotkin, 1967; Wynder et al, 1954).

There is also some suspicion that cervical cancer may be associated with venereal disease. This suspicion has been strengthened by the finding that increased levels of antibodies to genital herpes virus have been found in some women with cervical cancer, indicating that they were exposed to herpes. Papilloma virus and Chlamydia, which cause genitourinary warts and infections in both men and women, are also being looked at in this connection.

Type of contraception is related to cervical cancer incidence; more cervical cancer is seen among women who use oral contraceptives, less among those who use barrier methods. This may be because barrier methods protect against venereal infection, or because women who use oral contraceptives may be more sexually active.

The circumcision status of the man has been found not to be a risk factor.

Smoking is a risk factor although how it might be related biologically is unclear.

The effects of nutrition on risk are not well established. Intake of foods high in retinol and carotene has been found to exert a protective effect against some squamous cell tumors (the type that accounts for most cervical cancer), and two other studies have suggested that vitamin C and folicin–one of the B complex vitamins–are associated with decreased risk of cervical dysplasia and CIS.

Overall, the evidence suggests that cervical cancer is caused by a number of agents, not just one. The National Cancer Institute (Brinton et al) is now doing a case control study of 2,000 women–500 with CIS, 500 with cervical cancer and 1,000 controls–in Birmingham, Miami, Philadelphia, Chicago, and Denver that may help to shed more light on the causes of cervical cancer.

Risks for Major Cancers
Uterine Corpus (Endometrium)

Cancer of the uterine corpus, or endometrial cancer is the third most common cancer among U.S. women and accounts for about 9 percent of all cancers in American women (Young et al, 1981).

The uterus is a pear-shaped organ that lies in the abdomen between the bladder and the rectum. It consists of the cervix, the opening of the uterus into the vagina, and the corpus, sometimes called the body or womb. The corpus is composed of two layers of tissue. The spongy inside layer the endometrium, proliferates between menses and is shed during menstruation if fertilization has not occurred. The outside layer the myometrium, is a muscle capable of expanding during pregnancy to accommodate a growing fetus. Female sex hormones, including estrogen, prepare the uterus for pregnancy. Because most cancers of this site originate in the endometrium, cancer of the uterine corpus is usually referred to as endometrial cancer (Young et al, 1981).

After a large increase in the incidence of endometrial cancer in the 1970s, both the incidence and the death rate are now dropping (Austin et al, 1982). In U.S. white women, the annual incidence is 29.9 cases per 100,000, one of the highest in the world, and in U.S. black women, it is 14.6 (Young et al,

1981). Most women diagnosed with endometrial cancer are around age 60; the median age for white women is 61 and for black women, 64 (Young et al, 1981).

Some of the risk factors for endometrial cancer are the same as those for breast cancer; women at increased risk of developing breast cancer are also at increased risk of endometrial cancer. These risk factors include obesity, few or no children, early menarche, late age at menopause, and high socioeconomic status (de Waard, 1982). Most of the risk factors for endometrial cancer may be related to hormonal imbalances, especially excess estrogen production (Elwood et al, 1977).

Obesity has long been recognized as a risk factor for endometrial cancer. Obese women are twice as likely to develop endometrial cancer as women of normal weight, and this risk increases with increasing weight (Elwood et al, 1977). There is also some evidence that obese women who are tall (5 feet 7 inches and over) are at even greater risk (Elwood et al, 1977). Both diabetes and high blood pressure have also been associated with increased risk of endometrial cancer but as both illnesses are related to obesity, it is not clear if these are separate risk factors (de Waard, 1982).

Multiple births decrease risk. Women who have four or more children are one-third as likely to develop endometrial cancer as women who have no children

(Elwood et al, 1977). Women who have never had children, particularly women with a history of infertility, are at greatest risk. Studies of women with Stein-Leventhal syndrome, a rare illness characterized by multiple ovarian cysts, excessive estrogen production, and infertility, are helping scientists define possible reasons for the observed reproductive associations (de Waard, 1982).

Women of high socioeconomic status have an increased risk of developing endometrial cancer; diet and lifestyle may be contributing factors (de Waard, 1982).

Estrogen replacement therapy has been linked to endometrial cancer. Postmenopausal women who use estrogens are estimated to have a six- to seven-fold increase in risk (Antunes et al, 1979). The risk increases with increasing duration of use and dosage of replacement estrogens (Antunes et al, 1979). The use of estrogens for treatment of menopausal symptoms increased until about 1975, when their use decreased after reports associating menopausal estrogen with endometrial cancer (Jick et al, 1979). There was a subsequent decrease in endometrial cancer incidence (Austin et al, 1982).

Obesity has been linked to estrogen imbalance and there is a strong association between high levels of estrogen and development of endometrial cancer. Obese women, particularly after menopause, have higher levels of estrogens in their blood than women of normal weight. It is thought that this estrogen is produced in the excess fatty tissue (de Waard, 1982).

Recent evidence shows that use of birth control pills may decrease the risk of developing endometrial cancer (CDC, 1983). Women who use combination pills containing both estrogen and progesterone in each pill for at least one year have only half the risk of endometrial cancer as women who use other types of birth control pills or none. "Sequential" pills, for instance, which contain a series of 16 estrogen and five progesterone pills, appear to double the risk of endometrial cancer (CDC, 1983). The longer a woman takes the combination pill, the more this protection increases (Hulka et al, 1982). Childless women are protected even further by this pill and are two-and-a-half times less likely to develop endometrial cancer (Hulka et al, 1982).

Glossary

Age-adjusted. Cancer risk increases significantly with age. As the proportion of older individuals increases in any population, so, too, does the overall number of cancer cases. Data are age-adjusted mathematically to compare statistics over time in a given population, or to compare statistics among countries with different age proportions.

Benign. Not life-threatening.

Biopsy. Removal and examination, usually microscopic, of tissue or other material from the living body for purposes of diagnosis.

Carcinogen. Any cancer-causing substance or agent.

Cocarcinogen. Any agent that increases or augments the effect of a carcinogen.

Carcinoma. A cancer that arises in the epithelial cells that cover external and internal body surfaces.

Case-control studies. Those that compare data on individuals with an illness (cases) with apparently similar healthy individuals (controls), matched by age, sex, and other factors, in an effort to define risk factors for an illness.

Cohort. Any group of individuals selected for study.

Epidemiology. A science dealing with relationships of various factors that determine frequency, distribution and possible causes of a disease in a human community.

Incidence. New cases of a specific disease occurring during a certain period, usually expressed as new cases per 100,000 population per year.

Initiator. A substance or agent that can start the process of carcinogenesis.

Inverse association. Opposite in order or effect to that which is under consideration.

Latency or latent period. The incubation period of a disease, from exposure to disease development.

Lesion. Any morbid change in the structure of organs or parts.

Leukemia. Cancer of the blood-forming organs.

Lymphoma. A cancer that arises in lymph tissue.

Malignant. Tending or threatening to produce death; opposed to benign.

Metastasis. Spread of cancer cells from a primary tumor to sites elsewhere in the body.

Morbidity. Illness.

Mortality. Number of deaths occurring during a certain period, usually expressed as number of deaths per 100,000 population per year.

Mutagen. A chemical or physical agent that induces permanent, transmissible genetic change.

NCHS. National Center for Health Statistics. A Federal agency, part of the U.S. Public Health Service, that collects and analyzes data on health and disease.

Neoplasm. Any new tissue growth.

Population-based. Disease incidence and mortality data, for example, based on the exact count of a population in a given geographic location.

Promoter. A substance or agent that completes the carcinogenic process after initiation.

Precursor. Forerunner; sign or indication that precedes.

Predispose. To dispose or incline beforehand; to give a tendency to.

Prognosis. Forecast of the course of a disease; outlook for it.

Prospective. Describing a study that begins with a present status of individuals in a particular group and periodically reviews their status as time goes by.

Relative risk. A measure of the risk of disease in an exposed group compared with the risk in an unexposed group. A relative risk of 1.0 means risks in the two groups are the same. If, for example, risk is double for an exposed population, the relative risk is 2.

Retrospective. Describing a study that tries to ascertain data based on past events.

Risk/benefit. The relation between the risks and the benefits of a given treatment or procedure.

Sarcoma. A cancer that arises in connective and skeletal tissue, i.e. muscle, bone.

SEER. The National Cancer Institute's Surveillance, Epidemiology, and End Results program, begun in 1973. It monitors annual cancer incidence and survival in the United States. The original registries were made up of a 10 percent nonrandom sample of the population, representing diverse population subgroups. In 1983, SEER was expanded to represent 12 percent of the population in six states, four metropolitan areas, and Puerto Rico.

Survival. Usually expressed as a ratio: those who survive a disease per number of persons diagnosed with the disease in a given time period.

Synergism. Cooperative effects of two agents giving a total effect greater than the sum of the two effects taken independently.

USBC. U.S. Bureau of the Census. Census population counts are used for incidence and mortality rates and for the U.S. standard population.

References

Adamson RH, Sieber SM: Antineoplastic agents as potential carcinogens. *In* Origins of Human Cancer (Hiatt HH, Watson JD, Winsten JA, eds). Cold Spring Harbor Conferences on Cell Proliferation, pp 429–443, 1977.

Albores-Saavedra J, Alcantara-Vazquez A, Cruz-Ortiz H et al: The precursor lesions of invasive gallbladder carcinoma. Hyperplasia, atypical hyperplasia and carcinoma *in situ*. Cancer 45:919–927, 1980.

American Cancer Society: Cancer Facts and Figures, 1983. New York: ACS, 1982.

American Cancer Society: Cancer Facts and Figures, 1984. New York: ACS, 1983.

Antunes CMF, Stolley PD, Rosenshein NB et al: Endometrial cancer and estrogen use: Report of a large case-control study. N Engl J Med 300(1):9–13, 1979.

Archer VE, Gillam JD, Wagoner JK: Respiratory disease mortality among uranium miners. Ann NY Acad Sci 271:280–293, 1976.

Armstrong BK, Doll R: Environmental factors and cancer incidence and mortality in different countries, with special reference to dietary practices. Int J Cancer 15:617–631, 1975.

Arnold DL, Moodie CA, Grice HC et al: Long-term toxicity of orthotoluene sulfonamide and sodium saccharin in the rat. An interim report. Ottawa, Canada: National Health and Welfare Ministry, 1977.

Austin DF, Roe KM: The decreasing incidence of endometrial cancer: Public health implications. Am J of Public Health 72(1):65–68, 1982.

Axtell LM, Asire AJ, Myers MH, eds: Cancer Patient Survival: Report No. 5. DHEW Publ No. (NIH) 77-992. Washington, D.C.: U.S. Govt Print Off, 1976.

Beasley RP: Hepatitis B virus as the etiologic agent in hepatocellular carcinoma, epidemiologic considerations. Hepatology 2:218–268, 1982.

Beasley RP, Lin CC: Hepatoma risk among HBsAg Carriers. Am J Epidemiol 108:247, 1978.

Beebe GW, Kato H, Land CE: Mortality experience of atomic bomb survivors, 1950–74. Life Span Study, Report 8. Radiation Effects Research Foundation TR1–77, 1977.

Beebe GW, Kato H, Land CE: Studies of the mortality of A-bomb survivors. 6. Mortality and radiation dose, 1950–1974. Radiat Res 75:138–201, 1978.

BEIR. Advisory Committee on the Biological Effects of Ionizing Radiations (The BEIR Report). National Academy of Sciences-National Research Council. The Effects on Populations of Exposure to Low Levels of Ionizing Radiation. Washington, D.C.: U.S. Govt Print Off, 1972, 1980.

Berg JW: Can nutrition explain the pattern of international epidemiology of hormone-dependent cancers? Cancer Res 35:3345–3350, 1975.

Berg JW: The incidence of multiple primary cancers. I. Development of further cancers in patients with lymphomas, leukemias and myeloma. J Natl Cancer Inst 38:741, 1967.

Berk PD, Goldberg JD et al: Increased incidence of acute leukemia in polycythemia vera associated with chlorambucil therapy. N Engl J Med 304:441–447, 1981.

Bibbo M, Haenszel WM, Wied GL et al: A twenty-five-year follow-up study of women exposed to diethylstilbestrol during pregnancy. N Engl J Med 298:763–767, 1978.

Biggar RJ, Henle W, Fleisher G: Primary Epstein-Barr virus infections in African infants. 1. Decline of maternal antibodies and time of infection. Int J Cancer 22:239–243, 1978.

Bingham S, William TR, Cole TJ et al: Dietary fibre and regional large-bowel cancer mortality in Britain. Br J Cancer 40:456–463, 1979.

Bithell JF, Stewart AM: Pre-natal irradiation and childhood malignancy: A review of British data from the Oxford Survey. Br J Cancer 31:271–287, 1975.

Bjelke E: Dietary factors and the epidemiology of cancer of the stomach and large bowel. *In* Aktuelle Probleme der Klinischen Diatetik, Supplement zu "Aktuelle Ernahrungsmedizin." Stuttgart: George Thieme Verlag, 1978, pp. 10–17.

Blattner WA, et al: Geneology of cancer in a family. JAMA 241:259–261, 1979.

Blattner WA: Multiple myeloma and macroglobulinemia. *In* Cancer Epidemiology and Prevention (Schottenfeld D and Fraumeni JF Jr, eds). Philadelphia: W.B. Saunders, 1982, pp 795–811.

Blot WJ, Davies JE, Brown LM, Nordwall CW, Buiatti E, Ng A, Fraumeni JF Jr: Occupation and high risks of lung cancer in northeast Florida. Cancer 50:364–371, 1982.

Blot WJ, Fraumeni JF Jr: Cancer among shipyard workers. Banbury Rpt 9:37–49, 1981.

Blot WJ, Fraumeni JF Jr: Geographic patterns of oral cancer in the United States: Etiologic implications. J Chron Dis 30:745–757, 1977.

Blot WJ, Fraumeni JF Jr, Stone BJ: Geographic patterns of breast cancer in the United States. J Natl Cancer Inst 59:1407–1411, 1977.

Blot WJ, Fraumeni JF Jr, Stone BJ, McKay FW: Geographic patterns of large-bowel cancer in the United States. J Natl Cancer Inst 57:1225–1231, 1976.

Blot WJ, Harrington JM, Toledo A et al: Lung cancer after employment in shipyards during World War II. N Engl J Med 299:620–624, 1978.

Blot WJ, Morris LE, Stroube R et al: Lung and pharyngeal cancers in relation to shipyard employment in coastal Virginia. J Natl Cancer Inst 65:571–575, 1980.

Blot WJ, Winn DM, Fraumeni JF Jr: Oral cancer and mouthwash. J Natl Cancer Inst 70:251–253, 1983.

Blumberg BS, London T: Hepatitis B virus: Pathogenesis and prevention of primary cancer of the liver. Cancer 50:2657–2665, 1982.

Boice JD Jr, Greene MH, Killen JY et al: Leukemia following treatment with methyl-CCNU for gastrointestinal cancers. N Engl J Med 309:1079–1084, 1983.

Boice JD Jr, Land CE. Ionizing Radiation. In Cancer Epidemiology and Prevention (Schottenfeld D, Fraumeni JF Jr, eds). Philadelphia: W.B. Saunders 1982, pp 231–253.

Boice JD Jr, Land CE, Shore RE et al: Risk of breast cancer following low-dose radiation exposure. Radiology 131:589–597, 1979.

Boice JD Jr, Monson RR: Breast cancer in women after repeated fluoroscopic examinations of the chest. J Natl Cancer Inst 59:823–832, 1977.

Brian DD, Tilley BC, Labarthe DR et al: Breast cancer in DES-exposed mothers. Absence of an association. Mayo Clin Proc 55:89–93, 1980.

Brinton, LA, Blot WJ, Becker JA et al: A case-control study of cancers of the nasal cavity and paranasal sinuses. Am J Epidemiol 119:896–906, 1984.

Brinton LA, Hoover RN et al: Menopausal estrogen use and risk of breast cancer. Cancer 47:2517–2521, 1981.

Brinton LA, Hoover RN, Szklo M et al: Oral contraceptives and breast cancer. Int J Epidemiol 11:316–322, 1982.

Brinton LA, Stone BJ, Blot WJ, Fraumeni JF Jr: A death certificate analysis of nasal cancer among furniture workers in North Carolina. Cancer Res 37:3473–3474, 1977.

Buell P: Relative impact of smoking and air pollution on lung cancer. Arch Environ Health 15:291–297, 1967.

Cantor KP, Hoover R, Mason TJ, et al: Associations of cancer mortality with halomethanes in drinking water. J Natl Cancer Inst 61:979–985, 1978.

Carroll KK, Khor HT: Dietary fat in relation to tumorigenesis. In Lipids and Tumors (Carroll KK, ed). Progr Biochem Pharmacol, Vol 10. Basel: Karger, 1975, pp 308–353.

Case RAM, Hosker ME, McDonald DB et al: Tumors of the urinary bladder in workmen engaged in the manufacture and use of certain dyestuff intermediates in the British chemical industry. Br J Ind Med 11:75–104, 1954.

Cederlof R, Friberg L, Hrubec Z et al: The relationship of smoking and some social covariables to mortality and cancer mortality. A ten-year follow-up on a probability sample of 55,000 Swedish subjects age 18 to 69. Stockholm: Dept of Environmental Hygiene, The Karolinska Institute, 1975.

Centers for Disease Control: Long-term oral contraceptive use and the risk of breast cancer. JAMA 249:1591–1595, 1983.

Centers for Disease Control: Oral contraceptive use and the risk of ovarian cancer. JAMA 249:1596–1599, 1983.

Centers for Disease Control: Oral contraceptive use and the risk of endometrial cancer. JAMA 249:1600–1604, 1983.

Choi NW, Schuman LM, Gullen WH: Epidemiology of primary central nervous system neoplasms: II. Case control study. Am J Epidemiol 91:467–485, 1970.

Clemmesen J: On the etiology of some human cancers. J Natl Cancer Inst 12:1–21, 1951.

Coldman AJ, Elwood JM, Gallagher RP: Sports activities and risk of testicular cancer. Br J of Cancer 46:749–756, 1982.

Cole P, Hoover R, Friedell GH: Occupation and cancer of the lower urinary tract. Cancer 29:1250–1260, 1972.

Correa P: Precursors of gastric and esophageal cancer. Cancer 50:2554–2565, 1982.

Correa P, O'Conor GT: Epidemiologic patterns of Hodgkin's disease. Int J Cancer 8:192–201, 1971.

Correa P, Pickle LW, Fontham ETH, Johnson WD: Preliminary report on a case-control study of cancers of the lung, stomach, and pancreas in southern Louisiana. In Progress on Joint Environmental and Occupational Cancer Studies, September 9–11, 1981. Proceedings of the Second NCI/EPA/NIOSH Collaborative Workshop, Rockville, Maryland, printed April, 1982, pp 67–88.

Court Brown WM, Doll R: Mortality from cancer and other causes after radiotherapy for ankylosing spondylitis. Br Med J 2:1327–1332, 1965.

Cramer DW, Welch WR, Scully RE et al: Ovarian cancer and talc, a case-control study. Cancer 50:372–376, 1982.

Crump KS, Guess HA: Drinking water and cancer: Review of recent epidemiological findings and assessment of risks. Ann Rev Public Health 3:339–357, 1982.

Cuello C, Correa P, Haenszel W, et al: Gastric cancer in Colombia. J Natl Cancer Inst 57:1015–1020, 1976.

Cutler SJ, Young JL Jr (eds): Third National Cancer Survey: Incidence Data. Natl Cancer Inst Monogr 41, 1975.

da Silva Horta J, da Motta LC, Tavares MH: Thorium dioxide effects in man. Environ Res 8:131–159, 1974.

Day NE, Munoz N: Esophagus. In Cancer Epidemiology and Prevention (Schottenfeld D, Fraumeni JF Jr, eds). Philadelphia: W.B. Saunders, 1982, pp. 596–623.

Dean G, MacLennan R, McLoushlin H, Shelley E: Causes of death of blue-collar workers at a Dublin brewery, 1954–73. Br J Cancer 40(4): 581-589, 1979.

Decoufle P: Cancer risks associated with employment in the leather and leather products industry. Arch of Envir Health 34:33–37, 1979.

De Jong UW, Breslow N, Goh Ewe Hong J et al: Aetiological factors in oesophageal cancer in Singapore Chinese. Int J Cancer 13:291–303, 1974.

DES Task Force Summary Report, NIH Publ No. 81-1688. Bethesda, Md.: U.S. Dept of Health & Human Serv, September 21, 1978.

DeVesa SS, Silverman DT: Cancer incidence and mortality trends in the United States: 1935–74. J Natl Cancer Inst 60:545–571, 1978.

de Waard F: Breast cancer incidence and nutritional status with particular reference to body weight and height. Cancer Res 35:3351–3356, 1975.

de Waard F: Uterine corpus. In Cancer Epidemiology and Prevention (Schottenfeld D and Fraumeni JF Jr, eds). Philadelphia: W.B. Saunders, 1982, pp 901–908.

Doll R, Peto R: Mortality in relation to smoking: 20 years' observations on male British doctors. Br Med J 2:1525–1536, 1976.

Doll R, Peto R: The causes of cancer: quantitative estimates of avoidable risks of cancer in the United States today. J Natl Cancer Inst 66:1193–1308, 1981.

Dunn JE Jr, Levin EA, Linden G et al: Skin cancer as a cause of death. Calif Med 102:361–363, 1965.

Economic Research Service, U.S. Department of Agriculture. Tobacco Outlook and Situation, TS-183, March 1983. USDA, Washington D.C.

Ehrich M, Aswell JE, Wilkins TD: Alteration of the mutagenicity of human fecal extracts by hepatic microsomal enzymes. J Toxicol Environ Health 7:107–115, 1981.

Elwood JM, Cole P, Rothman KJ, Kaplan SD: Epidemiology of endometrial cancer. J Natl Cancer Inst 59(4):1055–1060, 1977.

Enstrom JE: Cancer and total mortality among active Mormons. Cancer 42:1943–1971, 1978.

Ernster VL, Selvin S et al: Prostate cancer: mortality and incidence rates by race and social class. Am J Epidemiol 107:311–320, 1978.

Falk H: Liver. In Cancer Epidemiology and Prevention (Schottenfeld D and Fraumeni JF Jr, eds). Philadelphia: W.B. Saunders, 1982, pp 668–682.

Fears TR, Scotto J: Changes in skin cancer morbidity between 1971–72 and 1977–78. J Natl Cancer Inst 69:365–370, 1982.

Fears TR, Scotto J: Estimating increases in skin cancer morbidity due to increases in ultraviolet radiation exposure. Cancer Investigation Vol 1, No. 2, 1983.

Findlay GM: Ultraviolet light and skin cancer. Lancet 2:1070–1073, 1928.

Fraumeni JF Jr: Persons at High Risk of Cancer. New York: Academic Press, 1975.

Fraumeni JF Jr, Blot WJ: Lung and pleura. In Cancer Epidemiology and Prevention (Schottenfeld D and Fraumeni JF Jr, eds). Philadelphia: WB Saunders, 1982.

Fraumeni JF Jr, Hoover R: Immunosurveillance and cancer: Epidemiologic observations. Natl Cancer Inst Monogr 47:121–126, 1977.

Fraumeni JF Jr, Kantor AF: Biliary Tract. In Cancer Epidemiology and Prevention (Schottenfeld D and Fraumeni JF Jr, eds). Philadelphia: W.B. Saunders, 1982, pp 683–691.

Gallo RC: Editorial: Gallo on T-cell leukemia-lymphoma virus. The Lancet 2:1083, November 13, 1982.

Gatti RA, Good RA: Occurrence of malignancy in immunodeficiency diseases. Cancer 28:89–98, 1971.

Geleprin A, Moses V, Fox G: Nitrate in water supplies and cancer. Illinois Med J 149:251–253, 1976.

Gilbert JB: Tumors of the testis following mumps orchitis: Case report and review of 24 cases. J Urol 51:296–300, 1944.

Glass AG, Fraumeni JF Jr: Epidemiology of bone cancer in children. J Natl Cancer Inst 44:187–199, 1970.

Gobar AH: L'abus des drogues en Afghanistan. Bull Stupefiants 28:1–12, 1976.

Gold E, Gordis L, Tonascia J, Szklo M: Risk factors for brain tumors in children. Am J Epidemiol 109:309–319, 1979.

Graham S, Dayal H. Rohrer T et al: Dentition, diet, tobacco, and alcohol in the epidemiology of oral cancer. J Natl Cancer Inst 59:1611–1618, 1977.

Graham S, Dayal H, Swanson M et al: Diet in the epidemiology of cancer of the colon and rectum. J Natl Cancer Inst 61:709–714, 1978.

Graham S, Gibson R, West D et al: Epidemiology of cancer of the testis in Upstate New York. J Natl Cancer Inst 58:1255–1261, 1977.

Graham S, Haughey B, Marshall J et al: Diet in the epidemiology of carcinoma of the prostate gland. J Natl Cancer Inst 70:687–692, 1983.

Greene MH: Non-Hodgkin's Lymphoma and Mycosis Fungoides. In Cancer Epidemiology and Prevention (Schottenfeld D and Fraumeni JF Jr, eds). Philadelphia: W.B. Saunders, 1982, pp 754–778.

Greene MH, Boice JD Jr et al: Acute non-lymphocytic leukemia after therapy with alkylating agents for ovarian cancer: A study of five randomized trials. N Engl J Med 307:1416–1421, 1982.

Greene MH, Clark WH Jr, Tucker MA et al: Precursor naevi in cutaneous malignant melanoma: A proposed nomenclature. Lancet, November 8, 1980, pp. 1024.

Greene MH, Goldin LR, Clark WH et al: Familial cutaneous malignant melanoma—an autosomal dominant trait possibly linked to the Rh locus. Proc Natl Acad Sci 80:6071–6075, 1983.

Greene MH, Hoover RN, Eck RL et al: Cancer mortality among printing plant workers. Environ Res 20:66–73, 1979.

Greene MH, Young RC et al: Evidence of a treatment dose-response in acute nonlymphocytic leukemias which occur after therapy of non-Hodgkin's lymphoma. Cancer Res 43:1891–1898, 1983.

Greenwald P: Prostate. *In* Cancer Epidemiology and Prevention (Schottenfeld D and Fraumeni JF Jr, eds). Philadelphia: W.B. Saunders, 1982, pp 938–946.

Greenwald P, Korns, RF, Nasca PL et al: Cancer in United States Jews. Cancer Res 35:3507–3512, 1975.

Grufferman S: Hodgkin's disease. *In* Cancer Epidemiology and Prevention (Schottenfeld D and Fraumeni JF Jr, eds). Philadelphia: W.B. Saunders, 1982, pp 564–582.

Grufferman S, Duong T, Cole P: Occupation and Hodgkin's disease. J Natl Cancer Inst 57:1193–1195, 1976.

Haenszel W, Kurihara M: Studies of Japanese migrants. I. Mortality from cancer and other diseases among Japanese in the United States. J Natl Cancer Inst 40:43–68, 1968.

Haenszel W, Kurihara M, Segi M et al: Stomach cancer among Japanese in Hawaii. J Natl Cancer Inst 49:969–988, 1972.

Hammond EC: Smoking habits and air pollution in relation to lung cancer. *In* Environmental Factors in Respiratory Disease (Lee DHK, ed). New York: Academic Press, 1972, pp 177–198.

Hammond EC: Smoking in relation to the death rates of 1 million men and women. *In* Epidemiological Approaches to the Study of Cancer and Chronic Diseases (Haenszel W, ed). Natl Cancer Inst Monogr 19, 1966, pp 127–207.

Hammond EC, Selikoff IJ, Lawther PL et al: Inhalation of Benzpyrene and cancer in man. Ann NY Acad Sci 271:116–124, 1976.

Hammond EC, Selikoff IJ, Seidman H: Asbestos exposure, cigarette smoking and death rates. Ann NY Acad Sci 330:473–490, 1979.

Harris RH, Page T, Reiches NA: Carcinogenic hazards of organic chemicals in drinking water. *In* Incidence of Cancer in Humans (Hiatt HH, Watson JD, Winsten JA, eds). Cold Spring Harbor, New York: CSH Laboratory, 1977, pp 309–330.

Harris RWC, Brinton LA, Cowdell RH et al: Characteristics of women with dysplasia or carcinoma *in situ* of the cervix uteri. Br J Cancer 42:359–369, 1980.

Hartge P, Hoover R, West DW et al: Coffee drinking and risk of bladder cancer. J Natl Cancer Inst 70(6):1021–1026, 1983.

Hartge P, Lesher L, McGowan L, Hoover R: Talc and ovarian cancer (letter). JAMA 250(14):1844, 1983.

Hecht SS, Chen CB, Ohmori T, Hoffman D: Comparative carcinogenicity in F344 rats of the tobacco-specific nitrosamines, N,nitrosonornicotine and 4-(N-methyl-N-nitrosamino)-1-(3-pyridyl)-1-butanone. Cancer Res 40:298–302, 1980.

Hempelmann LH, Hall WJ, Phillips M, Ames WR: Neoplasms in persons treated with X-rays in infancy: Fourth survey in 20 years. J Natl Cancer Inst 55:519–530, 1975.

Henderson BE, Benton B, Jing J, Yu MC, Pike MC: Risk factors for cancer of the testis in young men. Int J Cancer 23:598–602, 1979.

Henderson WJ, Joslin CAF, Turnvull AC et al: Talc and carcinoma of the ovary and cervix. J Obstet Gynecol Br Comm 78:266–272, 1971.

Herbst AL, Ulfelder H, Poskanzer DC: Adenocarcinoma of the vagina: Association of maternal stilbestrol therapy with tumor appearance in young women. N Engl J Med 284:878–881, 1971.

Hildick-Smith GY: The biology of talc. Br J Industr Med 33:217–229, 1976.

Holly EA, Weiss NS, Liff JM: Cutaneous melanoma in relation to exogenous hormones and reproductive factors. J Natl Cancer Inst 70:827–831, 1983.

Hoover R: Effects of drugs—immunosuppression. *In* Origins of Human Cancer (Hiatt HH, Watson JD, Winsten JA, eds). Cold Spring Harbor, New York: Proc of CSH Conferences on Cell Proliferation, 1977, pp 369–379.

Hoover R, Fraumeni JF Jr: Drugs in clinical use which cause cancer. J Clin Pharmacol 15:16–23, 1975.

Hoover R, Fraumeni JF Jr: Drug-induced cancer. Cancer 47:1071–1080, 1981.

Hoover R, Fraumeni JF Jr: Risk of cancer in renal transplant recipients. Lancet 2:55, 1973.

Hoover R, Gray LA, Cole P et al: Menopausal estrogens and breast cancer. N Engl J Med 295:401–405, 1976.

Hoover RN, Strasser PH et al: Artificial sweeteners and human bladder cancer. Lancet, April 19, 1980, pp. 837–840.

Horm JW, Asire AJ: Changes in lung cancer incidence and mortality rates among Americans: 1969–78. J Natl Cancer Inst 69:833–837, 1982.

Hounam RF, Williams J: Levels of airborne dust in furniture-making factories in the High Wycombe area. Br J Ind Med 31:1–9, 1974.

Hulka BS, Chambless LE et al: Breast cancer and estrogen replacement therapy. Am J Obstet Gynecol 143:638–644, 1982.

Hulka BS, Chambless, LE, Kaufman DG et al: Protection against endometrial carcinoma by combination-product oral contraceptives. JAMA 247(4):475–477, 1982.

Hyde JN: On the influence of light in the production of cancer of the skin. Am J Med Sci 131:1–22, 1906.

International Agency for Research on Cancer (IARC) monographs on the evaluation of the carcinogenic risk of chemicals to humans. Lyons, France:

Some anti-thyroid and related substances, nitrofurans and industrial chemicals. Vol 7, 1974.

Asbestos. Vol 14, 1977.

Some metals and metallic compounds. Vol 23, 1980.

Wood, leather, and some associated industries. Vol 25, 1981.

Chemicals, industrial processes and industries associated with cancer in humans. Vols. 1–20, Supplement 4, 1982.

Ichimaru M, Ishimaru T, Mikami M et al: Multiple myeloma among atomic bomb survivors in Hiroshima and Nagasaki, 1950–1976: Relationship to radiation dose absorbed by marrow. J Natl Cancer Inst 69:323, 1982.

Jain M, Cook GM, Davis FG, Grace MG, Howe GR, Miller AB: A case-control study of diet and colo-rectal cancer. Int J Cancer 26:757–768, 1980.

Jayant K, Balakrishnan V, Sanghvi LD, Jussawalla DJ: Quantification of the role of smoking and chewing tobacco in oral, pharyngeal, and esophageal cancers. Br J Cancer 35:232–235, 1977.

Jensen OM: Cancer morbidity and causes of death among Danish brewery workers. Int J Cancer 23:454–463, 1979.

Jick H, Walker AM et al: Replacement estrogens and breast cancer. Am J Epidemiol 112:586–594, 1980.

Jick H, Watkins RN, Hunter JR et al: Replacement estrogens and endometrial cancer. New Engl J Med 300(5):218–222, 1979.

Johnson FL, Feagler JR, Lerner KG et al: Association of androgenic anabolic steroid therapy with development of hepatocellular carcinoma. Lancet 2:1273–1276, 1972.

Jussawalla DJ: Epidemiological assessment of aetiology of oesophageal cancer in greater Bombay. International Seminar on Epidemiology of Oesophageal Cancer, Bangalore, India. Monogr 1, November 1971, pp 20–30.

Kato H, Tillotson J et al: Epidemiologic studies of coronary heart disease and stroke in Japanese men living in Japan, Hawaii and California: Serum lipids and diet. Am J Epidemiol 97:372–385, 1973.

Kelsey JL: A review of the epidemiology of human breast cancer. Epidem Reviews I:74–109, 1979.

Kelsey JL, Fischer DB, Holford TR et al: Exogenous estrogens and other factors in the epidemiology of breast cancer. J Natl Cancer Inst 67:327–333, 1981.

Kew MC, Gear AJ, Baumgarten I et al: Histocompatibility antigens in patients with hepatocellular carcinoma and their relationship to chronic hepatitis B virus infection in these patients. Gastroenterology 77:537–539, 1979.

Kinlen LJ, Shiel AGR, Peto J et al: A collaborative study of cancer in patients who have received immunosuppressive therapy. Br Med J 2:1461–1466, 1979.

Kirsner JB: Introduction: Inflammatory bowel disease—consideration of etiology and pathogenesis. In Colorectal Cancer: Prevention, Epidemiology and Screening (Winawer SJ, Schottenfeld D, Sherlock P, eds.) New York: Raven Press, 1980, pp 319–323.

Knox EG: Foods and disease. Br J Prev Soc Med 31:71–80, 1977.

Kolonel LN, Hankin JH, Lee J et al: Nutrient intakes in relation to cancer incidence in Hawaii. Br J Cancer 44:332–339, 1981.

Kolonel L, Winkelstein W Jr: Cadmium and prostate carcinoma. Lancet 2:566–567, 1977.

Knudson AG Jr, Meadows AT: Developmental genetics of neuroblastoma. J Natl Cancer Inst 57:675–682, 1976.

Kraybill HF et al: Evaluation of public health aspects of carcinogenic/mutagenic biorefractories in drinking water. Preventive Med 9:212–218, 1980.

Lew EA, Garfinkel L: Variations in mortality by weight among 750,000 men and women. J Chronic Dis 32:563–576, 1979.

Li FP: Cancers in children. In Cancer Epidemiology and Prevention (Schottenfeld D and Fraumeni JF Jr, eds). Philadelphia:W.B. Saunders, 1982, pp 1012–1024.

Li FP, Connelly RR, Myers M: Improved survival rates among testicular cancer patients in the U.S. JAMA 247(6):825–826, February 1982.

Li FP, Fraumeni JF Jr: Prospective study of a family cancer syndrome. JAMA 247:19, 1982.

Li FP, Fraumeni JF Jr: Rhabdomyosarcoma in children: Epidemiologic study and identification of a familial cancer syndrome. J Natl Cancer Inst 43:1365–1373, 1969.

Li FP, Fraumeni JF Jr: Soft-tissues sarcoma, breast cancer, and other neoplasms: A familial syndrome. Ann Int Med 71:747–752, 1969.

Li FP, Fraumeni JF Jr, Mantel N et al: Cancer mortality among chemists. J Natl Cancer Inst 43:1159–1164, 1969.

Lindqvist C: Risk factors in lip cancer: A questionnaire survey. Am J Epidemiol 109:521–530, 1979.

Lloyd JW, Decoufle P, Salvin LF: Unusual mortality experience of printing pressman. J Occup Med 19(8):543–550, 1977.

Lundin FE Jr., Wagoner JK, Archer VE: Radon Daughter Exposure and Respiratory Cancer: Quantitative and Temporal Aspects. NIOSH and NIEHS Joint Monogr No. 1. Springfield, Virginia: NTIS, 1971.

Lyon JL, Gardner JW, West DW: Cancer risk and lifestyle: Cancer among Mormons from 1967 to 1975. *In* Banbury Report 4: Cancer Incidence in Defined Populations (Cairns J, Lyon JL, Skolnick M, eds). Cold Spring Harbor, New York: CSH Laboratory, 1981, pp 3–30.

Lyon JL, Sorenson AW: Colon cancer in a low-risk population. Am J Clin Nutr 31:S227–230, 1978.

Mack TM, Paganini-Hill A: Epidemiology of pancreas cancer in Los Angeles. Cancer 47:1474–1481, 1981.

MacDonald PC, Siiteri PK: The relationship between the extraglandular production of estrone and the occurrence of endometrial neoplasia. Gynecol Oncol 2:259–263, 1974.

MacLennan R, Jensen OM, Mosbech J, Vuori H: Diet, transit time, stool weight, and colon cancer in two Scandinavian populations. Am J Clin Nutr 31:S239–242, 1978.

MacMahon B, Cole P, Lin TM et al: Age at first birth and cancer of the breast. A summary of an international study. Bull WHO 43:209–221, 1970.

MacMahon B, Yen S, Trichopoulos D et al: Coffee and cancer of the pancreas. New Engl J Med 304:630–633, 1981.

Mahboubi E, Sayed GM: Oral cavity and pharynx. *In* Cancer Epidemiology and Prevention (Schottenfeld D and Fraumeni JF Jr, eds). Philadelphia: W.B. Saunders, 1982, pp 583–595.

Malik MOA, Hidaytalla A, Daoud EH et al: Superficial cancer in the Sudan—a study of 1225 primary malignant superficial tumours. Br J Cancer 30:355–364, 1974.

Malik MOA, Zaki EL, Din ZA, El Masri SH: Cancer of the alimentary tract in the Sudan—a study of 546 cases. Cancer 37:2533–2542, 1976.

Mancuso TF, Brennan MJ: Epidemiological considerations of cancer of the gallbladder, bile ducts and salivary glands in the rubber industry. J Occup Med 12:333–341, 1970.

Mason TJ: Cancer mortality in U.S. counties with plastics and related industries. Environ Health Perspect 11:79–84, 1975.

Mason TJ, McKay FW, Hoover R, Blot WJ, Fraumeni JF Jr: Atlas of Cancer Mortality in U.S. Counties 1950–1969. DHEW Publ No. (NIH) 75-780. Washington, D.C.: U.S. Govt Print Off, 1975.

Matanoski GM, Sartwell P, Elliott EA: Hodgkin's disease and mortality among physicians. Lancet ii:926–927, 1975.

Matanoski GM, Seltser R, Sartwell PE et al: The current mortality rates of radiologists and other physician specialists: Specific causes of death. Am J Epidemiol 101(3):199–210, 1975.

McKay FW, Hanson MR, Miller RW: Cancer Mortality in the United States: 1950–1977. DHHS Publ No. (NIH) 82-2435, Natl Cancer Inst Monogr 59. Washington, D.C.: U.S. Govt Print Off, 1982.

McKusick VA: Mendelian inheritance in man. Catalogs of autosomal dominant, autosomal recessive, and X-linked phenotypes. Baltimore: The Johns Hopkins University Press, 1978, pp. 605–606.

McLaughlin JK, Blot WJ, Mandel JS et al: Etiology of cancer of the renal pelvis. J Natl Cancer Inst 71:287–291, 1983.

McLaughlin JK, Mandel JS, Blot WJ et al: A population-based case-control study of renal cell carcinoma. J. Natl Cancer Inst 72(2):275–284, 1984.

McMichael AJ, Hartshorne JM: Mortality risks in Australian men in occupational groups, 1968–78. Med J of Australia 1:253–256, 1982.

Medical Research Council (U.K.): The Hazards to Man of Nuclear and Allied Radiations. London: H.M. Stationery Office, 1956.

Mettlin C, Graham S, Priore R et al: Diet and cancer of the esophagus. Nutrition and Cancer 2:143–147, 1981.

Mettlin C, Graham S, Swanson M: Vitamin A and lung cancer. J Natl Cancer Inst 62:1435–1438, 1979.

Milham S: Occupational mortality in Washington State, 1950–1971. DHEW Publ No. (NIOSH) 76-175-C. Washington, D.C.: U.S. Govt Print Off, 1976.

Miller AB, Howe GR et al: Food items and food groups as risk factors in a case-control study of diet and colorectal cancer. Int J Cancer 32:155–161, 1983.

Miller RW: Cancer epidemics in the People's Republic of China. J Natl Cancer Inst 60:1195, 1978.

Miller RW, Epidemiology of leukemia. *In* Modern Trends in Human Leukemia III. New York: Springer-Verlag, 1979, pp 37–40.

Miller RW: Ethnic differences in cancer occurrence: Genetic and environmental influences with particular reference to neuroblastoma. *In* Genetics of Human Cancer (Mulvihill JJ, Miller RW, Fraumeni JF Jr, eds). New York: Raven Press, 1977, pp 1–14; Discussion pp 39–41.

Miller RW: Genetic and familial factors. *In* Medical Oncology. New York: MacMillan, in press.

Miller RW, Beebe GW: Infectious mononucleosis and the empirical risk of cancer. J Natl Cancer Inst 50:315–321, 1973.

Miller RW, Fraumeni JF Jr, Hill JA et al: Neuroblastoma: Epidemiologic approach to its origin. Am J Dis Child 115:253–261, 1968.

Moertel CG, Hagedorn AB: Leukemia or lymphoma and coexistent primary malignant lesions: A review of the literature and study of 120 cases. Blood 12:788, 1957.

Morrison AS: Cryptorchidism, hernia, and cancer of the testis. J Natl Cancer Inst 56:731–733, 1976.

Morrison AS, Buring JE: Artificial sweeteners and cancer of the lower urinary tract. N Engl J Med 302:537–541, 1980.

Morrison AS, Buring JE, Verhock WG et al: Coffee drinking and cancer of the lower urinary tract. J Natl Cancer Inst 68:91–94, 1982.

Morrison AS, Cole P: Epidemiology of bladder cancer. Urol Clin North Am 3:13–29, 1976.

Morrison AS, Cole P: Urinary tract. In Cancer Epidemiology and Prevention (Schottenfeld D and Fraumeni JF Jr, eds). Philadelphia: W.B. Saunders, 1982, pp 925–937.

Myers MH, Hankey BF: Cancer Patient Survival Experience: Trends in Survival 1960–63 to 1970–73. DHHS Publ No. (NIH) 80-2148. Bethesda Md.: Natl Inst of Health, June 1980.

NAS/NRC: The Biological Effects of Atomic Radiation: Summary Reports. Washington, D.C.: NAS/NRC, 1956.

National Toxicology Program, DHHS, USPHS, Research Triangle Park, NC, Tech. Report No. 289, 1984 (draft).

Newhouse ML, Berry G, Wagner JC et al: A study of the mortality of female asbestos workers. Br J Industr Med 29:134–141, 1972.

Nomura A: Stomach. In Cancer Epidemiology and Prevention (Schottenfeld D and Fraumeni JF Jr, eds). Philadelphia: W.B. Saunders, 1982, pp 624–637.

Olin GR, Ahlbom A: The cancer mortality among Swedish chemists graduated during three decades. A comparison with the general population and with a cohort of architects. Environ Res 22:154–161, 1980.

Palmer S, Bakshi K: Diet, nutrition, and cancer. Interim dietary guidelines. J Natl Cancer Inst 70:1151–1170, 1983.

Peto R, Doll R, Buckley JD, Sporn MB: Can dietary beta-carotene materially reduce human cancer rates? Nature 290:201–208, 1981.

Phillips RL et al: Mortality among California Seventh-Day Adventists for selected cancer sites. J Natl Cancer Inst 65:1097–1107, 1980.

Pickle LW, Greene MH, Ziegler RG et al: Colorectal cancer in rural Nebraska. Cancer Res 44:363–369, 1984.

Pike MC, Krailo MD, Henderson BE et al: Breast cancer in young women and use of oral contraceptives: Possible modifying effect of formulation and age at use. Lancet 8359:926–929, 1983.

Poiesz BJ, Ruscetti FW, Gazdar AF et al: Detection and isolation of type C retrovirus particles from fresh and cultured lymphocytes of a patient with cutaneous T-cell lymphoma. Proc Natl Acad Sci 77:7415–7419, 1980.

Pottern LM, Ziegler RG et al: Esophageal cancer among black men in Washington, D.C.: I. Alcohol, tobacco, and other risk factors; II. Role of nutrition. J Natl Cancer Inst 67:777–783; 1199–1206, 1981.

Prates MD, Torres FO: A cancer survey in Lourenco Marques, Portuguese East Africa. J Natl Cancer Inst 35:729–757, 1965.

Purtilo DT: Opportunistic non-Hodgkin's lymphoma in X-linked recessive immunodeficiency and lymphoproliferative syndromes. Semin Oncol 4:335–343, 1977.

Radl J, Sepers JM, Skvaril F et al: Immunoglobulin patterns in humans over 95 years of age. Clin Exp Immunol 22:84–90, 1975.

Rehn L: Blasengeschulste bei Fuchsin-Arbeitern. Arch Klin Chir 50:588–600, 1895.

Ries LG, Pollack ES, Young JL Jr: Cancer patient survival: Surveillance, Epidemiology, and End Results Program, 1973–79. J Natl Cancer Inst 70:693–707, 1983.

Ritchie JK, Allan RN, Macartney J et al: Biliary tract carcinoma associated with ulcerative colitis. Quart J Med 43:263–279, 1974.

Rosdahl N, Larsen S, Clemmesen J: Hodgkin's disease in patients with previous infectious mononucleosis: 30 years' experience. Br Med J 2(913):253–256, May 4, 1974.

Ross RK, Paganini-Hill A et al: A case-control study of menopausal estrogen therapy and breast cancer. JAMA 243:1635–1639, 1980.

Rothman K, Keller A: The effect of joint exposure to alcohol and tobacco on the risk of cancer of the mouth and pharynx. J Chron Dis 25:711–716, 1972.

Rotkin ID: Epidemiology of cancer of the cervix. III. Sexual characteristics of a cervical cancer population. Am J Public Health 57:815–829, 1967.

Schindler AE, Ebert A, Friedrick E: Conversion of androstenedione to estrone by human fat tissue. J Clin Endocrinol Metab 35:627–630, 1972.

Schoenberg BS: Nervous System. In Cancer Epidemiology and Prevention (Schottenfeld D and Fraumeni JF Jr, eds). Philadelphia: W.B. Saunders, 1982, pp 968–983.

Schottenfeld D, Warshauer ME: Testis. In Cancer Epidemiology and Prevention (Schottenfeld D and Fraumeni JF Jr, eds). Philadelphia: W.B. Saunders, 1982, pp 947–957.

Schottenfeld D, Winawer SJ: Large Intestine. In Cancer Epidemiology and Prevention (Schottenfeld D and Fraumeni JF Jr, eds). Philadelphia: W.B. Saunders, 1982, pp. 703–727.

Schreier HA, Sherry N, Shaughnessy E: Lead poisoning & brain tumors in children: A report of 2 cases. Ann Neurol 1:599–600, 1977.

Scotto J, Fears TR, Fraumeni JF Jr: Incidence of Non-melanoma Skin Cancer in the United States. DHHS Publ No. (NIH) 82–2433. Washington, D.C.: U.S. Govt Print Off, 1981.

Scotto J, Fears TR, Fraumeni JF Jr: Solar radiation. In Cancer Epidemiology and Prevention (Schottenfeld D, Fraumeni JF Jr, eds). Philadelphia: W.B. Saunders, 1982, pp 254–274.

Scotto J, Fears TR, Gori GB: Measurements of Ultraviolet Radiation in the United States and Comparisons with Skin Cancer Data. DHEW Publ No. (NIH) 76-1029. Washington, D.C.: U.S. Govt Print Off, 1976, pp 3.1.–3.10.

Scotto J, Fraumeni JF Jr: Skin (other than melanoma). In Cancer Epidemiology and Prevention (Scottenfeld D, Fraumeni JF Jr, eds). Philadelphia: W.B. Saunders, 1982, pp 996–1101.

Selikoff IJ, Hammond EC, Seidman H: Mortality experience of insulation workers in the United States and Canada, 1943–1976. Ann NY Acad Sci 330:91–116, 1979.

Shekelle RB, Liu S, Raynor WJ et al: Dietary vitamin A and risk of cancer in the Western Electric study. Lancet, November 18, 1981.

Shimkin MB: Contrary to Nature. DHEW Publ No. (NIH) 76-720. Washington, D.C.: U.S. Govt Print Off, 1977.

Shy CM, Struba RJ: Air and water pollution. In Cancer Epidemiology and Prevention (Schottenfeld D and Fraumeni JF Jr, eds). Philadelphia: W.B. Saunders, 1982, pp 336–363.

Silverberg E, Lubera JA: Cancer Statistics 1983. American Cancer Society, CA 33 (adapted from SEER data).

Silverman DT, Hoover RN, Albert S et al: Occupation and cancer of the lower urinary tract in Detroit. J Natl Cancer Inst 70:237–245, 1983.

Sinnhuber RO, Wales JH, Ayres JL et al: Dietary factors and hepatoma in rainbow trout (Salmo Gardneiri). 1. Aflatoxins in vegetable protein feedstuffs. J Natl Cancer Inst 41:711–718, 1968.

Smith EM: Epidemiology of oral and pharyngeal cancers in the United States: Review of recent literature. J Natl Cancer Inst 63:1189–1198, 1979.

Smith PG, Doll R: Mortality among patients with ankylosing spondylitis after a single treatment course with X-rays. Br Med J (Clin Res) 284(6314): 449–460, Feb 13, 1982.

Smith PG, Kinlen LJ, Doll R: Hodgkin's disease mortality among physicians. Lancet ii:525, 1974.

Sporn MB: Prevention of epithelial cancer by vitamin A and its synthetic analogs (retinoids). In Origins of Human Cancer (Hiatt HH, Watson JD, Winsten JA, eds). Cold Spring Harbor, New York: CSH Laboratory, 1977, pp 801–807.

Staszewski J: Migrant studies in alimentary tract cancer. In Current Problems in the Epidemiology of Cancer and Lymphomas (Grandmann E, Tulinius H eds). New York: Springer-Verlag, 1972.

Stern RS, Thibodeau LA, Kleinerman RA et al: Risk of cutaneous carcinoma in patients treated with oral methoxsalen photochemotherapy for psoriasis. N Engl J Med 300:809–813, 1979.

Stolley PD, Hibberd PL: Drugs. In Cancer Epidemiology and Prevention (Schottenfeld D and Fraumeni JF Jr, eds). Philadelphia: W.B. Saunders, 1982, pp 304–317.

Stott H, Fox W et al: Acute leukaemia after busulphan. Br Med J 2:1513–1517, 1977.

Swerdlow AJ, Stiller CA, Kinnier-Wilson LM: Prenatal factors in the aetiology of testicular cancer: An epidemiological study of childhood testicular cancer deaths in Great Britain, 1953–73. J Epid & Comm Health 36:96–101, 1982.

Szmuness W, Stevens CE, Ikram H et al: Prevalence of hepatitis B virus infection and hepatocellular carcinoma in Chinese-Americans. J Infec Dis 137:822–829, 1978.

Thomas DB: Non-contraceptive exogenous estrogens and risk of breast cancer: A review. In Breast Cancer Research and Treatment. The Hague: Martinus Nijhoff Pub, 1982, Vol 2, pp 203–211.

Thomas TL, Decoufle P: Mortality among workers employed in the pharmaceutical industry: A preliminary investigation. JOM 21:619–623, 1979.

Thomas TL, Waxweiler RJ, Moure-Eraso R et al: Mortality patterns among workers in three Texas oil refineries. JOM 24:135–141, 1982.

Thomas TL, White DW, Moure-Eraso R et al: Brain cancer among OCAW members in three Texas oil refineries. Ann NY Acad Sci 381:120–129, 1982.

Tseng WP: Effects and dose-response relationships of skin cancer and black-foot disease with arsenic. International Conference on Arsenic. Fort Lauderdale, Florida, 1976.

Tseng WP, Chu HM, How SW, et al: Prevalence of skin cancer in an endemic area of chronic arsenicism in Taiwan. J Natl Cancer Inst 40:453–463, 1968.

Tuyns AJ: Alcohol. In Cancer Epidemiology and Prevention (Schottenfeld D and Fraumeni JF Jr, eds). Philadelphia: W.B. Saunders, 1982, pp 293–303.

Tuyns AJ: Epidemiology of alcohol and cancer. Cancer Res 39:2840–2843, 1979.

Tuyns AJ, Pequignot G, Abbatucci JS: Oesophageal cancer and alcohol consumption. Importance of type of beverage. Int J Cancer 23:443–447, 1979.

915

Tuyns AJ, Pequignot G, Jensen OM: Le cancer de l'oesophage en Ille-et-Vilaine en fonction des niveaux de consommation d'alcool et de tabac. Des risques qui se multiplient. Bull Cancer 64:45–60, 1977.

Tuyns AJ, Pequignot G, Jensen OM: Role of diet, alcohol and tobacco in oesophageal cancer as illustrated by two contrasting high incidence areas in North Iran and west of Africa. In Frontiers of Gastrointestinal Research, Vol 4, Gastrointestinal Cancer: Advances in Basic Research (Rozen P, Eidelman S, Gilat T, eds). Basel: Karger, 1979, pp 101–110.

Tyroler HA, Andjelkovic D, Harris R et al: Chronic disease in the rubber industry. Environ Health Persp 17:13–20, 1976.

Urbach F: Geographic distribution of skin cancer. J Surg Oncol 3:219–234, 1971.

U.S. Department of Health and Human Services: The Health Consequences of Smoking: A Report of the Surgeon General. DHHS Publ No. (PHS) 82-50179. Washington, D.C.: U.S. Gov Print Off, 1982.

Vianna NJ, Greenwald P, Davies JNP: Extended epidemic of Hodgkin's disease in high school students. Lancet i:1209–1211, 1971.

Vianna NJ, Polan AK: Epidemiologic evidence for transmission of Hodgkin's disease. N Engl J Med 10:499–502, 1973.

Vianna NJ, Polan AK, Keogh MD et al: Hodgkin's disease mortality among physicians. Lancet ii:131–133, 1974.

Walrath J, Fraumeni JF Jr: Mortality among embalmers. Int J Cancer 31:407–411, 1983.

Waterhouse J, Muir C, Correa P et al (eds): Cancer Incidence in Five Continents, Vol. 3, IARC Scientific Publ No. 15. Lyon, France: International Agency for Research on Cancer, 1976.

Waterhouse J, Muir C, Powell J. et al (eds): Cancer Incidence in Five Continents, Vol. IV, IARC Scientific Publ No. 42. Lyon, France: International Agency for Research on Cancer, 1982.

Welton JC, Marr JS, Friedman SM: Association between hepatobiliary cancer and typhoid carrier state. Lancet 1:791–794, 1979.

Weiden PL, Lerner KG, Gerdes A et al: Pancytopenia and leukemia in Hodgkin's disease: Report of three cases. Blood 42:571, 1973.

Weiss NS: Ovary. In Cancer Epidemiology and Prevention (Schottenfeld D and Fraumeni JF Jr, eds). Philadelphia: W.B. Saunders, 1982, pp. 871–880.

Weiss NS, Sayvetz TA: Incidence of endometrial cancer in relation to the use of oral contraceptives. N Engl J Med 302:551–554, 1980.

Winn DM, Blot WH, Shy CM et al: Snuff dipping and oral cancer among women in the southern United States. N Engl J Med 304:745–749, 1981.

Winn DM, Blot WJ, Shy CM, Fraumeni JF Jr: Occupation and oral cancer among women in the South. Am J Ind Med 3:161–167, 1982.

Wittenmore AS, McMillan A: Lung Cancer Among U.S. Uranium Miners: A Reappraisal. J Natl Cancer Inst 71:489–499, 1983.

Wynder EL, Cornfield J, Schroff PD et al: A study of environmental factors in carcinoma of the cervix. Am J Obstet Gynecol 68:1016–1047, 1954.

Wynder EL, Hoffmann D. Tobacco. In Cancer Epidemiology and Prevention (Schottenfeld D and Fraumeni JF Jr, eds.). Philadelphia: W.B. Saunders, 1982, pp 277–292.

Wynder EL, Hultberg S, Jacobsson F et al: Environmental factors in cancer of the upper alimentary tract. A Swedish study with special reference to Plummer-Vinson (Paterson-Kelly) syndrome. Cancer 10:470–487, 1957.

Wynder EL, Mabuchi K, Whitmore WF Jr: Epidemiology of adenocarcinoma of the kidney. J Natl Cancer Inst 53:1619–1634, 1974.

Wynder EL, Mabuchi K, Whitmore WF: Epidemiology of cancer of the prostate. Cancer 28:344–360, 1971.

Young JL Jr, Heise HW, Silverberg E, Myers MH: Cancer Incidence, Survival and Mortality for Children Under 15 Years of Age. American Cancer Society, Professional Education Publication, 1978.

Young JL Jr, Miller RW: Incidence of malignant tumors in U.S. children. J Pediatr 86:254–258, 1975.

Young JL Jr, Percy CL, Asire AJ, eds: Surveillance, Epidemiology, and End Results: Incidence and Mortality Data, 1973–77. DHHS Publ No. (NIH) 81-2330, Natl Cancer Inst Monogr 57. Washington, D.C.: Govt Print Off, 1981.

Young RC, Knapp RC, Perez CA: Cancer of the ovary. In Cancer, Principles and Practice of Oncology (DeVita VT, Hillman S, Rosenberg SA, eds). Philadelphia: W.B. Saunders, 1982, pp. 884–913.

Zeil HK, Finkle WD: Increased risk of endometrial carcinoma among users of conjugated estrogens. N Engl J Med 293:1164–1167, 1975.

Ziegler RG, Morris LE, Blot WJ, Pottern LM, Hoover R, Fraumeni JF Jr: Esophageal cancer among black men in Washington, D.C. II. Role of nutrition. J Natl Cancer Inst 67:1199–1206, 1981.

PART V–
INDEX

A

Acoustic Neuroma Association, 55
Acoustic neuromas, 48
Acute leukemias, 868-69, 498, 498,
  877, 877 *See also* Leukemia
  diagnosis, 649
  treatment, 248-49, 649
  types of, 239-40
Adenocarcinoma
  colon-rectum, 172
  kidney, 215
  lungs, 261
  prostate, 344
  stomach, 380
Adult T-cell leukemia-lymphoma
  (ATLL), 199
AIDS (acquired immunodeficiency
  syndrome), 30
Air pollution and cancer, 835-36
Albinism, 368
Alcohol use and cancer, 312-13,
  838-39, 889-90
Alkylating agents, 245
American Cancer Society (ACS), vii,
  619, 683-84, 795
  Reach to Recovery Program, 82,
    140, 162, 449, 620
American Chemical Society, 332
American Joint Committee on
  Cancer, 387
American Society of Plastic and
  Reconstructive Surgeons, 140
Amputation, 32-34
Anemia, 238, 467-68
Angiosarcoma, 880
Aplastic anemia, 499
Aromatic amines, 15
Arteriogram, 31
Artificial sweeteners, 15
Asbestos and cancer, 263, 263,
  300-02, 835-36, 837, 855-56, 882

Asparaginase, 479
Association for Brain Tumor
  Research, 54
Astrocytomas, 46-47
Atomic Bomb Casualty Commission,
  242

B

Barium enema, 182
Basal cell carcinoma *See* Skin
  cancers
BCG (bacillus Calmette-Guerin), 20
Benign hyperplasia (BHP), 343-44
Benign tumors, 6
Benzene, 245
Biliary duct cancers, 864
Biliary tract cancers, 863-64
Bill of Rights for the Friends and
  Relatives of Cancer Patients, 588
Billroth, Theodore, 388
Biological response modifiers
  (BRMs) *See* Immunotherapy
Biopsy, 542
  See also Breast cancer — biopsy
  bone, 30-31
  cervix, 419
  endometrium, 423
  lymph nodes, 200
  mesothelium, 303
  oral cavity, 317
  prostate, 349
  skin, 284, 371
  testes, 400
Birth control pills, 417, 844
Bladder
  description and function, 13
Bladder cancer, 15-23, 899-900
  causes and prevention, 15-16
  classification and staging, 18-19
  diagnosis, 17-18
  incidence, 14-15

Erythropoietin, 214
Esophageal cancer, 874-75
    alcohol and, 838-39
    mortality rates, 807, 826
Estramustine, 483
Etoposide, 483
Ewing's sarcoma, 33-34
    childhood, 653, 870
Exocrine cancer
    types of, 330
Experimental treatments, 373,
547-49, 662-63
Eye
    description and function, 289
Eye cancer *See* Ocular melanoma;
Retinoblastomas

F

Familial polyposis, 176-77
Families and cancer, 575-89, 788-90,
614-16, 634-42
    emotional support, 577-79
Fat (dietary), 693, 841-42
Feline leukemia, 244
Fiber (dietary), 696
    colorectal cancer and, 174-75,
    842, 873-74
Fibrosarcoma of bone, 34
Fine needle aspiration, 349
Flow cytometry, 351
Floxuridine, 484
Fluorescein angiography, 290
Fluorouracil, 484
Food and Drug Administration
    (FDA), 15, 217, 356, 405
Fulguration, 20

G

Gallbladder cancer, 863
Gallo, Robert, 199
Gardner's syndrome, 332

Gastric cancer *See* Stomach cancer
Gastric polyps, 383
Gastroscopy, 385
Genetics and cancer, 847-48, 872
    See also specific hereditary and
    congenital disorders
Glioblastoma multiforme, 46
Gliomas, 46, 864-65
Gonadal aplasia, 399
Gonioscopy, 290
Graft-versus-host disease (GVHD),
504-06
Grieving, 784
GVHD *See* Graft-versus-host
disease

H

Hairy cell leukemia, 254
Hematuria, 16
Herbicide exposure and cancer, 29,
200
Hermaphroditism, 399
Hodgkin's disease, 195-209, 498-99,
650, 875-77 *See also* Lymphoma
    causes and prevention, 198
    classification, 196-98
    incidence, 198
    mononucleosis and, 876
    selected references, 209
    staging, 201
    symptoms, 200
    treatment, 202-03, 651, 845
Hormonal therapy, 545
    breast cancer, 148
    kidney cancer, 224
    prostate cancer, 355-57
    uterine cancer, 425
Hormone receptor assay test, 60,
148
Hormones and cancer risks, 843-45
Hospices, 790-91

N

O

Prostate
description and function, 343
Prostate cancer, 343-62
causes, 346-47, 893
clinical trials, 361
diagnosis, 348-49
incidence, 345-46, 892-93
mortality rates, 811, 826
recurrence, 361
screening and early detection,
347-48
staging, 349-53
statistics, 820-21
symptoms, 348
treatment, 353-61
types of, 344-45
Prostheses
bone, 32
breast, 122-24
eye, 294
oral cavity, 320
Proteins
in diet, 693
Pulmonary angiography, 270
Purcutaneous transhepatic
cholangiography (PTC), 334

R

Radiation exposure and cancer,
242-43, 848-51, 878-79, 883
Radiation therapy, 431-52, 632
aftercare, 450-52
benefits, 432
breast cancer, 64-65, 77-78,
85-101
cervical cancer, 421
colorectal cancer, 185, 188
cost of, 433-34
description of, 660-61
external, 433-38
hair loss in, 441-43
head and neck cancer, 446-48

implant therapy, 320, 438-40
internal, 433
intraoperative radiotherapy
(IORT), 390
kidney cancer, 223
mesothelioma, 304
nutrition during, 442-43, 449-50
oral cancer, 320-22
pancreatic cancer, 337-38
prostate cancer, 354-55
risks, 432-33
sexual activity and, 436, 445-46
side effects, 321-22, 354-56, 436,
439-50, 448-49, 633, 661-62, 700,
849-50
skin cancer, 373
stomach cancer, 390
Radical cystectomy, 21
Radical mastectomy, 72
Radical prostatectomy, 353-54
Radioactive drugs, 846-47
Radiotherapy See Radiation
therapy
Radium exposure and cancer, 29
Radon exposure and cancer, 263,
836, 837-38, 882-83
Rectal cancer See Colorectal
cancer
Recurrent cancer See Cancer,
recurrence of
Reed-Sternberg cell, 196
Rehabilitation Act of 1973, 610
Renal arteriography, 220
Renal cell carcinoma See Kidney
cancer
Retinoblastomas
childhood, 652, 870
Retrograde pyelogram, 220
Retroperitoneal lymph nodes, 402
Retropubic prostatectomy, 354
Rhabdomyosarcoma
childhood, 652-53
Ronald McDonald Houses, 685

S

Sarcomas, 5, 650, 653, 870
Schiller's test, 419
Schistosomiasis infections, 15-16
Schwannomas, 47-48
SCID See Severe combined
 immunodeficiency disease (SCID)
Seminomas, 401 See also Testicular
 cancer
 treatment, 403-04
Serum markers, 401-02
Severe combined immunodeficiency
 disease (SCID), 499
Sigmoidoscopy, 180
Skin
 description and function, 279-80,
 365-66
Skin cancer, 365-74 See also
 Melanoma
 causes and prevention, 369-70,
 858-59, 894-96
 detection and diagnosis, 370-71
 follow-up care, 374
 incidence, 366-67, 894
 investigational therapies, 373
 staging, 371
 surgical treatment procedures,
 371-73
 types of, 280-81, 366
Skin graft, 372
Small cell lung cancer (SCLC), 261
 treatment, 273-75
Smokeless tobacco
 oral cancer, 312-13
Smoking and cancer, 855-56
 bladder, 15, 900
 kidney, 216, 901
 larynx, 881-83
 lungs, 263-66, 859-60, 881-83
 oral cavity, 312-13, 860
 pancreas, 331

Soft tissue sarcomas
 causes and prevention, 29-30
 children, 35-36
 detection and diagnosis, 30-31
 incidence, 28
 lung metastasis, 30
 treatment, 34-36
 types of, 28
Solar radiation See Ultraviolet
 (UV) radiation
Spinal tap See Lumbar puncture
Squamous cell carcinoma See Oral
 cancer; Skin cancer
Stomach
 description and function, 377-79
Stomach cancer, 377-94
 causes and prevention, 381-84,
 896-97
 clinical trials, 392-93
 diagnostic procedures, 385-87
 incidence, 380-81, 896
 mortality rates, 812, 826-27
 staging, 387-88
 statistics, 820-21
 surgical procedures, 388-90
 symptoms, 384-85
 types of, 379-80
Stomach ulcers, 384
Streptozocin, 490
Stress, 473-75
Sun exposure See Ultraviolet (UV)
 radiation
Suncreens, 283
Surgery, 543, 656-57 See also
 treatment of specific cancer types

T

Tamoxifen, 490
Teenagers
 cancer and, 679-80, 766-68
Testes
 description and function, 397-98